The Palgrave Handbook of Innovative Community and Clinical Psychologies

"This clear, accessible, manual, written by authors overwhelmingly committed to transparency about how their work was done, will appeal to clinical psychologists keen to engage in reformist community activism and, as an inscription of an increasingly dominant 'humanist community psychology' thesis, will stimulate engagement with its critical antithesis."

—David Fryer, *University of Queensland, Australia*

"This book will be essential reading for all those who want to put into practice community psychological ideas and who want to work differently to enhance social and psychological wellbeing. It gives us hope that other ways of working to build better worlds are possible."

—Carolyn Kagan, *Manchester Metropolitan University, UK*

"If you are looking for inspiration about how psychology can be used to address structural inequalities and injustices, then this book is for you. You will not find here the kind of psychology that favours quantification and experiment; traditional psychology and mental health practice are seen as too often colluding with and failing to ameliorate distress and disadvantage. What you will discover are many examples of creative ideas and ways of collaborating with community groups drawn from around the world, including from African and Asian countries. At the same time, chapter authors do not flinch from acknowledging and reflecting on the struggles and challenges involved in practising psychology in this new way."

—Jim Orford, *Emeritus Professor of Clinical and Community Psychology, the University of Birmingham, England*

Carl Walker • Sally Zlotowitz • Anna Zoli
Editors

The Palgrave Handbook of Innovative Community and Clinical Psychologies

palgrave
macmillan

Editors
Carl Walker
School of Applied Social Science
University of Brighton School of Applied Social Science
Brighton, UK

Anna Zoli
School of Applied Social Science
University of Brighton School of Applied Social Science
Brighton, UK

Sally Zlotowitz
MAC-UK & Art Against Knives
London, UK

ISBN 978-3-030-71189-4 ISBN 978-3-030-71190-0 (eBook)
https://doi.org/10.1007/978-3-030-71190-0

Cover Illustration: philsajonesen/gettyimages

This Palgrave Macmillan imprint is published by the registered company Springer Nature Switzerland AG.
The registered company address is: Gewerbestrasse 11, 6330 Cham, Switzerland

In memory of Tod Sloan.
Sally Zlotowitz
My parents, Carol and Sheldon Zlotowitz, for their endless support.
And to the young people and staff of the pioneering charity MAC-UK, where I learnt how to put social justice at the heart of my practice.
For Eve
Dancing silently
Anna Zoli
"To you, who never stop believing in peace, freedom, and justice."

Contents

1 **Introduction** 1
Sally Zlotowitz, Carl Walker, and Anna Zoli

Part I Clinical Psychology and Political Activism 17

2 **Building Alliances with Marginalised Communities to Challenge London's Unjust and Distressing Housing System** 19
Nina Carey, Sally Zlotowitz, Samantha James, Aysen Dennis, Thomas Gillespie, and Kate Hardy on behalf of The Housing & Mental Health Network

3 **Growing a Movement: Psychologists for Social Change** 31
Psychologists for Social Change

4 **Getting off the Fence and Steppin' Outta the Clinic Room** 51
The Walk the Talk Crew

5 **Taking a Position Within Powerful Systems** 69
James Randall, Sarah Gunn, Steven Coles, and With thanks to Gary H.

6 **Supporting Activists and Progressive Social Movements** 101
Tod Sloan and John Brush

7 **Statactivism and Critical Community Psychology: Using Statistical Activism to Resist Injustice in the NHS and Higher Education** 121
Carl Walker and Anna Zoli

Part II Working in Radical and Disruptive Spaces 139

8 **Reflexively Interrogating (De)colonial Praxes in Critical Community Psychologies** 141
Nick Malherbe, Shahnaaz Suffla, and Mohamed Seedat

9 **Options: Conversation in Collaboration** 159
Hannah Denton, Mark Haydon-Laurelut, Duncan Moss, Angela Paterson Foster, and Jan Shepherd

10 **Protesting Against Property Foreclosures in a Fragmentized Socio-Political Sphere: An Action-Oriented Model** 179
Andreas Vavvos and Sofia Triliva

11 **'We the Marlborough': Elucidating Users' Experience of Radical, Informal Therapeutic Practices Within a Queer Community Pub** 201
Charlotte Wilcox and Rebecca Graber

12 **The Evolution of the Community Psychology Festival** 223
Miltos Hadjiosif and Meera Desai

13 **The Define Normal Project** 239
Danny Taggart, Cheryl Nye, Jessica Taylor, Jacob Solstice, Matthew Harrison, Rebecca Bryant, Stacey Clark, and Wendy Franks

14 **Rewriting the Space Between a University and a Healthcare Provider: The Model of Converge** 259
Emma Anderson, Adam Bell, Paul Birch, Lucy Coleman, Paul Gowland, Matt Harper-Hardcastle, Eloise Ingham, Bekhi Ostrowska, and Kev Paylor

15 **The Jannah Tree: An Islamic Faith–Inspired Metaphor and Spiritual Framework for Healing, Co-created by British-Pakistani Women Through Cyberspace Technology** 277
Rukhsana Arshad

Part III Transformative Change Work 301

16 **Towards Social Inclusion: Creating Change Through a Community-Developed Model of Person-Centred Reviews (PCRs) to Support Children with Special Educational Needs and Disabilities (SEND)** 303
Nick Hammond and Nicola Palmer

17 **Overcoming Marginalisation and Mental Distress Through Community Supported Agriculture: The *Streccapogn* Experience in Monteveglio, Italy** 325
A. Zoli, J. Akhurst, S. Di Martino, and D. Bochicchio

18 **Community-Based Service Learning During Clinical Psychology Training: Working at the Critically Reflective Interface** 347
Jacqueline Akhurst and Carol Mitchell

19 **Health Inequities of Silent Roma Ranks from a Social Justice Perspective** 375
Daniela E. Miranda, Marta Escobar-Ballesta, Emilio Vizarraga Trigueros, María Jesús Albar Marín, and Manuel García-Ramírez

20 **'I Am Not Disabled, I Just Need Some Help': Are Critical Community Psychology Approaches a Promising Way to Engage with People with Learning Disabilities?** 403
Michael Richards

21 **Marginalised Youth Navigating Uncertainty: Reflections on Co-construction and Methodology in Nepal** 425
Vicky Johnson, Andy West, Sumon Kamal Tuladhar, Shubhendra Man Shrestha, and Sabitra Neupane

22 **Finding Safety in Trauma Recovery at a South African State Care Centre for Abused and Neglected Youth** 447
Sharon Johnson

23 **Collaborating with Social Justice Activists in Ghana's Fight Against Modern Slavery: A Case Study of Challenging Heights** 473
Kate Danvers

24 **Community-Based Participatory Research (CBPR) as an Emancipatory Modality Promoting Social Transformation, Empowerment, Agency, and Activism** 497
Naiema Taliep, Samed Bulbulia, Sandy Lazarus, Mohamed Seedat, and Building Bridges Team

Part IV Creativity and Social Change 521

25 **The Value of Togetherness Across Cultures** 523
Kelly Price, Hayley Higson, and Ndumanene Devlin Silungwe

26 **Linking Space, Place, and Relational Well-being in Co-productive Ways** 545
Jenny Fisher, Rebecca Lawthom, Leanne Rimmer, Andrew Stevenson, and The Manchester Street Poem Collective

27 **Mediating the Effects of Austerity with Creativity, Compassion and Community-Based Approaches** 559
Hayley Higson, Ste Weatherhead, and Suzanne Hodge

28 **Writing Stories of and from the Future: Fostering Personal and Socio-Political Action** 577
Nicholas Wood and Anneke Sools

29 **The Legacy of Art Making: Agency, Activism and Finding the World** 597
Olivia Sagan

30 We Tell Our Own Stories: Older Adults as Expert Researchers 615
Erin Elizabeth Partridge

31 'We Can Speak but Will There Be Any Change?' Voices from Blikkiesdorp, South Africa 631
Rashid Ahmed, Abdulrazak Karriem, and Shaheed Mohammed

32 Conclusion 653
Carl Walker, Sally Zlotowitz, and Anna Zoli

Index 665

List of Figures

Fig. 3.1	The origin of PSC	32
Fig. 4.1	Affecting policy change	60
Fig. 5.1	The poster	75
Fig. 7.1	Publicity for the survey	131
Fig. 12.1	Images from the festival	234
Fig. 12.2	Wristband from the third Community Psychology Festival	234
Fig. 13.1	Professional-generated formulation	244
Fig. 15.1	Sketch of The Jannah Tree	287
Fig. 15.2	Photo of original comissioned Art -Author's impression of The Jannah Tree blossoming	291
Fig. 18.1	Comparison of three models of community psychology-based interventions	351
Fig. 19.1	Community mobilization process for local Roma health governance	381
Fig. 19.2	Map of identified Roma assets in Polígono Sur. This example presents density of Roma population in the area and community resources. The darker gradient reflects high density of Roma and icons represent different resources available in the district	387
Fig. 19.3	Weekly meetings to build advocacy capacity among Roma neighbors	388
Fig. 19.4	Photograph of trash bins and discussion excerpt from group reflection: "We live amongst trash and its saturating. Why? Because it's not only the trash but what surrounds it. It is not the same waking up in the morning and see a park all clean than it is waking up surrounded by trash and that influences your mental state. Why? It is really depressing, you can't even go downstairs in the summertime…the insects, the cockroaches"	390

Fig. 19.5 Photograph of mailboxes and excerpt from group reflection: "These are the mailboxes of my building…it has been like this for years…, we have to go to the post office to pick up mail since they do not come here" 390
Fig. 19.6 Photograph of commercial spaces and excerpt of group reflection: "There are no shopping spaces in the area. So what do people do? They build informal shops outside apartment building or in their homes…spaces for real shops have no activity, so the physical state is undesirable…the roofs break when it rain, they are full of insects, cockroaches, rats…we are talking about spaces where people sell food and where people go to have a cup of coffee" 391
Fig. 19.7 Photograph of an empty space near neighbors' apartment building and group excerpt: "This used to be a football field… I used to look out the window to watch people play and go with my son. Later they removed it to build a park but they never did and this is how it was left…a space filled with trash, rats, insects and broken bottles" 392
Fig. 19.8 Group reflection between Roma neighbors, university-community partnership, and key health providers 394
Fig. 19.9 The recent PS Sur initiative "*3000* DeSCencias" led by the Roma community-based organization, Studio 41013. Flamenco music and dance were used by PS Roma neighbors to tell their stories and defend their rights as citizens. This is an example of using community strengths as a source for liberation 395
Fig. 20.1 Some of the young men I worked with expressing their frustrations in life through photography (see Lawthom et al., 2012) 405
Fig. 20.2 A photograph presenting one side of the community exhibition where poetry and photography were displayed, created by the men who participated in Project 1 (also see Richards et al., 2018) 410
Fig. 20.3 A comic strip that presents the men discussing aspects of the project 412
Fig. 20.4 Andrew's art work depicting himself brushing his teeth 413
Fig. 20.5 One of the producers of the radio shows in the studio preparing to go live on air 415
Fig. 21.1 Nepalese researcher presenting research to the National Reference Group 437
Fig. 21.2 Co-production with young people 439
Fig. 22.1 Connecting with nature at the sea and feeling safe and comfortable with my "big brother" 459
Fig. 22.2 Connecting with nature…tending these plants like we are being tended and growing in this place 460

Fig. 22.3 (a) and (b) Transforming the place that we are living in…as the staff of the centre are transforming us 460
Fig. 22.4 Shakespeare pushing up daisies at the inn: YCEC counsellor (male) 461
Fig. 22.5 Portability of skills (work skills) 462
Fig. 22.6 Trusting is a big issue in training (belonging) 463
Fig. 22.7 Taking care of nature as a transferable skill to taking care of self (belonging) 464
Fig. 22.8 Mastery skills for self-image, with a "can do" attitude 465
Fig. 22.9 Fishing…a positive recreational activity—Occupational therapist (female) 466
Fig. 22.10 This picture shows (to) me that the boys are now being exposed to other possible recreational activities that (is) are available to them other than substance (abuse) and gangsterism 466
Fig. 22.11 The look on his face as he learns how to use the fish line and preparing to go and catch fish shows that he is a bit (in) shock, as he probably didn't think that he would ever do this, as well as happy learning a new activity skill 467
Fig. 22.12 On the quayside—Admin Clerk (female) 467
Fig. 22.13 I have chosen this pic because I can see the care shown from one boy to the other. I get the sense that the one boy is telling the other boy to be careful not to fall in the water 468
Fig. 23.1 Children working on Lake Volta 479
Fig. 23.2 Challenging Heights model of change 481
Fig. 23.3 Challenging Heights staff help to reunite a family in Winneba 484
Fig. 23.4 The holistic approach 485
Fig. 24.1 Transforming spaces and places: Illustrations of community activism in Erijaville 510
Fig. 24.2 Community activist researchers participating in the University of South Africa Research & Innovation Week 512
Fig. 26.1 Ecological metaphor of multiple systems of analysis 548
Fig. 27.1 Conceptual diagram of themes 562
Fig. 27.2 Compassionate formulation and neo-liberal ideology 570
Fig. 30.1 Communication mural. The mural was painted on unstretched canvas and then stretched and hung when complete, in order to enable more people to participate 616
Fig. 30.2 Traditional research dynamics. In traditional research methods, the researcher holds the methods tightly. The researcher has the initial ideas, asks the questions, and receives recognition for the produced knowledge. The research subjects provide data, but do not receive anything back. The barrier between researcher and research subjects is strong; the relationship is unidirectional 617

Fig. 30.3 Participatory research dynamics. In this model of research, the researcher and participants are on the same level; they share in the inquiry, findings, and knowledge creation. The researcher offers methods with an open hand. Data and knowledge flow in an omnidirectional manner between stakeholders 617

List of Tables

Table 5.1	The two core issues with diagnostic classification as identified in the Position Statement (DCP, 2013)	74
Table 5.2	Advantages and disadvantages to clinicians of attempting to integrate diagnostic stances with other approaches	83
Table 5.3	Advantages and disadvantages to clinicians of attempting to question diagnostic stances	86
Table 5.4	Advantages and disadvantages to clinicians of assuming protesting or activist stances	91
Table 10.1	Key events in this research initiative and in Greek politics	183
Table 10.2	Debtor's stories in the public space	192
Table 11.1	Participant demographics	206
Table 11.2	Theme descriptions and exemplar quotes	208
Table 19.1	Key health providers' narratives regarding PS Roma health	383
Table 19.2	Evaluation Index for local Roma health assets in Polígono Sur	385
Table 19.3	Sample of health providers and organizational Roma sensitivity by asset type	386
Table 19.4	Empowering Roma community settings-specific commitments, strategies, and recommendations	395

List of Boxes

Box 3.1	The Influence of David Smail	35
Box 3.2	Liberation Psychology Influence	36
Box 3.3	Liberation Psychology Influence	36
Box 3.4	Influence of Gene Sharp	41
Box 3.5	The Influence of the Survivor and Social Justice Movements	43
Box 5.1	An Example of Questioning Diagnosis Beyond the Clinic Room	85
Box 5.2	An Example of Networks Set up Through and for Protest and Activism	90
Box 23.1	Voices of Survivors (Osabutey, 2015)	478
Box 26.1	'Streets of Resilience': Exploring Resilience in Street-Connected Young People in Guatemala City	550
Box 26.2	Co-production Research in Action: A Case Study in Homelessness	551
Box 26.3	Place-Making with Older Adults	553

1

Introduction

Sally Zlotowitz, Carl Walker, and Anna Zoli

It's probably not right to start this book by saying we gave it the wrong title but we have questioned the title along the way. After all, we are aware that many of the ideas contained in this book are not 'new', nor do they belong to or can be owned by the discipline of 'psychology'. That is of course not meant as a slight to our authors, but an acknowledgement of the many visible and invisible people who have paved the way for this book and these practices; potentially people who have been marginalised by the dominant psychological culture, which is Euro-American centric, English-speaking, individualistic and values positivist, quantitative science (see Katz, 1985; McDermott, 2001; Naidoo, 1996). People who remain 'unsung' in our psychological history. After all, mainstream Western psychology celebrates and teaches, at all levels of education, experimental science, reductionism and the institutionalised removal of people's social context (Bulhan, 1985). It is a cliché now to say it, but it remains true that the psychology heroes we learn about in psychological curriculums are white men conducting experiments with white North American students (Henrich et al., 2010). In the UK, historically we owe our

S. Zlotowitz
MAC-UK & Art Against Knives, London, UK

C. Walker (✉) • A. Zoli
School of Applied Social Science, University of Brighton, Brighton, UK
e-mail: c.j.walker@brighton.ac.uk; a.zoli@brighton.ac.uk

C. Walker et al. (eds.), *The Palgrave Handbook of Innovative Community and Clinical Psychologies*, https://doi.org/10.1007/978-3-030-71190-0_1

more radical liberation and critical psychology ideas to the international critical thinkers of South America and South Africa (e.g. Freire, 1972; Martín-Baró, 1996; Maldonado-Torres, 2017), and to the psychiatric survivor movements (see Adame et al., 2017; Morrison, 2013), critical psychiatry (e.g. Rapley et al., 2011), post-colonial scholars (e.g. Césaire, 2000; Fanon, 1967), activist groups (e.g. Recovery in the Bin), feminist and race scholars and activists (e.g. Crenshaw, 1991; Hooks, 2000), most of whom remain marginal in our psychology curriculums but provide inspiration for this work (the above is of course a tip of the iceberg list).

However, perhaps what is unique is the application of these ideas in current times, within our current contextual challenges. Here our authors and their collaborators are bringing to life ways which we can change thinking and practice that address the realities, challenges and suffering of a post-financial crash and a hyper-neoliberal global system.

The Current Context in the UK and Beyond in 2019

Since the financial crash in 2009, the UK and other parts of Europe, have experienced the 'violence' of neoliberal, ideological power through the austerity policies implemented, demanding a reduced state and public spending with accompanying privatisation and an ongoing marketisation of our public services (Cooper & Whyte, 2017). Professor Philip Alston, the United Nations Special Rapporteur on extreme poverty and human rights came to visit the UK in 2018 on a fact-finding mission and found that '*14 million people, a fifth of the population, live in poverty. Four million of these are more than 50% below the poverty line, and 1.5 million are destitute, unable to afford basic essentials…For almost one in every two children to be poor in twenty-first century Britain is not just a disgrace, but a social calamity and an economic disaster, all rolled into one.*'

These powerful social and economic forces have also generated opportunities for anti-immigration sentiment, growing racism and hate crime and the scapegoating of the unemployed, those suffering psychological distress or living with disabilities who have experienced changes to social security systems as cuts and policy changes have created harmful and callous welfare systems, such as 'fit for work' assessments and coercive psychological approaches to 'getting people into work' (Cooper & Whyte, 2017; Friedli & Stearne, 2015). The degree of human suffering created by this welfare reform has exacerbated distress and increases in suicide by people with disabilities, as reported by activist groups such as 'Disabled People Against the Cuts' and recorded in the academic and non-fiction literature (e.g. Barr et al., 2015b; O'Hara, 2015). Moreover, women from the most marginalised and poorest communities in the UK have suffered disproportionately from austerity, notably those from Black and Asian communities (Hall et al., 2017) and austerity has exacerbated place-based health and social inequalities.

Additionally, in the UK, public and community spaces have been sold off by local government in response to austerity (Wheatly, 2019), meaning there are fewer non-commercialised places and spaces for people to meet, alongside huge inequalities in land ownership and wealth (Monbiot et al., 2019). Housing has become unaffordable for the many as gentrification takes hold in many of our cities (Minton, 2017), and the austere changes to housing policies since 2010, has led to homelessness vastly increasing, with rough sleeping rising by 165% in England and the use of temporary accommodation by 71% (Fitzpatrick et al., 2019).

This is not just in the UK. Several of the authors in this book write from Europe and South African perspectives and describe similar increasing distress from socio-economic inequalities. For instance, Vavvos and colleagues describe their role as action-orientated researchers and community psychologists within a coalition in Greece that acted to resist the evictions caused by an enforced national austerity programme. Similarly, our South African colleagues, Ahmed, Karriem and Mohammed, describe in their chapter of this book how the pursuit of a neoliberal, free-market economic system in South Africa has done little to transform the vast inequities, including across race and class lines, that still plague South Africa in the post-Apartheid era. They describe that although some gains have been made, poverty increased between 2011 and 2015, with 2.5 million more people in poverty, informal housing settlements have increased and a class divide in healthcare access remains extensive.

Many manifestations of distress have risen in response to these sociopolitical contexts. The chapters in this book document more international examples. In the UK, academics and campaigners have documented rising suicide rates, self-harm and rise in mental health problems for those in the most deprived areas (Barnes et al., 2016; Barr et al., 2015; Mattheys et al., 2018); this is reflected in treatments too. In the UK in 2016, there were 64.7 million antidepressant items prescribed compared to 31.0 million in 2006 (NHS Digital, 2017), with a disproportionate use of psychiatric drugs within low-income communities (EXASOL, 2017). Levels of loneliness in the UK are reported as almost a fifth of the population, up to 9 million people (British

Red Cross & Coop, 2016), whilst there has also been a significant rise in knife crime (Wilkinson, 2019) and a 26% increase in the number of children placed on a child protection plan (children's safeguarding services) between 2010–2011 and 2017–2018 (National Audit Office, 2019). Behind these issues lies so much pain and suffering for individuals, families, communities and the nation.

Responding to Rising Distress

David Smail famously stated that we cannot escape the clinic. That, while it is clear that the clinic is far from the most appropriate site to address the psychological distress and suffering that people experience, it would be a callous society that stood back and offered nothing. Smail implicitly recognised a need to acknowledge the modesty of the therapeutic contribution so long as people continued to labour under a global corporate plutocracy that depends for its very survival on the unremitting exploitation of mass of consumers rendered incapable of accurately criticising their condition (Smail, 2005).

While being mindful of the fundamental sense in Smail's observation, this book is an account of those who have sought, in one or another to escape the clinic. The authors and practitioners within have, through their own practices, some modest, others more radical, sought alternate terrains in order to conduct what they consider to be legitimate psychologies of distress. For many, the recognition of the ordinary humanity of the therapeutic relationship, and its role as a source of solidarity, has been the launch pad to engage in relational, spatial, political and rights-focused distress work. If there is one key element that ties together the contributions in this handbook it is an increasing understanding that suffering is social and the diagnostic tools and assumptions of mainstream psychiatry and psychologies too often fail to do justice to the complex realities of distress (Moloney, 2013). This realisation is not only grasped by the endeavours of the authors and practitioners in this book. There has been repeated and multiple calls for more operationalisation of systems thinking in both the design of interventions which address health inequality and their evaluation (Hernández et al., 2017).

However, the projects and practices contained in this book still stand largely against the individualising tide. For those experiencing mental health problems, recent years have seen a year-on-year increase in the provision of primarily individually focused mental health interventions; psychiatric medication and psychological therapy are still the default interventions in mental health

(Harper, 2016). Indeed the Healthcare Commission (2007) noted that 92 % of their service-user sample had taken medication. Sloan (2010) was concerned that psychology has systematically made itself irrelevant to debates in economics and politics because it has failed to include broad socio-economic concepts in the education of psychology professionals. This mode of practice is most certainly still the dominant model in the training and practice of psychologists of distress and remains directly connected to the wider forces of colonialism, capitalism and injustice. As Malherbe and colleagues in Chap. 8 describe, other forms of knowing have been subjugated:

> *Certainly, colonised peoples and their knowledge system are unable to sufficiently meet the 'requirements of respectability'—or what is sometimes referred to as the master codes* (Mbembe, 2001)*—of a colonial world that is made largely in the image of wealthy, white, cisgendered, heterosexual, male able bodies.*

There are a number of ways to construct the key sites for action when creating health responses. Such constructions legitimise what we consider to be appropriate responses to the constructed problem. Rather than contextualise the suffering that has characterised many peoples' lives as the result of political and economic and political ideology, 'mental health' has been substantially viewed as an individual issue that requires psychological or pharmacological intervention.

However, we would argue that most, if not all, of the work in this book points towards ways in which the disciplines of critical community psychology and clinical psychology, often related in many countries, and in the UK in particular, are currently experiencing innovations that could be characterised as moving from the individualising practice realm toward an altogether more contextualising orientation. As the chapters in this book demonstrate, this requires fundamental shifts at all stages of our approach—from research methodologies, how we understand impact and for who, to the construction and legitimisation of different sites for action and responses to differently constructed 'problems'. This book seeks to document new opportunities to challenge local, national or global political, social and economic systems at different scales. We hope the reader will see this book as an inspiring manual containing opportunities to practice differently in the UK and beyond, as ways of resisting and challenging these forces.

Moving from the Marginal to Mainstream: The Opportunities and Challenges

These innovations are also timely because 'mental health awareness' is becoming a zeitgeist. In the UK in 2019, everyone is talking about mental health or is pressing for people to be talking about it. The wellness industry, the mindfulness industry, mental health in the workplace they have all taken off as large-scale, capitalist industries. Similarly, tech companies are releasing mental health apps, data, videos and animations and so forth and the cash strapped service commissioners and policy-makers are wondering if digital solutions can fill the mental health treatment gap (e.g. Hollis et al., 2015). Digital entrepreneurs are perceived as key to the future of the nation's well-being (e.g. see Cook, 2019, article in 'Elite Business Magazine'). We do not need to critique the wellness industries here when others, like academic Will Davies, have exposed their weaknesses (Davies, 2015) and it is not to say digital healthcare doesn't have a role, however, we believe that as practitioners, students, psychologists, therapists, academics and related roles, we need to take responsibility for the role our professions have had in individualising distress and how this has been mainstreamed and work hard to counteract this. The evidence for the social determinants of mental health are robust, the social and economic conditions people live in are paramount (World Health Organization, 2014), yet the mainstream narratives and spending do not represent this, focusing on ameliorative interventions (Johnston et al., 2018; Thomas et al., 2018). We need to shift from responsibilising 'clients' through over-emphasising the individualistic and intra-psychic notions to responsibilising ourselves as practitioners, researchers and so forth for being complicit in making the political personal, whilst also recognising that our own practice also happens in context and driven by wider systems. This responsibility-taking may involve some discomfort, indeed, it necessitates some discomfort as we try and bring these 'new' ways of working from the marginal to the mainstream.

Whilst this means we are encouraging many applied psychologists (including clinical, counselling, educational etc.) to take up ideas from critical community and liberation psychology and take inspiration from these chapters, where this does happen, these approaches can become 'add ons' to the mainstream clinical teaching, perhaps even 'nice to haves' in students' final lectures before qualifying. As Ahmed and colleagues explain in their chapter in this book, this conjunction applies in South Africa too, drawing on their example of trying to facilitate a community psychology project as part of clinical psychology programme and the inherent tensions and limitations of this.

It is important that we acknowledge the differences and tensions between the philosophies of these fields and understand the risks of putting them together, including within this book. These differences become clear from quotes such as '*clinical psychology has its foundations in modernity, privileging rationality, and the belief in continual scientific and technological progress* (in Van De Mwere & Weatherall, 2019, p. 2).' This aspect of our UK professional training and the evidence-based discourse dominates thinking. Anecdotally, pejorative statements and concerns are raised by colleagues about 'less qualified' practitioners or misuse of protected titles far more frequently than statements about the over-individualising nature of any practice. In addition, knowledge that seems self-evident becomes legitimate evidence only through (expensive) experimental science or neuroscience. For instance, articles in newspapers report on neuroscience studies encouraging us to go into nature because of the benefits to our brains (Johnston, 2013). Experimental psychology books, careers and research funding are dedicated to how poverty impacts on our limited cognitive 'bandwidth' (Mullainathan & Shafir, 2013). Poverty creates scarcity and overloads cognitive bandwidths, which means that 'interventions' on people in poverty might fail. In other words, in the field of psychology, it is these repeated experiments on students in lab-induced 'scarce' experimental conditions that becomes the legitimate evidence required to confirm that living in poverty might be genuinely hard, rather than the lived experience of millions.

Nor does current mental health training consider the 'social pathologies of contemporary civilisation' as in sociology (Keohane & Petersen, 2013). For instance, our disconnection from nature and the non-human world is rarely taken as a serious affliction and it is incredible how little UK clinical psychology (and again clinical can be exchanged here with counselling, educational, other forms of applied psychology and many forms of therapy) is attuned to structural and social forces, planetary health or takes a political stance.[1] We are engaged in veteran mental health programmes and research, but there is little said about war or other forms of violence. We have spread the mantra of 'trauma-informed' practice whilst we fear that in our workplaces we could be viewed as stepping outside of rationality if we challenge social adversity itself. It is in this context that Psychologists for Social Change (originally Psychologists Against Austerity) developed in the UK and their chapter in the book outlines

[1] Arguably this is changing in the UK and there is a growing number of psychologists engaging with policy, climate justice and social change.

their origins, strategy and approach to mobilising psychologists for political activism.

The spiritual dimensions of our humanity are also separated out within clinical practice. Spiritual practices are not easily integrated into Western psychological therapy, except perhaps when conceptualised as 'coping mechanisms'. Mindfulness has for instance become mainstream but a side effect of this isolated practice has been to reinforce the notion of self-improvement and coping better with intense employment and education systems rather than necessarily resist or transform them (Purser, 2019). Although mindfulness can of course be beneficial, if wider mental health practice ignores the social context of neoliberalism and a fake meritocracy, spiritual practices like mindfulness can be misused for personal gain or career and business development. A moving chapter in this book, 'The Jannah Tree' by Rukhsana Arshad, outlines an innovative approach to reintegrating the spiritual with the clinical in a meaningful way by creating online communities and drawing on metaphors and images from the Islamic faith. This chapter demonstrates how relatively small co-creation processes and changes in the therapeutic process can be of significant value to a culturally excluded group and be more focused around lived experience than technicalities.

The positionality of applied psychologists as 'neutral' must be understood systemically. 'Evidence-based practice' is the UK's healthcare system's only way of knowing despite this evidence being in and of itself, shaped by historical, cultural and sociological stories (Thomas et al., 2018). Far more research funding is available for biomedical ways of knowing about health than socially contextualised or co-created knowledge (Jones & Wilsdon, 2018). As a result clinicians have become accountable to these practices and systems, more than they are to those they serve. Indeed, psychologists in our National Health Service (NHS) have even been penalised simply for advocating for their service users in terms of their housing and social security needs because this is not considered in line with legitimate practice.

This over-emphasis on positivist science within mental health and a concordant superior belief in its methods and techniques, mean it is possible clinical psychology and its systems will inevitably compromise community psychology practice. For instance, social justice values can be compromised, and clinical psychologists can be forced into more comfortable positions that don't challenge power. It is so often the case that people seem more interested in brains than poverty and it is easy to be seduced by that. Yet all manner of large-scale social forces and discreet local social experiences can come to be translated into distress and misery; we must attend to these. Herein lies the tensions for those trained in clinical psychology wanting to take a different positionality and a number of chapters in the first part of this book explore this head on as they bring the political into clinical psychology.

Academic colleagues from counselling psychology have reflected on the importance of stewardship of concepts like 'intersectionality', creating guidelines to ensure its radical roots and authorship are not watered down or lost as the ideas move into the mainstream (Moradi & Grzanka, 2017): for example, ensuring that 'intersectionality' is accurately recorded with its historical roots in Black feminism and women of colour social justice activism. Similarly, as practitioners we must be stewards of the radical roots of the fields of community and liberation psychologies. It is so much more than another technique. It is a sociohistorical way of understanding the world that permeates what we might consider important knowledge and ways of knowing in the context of power relations (Montero et al., 2017). It is about being directly accountable to marginalised people in a meaningful way, whatever form that might take. The chapters in this book bring to life some helpful thinking about authentic accountability. For instance, in Chap. 24, Taliep and colleagues bring to life structures and processes of community-based participatory research which ensured the teams were accountable to the community.

The Everyday Challenges of Working Differently

Without wanting to become too mired in professional naval-gazing, it is worth briefly exploring the tensions and dilemmas that can arise when as practitioners we try to work from a social justice and critical community psychology framework. Dilemmas in which there are often no straightforward answers, such as: whether to participate in events led by institutions we may not completely agree with? Whether to work for such institutions and try and change them from the inside? Or when working with communities, dilemmas such as: are we undermining community activists and bringing too much of our own 'psychology' agenda and rituals? If we are given platforms, and choose to speak about marginalised communities, are we making assumptions about what those people might say or are we helpfully speaking out? Is any research done 'on' communities useful for the greater good? In Sally's work at MAC-UK (www.mac-uk.org), a charity transforming services for excluded young people in London, there are multiple dilemmas every day. The work involves supporting other youth mental health services to embed the principles of community psychology and co-production into their design and delivery (Zlotowitz et al., 2016; Durcan et al., 2017). The questions arise of how do you best bring people onto the journey of working differently? How do you negotiate and compromise within statutory services? How do new ways of working interact with a conventional system? It requires consistent reflective and reflexive practice, diverse teams and critical friendships to support with thinking through these sorts of dilemmas.

Dialogue is key and spaces are needed to build trust with colleagues, activists and those we work with to allow for this real dialogue. Within many of the chapters in this book the authors have been generous enough to cover their own dilemmas, tensions, mistakes and challenges in this work. This is what makes it so useful. It is important to know that we all struggle, that we are often drowning in the grey areas, that we all have blind spots and can get it wrong in practice. Collective solidarity and generosity towards colleagues, students and those in different agencies are all part of the change required. And yet, at the same time, it is also true that is the responsibility of those with privilege to understand our impact and do what we can to ensure our work does not replicate social inequities. This requires constructive collective thinking like that provided by the authors in this book.

Possible Futures

'Global mental health' initiatives and movements have led to some uncritically transposing Western values onto other societies (Bracken et al., 2016) and without considering learning in the other direction. Yet bold ideas about what constitutes good health and well-being are emerging out of the climate and social justice movements, for instance, the 'sumak kawsay' concept which originates in South America indigenous cultures and has been enshrined in the constitutions of Ecuador and Bolivia (Gudynas, 2011). As explained by the writer Oliver Balch in the UK's *Guardian* newspaper (2013), 'Buen Vivir' (the Spanish translation) challenges so many elements of the Eurocentric dominant culture:

> *A defining characteristic of buen vivir is harmony… harmony between human beings, and also between human beings and nature. A related theme is a sense of the collective. Capitalism is a great promoter of individual rights: the right to own, to sell, to keep, to have. But this alternative paradigm from South America subjugates the rights of the individual to those of peoples, communities and nature.*

Many other indigenous cultures around the world have wonderfully variegated vocabularies to express similar concepts about ways of life that value togetherness, diversity, reciprocity and care for life, that is the African *Ubuntu* philosophy (Mabovula, 2011) or *utu* and *mana* in Māori culture (Metge, 2002; Henare 2001). Our colleagues in South Africa are doing thought-provoking work with excluded young people through nature-based practice, traditional rites of passage and wilderness work (this work is not represented in this book but take a look at https://usiko.org.za/ and Naidoo et al., 2017). Many of our South African colleagues in this book are arguing for a decolonised approach to research, services and models in improving their communities' health and reducing structural and physical violence—resisting the medical and psychological models of Europe and the US. These bigger picture visions which link the social, economic and ecological to human welfare are gaining traction in the Global North. The well-being economy alliance (https://wellbeingeconomy.org/) is pulling together the different innovations, governments and organisations working to redefine progress according to concepts such as planetary health, degrowth, economic indicators beyond GDP, community wealth building, the regenerative economy and other new economies. Our hope is that the work outlined in this book will contribute to these bigger visions and movements, providing practical, smaller scale examples of how we can slowly move towards them in the work we do as psychologists and ways that we can contribute (e.g. Zlotowitz & Lloyd, 2019). We hope this will help us make steps towards a new era in psychological practice and thinking.

About This Book

When we asked for submissions for this book our ambition was for that it could partly act as a platform for more marginalised voices and guard against the 'ivory towers'. That included our younger colleagues, those based in non-European countries, those from marginalised communities and with direct experiences of oppressive structural forces, like inequality, poverty, violence, racism, sexism, ableism, heterosexism and so forth. We encouraged authors to include the voices of participants from projects or services and to be practical, creative and accessible wherever possible. We wanted to humanise our authors and their work with photos and stories. Our hope was, and is, that this book might appeal to community activists and be a useful tool to a range of practitioners and citizens. Unsurprisingly, it was difficult to realise this aim—the language and rituals of psychology are still strong within the book and therefore it is unlikely to be inclusive and accessible. Nonetheless, we are grateful to our authors and contributors for thinking with us about this process and putting extra time into creative processes which we hope has made some difference.

The chapters feature activities in which the traditional remits of community and clinical psychology (and other psychologies) have been subverted, altered, stretched, changed and reworked in order to reframe practice around human rights, creativity, political activism, social change, space and place, systemic violence, community transformation, resource allocation and radical practices of disruption and direct action. As Editors, we understand that readers will have different perspectives about the degree to which each case example breaks away from traditional remits. People are beginning in different contexts and working within different systems and there is often tension between what is and what seems possible. What we hope is that the tensions are named, are clear and will encourage dialogue with each other and across countries as we build a movement of practice.

We have loosely split the chapters into the following themes: clinical psychology and political activism, working in radical and disruptive spaces, transformative change work, creativity and social change. These are not 'hard' distinctions, there is certainly overlap and difference within and across the categories, but these themes we hope provide a pragmatic structure. Beginning with the part 'Clinical Psychology and Political Activism' the first three chapters outline how through collective and political action outside of services, clinical psychologists can challenge the social determinants of mental ill-health (e.g. housing, austerity) and the opportunities and limitations of this. This part includes a discussion of the ways in which acts of resistance from inside the clinical system can move practice away from damaging models and on activism and psychology in a broader sense with some ideas for creating and sustaining activism. The part 'working in radical and disruptive spaces' includes a host of different approaches, from disrupting individual therapeutic methods in the UK through to decolonial practice with community groups in South Africa, co-creation of support through online communities and the 'opening up' of university spaces for those experiencing mental distress. The third part 'transformative change work' contains an exciting range of innovative approaches to research and practice from work based in many different countries. The chapters are full of thoughtful ways of partnering with marginalised groups to create better services, social conditions, platforms for resistance and self and community expression. Finally, the fourth part on 'creativity and social change' offer examples of creative methods and outputs, from poetry, creative writing to photography, documentary-making and other arts, to inspire action on incredibly difficult experiences, like homelessness, the effects of austerity and poverty or mental ill-health. For us all these chapters create a huge amount of hope for a better way of connecting and creating social change.

References

Adame, A. L., Morsey, M., Bassman, R., & Yates, K. (2017). A brief history of the psychiatric survivor movement. In *Exploring identities of psychiatric survivor therapists*. Palgrave Macmillan.

Balch, O. (2013). *The Guardian*. Retrieved October 10, 2019, from https://www.theguardian.com/sustainable-business/blog/buen-vivir-philosophy-south-america-eduardo-gudynas

Barnes, M. C., Gunnell, D., Davies, R., Hawton, K., Kapur, N., Potokar, J., & Donovan, J. L. (2016). Understanding vulnerability to self-harm in times of economic hardship and austerity: A qualitative study. *BMJ Open, 6*(2), e010131.

Barr, B., Kinderman, P., & Whitehead, M. (2015a). Trends in mental health inequalities in England during a period of recession, austerity and welfare reform 2004 to 2013. *Social Science & Medicine, 147*, 324–331.

Barr, B., Taylor-Robinson, D., Stuckler, D., Loodstra, R., Reeves, A., & Whitehead, M. (2015b). First, do no harm': Are disability assessments associated with adverse trends in mental health? A longitudinal ecological study. *Journal of Epidemiology and Community Health., 0*, 1–7.

Bracken, P., Giller, J., & Summerfield, D. (2016). Primum non nocere. The case for a critical approach to global mental health. *Epidemiology and Psychiatric Sciences, 25*(6), 506–510.

British Red Cross & Coop. (2016). Trapped in a bubble: An investigation into triggers for loneliness in the UK.

Bulhan, H. A. (1985). *Frantz Fanon and the psychology of oppression*. Plenum Press.

Césaire, A. (2000). *Discourse on colonialism* (New ed.). New York University Press.

Cook, L. (2019). *Elite Business Magazine*. Retrieved October 10, 2019, from http://elitebusinessmagazine.co.uk/people/item/ten-uk-startups-paving-the-way-to-better-mental-health

Cooper, V., & Whyte, D. (2017). *The violence of austerity*. Pluto Press.

Crenshaw, K. W. (1991). Mapping the margins: Intersectionality, identity politics, and violence against women of color. *Stanford Law Review, 43*, 1241–1299.

Davies, W. (2015). *The happiness industry: How the government and big business sold us well-being*. Verso Books.

Durcan, G., Zlotowitz, S., & Stubbs, J. (2017). *Meeting us where we're at: Learning from INTEGRATE's work with excluded young people*. Centre for Mental Health.

EXASOL. (2017). EXASOL analyzes: research shows that over 64, prescriptions of antidepressants are dispensed per year in England. Visualised for the first time.

EXASOL. Available at https://www.exasol.com/en/company/newsroom/news-and-press/2017-04-13-over-64-million-prescriptions-of-antidepressants-dispensedper-year-in-england/

Fanon, F. (1967). *Black skins, white masks* (R. Philcox, Trans.). Grove.

Fitzpatrick, S., Pawson, H., Bramley, G., Wood, J., Watts, B., Stephens, M., & Blenkinsopp, J. (2019). The homelessness monitor: England 2019. *Crisis*. https://www.crisis.org.uk/media/240419/the_homelessness_monitor_england_2019.pdf

Freire, P. (1972). *Pedagogy of the oppressed* (M.B. Ramos, Trans.). Herder and Herder (Original work published 1968).

Friedli, L., & Stearn, R. (2015). Positive affect as coercive strategy: Conditionality, activation and the role of psychology in UK government workfare programmes. *Medical humanities, 41*(1), 40–47.

Gudynas, E. (2011). Buen Vivir: Today's tomorrow. *Development, 54*(4), 441–447.

Hall, S. M., McIntosh, K., Neitzert, E., Pottinger, L., Sandhu, K., Stephenson, M. A., Reed, H., & Taylor, L. (2017). *Intersecting inequalities: The impact of austerity on Black and Minority Ethnic women in the UK*. Runnymede and Women's Budget Group.

Harper, D. (2016). Beyond individual therapy: Towards a psychosocial approach to public mental health. *The Psychologist, 29*(June), 440–444.

Healthcare Commission, Britain, G., Kennedy, I., & Walker, A. (2007). *State of healthcare 2007: Improvements and challenges in services in England and Wales*. Stationery Office.

Henare, M. (2001). Tapu, mana, mauri, hau, wairua: A Maori philosophy of vitalism and cosmos. In *Indigenous traditions and ecology: The interbeing of cosmology and community* (pp. 197–221). Harvard University Press for the Centre for the Study of World Religions.

Hernández, A., Ruano, A. L., Marchal, B., San Sebastián, M., & Flores, W. (2017). Engaging with complexity to improve the health of indigenous people: A call forthe use of systems thinking to tackle health inequity. *International Journal for Equity in Health, 16*(1), 1–5.

Henrich, J., Heine, S. J., & Norenzayan, A. (2010). The weirdest people in the world? *Behavioral and Brain Sciences, 33*(2–3), 61–83.

Hollis, C., Morriss, R., Martin, J., Amani, S., Cotton, R., Denis, M., & Lewis, S. (2015). Technological innovations in mental healthcare: Harnessing the digital revolution. *The British Journal of Psychiatry, 206*(4), 263–5.

Hooks, B. (2000). *Where we stand: Class matters*. Psychology Press.

Johnston, I. (2013). *The Independent*. Retrieved October 10, 2019, from https://www.independent.co.uk/news/science/human-brain-hard-wired-for-rural-tranquillity-8996368.html

Johnstone, L., Boyle, M., Cromby, J., Dillon, J., Harper, D., Kinderman, P., Longden, E., Pilgrim, D., & Read, J. (2018). *The power threat meaning framework: Towards the identification of patterns in emotional distress, unusual experiences and troubled or troubling behavior, as an alternative to functional psychiatric diagnosis.* British Psychological Society.

Jones, R., & Wilsdon, J. (2018). *The biomedical bubble: Why UK research and innovation needs a greater diversity of priorities, politics, places and people.* NESTA.

Katz, J. (1985). The sociopolitical nature of counselling. *Counselling Psychologist, 13*, 615–624.

Keohane, K., & Petersen, A. (Eds.). (2013). *The social pathologies of contemporary civilization.* Routledge.

Mabovula, N. N. (2011). The erosion of African communal values: A reappraisal of the African Ubuntu philosophy. *Inkanyiso: Journal of Humanities and Social Sciences, 3*(1), 38–47.

Maldonado-Torres, N. (2017). Frantz Fanon and the decolonial turn in psychology: From modern/colonial methods to the decolonial attitude. *South African Journal of Psychology, 47*, 432–441.

Martín-Baró, I. (1996). *Writings for a liberation psychology* (A. Aron & S. Corne, Eds.). Harvard University Press.

Mattheys, K., Warren, J., & Bambra, C. (2018). "Treading in sand": A qualitative study of the impact of austerity on inequalities in mental health. *Social Policy & Administration, 52*(7), 1275–1289.

Mbembe, A. (2001). *On the postcolony.* University of California Press.

McDermott, D. (2001). Parenting and ethnicity. In *Handbook of diversity in parenting education: The changing faces of parenting and parent education* (pp. 73–96). Academic Press.

Metge, J. (2002). Returning the gift—Utu in intergroup relations: In memory of Sir Raymond Firth. *The Journal of the Polynesian Society, 111*(4), 311–338.

Moloney, P. (2013). *The therapy industry: The irresistible rise of the talking cure, and why it Doesn't Work.* Pluto Press, London.

Minton, A. (2017). *Big capital: Who is London for?* Penguin.

Monbiot, G., Grey, R., Kenny, T., Macfarlane, L., Powell-Smith, A., Shrubsole, G., & Stratford, B. (2019). Land for the Many: Changing the way our fundamental asset is used, owned and governed. *The Labour Party.* Retrieved October 10, 2019, from http://labour.org.uk/wp-content/uploads/2019/06/12081_19-Land-for-the-Many.pdf

Montero, M., Sonn, C. C., & Burton, M. (2017). Community psychology and liberation psychology: A creative synergy for an ethical and transformative praxis. In M. A. Bond, I. Serrano-García, C. B. Keys, & M. Shinn (Eds.), *APA handbook of community psychology: Theoretical foundations, core concepts, and emerging challenges* (pp. 149–167). American Psychological Association.

Moradi, B., & Grzanka, P. R. (2017). Using intersectionality responsibly: Toward critical epistemology, structural analysis, and social justice activism. *Journal of Counseling Psychology, 64*(5), 500–513.

Morrison, L. J. (2013). *Talking back to psychiatry: The psychiatric consumer/survivor/ex-patient movement.* Routledge.

Mullainathan, S., & Shafir, E. (2013). *Scarcity: Why having too little means so much*. Macmillan.

Naidoo, A. V. (1996). Challenging the hegemony of Eurocentric psychology. *Journal of Community and Health Sciences, 2*(2), 9–16.

Naidoo, A. V., Zygmont, C., & Philips, S. (2017). Harnessing the power of ecopsychology in community work. In *Emancipatory and participatory methodologies in peace, critical, and community psychology* (pp. 77–89). Springer. Journal of Community and Health Sciences, 2(2), 9–16.

National Audit Office. (2019). *Pressures on children's social care*.

NHS Digital. (2017). Prescriptions dispensed in the community, statistics for England–2006–2016 [PAS].

O'Hara, M. (2015). *Austerity bites: A journey to the sharp end of cuts in the UK*. Policy Press.

Purser, R. E. (2019). *McMindfulness, how mindfulness became the new capitalist spirituality*. Repeater Books.

Rapley, M., Moncrieff, J., & Dillon, J. (Eds.). (2011). *De-medicalizing misery: Psychiatry, psychology and the human condition*. Springer.

Smail, D. J. (2005). *Power, interest and psychology: Elements of a social materialist understanding of distress*. PCCS books.

Sloan, T. (2010). Globalization, poverty and social justice. In G. Nelson & I. Prilleltensky (Eds.), *Community psychology: In pursuit of liberation and well-being* (2nd edn) (pp. 309–329). New York: Palgrave Macmillan.

Thomas, F., Hansford, L., Ford, J., Wyatt, K., McCabe, R., & Byng, R. (2018). Moral narratives and mental health: Rethinking understandings of distress and healthcare support in contexts of austerity and welfare reform. *Palgrave Communications, 4*(1), 1–8.

Van Der Merwe, H., & Wetherell, M. (2019). The emotional psychologist: A qualitative investigation of norms, dilemmas, and contradictions in accounts of practice. *Journal of Community & Applied Social Psychology, 30*, 1–19.

Wheatly, H. (2019). The mass sell-off of public land is driving the housing crisis. *The Huffington Post*. Retrieved October 10, 2019, from https://www.huffingtonpost.co.uk/entry/housing-crisis-public-land_uk_5c811055e4b0a135b5199d5d

Wilkinson, E. (2019). How medical teams are coping with rising knife crime. *BMJ, 364*, l104.

World Health Organization and Calouste Gulbenkian Foundation. (2014). *Social determinants of mental health*. World Health Organization.

Zlotowitz, S., Barker, C., Moloney, O., & Howard, C. (2016). Service users as the key to service change? The development of an innovative intervention for excluded young people. *Child and Adolescent Mental Health, 21*(2), 102–108.

Zlotowitz, S., & Lloyd, J. (2019). Beyond the individual in mental health and wellbeing. *Stir to Action magazine*: 'Playground for a new economy', issue 26.

Part I

Clinical Psychology and Political Activism

> I pondered [...] what effect poverty has on the mind; and what effect wealth has on the mind; [...] and I thought how unpleasant it is to be locked out; and I thought how it is worse perhaps to be locked in. (Virginia Woolf, *A Room of One's Own*)

This section presents a range of contributions positioned to fill the gap between the narrow space of individual clinical psychologies and political activism call for mobilising towards social justice. In their chapters, the authors acknowledge that clinical interventions are often too limited in scope, and therefore the increasing need to serve a wider range of different people within their community contexts is an open challenge for contemporary psychologies. All the chapters contained in this section embrace a common vision that clinical psychology can better tackle mental distress by going beyond the therapeutic room and the *modus operandi* of profit-based healthcare provision. In fact, whilst an increasing number of *psy* professionals are aware of how structural inequalities impact individual mental health, in this section authors call for an explicit engagement of such professions with political activism for social justice.

In Chap. 2, for example, Carey et al. argue how the *psy* professionals can support collective action for social justice, through the example of their collaborative work with housing activists and groups to raise awareness and take action against London's unjust housing system. Following a similar ethos, in Chap. 3, Psychologists for Social Change outline how the homonymous movement was born and developed in the UK, gathering a heterogeneous group of *psy* professionals and like-minded people, in order to enact meaningful social change for those affected by structural social inequalities. In Chap. 4, the Walk the Talk Crew presents an initiative where the authors, as clinical psychologists themselves, embarked on a hundred miles journey to literally step out of the clinic room, and engage in person with the lives of those they encountered in the journey.

Moving from the outdoors to the indoors, in Chap. 5, Randall, Gunn, and Coles explore how clinical psychologists working within the constraints of imposed psychiatric diagnosis can challenge such powerful and dominant discourses by integrating alternative approaches, learning how to question diagnosis, and ultimately building alliances with the public and political activists. Interestingly, in Chap. 6, Sloan and Brush identify in working with activists an important chance for the '*psy*-workers of the world' to help activism within social movements. In Chap. 7, Walker and Zoli argue how academics in the *psy*-related disciplines, as well, have an important role to play in bridging the gap between professionals, scholars, and citizens. Here they provide a critical account of how the militant methodology of 'statactivism' can be used to subvert dominant representations of reality, which hide and deny the ongoing marketization of healthcare and Higher Education in the UK.

To conclude, the quote by Virginia Woolf opening this section represents the dilemma between who is 'locked in' (*psy* professionals and service users) and who is 'locked out' (activists, and people who cannot afford therapies and healthcare). Such a *status quo* is painful and subjugating both for who is 'locked out' unable to access services and unheard by *psy* professionals and policymakers, and for who is 'locked in' torn between privilege and thirst for change. The full chapters will show in detail why it is necessary for clinical psychologies and related services to meet political activism and provide ideas on how to do it.

2

Building Alliances with Marginalised Communities to Challenge London's Unjust and Distressing Housing System

Nina Carey, Sally Zlotowitz, Samantha James, Aysen Dennis, Thomas Gillespie, and Kate Hardy on behalf of The Housing & Mental Health Network

Aysen's Story

Aysen Dennis is a housing activist from the Aylesbury estate in Southwark, London. She started the Aylesbury campaign to resist the 'regeneration' of the large council estate back in 1999. A 'regeneration' which would see her displaced from the estate, or at best under the control of a housing association with inevitable rising rents. Aysen's life and the lives of her community have been immeasurably changed by the UK's unjust housing system. A system in which local and national government policies privilege the story of 'economic development' and powerful business over the views and experiences of local communities. Aysen summarises this as, 'they don't think working class people deserve to live in zone 1 of London.' The campaign has fought against

---

Dedication: we would like to dedicate this chapter to all the housing activists in Focus E15 and other London campaigns who devote so much of their time in the struggle for a just housing system and for which there is little recognition or paid work. Their support for those most affected by the unfair housing system simply cannot be quantified.

N. Carey
Homerton University Hospital NHS Foundation Trust/ East London NHS Foundation Trust, London, UK

S. Zlotowitz (✉)
MAC-UK & Art Against Knives, London, UK

C. Walker et al. (eds.), *The Palgrave Handbook of Innovative Community and Clinical Psychologies*, https://doi.org/10.1007/978-3-030-71190-0_2

such 'social cleansing' through many tactics including direct action, legal action and the occupation of unused buildings. In other ways, Aysen's resistance has been through her optimism and humanity: making links with neighbours, creating relationships and a sense of community, supporting and advocating for those who have no voice or are afraid of the authorities; mostly those from BAME communities.

All of this action and housing insecurity, which includes according to Aysen 19 years of lived experience of witnessing evictions, empty buildings, boarded up areas, security guards, stigma, community blaming, the withholding of maintenance repairs by the authorities, mistrust and fighting against powerful others, takes its toll on a community's psychological health. It is no surprise that individuals might feel distressed, given that we know insecurity is linked to good mental health (McGrath et al., 2015). It is also easy to see that the typical 'prescriptions' for mental health would be no replacement for solidarity, community cohesion and your own secure and personal place you can call 'home.'

Aysen, like all the housing activists we meet, is a true force of determination and deeply passionate about equality and justice. She has started working alongside the 'Housing and Mental Health Network' to mobilise mental health[1] professionals, calling on us to do our part in changing this unjust system, speaking out against social cleansing and speaking up for oppressed communities.

'The Housing and Mental Health Network'

A group of us set up a network made up of community members, academics, community and clinical psychologists, trainee clinical psychologists, teachers, students, artists and many more. We wanted to recognise the profound impact

S. James • A. Dennis
Fight for Aylesbury Campaign, London, UK

T. Gillespie
Global Development Institute, University of Manchester, Manchester, UK
e-mail: thomas.gillespie@manchester.ac.uk

Kate Hardy on behalf of The Housing & Mental Health Network
University of Leeds, Leeds, UK
e-mail: K.R.Hardy@leeds.ac.uk

[1] We note that the use of the term 'mental health' can be problematic, but the network honours the local communities who use this term to describe their experiences.

that the UK's unjust housing system has on the psychological health and wellbeing of our communities. These injustices are described below and are a result of neoliberal economic, financial and social policies which have led to gentrification, 'social cleansing' and huge shortages of council homes and affordable housing (Elmer & Dening, 2016; Watt & Minton, 2016). We had a shared goal of resisting these injustices to improve wellbeing at the community level and prevent the development of distress resulting from housing inequality and insecurity.

We worked together with other housing activists and groups to raise awareness and take action against London's unjust housing system through organising and speaking at events, participating in grassroots resident-led campaigns, doing *useful* (usually action) research, advocacy, creative productions and developing policy briefings and other informational materials. We campaigned about the structures, systems and policies that maintain housing insecurity, are profoundly coercive and that displace people from their communities. Our message is that good psychological health is a product of social justice, including adequate and secure housing and a connection to our community (Anderson et al., 2003; Marmot & Bell, 2012; Wilkinson & Pickett, 2011).

The Unjust Housing System in London

In the context of the UK, and particularly London, neoliberalism, privatisation and financialisation of the housing system has ensured a system that is rigged towards property developers and the already rich in combination with the reduction of social housing stock and a housing crisis for the poorest (Minton, 2017; Watt & Minton, 2016). These policies have included: the selling off of council housing under Prime Minister Margaret Thatcher in the 1980s onwards; the limitation of local authorities to build social housing; the austerity policies after the financial crash of 2007–2008 that grew inequality in London and undermined wages of the poorest and of course the buying of London property for investment and profiting purposes by the global rich and elite (for fuller overviews see Edwards, 2016 and Watt & Minton, 2016). As Beswick et al. (2016) state: '*London is now the unrivalled king of the global property league for the super-rich, with prime property values rising faster than any major city in the last decade* (Knight Frank, 2015)' (p. 321). Indeed, Edwards (2016) quotes a study suggesting that just 189,000 families own nearly two-thirds of the UK's 60 million acres and a further 40,000 families own three quarters of that (Cahill, 2001).

In addition, corporate power has also contributed to the housing crisis. The campaigning organisation, 'Debt Resistance UK,' has shown how corporate banks have loaned local authorities harmful 'LOBO' loans that result in huge interest rates and council tax being used to directly pay off these loan interests. Debt Resistance UK estimates that approximately 80% of Newham's publicly raised council tax is being used to pay loan interest; money going straight to corporate banks. As they state on their website, 'Debt is a tool to uphold the status quo, part of a system that distributes wealth from the majority and public to the super-rich' (http://debtresistance.uk/). (And on the back of the public 'bail-out' of the corporate banks.) Newham is not alone, hundreds of councils across the UK hold LOBO loans and as a result citizens are paying huge amounts in interest across the UK and Debt Resistance UK are encouraging local action to challenge these corporate debts (see http://lada.debtresistance.uk/).

Meanwhile, 'affordable' homes, otherwise known as 80% of the market rate, are deeply unaffordable to local people (Elmer & Dening, 2016; e.g. this definition includes monthly rents of £1500 and one-bedroom flats sold at £450,000). Although gentrification has been promoted in policies as a way to decrease segregation in communities, research suggests it results in inner cities being claimed by the middle classes to the detriment of the communities that are assumed to be helped by the process (Lees, 2008). When areas are 'regenerated', homes are often demolished, and existing residents forced to move out of an area (Elmer & Dening, 2016). When people are displaced, not only are they moved away from their friends, family and networks, they are often not allocated a permanent home and may end up homeless. There are many ways a person can be legally categorised as homeless, including not having accommodation available, the accommodation being uninhabitable, or a person being at risk of violence by continuing to live in their accommodation (Shelter, 2010).

As a network, we believe that a permanent home is a human right. We are becoming increasingly concerned about the number of households, including families with children, who are being placed in temporary accommodation, up by 60% since 2011 according to recent government statistics (House of Commons, 2018). Temporary accommodation can include hostels, bed and breakfast hotels, registered social landlords and local authority accommodation or private rented properties which can be arranged through the local authority. People do not get to choose which type of accommodation they are placed in, and there are huge variations in the quality of these homes (Shelter, 2010).

By the end of December 2017, 78,930 households in England were in temporary accommodation, and these households included 120,510 children. Sixty-nine per cent of these households were in London. There has also been an increase in the number of families with children who have been placed in B&B style temporary accommodation from 740 in 2010 to over 2000 in 2017 (House of Commons, 2018). This is shocking considering at a conservative estimate there are over 200,000 empty homes in England and the number is rising, many of them left purposefully empty by foreign investors in London or owners cannot afford to renovate them (Action on Empty Homes, 2019).

The Impact of Injustices in the Housing System

It may come as no surprise that distress named as stress, depression, panic attacks and insomnia has been attributed to difficulties people face going through the social housing system (Thompson et al., 2017). In fact, research from a range of cities suggests that families pay a particularly high price for housing instability. Longitudinal research has demonstrated that mental health problems are higher in mothers who have experienced housing instability in comparison to a control group of families of low socioeconomic status in stable housing (Vostanis et al., 1998). Children are also hugely impacted, and those who have experienced homelessness have often experienced traumatic events such as witnessing domestic violence, being separated from parents or being threatened with being separated from their parents (Herbers et al., 2014). This may be particularly relevant in current cases where social care agencies threaten to remove children from their families as a result of homelessness, as the agencies only have a duty to the child.

Samantha James is a teacher in a London secondary school and a member of the Housing and Mental Health Network. She writes about her experience of working with pupils facing homelessness: *As a teacher, you quickly learn behind every student is a story. The 'quiet ones' who 'get on with it' in at 7:30am to prepare before school are also carers for parents, maybe grieving the loss of loved ones or survivors of domestic violence. The loud ones, impulsive and (mostly) quick witted shouting out in class because when you're one of seven children at home; you shout to be heard, listened to. Knowing your students is the concrete used as the foundations of your practice. But what about when you know your student has an unfit home environment or is in fact, homeless?*

For children to thrive they need safety, security and consistency. Abstracts enabled by one, single entity: a home. You need look no further than Maslow's hierarchy of needs to recognise the fundamental importance of shelter to allow students to be cognitively prepared for the process of learning. In fact, a report commissioned by Shelter, found "Homeless children are more likely to have behavioural problems such as aggression, hyperactivity and impulsivity, factors that compromise academic achievement and relationships with peers and teachers."

How Did the Network Begin?

The network was established in April 2017, launched at a meeting in East London following the findings from a Participatory Action Research (PAR) project undertaken by campaign group Focus E15 and two researchers (see Hardy & Gillespie, 2016 for the full research report).

Drawing on the experiences of people from the Focus E15 campaign group threatened with displacement from their home borough of Newham, East London to places such as Hastings, Birmingham and Manchester, the research examined the experiences of people facing homelessness and displacement. Activists from the Focus E15 campaign, some of whom were struggling with homelessness, were trained as researchers and conducted 64 structured interviews with participants who had approached Newham Council with a housing need in the previous year.

Amongst other findings, a key and striking outcome of the research was the demonstration of a dramatic detrimental impact on people's mental health. In sum, 89% of respondents report worsening mental health as a result of their housing situation (Hardy & Gillespie, 2016). The research informed Focus E15's decision to launch their 'Housing Is a Mental Health Issue' campaign and led to a realisation that stronger networks needed to be built between activists, campaigners, practitioners and academics working on the intersection of wellbeing and housing. The launch event was the first step towards developing this community in order to generate and share knowledge and campaign for housing and health justice for the most marginalised.

What Have We Been Doing So Far?

Since we set up, we have been hosting monthly meetings where we plan events and invite speakers in to learn more about particular issues. Working jointly with other activists and activist groups is a very important part of our work, such as Focus E15 and Medact. For example, we hosted a screening of the film

Dispossession directed by Paul Sng, which sheds light on the long-term failure to maintain council estates resulting in widespread demolition and 'regeneration' projects. The film follows residents who have been pushed out of their homes as a result of this process and the many communities that have been fighting tirelessly to protect their homes. We showed the film at a community cinema in Hackney in London and was followed by a Q&A panel with Paul Sng and a number of housing activists. We promoted the event through many psychologist networks and platforms (e.g. on psychologist Facebook groups), plus our own social networks and in local community spaces, reaching people who might be concerned by the issues but unsure how to respond. Over 300 people attended, and it was an important opportunity to inform a large number of people about the difficulties faced by people living in social housing.

We have also written letters to the media to shed light on the impact of the housing system on mental health, such as an open letter to the *Evening Standard* which stated the importance of finding permanent homes for ex-residents of the Grenfell tower. This was shared and signed widely on social media by psychologists and many others, which showed us how many people have been concerned about the wellbeing of Grenfell residents.

We have also been able to join events by other activist groups to offer a mental health lens, for example when joining Focus E15 mothers' event on child homelessness to speak on their panel. This was a successful event which demonstrated the effectiveness of mental health practitioners joining people with lived experience of housing insecurity to spread awareness and encourage action. We were also joined by the *Please Hold* theatre group at the community psychology festival in 2017 in Bristol in the UK. They performed a powerful spoken word piece based on their own experiences of housing insecurity, which was a creative way to draw people in and mobilise people into action. This type of joint work must be conducted thoughtfully, ensuring activists are not used to further professionals' interests or that 'professional voices' are not viewed as 'legitimising' the lived experience voices.

Our Hoped for Aims and the Realities of Organising

In 2018, we hoped to run a campaign about the misuse and overuse of temporary accommodation. We started to focus on this and plan our campaign with the following aims:

- To raise awareness of the impact of being placed in temporary accommodation on the mental health of families.
- To work towards putting an end to any family being placed in temporary accommodation for more than six weeks.
- To support local campaigns to empower residents of temporary accommodation to resist temporary accommodation and improve the conditions of any temporary accommodation they are in.
- To mobilise mental health and social care professionals to get involved in the campaigns and work towards social change (potentially taking direct action through their job roles if required, e.g. refusing to facilitate 'parenting' sessions for families in temporary accommodation).

Despite having good numbers of people attending meetings regularly, and a wonderful person doing some overall coordinating work, we struggled to make this campaign a reality. Many of us were volunteers doing this in our spare time and at times it became difficult to keep momentum going and to effectively absorb new members of the network. Indeed, as we write in 2019, we are less active as a network although still all connected via the social media app, 'WhatsApp' which has been a key organising tool. Partly this was also a response to changes in context: the European Union referendum and the outcome to 'leave' the EU ('Brexit') took over the political agenda of the UK in 2016 and it has been difficult to get any other political issues on to the national agenda. Austerity has continued, indeed worsened over the years, and so local government has continued to struggle to meet its housing duties, with ever growing social housing waiting lists. Members of the network have also been involved in these struggles. Nonetheless, activity does continue. Two trainee clinical psychologists (including author Nina Carey) have or are completing research theses on the topic of temporary accommodation or related issues in order to drive our knowledge of the impact. Other members have supported newly forming provision for single mothers. An organisation called 'The Magpie Project' in Newham in London (https://themagpieproject.org) arose around the same time to provide childcare, solidarity and support for the local mums in temporary accommodation. One of the Magpie's founders came and spoke at a community psychology event and it led to a series of connections being made. Invited by the group, psychologists volunteered to provide reflective spaces for staff and share psychological knowledge about social adversity, trauma and good practices in peer support and psychosocial accompaniment.

It is useful when these types of connections are made organically and so psychologists (and those of other backgrounds too) are invited in directly by community groups. However, it's important to stay reflexive about being clinical psychologists (or counselling, educational psychologists etc.) in these community spaces, making sure we do not 'over-professionalise' the nature of this community support (e.g. insisting on 'evidence-based' therapies only), checking in about what the mums, volunteers and staff really want (not assuming what we might think they want or need) and that we interact as humans not professionals in these spaces. Acting as 'professionals' is so embedded in our cultural norms it can be difficult to unpick; it doesn't mean losing all boundaries but an awareness that people's experiences of institutional services can be dehumanising. From these mums' perspectives, for instance, they are fully aware that professionals (who are often white and middle class) may see them primarily through a lens of 'poor parenting', 'unhelpful' thoughts or 'poor coping'. As Sonn (2004) outlines it is part of our work as psychologists in any context to pay attention to our multiple social identities in order to *'reveal the different positions of power and privilege we occupy in different contexts and how these can work in empowering and disempowering ways'* (p. 7). See that paper for a more detailed example of this process in practice.

In 2019, the London branch of the health professional campaigning organisation, 'Medact' (https://www.medact.org), invited members in to talk on the impact of temporary accommodation on mental health, with a view to launching their own housing campaign with an emphasis on both physical and mental health impacts. With this development came the opportunity for our original campaign aims to be realised and the network's members could now support Medact's campaign, who as an established organisation, fortunately have more funding, resources and infrastructure for organising.

As our resources and capacity reduced, we started to see the network role as one of supporting the wider housing movement and this work continues. For example, by making connections between different groups, creating platforms to reach new audiences, supporting activists and conducting research. Movement-building training by the New Economy Organisers Network (NEON) in the UK (https://neweconomyorganisers.org/) emphasises the different roles groups can have in the 'ecology' of a movement. Certainly the Housing and Mental Health network has played a small role within the ecology of London's housing movement, highlighting the very real distress caused by the system (for impressive groups in the movement have a look at the Radical Housing Network, the various estate-specific housing campaigns, e.g. Cressingham Gardens, Renter's Union, Defend Council Housing, Grenfell Action Group) and our contribution though small was welcomed and appreciated.

Just Do It!

We would encourage other mental health professionals to engage with other movements and offer their contribution with humility and passion as our members did. To maximise impact and to be sustainable, this may require finding ways of bringing these conversations into workplaces, such as the NHS or local authorities. There is so much robust evidence to support the link between health, mental health and social determinants that it should be part of psychologists' roles to find local or regional structural issues that are affecting the community's health and act on them. Potentially linking up with local public health practitioners or community groups and inviting them to speak could be one way of opening the conversation to these issues whilst working in traditional mental health services. After all, these opportunities have to be proactively created otherwise the status quo just continues. Don't wait for leaders—become them!

References

Action on Empty Homes. (2019). Empty homes in England. Retrieved September 29, 2019, from https://www.actiononemptyhomes.org/Handlers/Download.ashx?IDMF=68fa9a2d-83f5-4ca4-936b-a8d8248484c0

Anderson, L. M., Scrimshaw, S. C., Fullilove, M. T., & Fielding, J. E. (2003). The Community Guide's model for linking the social environment to health. *American Journal of Preventive Medicine, 24*(3), 12–20.

Beswick, J., Alexandri, G., Byrne, M., Vives-Miró, S., Fields, D., Hodkinson, S., & Janoschka, M. (2016). Speculating on London's housing future: The rise of global corporate landlords in 'post-crisis' urban landscapes. *City, 20*(2), 321–341.

Cahill, K. (2001). *Who owns Great Britain?* Canongate.

Edwards, M. (2016). The housing crisis and London. *City, 20*(2), 222–237.

Elmer, S., & Dening, G. (2016). The London clearances. *City, 20*(2), 271–277.

Hardy, K., & Gillespie, T. (2016). Homelessness, health and housing: Participatory action research in East London. Unpublished report. Retrieved May 30, 2018, from http://www.e15report.org.uk/

Herbers, J. E., Cutuli, J. J., Monn, A. R., Narayan, A. J., & Masten, A. S. (2014). Trauma, adversity, and parent–child relationships among young children experiencing homelessness. *Journal of Abnormal Child Psychology, 42*(7), 1167–1174.

House of Commons. (2018). *Households in temporary accommodation* [Online]. Retrieved May 30, 2018, from https://researchbriefings.parliament.uk/ResearchBriefing/Summary/SN02110

Knight Frank. (2015). Global Development Report 2015: Prime residential development trends and insight. Retrieved January 10, 2016, from http://www.knightfrank.com/research/global-developmentreport-2015-3229.aspx

Lees, L. (2008). Gentrification and social mixing: Towards an inclusive urban renaissance? *Urban Studies, 45*(12), 2449–2470.

Marmot, M., & Bell, R. (2012). Fair society, healthy lives. *Public Health, 126*(Suppl 1), S4–S10.

McGrath, L., Griffin, V., & Mundy, E. (2015). *The psychological impact of austerity: A briefing paper*. Psychologists Against Austerity.

Minton, A. (2017). *Big capital: Who is London For?* Penguin.

Shelter. (2010). *Supporting homeless children Guidance for children and family services.* Retrieved May 30, 2018, from https://england.shelter.org.uk/__data/assets/pdf_file/0007/269512/GP_Briefing_Supporting_homeless_children_Children_and_family_services.pdf

Sonn, C. (2004). Negotiating identities across cultural boundaries: Complicating cultural competence with power and privilege. *Critical Psychology*, 11, 134–149.

Thompson, C., Lewis, D. J., Greenhalgh, T., Smith, N. R., Fahy, A. E., & Cummins, S. (2017). "I don't know how I'm still standing" a Bakhtinian analysis of social housing and health narratives in East London. *Social Science & Medicine, 177*, 27–34.

Vostanis, P., Grattan, E., & Cumella, S. (1998). Mental health problems of homeless children and families: Longitudinal study. *BMJ, 316*(7135), 899–902.

Watt, P., & Minton, A. (2016). London's housing crisis and its activisms: Introduction. *City, 20*(2), 204–221.

Wilkinson, R., & Pickett, K. (2011). *The spirit level: Why greater equality makes societies stronger*. Bloomsbury Publishing USA.

3

Growing a Movement: Psychologists for Social Change

Psychologists for Social Change

In any social campaign or movement there will be multiple stories of origin and each of us will carry a version of that story into the group. Our personal stories are part of the wider social narrative in that they spring from the cultural, political and economic landscapes we occupy. Political activism is forged at points of social fracture—those points where things are going so badly wrong for so many that the need for change outweighs the obstacles to organising and action. When we come together and share our personal experiences, we can recognise the connectedness of those stories (Fig.3.1). But when we start to organise together and join our actions in solidarity with a wider community of people with a shared desire for change, we build a movement through which we can recognise our collective power and agency.

An Introduction to Psychologists for Social Change

Psychologists for Social Change (P.S.C.) is a national activist network, comprising several connected but autonomous local groups which have differing structures and emphases. What unites us is a body of psychological knowledge, a set of core values and a desire to integrate social and political action into the culture

Psychologists for Social Change (✉)
London, UK
e-mail: psychologychange@gmail.com

C. Walker et al. (eds.), *The Palgrave Handbook of Innovative Community and Clinical Psychologies*, https://doi.org/10.1007/978-3-030-71190-0_3

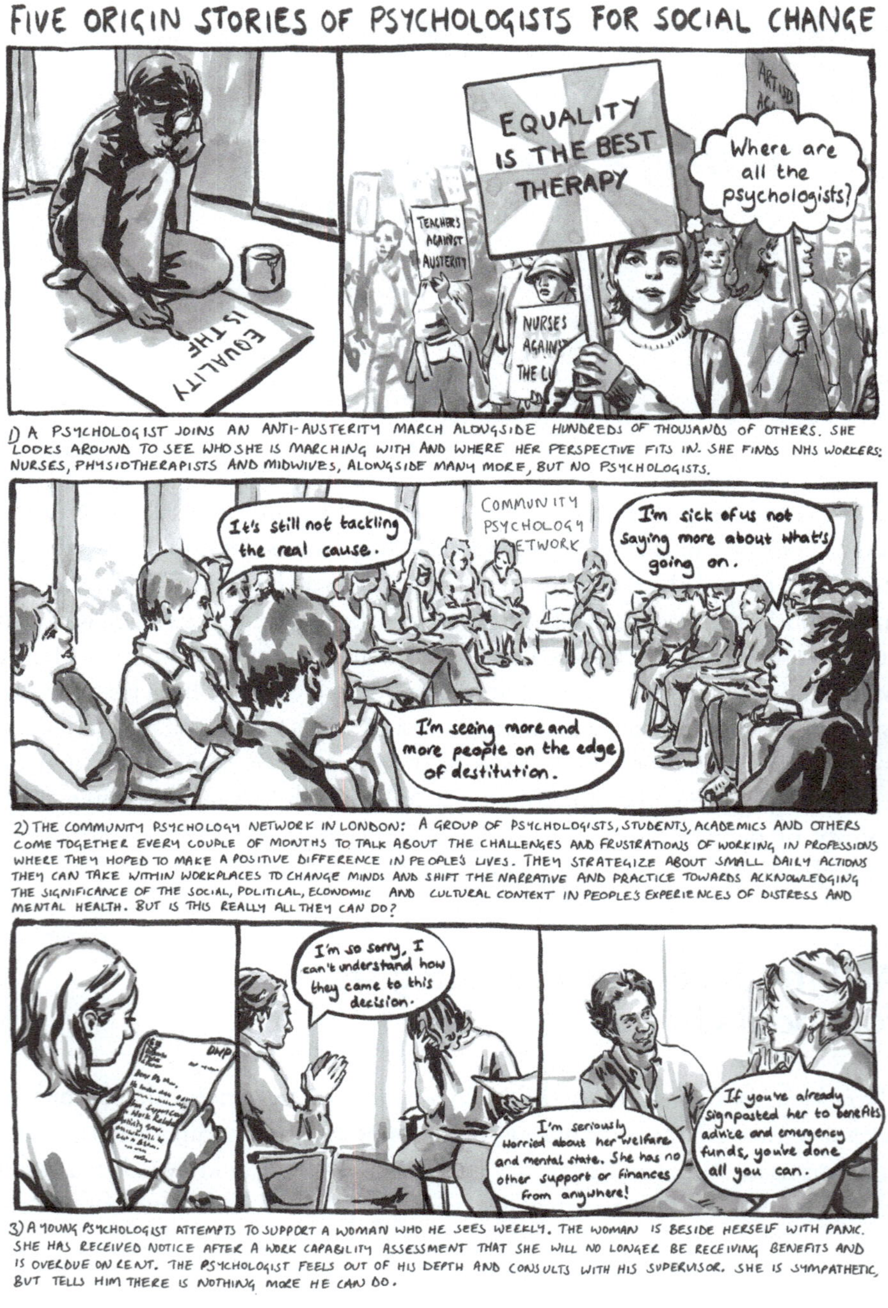

Fig. 3.1 The origin of PSC

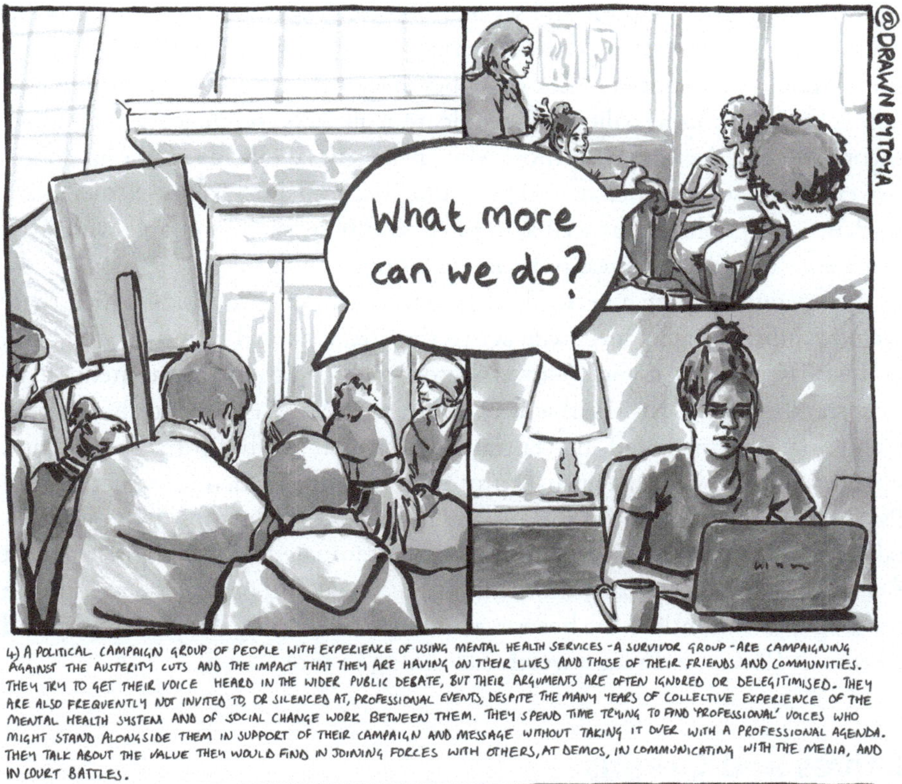

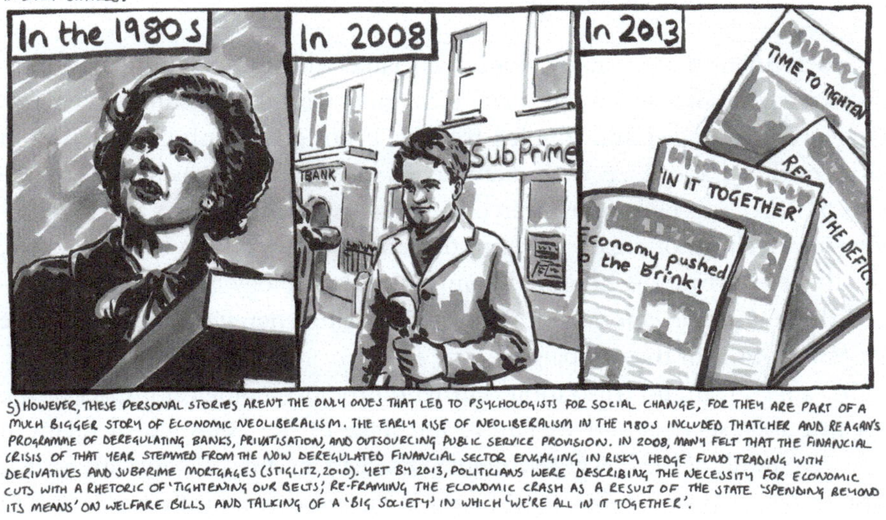

Fig. 3.1 (continued)

of Psychology as a discipline and set of professions. We argue that it is our ethical duty as psychologists to draw attention to the social context of distress and the psychological consequences of policy decisions. The term 'psychologists' here is broad; we are a coalition of people from all areas and stages of psychology theory and practice, as well as those who are largely sat outside of it. Our collective encompasses senior chartered psychologists, academics, trainees, therapists, students and graduates, as well as connected others, such as people with lived experience of mental distress or social exclusion.

We operate through a network of autonomous local groups, of which there are now approximately seventeen across the UK, Channel Islands and Ireland, and with several thousand followers across each of various social media platforms and mailing lists. In this way, P.S.C. embodies a model of horizontal, technologically mediated, de-centralised activism. We both draw upon, and operate outside of, the usual professional and academic structures of Psychology. The creation of this organisation was, for the most part, accidental. P.S.C. was born in 2014 as a single-issue campaign: Psychologists Against Austerity (P.A.A.). The early motivations, decisions and practices developed in those first few months have been instrumental in shaping the philosophy and culture of P.S.C., and so are worth examining in more detail.

Drives and Origins

It is no accident that so many words associated with campaigning are full of affective vigour. We talk about social movements, of momentum and energy, being swept to power and toppled from it. Emotion is central to the origin stories outlined above. As with many social justice campaigns, the establishment of P.S.C. was born of frustrated energy—with both politics and psychology—and feelings of anger, fear and powerlessness. Working as a collective, initially drawn from the London Community Psychology Network, we translated those negative emotions into an invigorating energy that propelled the first few months of the campaign.

Our anger, fear and frustration centred on the psychological impact of the cuts to public services and welfare in the wake of the 2008 global financial crisis. As a result of the UK government's choice to enforce 'austerity measures', the number of people using food banks increased dramatically from 25,899 people in 2008 to 1,084,604 in 2015 with the most commonly reported explanation of their use being problems with benefit payments (Cooper et al., 2014). This was just one of a vast number of examples of the catastrophic consequences on those affected. Mental health services were being doubly impacted by increased need and reduced resources; the experiences of practitioners and service users within this environment acted as another powerful driver to action. Our members felt a deep frustration and anger at the seemingly monolithic austerity narrative of 'we're all in this together' and the increasingly punitive narratives towards welfare claimants and people with disabilities (Afoko & Vockins, 2013). A secondary frustration was with Psychology itself. There was a lack of a visible response by the profession to these conditions that were so severely affecting our clients and working conditions. Added to that, Psychology and psychological research was being used to support and frame harmful narratives such as those that suggest that employment, under any circumstance, is good for mental health. We knew that actually this relationship was very complex, and that employment is not beneficial in every circumstance (Frayne, 2019). This toxic political soup gave the initial impetus for, and formed the content of, the Psychologists Against Austerity campaign.

In 2014, the relative silence of psychologists in the growing clamour of objections to the cuts to public services in the UK was notable. Nurses, speech therapists, doctors and midwives all had visible, loud campaigns from 2010 onwards, whilst psychologists did not. A desire to right this was one of the sparks that started P.A.A. as an idea and campaign. We were, of course, far from being the first set of psychologists to point out the lack of social and political engagement in psychology; as a group we were all influenced by critical and community approaches to psychology and mental health (Parker et al., 1996; Kagan et al., 2011; Nelson & Prilleltensky, 2010; Smail, 1993), which in many ways formed the backdrop of our collective thinking and culture. David Smail (1993; Fig 3.2) in particular was discussed in our early meetings. We also referred to the ideas of Paulo Freire (Box 3.1) and Gene Sharp (Box 3.2) in thinking through our organising processes and strategies,

Box 3.1 The Influence of David Smail

Our Influences and Theories of Social Change

We are sometimes asked about our theories of change and how that informs our strategy and activities. Like our origins as a group, there were multiple strands of influences that were grounded in broader movements and theoretical and practical approaches to social action. It is worth acknowledging some specific theoretical influences that informed our values, helped shape our political activity and enabled us to think more critically about our own activities.

David Smail (23 April 1938–3 August 2014)

David Smail was a British Clinical Psychologist credited for his advancement of a social materialist explanation of mental distress. He was critical of the ways in which psychotherapy and clinical psychology often focused on the internal worlds (i.e. the thoughts, feelings, drives, traumas, etc.) of individuals. Smail suggested that we must also look towards societal causes of distress such as inequalities in material wealth. By not concerning itself with issues such as the spread of power within societies, Smail argued that traditional clinical psychology and psychotherapy became complicit in these power imbalances and restricted the extent to which they could alleviate distress.

Box 3.2 Liberation Psychology Influence

Paulo Freire (19 September 1921–2 May 1997)

Freire was a Brazilian educator and leading figure in the critical pedagogy/education movement. For Freire, the process of developing a critical awareness of one's social reality was the key to positive social change and learning. He termed this process 'concientización'. Freire argued that we all acquire dominant social myths, and so to learn must engage in critically examining these myths, by using a reflection-action-dialogue cycle of identifying problems and needs in our social environment. Freire termed the interconnected practice of the three elements of reflection, action and dialogue as 'praxis'. Praxis enables us to see how the world and our position in it is not inevitable but historically and politically shaped, and to recognise ourselves as social and cultural actors and creators with a shared collective agency to transform the world around us. Thus, in acting to transform the world around us, we simultaneously develop and transform ourselves too, as collaborative learner-teacher-actors in society.

Box 3.3 Liberation Psychology Influence

Ignacio Martín-Baró (7 November 1942–16 November 1989)

Martín-Baró was a Spanish-born priest and scholar of philosophy, theology, literature and social psychology. He is seen as the founder of Liberation Psychology, which strives to provide a framework through which psychology can reduce its complicity with structural inequalities and oppression. This could be seen in contrast to Martín-Baró's critique of mainstream psychology as a discipline which asserts itself as value-neutral and universal and has limited societal relevance. For Martín-Baró, a psychologist's key task was to facilitate communities' understandings of their own psychologies as driven by their socio-political, cultural and historical contexts, rather than to impose an understanding onto them. Freire's 'concientización' is often seen as an important part of this process.

as well as the Survivor movement and social justice movements (Box 3.3) when considering our values and structures.

Our ability to access and disseminate research also acted as a facilitator and driver in our initial strategising. We were aware of huge amounts of research which supported our position that poverty, both absolute and relative, is a strong predictor for the development of mental health difficulties (Marmot & Bell, 2012; Melchior et al., 2009; Rogers & Pilgrim, 2010; Stuckler et al., 2009; Buckner, 2008). We also wanted to make the social determinants of health, and particularly the link between social inequality and poor mental health, more visible (Cromby et al., 2013; Friedli & World Health Organization, 2009; McGrath et al., 2016; Pickett & Wilkinson, 2010; Rogers & Pilgrim,

2003; Smail, 1993; Smail, 2005; Wilkinson & Pickett, 2010). For example, the work carried out by Wilkinson and Pickett (2010) supported our theoretical assumptions regarding the material conditions of distress. The authors stated that high income inequality was consistently found to have a negative impact on societies and individuals that was above and beyond the impact of the overall wealth of those societies. A comparison of national surveys across twelve 'economically developed' countries found that more unequal countries had worse outcomes on a range of measures including mental health, life expectancy, education, physical health, imprisonment and more. The epidemiological analysis found that levels of mental health diagnoses were three times higher in countries with high levels of income inequality.

In a short space of time we had a name, a website, a publication, a social media presence, a network of P.S.C. groups across the UK and invitations to speak in a wide variety of contexts. Importantly we had connected to other groups working in the same area, such as Disabled People Against Cuts, Black Triangle Campaign, Mental Health Resistance Network, Economists Against Austerity and Boycott Workfare. A significant challenge since this point has been to work out how to best utilise, embed and make sustainable the energy, connections and culture created in the run up to the election in 2015. In many ways, the impact and experience of forming P.A.A./P.S.C. outstripped our initial expectations and aims. As well as being surprised by the reach we had as a group, we also found that the acts of organising and taking action had value in themselves: in strengthening relationships, breaking the cycle of helplessness and inaction, and contributing towards larger movements in unforeseen ways. For example, although some of the requests we made in our petition or letters were not met, the process of writing these and gathering large numbers of supporters was an important aspect of building our movement and making our intentions clear.

Strategy Formation

Frustration and anger were perhaps the initial drivers to action, but formulating a campaign from these drivers required strategy. We considered which strengths and resources we had as psychologists that could be of use to the wider anti-austerity movement, and any psychological elements we could add to the relatively crowded field of austerity campaigning. We realised at this point that there were two parts to what we wanted to achieve:

1. Make a space to encourage psychologists to speak out and take action about austerity;
2. Contribute psychological knowledge and forms of evidence to the wider debate about austerity.

These were translated into the two strands of work which are still central to P.S.C. today: mobilising psychologists and mobilising psychological knowledge to take a stand against psychologically damaging policies and social injustices.

These ideas helped us to develop P.S.C. as a political-pedagogic project in which we ourselves are the learner-teachers through our collaborative political action and dialogue with each other and with other allied groups and organisers.

Looking Inwards: Mobilising Psychologists

We found many barriers to psychologists taking action beyond that of a politically engaged citizen. Many psychologists expressed nervousness at voicing political opinions based on clinical experience. Their worries ranged from concerns about backlash at work, to not wanting to be a political figure within a therapy room, to not thinking that they had the knowledge or skills to be a political advocate. One of our aims as P.S.C. was to counter these barriers, for example, by having a collective voice through which people could speak and take a political stand without being individually named.

This was crucial as many people have identified a culture within psychology, both academic and applied, which prioritises scientific and therapeutic neutrality, and thus downplays the role of social and political context in the production of psychological knowledge. The notion of scientific neutrality coupled with the overall tendency to individualism means that much of psychology training and education does not link psychological theory and practice with social, material and political context (Boyle, 2014). Instead it can reinforce individualising messages that are inaccurate and can leave people feeling blamed, which is ultimately harmful. This can, we argue, lead to personal barriers towards taking political action. Yet as Ian Parker et al. (1996) has argued, no position, not even a scientific one, is politically neutral; being silent is an implicit position as much as speaking out. Paulo Freire extends this idea, stating that "washing one's hands of the conflict between the powerful and the powerless means to side with the powerful, not to be neutral" (Freire, 1985: 122).

For this reason, P.S.C. extends the definition of ethical practice to include advocating on macro-level issues which impact on mental distress and wellbeing in our communities and workplaces. This was a key reason for centring psychology in the original name and focus of our campaign. In explicitly coupling 'psychologists' with a political position, 'against austerity', we aimed to implicitly reframe psychology. We model a politically engaged Psychology, one which proposes that psychologists' ethical and professional duty extends beyond the clinic, school and prison (British Psychological Society, 2009; Miell, 2014). We encourage psychologists to challenge social and economic policies that have deleterious psychological effects and argue that this should be an integral part of a psychologist's role and ethical code of practice. We aimed, therefore, to build an alternative narrative and model for psychologists, including those with greater power in the system (e.g. those with more influence or seniority), to draw upon.

We sought to identify and dismantle barriers that were preventing psychologists from thinking of their work, or themselves, as political. For example, our annual 'Week of Action' in the run up to local or national elections provides a daily framework of actions for psychologists to take within their everyday lives. These might include starting a conversation about austerity, contacting a local paper or a radio call-in, sharing a P.S.C. briefing paper, joining a demonstration in solidarity with allied groups or asking a question at election hustings. We have delivered workshops on clinical psychology training courses, taught undergraduate psychology students, spoken at conferences and Community Psychology festivals, and written in psychology publications. We encourage people to be politically active in whatever ways they feel able, even if they are unable to be directly involved in our group's activities or attend meetings. Examples range from rallying people to join protest demonstrations in solidarity with allied campaign groups or wider anti-austerity movement mobilisation calls, to writing to a newspaper or Member of Parliament (M.P.), signing an open letter or petition or helping out with regular tasks such as managing our social media.

Looking Outwards: Mobilising Psychological Knowledge

A central observation which shaped our work was the scarcity of well-evidenced psychological knowledge and experience in policy and political discourse. For example, austerity was being discussed in general economic or political terms, or as personal experience relatively disconnected from the dominant political discourse. We wanted to bring these together and encapsulate the visceral lived experience of austerity, as well as draw upon our positions as witnesses to the distress that it causes. We hoped to draw greater attention to the hidden human costs of austerity, as well as the long-term disadvantages to the economy which may result from these. In 2015, P.S.C. published its first briefing paper on the psychological impact of austerity (Psychologists Against Austerity, 2015). By bringing the psychological into the debate, our intentions were to *challenge* the culture of a 'neutral' psychology. However, we also *drew upon* this perception of psychology, making it clear that our position was evidence based and well researched.

The paper used research to provide an accessible overview of how the emotional wellbeing of societies and individuals is determined by multiple interacting factors. We conceptualised the impact of austerity policies on mental health in terms of five 'austerity ailments', which were shame and humiliation, fear and distrust, instability and insecurity, isolation and loneliness and finally, being trapped and humiliated. To take one example, that of the *instability and insecurity* 'ailment', the research outlined in our briefing paper stated that job insecurity is as damaging for mental health as unemployment. The paper argued that work is no longer a guarantee of stability and linked this to evidence which suggests that this insecurity is associated with mental distress (Shinn & Weitzman, 1996). By bringing together research, case studies and findings from other organisations, the document provided our colleagues, fellow activists, M.P.s and wider network with an accessible and easy to use evidence base to support their efforts to bring to light the social context in which distress arises.

In a similar vein, we sought to gather the everyday psychological knowledge from people's lived experiences—both that of practitioners working in services and the knowledge from direct personal experiences in people's lives and communities. Drawing inspiration from the *Everyday Sexism Project* (www.everydaysexism.com), which catalogues instances of sexism experienced on a day to day basis, we created an online platform called *Everyday Austerity* (http://www.psychchange.org/everyday-austerity.html): via our website people can write their stories of how economic cuts have impacted them or those they work with, their communities, services and people they care about. People are invited either to contribute anonymously or to choose how they wish to be identified. *Everyday Austerity* has become a crowd-sourced online public resource of over forty testimonies from various perspectives: those with personal experience of using services, people with disabilities, psychologists,

Box 3.4 Influence of Gene Sharp

Gene Sharp (21 January 1928–28 January 2018)

Early on in the P.S.C. journey, we decided to hold a screening of Ruaridh Arrow's film *How to Start a Revolution*, which documents the work of Gene Sharp, an American academic who has been described as the world's leading scholar of non-violent resistance. Sharp documented and analysed hundreds of cases of non-violent action that have been used throughout centuries and in current ongoing political struggle.

One of Sharp's key ideas was people power. He saw that the power of any regime or government relies on the obedience and co-operation of people and institutions in society. If people cease to accept the status quo and begin to resist, then the balance of power shifts. Sharp described these sources of a regime's power as its pillars of support. He talked about analysing the pillars holding up a particular regime or system, and how to strategically identify those which can be most effectively challenged so that the foundation can no longer support the regime. While some of the pillars use coercive force, such as law enforcement or the military, others, like the media, education system and religious institutions, exert influence over culture and popular opinion. His writings are translated into more than fifty languages and referred to by movements around the world, from political dissidents resisting dictatorship to women's rights groups and people involved in anti-corruption and anti-capitalist struggles.

P.S.C. members started to envisage a movement in which growing numbers of psychologists were mobilised and came together to fight against the so-called austerity policies. We thought about the pillars which were holding up austerity, such as political and media narratives, and how psychologists might be able to contribute our particular forms of knowledge to help the anti-austerity movement in reframing these narratives.

psychotherapists and other practitioners, those working within organisations supporting people financially or in other ways, family members and people who identify themselves simply as concerned citizens or workers. Since this beginning, P.S.C. has published two other briefing papers (Psychologists Against Austerity, 2016; Psychologists for Social Change, 2017) and various open letters, petitions and position statements, attracting varying levels of interest from the media, politicians and the public.

Partnerships and Solidarity

Central to the P.S.C. ethos is the principle of working collaboratively and in solidarity with people with different forms of expertise in our campaign areas. We aim to actively learn from those with other skills and knowledges, build relationships and partnerships, and join in solidarity to support others' campaigns and actions.

Building relationships and networks with others who are taking action or speaking out about relevant issues is key to developing a community of solidarity as well as to successfully mobilising psychological knowledge and feeding into the broader movement. It is through these alliances and mutually supportive relationships with other groups and organisers that there is the potential to build collective power for broader social and political change.

Equally, it is through meaningful exchange and dialogue with others with different kinds of expertise and perspectives that we can gain a fuller understanding of campaign areas in order to make informed decisions about our course of action as a group, including decisions about our campaign focus, which specific demands to make and which strategies to use. These relationships are also integral to becoming aware of the complexities, nuances and sensitivities that will exist within some political issues.

In line with this central value, we realised a valuable rule of thumb when embarking on a new campaign area was to strive to first seek out and attend to the views of those who were most directly impacted by the issues, and those groups who were already politically active or speaking out about the issues (often these will be the same people!). Sometimes where mistakes have been made in our approach, it has been through not having a full enough awareness of some different angles of an issue, such as the way it might impact on or be interpreted by a particular group. It is also important to acknowledge those who have been working on an issue and paving the way ahead of us—and to be aware of the giants on whose shoulders we are standing with our own organising efforts.

Social media can be used to nurture and build new relationships, as well as to share knowledge and influence those who are important to specific campaigns. Spreading the word about other groups' campaigns and actions is another way to show solidarity and support even if we are unable to attend protest actions in person. It can also be helpful to invite people from our partner organisations to attend and speak at a meeting or other type of planned event, and to attend the meetings and political actions of these other groups.

These ground-level actions also informed us of the key issues our communities cared about. Being present in the media, offering to do interviews, write articles, give talks to local political parties, conferences and student groups, and join our partners in marches, protests and 'thunderclap' Twitter campaigns all played the dual role of influencing a public narrative and wider views and helping to increase our visibility as a group, which ultimately led to a rapid expansion of P.S.C. to various parts of the UK and even a group set up in Finland.

Box 3.5 The Influence of the Survivor and Social Justice Movements

The survivor movement is an activist movement which has been active for several decades and which has gained particular momentum from the 1970s onwards. It is made up of groups of individuals who currently access or have previously accessed mental health services, often defining themselves as 'survivors' of the psychiatric system. Many of the beliefs behind the movement's aims inspired or resonated with our own perspectives on mental health systems and the sociocultural context of distress. Examples of these aims included the 'demedicalisation' of distress and highlighting the social and political causes of mental distress (e.g. Rapley et al., 2011; McKenna, 2016).

Social justice movements have, by definition, been around as long as politics and activism, but have seen a particular rise during the twentieth and twenty-first centuries. Some of these movements include the civil rights, workers' rights, gender equality, anti-racism and LGBTQ+ movements. One of the key markers of social justice movements is their focus on power and oppression.

Reflecting the strong links between distress and inequalities, many of the activist groups that we were inspired by had both survivor and social justice elements.

Adapting to Changing Contexts: Creating an Umbrella Name

Following the vote to leave the European Union in 2016, the political narrative in the UK began to shift. Brexit became the dominant political issue in British politics, and the key architects of austerity policies were no longer in power. Whilst the realities of austerity continued, for example with further cuts to public services and restrictions in benefits, the political discourse had altered. At the same time, reflecting on our activities to date, we concluded that the range of activities carried out nationally was wider than a response to austerity. A better way to capture our range of activity and overall mission was to think of our remit as a more general commitment, that of mobilising psychologists and psychology for social justice. We hence decided to adopt an umbrella name of 'Psychologists for Social Change' whilst keeping 'Psychologists Against Austerity' as a subsidiary campaign. Each regional P.A.A. group was able to decide whether to adopt the P.S.C. banner or continue as P.A.A. There are now multiple different areas of campaign focus with new members continuing to join us every month, sometimes bringing with them particular issues of concern that develop into new campaigns or working groups.

Culture and Organising Methods

Our early campaigning was focused around a specific event: the 2015 General Election; and around a particular topic: austerity. The group was small, and meetings were relatively easy to organise, sometimes happening as frequently as weekly in the immediate run-up to polling day. Since then, we have continued to meet regularly, except for occasional brief post-election hiatuses, which we use to recuperate. It is often the promise of re-engaging with valued social relationships as much as a renewed energy which inevitably draws the group back together after a few weeks. Most P.S.C. groups operate with a regular monthly or bi-monthly meeting, with smaller 'working groups' organising additionally outside of those times. As different groups respond to their different contexts, there has been variety in activities nationally, in terms of topic, approach and focus.

P.S.C. South West, for instance, decided early on to focus on the experiences of benefits claimants negotiating an increasingly hostile and sparsely resourced system. In response, the group set up a regular benefits clinic in collaboration with the Citizens Advice Bureau which offers a one-hour assessment with a psychologist, who can then provide a medical evidence letter to support benefit claims. This is an example of how psychologists can consider utilising their direct clinical skills outside of usual contexts, providing a resource which can materially improve people's lives. Realising a wider lack of knowledge and skills amongst psychologists about the benefit system, the South West group have also provided training in local NHS Trusts on how to write good-quality medical evidence letters.

Other groups have turned their focus outwards, to public persuasion. In the North East, a key organising method has been a regular street stall raising awareness of austerity and its impacts. Many P.S.C. groups have been led by local concerns and joined forces with local community activism, such as housing activism in the North West or marriage equality in Northern Ireland. London P.S.C. has continued to be led by our frustrations and interests, as well as actively responding to what is happening politically and through our relationships with allied campaign groups. We have aimed to remain open to new ideas and directions. Recently, for example, a new London P.S.C. member used her skills as a writer to set up and edit a monthly blog. We have experimented with various digital communication tools to keep in touch between meetings, most of which have served our campaigning purposes for at least a brief period, and none of which have been perfect.

P.S.C. has increasingly had to balance its aim of growing a movement against the necessity of ensuring that its existing cultures and structures are transparent, welcoming and flexible enough to support this. We value and have endeavoured to maintain our flattened hierarchy, partly in the hope that it may empower newcomers to take on new roles and challenges. However, it has also sometimes left them unsure who to turn to for advice or support in setting up campaigns or working groups. The different groups in P.S.C. have managed this challenge differently; some have organised with formal roles in the group to give clarity and structure, others have preferred a more fluid approach. Some groups rotate roles monthly to share the labour of tasks. We have also had to consider ways in which our organising methods may exclude particular groups. For example, London P.S.C. originally, and organically, started out meeting in pubs, which seemed to provide an informal, equalising setting for discussions, especially as our meetings included some very experienced psychologists and others at the start of their careers. However, we realised this meeting place excluded some other groups, such as certain religious or cultural groups, people who require disabled access or those with hearing difficulties. We, therefore, moved to university spaces, which had initially been rejected due to associations with elitism; this has proved to be largely successful. These considerations are all ongoing dilemmas which various P.S.C. groups continue to manage in different ways.

Case Study #1
Clinical Psychology Trainee in the North of England: Getting Involved in P.S.C. from a Distance

During my Clinical Psychology training, it quickly became clear to me that although psychological interventions could be helpful, people's life circumstances—poverty, domestic violence, housing instability, discrimination—were often working against them. More needed to be done, but how?

I first met Psychologists for Social Change (P.S.C.) at the London anti-austerity march in June 2015, at a time when I was keen to channel my frustrations into positive action. It was a chance to network with people who understood that psychologists need to be more than a sticking plaster for policies and politics which actively create psychological distress. Being linked to P.S.C. has fostered hope, solidarity and co-ordinated action. The group also assesses evidence on the impact of austerity, raises awareness, organises events, shares knowledge and expertise and, most importantly, elevates the power of individual voices. I have used all of these elements in some form or another over the past several years. P.S.C. consistently reminds us that wellbeing is not simply situated in our heads, but in our worlds.

There are some challenges to being part of P.S.C. As the work is voluntary, it takes some careful organisation to dedicate time to different projects. Many of the groups and events are located in the South of England, meaning that involvement can require long travel, and communication across the diverse range of P.S.C. groups can be tricky. However, it is all worth it to be part of this crucial and growing movement—*"equality is the best therapy"!*

Case Study #2
Trainee Clinical Psychologists Starting up Local P.S.C. Groups in Wales

Psychologists for Social Change Wales was established in March 2016 by a group of Trainee Clinical Psychologists. It has since divided into North and South Wales. The group was shaped from frustration witnessing the incremental increase of social adversity as the result of austerity cuts to services we already saw as struggling. There was also lack of inclusion in clinical teaching on the role of social adversity in mental health problems, and of ways of working that support Clinical Psychologists to embed this understanding within their practice. It is not within the British Psychology Society (B.P.S.) course requirements to provide teaching on these aspects of mental health. Principally, Charlotte Church's 2015 anti-austerity march mantra "I'm mad as hell and I'm not taking it anymore" captures the essence of the group's formation.

Wales operates as a devolved Government. 'Devolution' refers to the statutory granting of powers from central government to regional administration. The subsequent varying levels of devolved powers mean there are different local needs in terms of social policy, reform and culture. In Wales, we currently have a coalition Labour (majority) and Liberal Democrat government who support the ending of austerity policies. Mark Drakeford, Assembly Member (A.M.), Cabinet Secretary for Finance has called for the UK Government to end unnecessary austerity policies, but out of respect for the power-sharing agreement, the Welsh government has not gone further and rejected the UK budget provided for Wales. As a group, this means we further encourage and pressure the Welsh government to reject austerity-imposed budget cuts. However, the greater alignment between the values of P.S.C. and the Welsh government means we have more opportunity to influence through information sharing and relationship building, with open channels of communication. For example, in the autumn of 2018 we held a 'Social Adversity and Mental Health' event sponsored by a Labour Committee Chair and in early 2018 we held a similar event with the Leader of the Welsh Nationalist party, Plaid Cymru, which was sponsored by the Division of Clinical Psychology Wales. These are opportunities for us to build relationships in order to influence the narrative around poverty, structural inequality and mental health in Wales.

It has taken us some time to understand what the local need for the group is and this is still taking shape. One of the group's biggest challenges was navigating the world of politics: what are the rules of engagement; how do you effect change; and who stands for what. Because we were new to political organising, we were somewhat daunted by this and it remains one of our main barriers. It has been through building up networks with local organising groups, such as the Cardiff People's Assembly, and with other professional bodies, such as the British Association of Social Workers Cymru, that we have begun to gain confidence and get a sense of how to position ourselves. Largely this has focused on supporting discussion around how health and social services need to change to better address social and childhood adversity and trauma. We have also been attending meetings, marches and conferences organised by other local groups. This has helped others to know what we stand for as a group and provided opportunities to build partnerships and share information, and for us to learn from other groups with similar grassroots organising experience. For example, we produced T-shirts with the slogan 'Equality Is the Best Therapy' that members and others can purchase and wear to highlight the role of structural inequalities in mental distress.

Some members also worried about consequences from asserting a political position. The small world of Wales means that networks are interconnected and can cross personal and professional planes. Anxieties about this are heightened because when our group started it was mostly made up of trainees, and, although we have crossed the bridge into the post-qualification world, there is still a sense of vulnerability as newcomers to the field. We invited a local Politics student to help us feel more equipped in understanding politics in Wales. We also decided to start with peripheral actions and joined in other campaigns, such as supporting a Llamau 'End Youth Homelessness' event and running fundraising activities to support their fight against homelessness. Such activities are not direct P.S.C. actions but helped us build confidence and networks in our early days.

Building a Movement: Key Lessons

Drawing on our combined experience across P.S.C., we have reflected on our core lessons learnt. These we hope will help to guide others in how to start, and maintain, a grassroots campaign or organisation:

- The personal is political. Give yourself permission to have opinions and to share them in a professional context and vice versa, within professional and ethical guidelines.
- Connect. By attending a P.S.C. meeting, a community organising meeting or the gatherings of any politically active organisation, the actions you can take will emerge. Building alliances is the way to find out what's already going on and how you can best be of help.
- Act. Every action counts, the examples we mention in the chapter are just an idea. Draw on your strengths and build on what you already know. Act within your professional role and outside of it whilst harnessing strengths from both sets of experiences.
- Communicate. Use different methods to get your messages out there and connect with each other: social media, meetings, events, demos, traditional media...
- You have the skills. As people, we each hold skills that are crucial to bringing activism into our work. Whether it might be time, writing, talking, organising, painting—groups and individuals can harness these skills and assets to better the lives of others.
- Get organised. Think about your processes: how you are meeting, who does what, how decisions are made and how you communicate with each other. Keeping on top of these is important work and should be valued and shared.
- Be brave, humble and aware. If you are speaking or importantly, not speaking, from a position of power, be aware of how you can cause more harm than good by talking over people, not listening and thinking you have all the answers. Remember that your own worldview will always have limitations and that, in some cases, other activist groups may have been working in the area for much longer than you.
- Collectivise. Join up with other groups for increased power and impact. Between you, you may also have a greater set of skills to draw upon.
- Solidarity is key. Listen to and be guided by those who are most impacted by the issues you are campaigning on.
- Be visionary. Think big, remember why you were inspired to action in the first place and keep the long term in mind.
- Be responsive as well as strategic. Identify goals and be realistic about the resources (time, energy, finances, knowledge) of your group. Remember to balance being focussed with being able to respond to new developments (e.g. the publication of a government paper).

- Be reflective. Keep checking in with whether the direction things are going is in line with your values. Learn from mistakes and take the time to research new issues before parachuting in as a privileged group.
- Look after each other. Be mindful of the varying demands that may be on different members of your group. Personal relationships with others in your group may also help sustain you through some of the more challenging aspects of social activism.

With thanks to Tamsin Curno, Jennifer Daffin, Meera Desai, Carl Harris, Cheyann Heap, Laura McGrath and Rachel H. Tribe for contributions to this chapter.

References

Afoko, C., & Vockins, D. (2013). *Framing the economy: The austerity story*. New Economics Foundation.

Boyle, M. (2014). *Is clinical psychology fearful of social context?* [Video File]. Video retrieved from https://www.youtube.com/watch?v=Kt4JcTDPUoc&t=3s

British Psychological Society. (2009). *Code of ethics and conduct*. BPS.

Buckner, J. C. (2008). Understanding the impact of homelessness on children challenges and future research directions. *American Behavioral Scientist, 51*(6), 721–736.

Cooper, N., Purcell, S., & Jackson, R. (2014). *Below the breadline: The relentless rise of food poverty in Britain*. Retrieved from http://www.church-poverty.org.uk/breadline/read/belowbreadlinereport/view

Cromby, J., Harper, D., & Reavey, P. (2013). *Psychology, mental health and distress*. Palgrave Macmillan.

Frayne, D. (2019). *The work cure: Critical essays on work and wellness*. PCCS Books.

Freire, P. (1985). *The politics of education: Culture, power and liberation* (p. 122). Macmillan.

Friedli, L. & World Health Organization. (2009). *Mental health, resilience and inequalities*. WHO Regional Office for Europe.

Kagan, C., Burton, M., Duckett, P., Lawthom, R., & Siddiquee, A. (2011). *Critical community psychology* (1st ed.). Wiley-Blackwell.

Marmot, M., & Bell, R. (2012). Fair society, healthy lives. *Public Health, 126*, S4–S10.

McGrath, L., Walker, C., & Jones, C. (2016). Psychologists against austerity: Mobilising psychology for social change. *Critical and Radical Social Work, 4*(3), 409–413.

McKenna, D. (2016). *Welfare reforms and mental health*. Retrieved from https://recoveryinthebin.org/2016/03/10/welfare-reforms-and-mental-health-resisting-sanctions-assessments-and-psychological-coercion-by-denise-mckenna-mental-health-resistance-network-mhrn/

Melchior, M., Caspi, A., Howard, L. M., Ambler, A. P., Bolton, H., Mountain, N., & Moffitt, T. E. (2009). Mental health context of food insecurity: A representative cohort of families with young children. *Pediatrics, 124*(4), e564–e572.

Miell, D. (2014). President's column. *The Psychologist, 27*(10), 770–775.

Nelson, G., & Prilleltensky, I. (2010). *Community psychology: In pursuit of liberation and wellbeing*. Palgrave.

Parker, I., Georgaca, E., Harper, D., McLaughlin, T., & Stowell-Smith, M. (1996). *Deconstructing psychopathology*. Sage.

Pickett, K. E., & Wilkinson, R. G. (2010). Inequality: An underacknowledged source of mental illness and distress. *The British Journal of Psychiatry, 197*(6), 426–428.

Psychologists Against Austerity. (2015). *The psychological impact of austerity*. Retrieved from https://psychagainstausterity.files.wordpress.com/2015/03/paa-briefing-paper.pdf

Psychologists Against Austerity. (2016). *Improving public discussion about inequality: A briefing paper*. Retrieved from http://www.psychchange.org/uploads/9/7/9/7/97971280/talking-about-inequality.pdf

Psychologists for Social Change. (2017). *Universal basic income: A psychological impact assessment*. PAA: London.

Rapley, M., Moncrieff, J., & Dillon, J. (2011). *Demedicalising misery: Psychiatry, psychology and the human condition*. Palgrave Macmillan.

Rogers, A., & Pilgrim, D. (2003). *Inequalities and mental health*. Palgrave Macmillan.

Rogers, A., & Pilgrim, D. (2010). *A sociology of mental health and illness*. McGraw-Hill Education.

Shinn, M., & Weitzman, B. C. (1996). Homeless families are different. *Homelessness in America*, 109–122.

Smail, D. (1993). *The origins of unhappiness*. Constable.

Smail, D. J. (2005). *Power, interest and psychology: Elements of a social materialist understanding of distress*. PCCS Books.

Stuckler, D., Basu, S., Suhrcke, M., Coutts, A., & McKee, M. (2009). The public health effect of economic crises and alternative policy responses in Europe: An empirical analysis. *The Lancet, 374*(9686), 315–323.

Wilkinson, R., & Pickett, K. (2010). *The spirit level: Why equality is better for everyone*. Penguin.

4

Getting off the Fence and Steppin' Outta the Clinic Room

The Walk the Talk Crew

During the last decade, politics around the world has seen a significant shift to the right (Leahy, 2018; Malik, 2018; Shuster, 2016) following the world financial crisis that started in 2007 with the US subprime mortgage market collapse. We have witnessed more polarisation in debates, coupled with an increase in extreme views and evangelism on both sides of the political fence (Lee et al., 2018; Pew Research Center, 2014; Townsend, 2018). There have been an increasing number of political protests, and a marked increase in terrorism-related incidents from between 1000 and 2000 per year around the year 2000 to a peak of nearly 17,000 in 2014 (Roser, 2017). The media reporting of our world—particularly in new and social media spheres—has reflected, and arguably driven, the social polarisation that this combination of economic instability and emphasis on terror attacks has fuelled (Lee et al., 2018; Lewis, 2018). Many western nations have found their populace turning their attention inwards (European Commission, 2017; Kagan, 2018) while far right groups have flourished in both the USA and Europe (Jones, 2018; Townsend, 2019).

The rise of social media has provided a loudspeaker to many who had previously struggled to make their voice heard—a great boon to both groups and individuals who wish to stand up for those who have suffered as a result of their status in society. However, these loudspeakers broadcast with little of the

The Walk the Talk Crew (✉)
Lancaster, UK
e-mail: stephen.Weatherhead@liverpool.ac.uk

C. Walker et al. (eds.), *The Palgrave Handbook of Innovative Community and Clinical Psychologies*, https://doi.org/10.1007/978-3-030-71190-0_4

social or legal censorship we have previously relied upon to moderate some messages. In what have become perilous times for many in society as inequality for many groups has grown (Partington, 2018; Sowels, 2018) and fiscal policy has become largely driven by austerity (Goodman, 2018), activism is urgently needed to redress the issues our political polarisation has caused. This is an environment that is full of opportunity for activists to inform and influence with unprecedented reach. It also brings with it many dangers where both message and actions can rapidly be miscast by authorities and the general public.

Social media is regularly portrayed as being primarily an echo chamber for poorly informed opinions (Robson, 2018), a reputation which spawned the derogatory terms clicktivist and slacktivism. This is highlighted by the numerous political advocacy issues that rapidly gain momentum in the online sphere but fail to drive people to take action beyond the use of a single mouse click (Taylor, 2014). However, the grassroots mobilisation which drove the success of the occupy movement in 2011, Black Lives Matter in 2013, and the Donald Trump and Bernie Sanders campaigns in the 2016 US election showed that social media campaigns have the ability to influence action beyond the computer screen. Perhaps not surprisingly, what appears to drive success in converting exposure on social media and harnessing a 'twitterstorm' to drive physical action is personal resonance and a sense of grievance (Moyer, 2017).

This social media arms race is one which is shared by both the political left and right, terrorist, extremist and activist groups (Donovan, 2019). In many cases, the messages could not be more different but the approaches the groups take have developed many commonalities. It is perhaps inevitable that as a result of the electronic activities of various dissenting groups becoming more comparable, governmental organisations are now blurring their definitions of terrorism and extremism with activism becoming part of a melting pot of what are seen as 'potential threats' (Monaghan & Walby, 2012). The approaches to these threats are also worryingly homogeneous with non-violent protesters being treated as security threats and investigated by security services (Byrne, 2017). This issue is not limited to policing. Resisting extremism in any form is increasingly becoming portrayed in the media as a form of extremism itself and denounced as an attack on free speech. A social boundary has been constructed by many nation states, through both legislation and rhetoric, to define acceptable dissent not just by action but also by source (Salter, 2011). While it would generally be agreed that, when not in extremism, the actions of dissenters need limits, the freedom for those in power to silence groups based on message certainly raises significant concerns for freedom of expression.

What of the oppressed and silenced; the activists who are challenging the status quo in order to stand up for equality? People who stand up against the system often do so at great personal risk. Consider, for example, the person on benefits protesting against DWP policy or a person seeking asylum campaigning for better refugee care. These activists for social justice and others like them are in a position of attempting to balance risk and reward while seeking to implement a form of responsible activism which can be effective in an environment hostile to any challenge to power. There will always be a need for activist groups who are truly representing those who have been denied power and address those who hold it. Our world would be a significantly poorer place were it not for those who have had the courage to use their voice in the name of others. The current technological environment provides us with a greater reach to our voices than ever before but with the potential for significant backlash (Pew Research Center, 2018). However, this has always been the case for those who speak truth to power, be it against slavery, voting rights, apartheid, animal rights or green issues (Kurtz, 2010; Potter, 2011; Watts & Vidal, 2017). What we must hold close is that the courage to do what we believe is right continues to have the potential to overcome.

In psychology, one of the professional barriers we have to overcome in making a difference beyond 1:1 therapy is that of territorialism. We have an array of professional psychology groupings, counselling, clinical, occupational, community… the list is huge. Whilst this chapter places itself primarily in clinical and community psychology, we do not feel an ownership of any of the spaces in which we work. We are novices, temporary features of an ever-changing landscape. There have always been psychologists who work beyond 1:1 therapy, so in writing a chapter about the role of clinical psychologists in affecting social change, we recognise that we are 'standing on the shoulders of giants'. Sometimes the falling of a giant leads to a visible response; it feels as though the impact of the death of David Smail has reverberated across the clinical psychology community. Many of us who have been inspired by David, now feel a responsibility to continue to develop his work. This, combined with the shocks and after-shocks of austerity measures in the UK, and the rise of right-wing politics across Western Europe and the USA, has led to closer collaboration with the people affected by socio-economically oppressive policies. There has been a need to become more visible and present within our communities. If ever there was a time to unite and affect change for the psychological wellbeing of our communities, it is now.

Walk the Talk

In 2015 a number of us united to walk together from the British Psychological Society office in Leicester to the London office, a journey of just over 100 miles. We slept rough along the way and called at food banks, homeless shelters, mental health services and other spaces in order to gather testimonies of people affected by homelessness, food poverty and the welfare system. Our idea started in dialogue and was shared by word of mouth as the plan formed. Support grew via our social media presence and as more people 'joined the conversation' about #walkthetalk2015 the idea began to develop its own momentum. More information, video testimonies and resources can be accessed via the Walk the Talk website—http://walkthetalk2015.org/.

Our goals were simple; we wanted to get out of the clinic room, and show a desire to make a difference, and do what we could to influence the policy landscape which holds more than 20% of the population in poverty. 'Mainstream' media coverage and an invitation to Westminster to meet with Luciana Berger, the then Shadow Minister for Mental Health, suggest those goals were achieved. However, this doesn't tell the full story of the journey, a journey that wasn't really ours; we were just finding a way to walk alongside the people who were living the tremors that came with the earthquake of Political decisions, people who are too often silenced. Within the story of the journey, there is a tale in itself. As James, one of the group who walked the whole 100+ miles, testifies in his 'psycho-logical analysis' he had already made a very similar journey but because he lacked professional standing, he was unable to gain political influence.

Psycho-Logical Analysis

By James McLean

When I first heard that a bunch of psychologists were planning to walk from Leicester to London along 'A' roads to raise awareness of the impact of benefits changes and sanctions on the mental health of their clients and people across the country, I knew I had to bring a bit of 'mental' to their campaign. I found out through my psychologist Dr Suzanne Elliott who had helped me through some of my own difficulties and who was going to join us for a day of the five day walk. She told me about it because three years earlier I had taken a very similar pilgrimage to London from Leicester to raise awareness of the rise in homelessness (at the time I had done it homelessness stood at 50000 across the UK). Homelessness had risen to over 100,000 by the time we were walking to London. It was very extra-ordinary for professionals in a sometimes unfairly maligned field of medicine to take such extreme steps and to essentially potentially put their professional careers at risk. A group of twenty or so of us or 21 if you include our mascot Stormy Weathers (a toy storm trooper) set off from the BPS offices in Leicester and we set off to someone playing the bagpipes no less. The organiser Dr Steven Weatherhead (our drill sergeant) was apprehensive of me coming along as I turned up with a luggage trolley, a swivel-chair and various mascots. He need not have worried this was not my first rodeo and, to be fair to him, ***I*** *would have been concerned if I had turned up to* **my** *event. This was an eclectic mix of people from the field of psychology including academics, clinical psychologists and people with varying degrees and of psychological problems (plus someone from international rescue, true story). I would have said beforehand that I was the worst of those but now I worry for my psychologist friends mental health and sanity (I mean, seriously, walking along 'A' roads? all the way to London?! I have psychological problems, I have an excuse!). The journey itself taught me and them a few things:*

- *Psychologists don't always sit on the fence*
- *Never take directions from anyone from International Rescue… (I brought a compass and I genuinely do believe I was the sanest and most decisive of the group).*
- *Never expect a psychologist to make a definite decision without at least a half hour debate.*
- *Also "Never doubt that a small group of committed, determined citizens can change the world. Indeed, it is the only thing that ever has" Dr Margaret Mead circa 1930's.*
- *"You have got to challenge to change and be that change to inspire meaningful change" James McLean circa 40 seconds ago.*

We talked a lot with James over the course of the walk about how in taking this kind of action we are amplifying each other's voices; it is a reciprocal process. At times James talked of his experiences of being silenced in the past and watched this change as the Walk the Talk Crew alliance grew. Likewise, those of us with some 'role power' (Proctor, 2002) as professional psychologists frequently felt that the Walk the Talk Crew were given the opportunity to share our perspectives partly because of the alliance we had with those with lived experience. So whether it's Voltaire, Spiderman, or someone else who first said that "with great power comes great responsibility", we as psychological professionals have to act. Whether we like to admit it or not, the psychological professions have standing at an individual, community and societal level. We, therefore, have a responsibility to use that standing in order to influence social policies.

During Walk the Talk, we gathered testimonies through meeting and talking with people at various projects set up to address homelessness, food poverty or welfare reforms during Walk the Talk. We were given consent to share these testimonies on social media and via our website. They also formed part of the evidence we presented to the Shadow Minister for Mental Health, some examples follow.

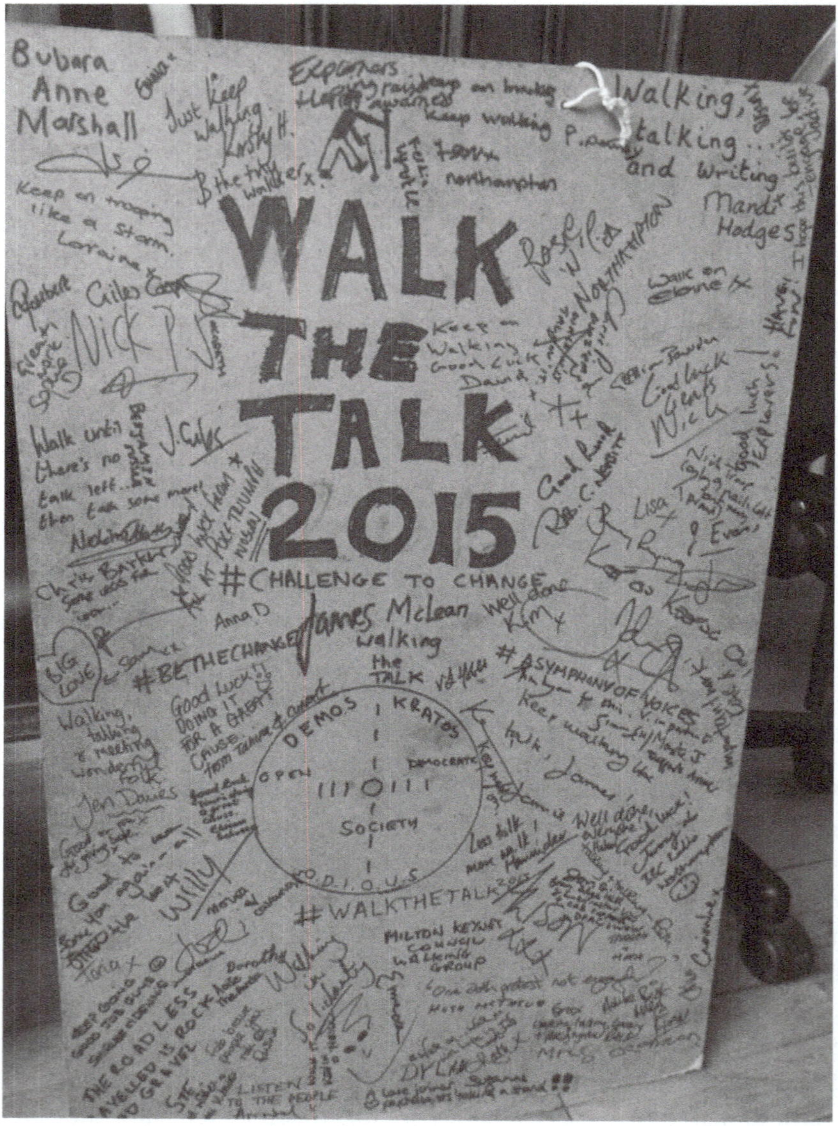

Phillipa told us about the impact of the so-called Bedroom Tax on her relationships and her own survival:

> *One of my friends is homeless and if I ever help my friend and let him sleep on the sofa I will get in trouble for that, see, so if you go and help someone you get in trouble as well, because he is staying at yours if you help them out. They just basically class you as having someone live with you and they put full rent on you and then they back*

date you to when you were helping him thinking that he's living there and he's not and then you've got to pay back all the rent from when that time was.

And it's like this bedroom tax that's what highers up your rent and all this lot so if you're in arrears you've got to pay off all that before you even think about getting any food. They expect the money to be with them and if you haven't go no money for food, they don't really care.

I've gotta find ways to pay it, I've got to ask my mum or I've gotta ask friends, and then when I do get my money in I've gotta pay back them. And you've gotta pay your rent as well, so by the time you've done that you've got no money for food or gas or electric, they don't really care, they don't care at all.

The council didn't tell me for 6 months that I had to pay the bedroom tax, that's why I've got the arrears.

When we spoke to Dennis, he wanted to impress on us how complicated the benefits system is, and the real-life problems caused by a lack of cohesion in the system:

If you put in a claim for ESA, let just say for example it takes 3 weeks to process that, and if you're declined for the ESA claim, then you need to start a new claim of Job Seekers Allowance so potentially then that's 3 weeks when you're waiting for your benefit to get declined which you're not getting money, so essentially what you're doing is the Government is stopping you from getting money from the date when you initially start your claim. If ESA and JSA were both in the same department, if you're applying for ESA and you get declined they just automatically send you onto JSA then so that you get your money from the start date.

You don't get any money while you're waiting for the claim to be processed. They do say that it takes up to 14 working days which is almost 3 weeks. So you have to go without money through that period. You are entitled to short term benefit advance, but then that is only a minimum amount of money as well it could be £20 or £30 it's what they deem a suitable amount to live on but we all know that £20 or £30 doesn't go very far in this day and age, so, yeah that's something that needs to be looked at I think.

*the specifics of these arrangements may have changed since 2015 when Dennis told us about his experiences.

Theresa told us about the impact that social policy and cuts to public sector services have on the ability for people to connect with community and a meaningful life:

There have been such a lot of cuts around Camden, wards have been closed, everything. They've started now that it's- you can't come here unless you're funded. You can't just come as a day centre or a drop in. You have to have personal income and you've got to wait until that's sorted out for you, and that takes months. And in the mean time people have got nowhere to go, in hospitals, turned away, nothing to do. So it's really about the cuts and of course the stigma. But we have to live with that, but it's really trying to improve the quality of life for people with mental health problems.

It's important because it's a place where we can all come and we've all got a mental health problem and we're all comfortable with each other and whatever's going on it stays in the centre. And that's how it is. It's good to have someplace to come where you can be yourself, meet your friends, a lot of volunteers work here, the place is nearly run by volunteers. Even if you don't feel like going out it's good that you've got some place to go.

I suffer with mild autism, which is coping with anxiety. And for me I need to be in an environment that is suitable and instructive and there's sustainability in the environment and if that's not the case then it's not the right environment for me.

John, who works at the food bank we visited, told us about how the demand for food banks has grown over the years and how the work of food banks is so much broader than providing food:

The food bank here has been going for this is our 11th year. The growth has been really quite exponential. When we first started we gave out 1000 food parcels in a year, we now give out 1000 each month. Some of that you can put down to the profile of food banks across the country has been escalated by political debate by need being identified, so there are far more food banks than there ever were in 2004. But we as a local grass roots organisation, we weren't asked to be set up by Government, we don't get Government money, we're supported entirely by the good will and the support of people in the community. They give us the food they give us their time as volunteers and thankfully they give us money as well. And that combination has kept us going and growing. As the need has escalated, and I suppose the biggest development has been in the last 3 or 4 years, we've gone from 9000 to 14000 food parcels, we've had to really ratchet up where we get the food from.

But the fact remains that nobody actually want to come to a food bank in my experience. There is a stigma. They feel nervous, they feel shy, worried, angry sometimes. And when they do come they are always grateful for what they get. Most of the people we see, things have broken down in their lives. Sometimes through their own fault, most times through not their own fault. They perhaps don't always have the skills and the competencies to cope with the kind of things that life throws at them; bureaucracy particularly is something a lot of people don't understand. And I think the gap between when something goes wrong in somebody's life and when the state can come in and intervene and help has got wider. I suppose the difficulty is that there are people that live their life in a way that they're almost in continual crisis, and they're the more, they're the people with enduring problems of one sort or another that we're not really geared up to help. But as a charity, our default position is to help and we will help, but we work a lot with other agencies, so the Citizen's Advice Bureau, the local authorities, the social services but also churches, also doctors surgeries, schools, all of the other charities that provide support to people in the community. And if we didn't do that we'd be very irresponsible I think, because we're not like an open door where you just come and get food whatever the circumstances, there needs to be a path that somebody's on to sorting out their problems, because unless they sort those problems out, that dependency and that link is not going to be broken.

We collected and shared these narratives and offer them here in order to ground the knowledge we present in lived experience. This has always been essential critical community psychology praxis, but may be even more important in the 'post-truth' era when 'expertise' is dismissed by sections of the political elite. As psychologists we have 'role power' (Proctor, 2002) that affords us a platform to speak. However, as Gupta (2019) commented, if we speak only from a position of 'expert by qualification' we are less easy to identify with and our voice and therefore the knowledge, too, is diminished. Speaking with a collective voice which is rich with a range of experiences, including those of 'Experts by Experience', amplifies all our voices and the narrative reaches further, so is arguably more powerful and more likely to contribute to social change.

The advancement of social media has perhaps made it easier than ever to affect policy change (see Fig. 4.1). We can all engage with mainstream media, social media, and blogging. Although engaging in this way can seem inconsequential, Fig. 4.1 shows how it can often act as a pre-curser to service innovations and empirical research, which can then in turn directly affect policy change. This is all set within the context of the often conflicting perspectives of The Houses of Parliament and Lords, and activist individuals and groups. It is important that we show an awareness of the contexts depicted in Fig. 4.1; listen to all voices, and find mechanisms for influence. There are many ways we can do this, but the main message is that we must do it. If we do not act and speak where others' voices are not being heard, then we are in many ways complicit in oppressions and marginalisations.

We are familiar with the 'hero-innovator' within leadership literature, which has of course been updated in various leadership frameworks. Perhaps the time has come to embody more action-focussed approach. In doing so we would advocate four elements to theory and practice development:

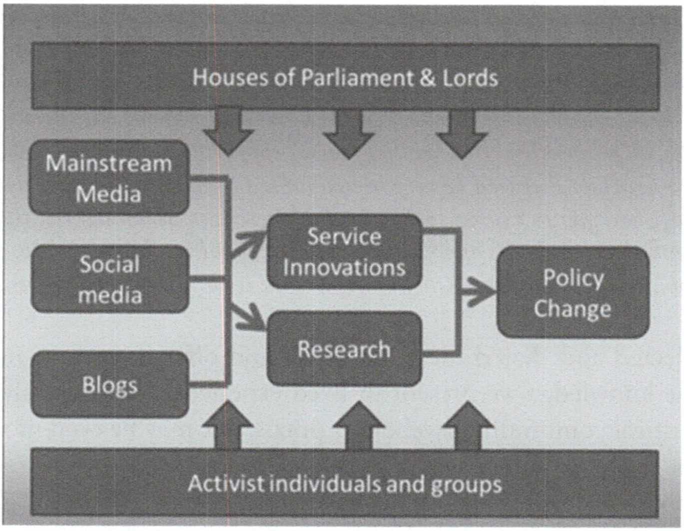

Fig. 4.1 Affecting policy change

1. Innovation
2. Influencing
3. Activism
4. Agitation/Resistance

Argue that innovation in itself isn't enough to affect social change, we must also consider the potential impact of our methods for disseminating those innovations. Whether we are working from a position of ego or altruism, our goal is to affect change in some form. Is there any point in psychology if it doesn't have some form of influence? Yes, we can influence on an individual level, but if we are to make direct therapy redundant (which should be the ultimate goal) then our influence needs to be at a societal level. Perhaps the only way to do this is to embrace activism and agitate in order to resist and challenge oppressive practices.

We need to question the relative reluctance of professional bodies to 'bite the (Political) hand that feeds them' and take an action-orientated approach to social change. We must involve the next generation of psychologists as early as possible in order to embed the notion that working visibly with our communities is a regular part of what is expected of psychologists. We must find ways to reduce the potential of repeating the mistakes of silence and collusion that our professions have made in the past.

Action-Focussed Teaching

Every year we facilitate teaching to Leicester DClinPsy trainees about disempowerment, gender and social action. This teaching attempts to bring the 'social action' element of the community psychology curriculum to life by making it a bit more 'action'. We get out of the classroom and utilise the teaching day and the trainee group as a resource to local people. Over the years we have built relationships with community groups in Braunstone, a residential area within the city of Leicester.

Until the 1920s, Braunstone was mainly farmland. However, the population of Leicester increased and in 1936 a large social housing estate was built in Braunstone as part of a 'slum clearance' programme. Currently, within the wider Leicester community, Braunstone is seen as a deprived area and has been associated with negative views and unhelpful discourses.

In 2016, the cohort of trainees we taught planned a walk collecting stories about the impact of homelessness, food poverty and welfare reforms to support the work of #walkthetalk2015 and Psychologists Against Austerity (PAA).

We visited four different community support organisations in Braunstone. They told us about:

- the impact of the current climate on staff: housing support staff on long-term sick due to being distressed by having to turn people away and 'gate-keep' resources
- reductions in staff by as much as 50% due to cuts to voluntary sector funding
- navigating hostile, complicated and ever-changing systems to get support
- running out of energy for seeking support due to being turned away so frequently
- feeling that their voices were not heard by those in power
- the impact of benefits 'sanctions'; examples including residents being able to eat, becoming emaciated and experiencing many physical health problems
- fleeing domestic violence but also having mental health problems and following cuts in refuge provision locally, being placed in a mixed homeless hostel where violent men and other offenders were housed
- fear about the imminent transition to Universal Credit (UC) and concern about having to make difficult choices (e.g. between paying for school uniforms or shoes for their children) at the same time as saving enough of the UC payment for rent
- worries about the future for their children, 'things are getting worse'

One woman from the community was moved to email us afterwards to say that government "pledges to support victims and survivors of childhood abuse are meaningless when they close down all the services survivors rely on to recover and feel part of society as adults. When they close hostels, refuges, cut benefits, cut restorative justice services, mental health services, it's abuse survivors who suffer… living in poor conditions, using food banks, no heating, no disability care, no emotional support, no hostel places, isolation…" We were all moved by the stories that were shared with us that day, and were humbled that the community felt able to share them with us.

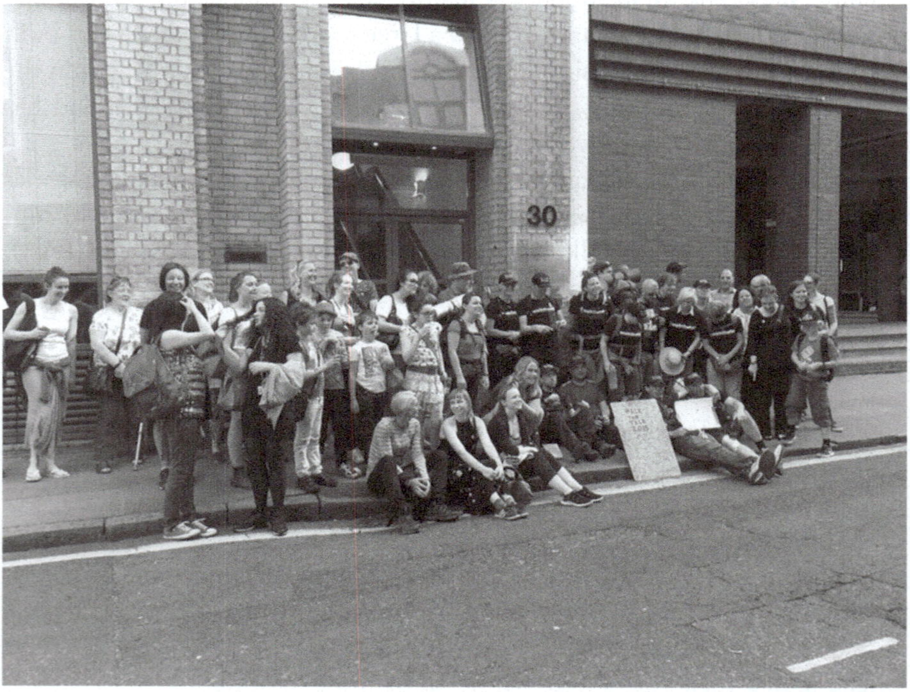

Trainees and facilitators collated the stories from local residents into a document. We discovered that we had heard stories relating to all five of the themes identified by PAA in their briefing paper about the psychological consequences of austerity (https://psychagainstausterity.wordpress.com/psychological-impact-of-austerity-briefing-paper/). We used these themes to structure a dossier of evidence which was taken by the #Walkthetalk2015 collective to the meeting with Luciana Berger MP. Psychologists and activists with lived experiences of homelessness, the benefits system, food poverty and mental health services travelled to meet the MP. During the meeting she listened to first-hand accounts of these things and copies of the dossier were left with her. At the meeting, she pledged to use the individual stories she had heard that day and those contained in the dossier to hold the Government to account. She told us that personal accounts were particularly powerful during parliamentary debates because the Government were less able to respond dismissively to questions if they were based on a constituent's experience.

We have begun to spread the word about this way of teaching to other DClinPsy courses, through a blog (psychologycultures@wordpress.com) and at the UK Group of Trainers conference. Each year the teaching adapts to the requests and challenges being faced by the Braunstone community through an ongoing dialogue with community leaders and grassroots organisations. Last year, the teaching took the form of a dig alongside local residents on a growing project in Braunstone which was then used to grow fresh veg for the local food share.

The social action teaching day is exhausting; although perhaps more emotionally than physically. One of the side effects of work at the level of the social context can be feelings of being overwhelmed by the extent of the marginalisation and powerlessness of oppressed groups. This is another reason why we would advocate for working as part of a collective. It is then possible to share the impact and hope that the sense of being overwhelmed hits individuals in the collective at different times so that the rest of the collective can support and re-energise those who are struggling. As trainers we have very much appreciated and been re-energised by the investment that trainees have given to these teaching days, even if they are not convinced by community psychology initially. Over the course of offering this teaching, we have been struck by how willing trainees are to suspend any scepticism about this different approach and take up our invitation to work with communities. Some have even reported to us that their opinions about CP changed on the basis of just this one day stepping out of the classroom; this is humbling to witness. Trainees' time, energy and enthusiasm for critical analysis and social justice is a resource that can be utilised and very much appreciated by communities if care is taken to ensure that we are walking alongside them.[1]

[1] An earlier version of this account of the social action teaching was published here: https://psychologycultures.wordpress.com/2016/05/09/taking-social-action-with-trainees-walking-and-talking-in-the-name-of-social-justice/.

The psychologists walking 100 miles to fight austerity's impact on mental health

Psychologists embark on a mental health march to raise awareness of the devastating effect that cuts are having on their patients

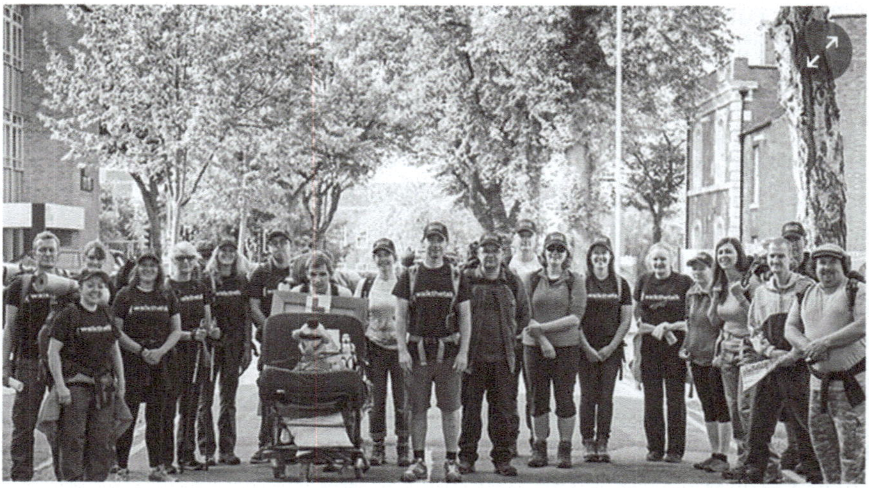

How to... Get off the Fence

We hope we have not sanitised this work in the telling or made it sound easy. It can be complex, murky, overwhelming, time consuming, draining and heartbreaking. It can also be moving, energising, growthful, humbling, inspiring, hopeful and immensely rewarding. For these reasons we urge readers to get off the fence and 'step out' today. We offer the following ideas for you to take with you on your journeys:

- Find allies: join an existing network, or create one. Don't be a hero, share the impact as well as the joy.
- Say yes! Engage with mainstream media, social media and blogging.
- If you don't have it, make sure you acquire 'street level' knowledge: psychologists are often seen as aloof and even those of us who do not consider ourselves to be academics can be viewed as confined to or hiding in 'ivory towers'.

- Challenge to change: Be bold. Use the power you have (the title clinical psychologist, for example, comes with some power which we can utilise in our social justice work). Do not be afraid to be seen or heard. Act and speak where others' voices are silenced; this can include creating opportunities or platforms on which silenced voices can take centre stage. None of us have lost our jobs over this; as a profession we need to be mindful of falling into self-policing away from social action.
- Reach out beyond the boundaries of your professional group: there is no need to compete with those who are working towards the same goals, choose your battles… there are plenty of them.
- Acknowledge those who have inspired you and stand on their shoulders: we are growing their ideas, we cannot be sure where this will go, we are all novices, our influence in this world is temporary, tread gently, and invest your time with passion.
- Welcome new connections: allow others to stand on your shoulders, including those who are otherwise invisible/d.
- Get out of the clinic room: meet people in communities with expertise relating to the issues you are taking action about, walk alongside them, listen and learn from them. Take action in public spaces where it can reach communities and the wider social context (there's no reason why your action can't take place in a university, but make sure you involve and invite the local community; make it free and accessible).
- Be the change: know yourself and take a stand for something you passionately care about.

References

Byrne, M. (2017). I was detained for protesting Trump. Here's what the Secret Service asked me. *The Washington Post*. https://www.washingtonpost.com/news/posteverything/wp/2017/08/23/i-was-detained-for-protesting-trump-heres-what-the-secret-service-asked-me/

Donovan, J. (2019). How Hate Groups' Secret Sound System Works. *The Atlantic*. https://www.theatlantic.com/ideas/archive/2019/03/extremists-understand-what-tech-platforms-have-built/585136/

European Commission. (2017). *Report from the Commission to the Parliament and the Council on Trade and Investment Barriers*. http://trade.ec.europa.eu/doclib/docs/2018/june/tradoc_156978.pdf

Goodman, P. S. (2018). In Britain, Austerity Is Changing Everything. *The New York Times*. https://www.nytimes.com/2018/05/28/world/europe/uk-austerity-poverty.html

Gupta, V. (2019, March 09). I find it difficult to identify with the "Expert by qualification" when they talk about mental health. Understand their expertise in the area but something about those with lived experiences and the "Expert by Experience" seems to resonate and feels more authentic and powerful. https://twitter.com/TheTealTigerUK/status/1104464950133702656Jones, S. G. (2018). *The Rise of Far-Right Extremism in the United States*. https://www.csis.org/analysis/rise-far-right-extremism-united-states

Jones, S. G. (2018). *The rise of far-right extremism in the United States*. Retrieved from https://www.csis.org/analysis/rise-far-right-extremism-united-states

Kagan, R. (2018). 'America First' Has Won. *The New York Times*. https://www.nytimes.com/2018/09/23/opinion/trump-foreign-policy-america-first.html

Kurtz, L. (2010). *The Anti-Apartheid Struggle in South Africa (1912-1992)*. https://www.nonviolent-conflict.org/anti-apartheid-struggle-south-africa-1912-1992/

Leahy, J. (2018). Brazilians elect Jair Bolsonaro in shift to the right. *Financial Times*. https://www.ft.com/content/350781a4-da33-11e8-9f04-38d397e6661c

Lee, C., Shin, J., & Hong, A. (2018). Does social media use really make people politically polarized? Direct and indirect effects of social media use on political polarization in South Korea. *Telematics and Informatics, 35*(1), 245–254.

Lewis, H. (2018). How Britain's political conversation turned toxic. *New Statesman*. https://www.newstatesman.com/politics/uk/2018/08/how-britain-political-conversation-turned-toxic

Malik, K. (2018). Sweden's shift to the right has been decades in the making. *The Guardian*. https://www.theguardian.com/commentisfree/2018/sep/09/sweden-elections-far-right-tolerance

Monaghan, J., & Walby, K. (2012). Making up 'Terror Identities': security intelligence, Canada's Integrated Threat Assessment Centre and social movement suppression. *Policing and Society, 22*(2), 133–151. https://doi.org/10.1080/10439463.2011.605131

Moyer, J. (2017). The End of Slacktivism? *New America Weekly*. https://www.newamerica.org/weekly/edition-164/end-slacktivism/

Partington, R. (2018). How unequal is Britain and are the poor getting poorer? *The Guardian*. https://www.theguardian.com/inequality/2018/sep/05/qa-how-unequal-is-britain-and-are-the-poor-getting-poorer

Pew Research Center. (2014). *Political Polarization in the American Public*. http://www.pewresearch.org/wp-content/uploads/sites/4/2014/06/6-12-2014-Political-Polarization-Release.pdf

Pew Research Center. (2018). *Activism in the Social Media Age*. http://www.pewinternet.org/2018/07/11/activism-in-the-social-media-age/

Potter, W. (2011). *Green is the New Red: An Insider's Account of a Social Movement Under Siege*. City Lights Books.

Proctor, G. (2002). *The Dynamics of Power in Counselling and Psychotherapy: Ethics, Politics and Practice*. PCCS Books.

Robson, D. (2018). The myth of the online echo chamber. http://www.bbc.com/future/story/20180416-the-myth-of-the-online-echo-chamber

Roser, M. (2017). Terrorism – Our World in Data. https://ourworldindata.org/terrorism/

Salter, C. (2011). Activism as terrorism: the green scare, radical environmentalism and governmentality. *Anarchist Developments in Cultural Studies, 1*, 211–238.

Shuster, S. (2016). European Politics Are Swinging to the Right. *Time*. http://time.com/4504010/europe-politics-swing-right/

Sowels, N. (2018). *An up-to-date account of economic inequalities in Britain since 2008*. https://blogs.lse.ac.uk/politicsandpolicy/an-up-to-date-account-of-economic-inequalities-in-britain-since-2008/

Taylor, A. (2014). Was #Kony2012 a failure? *The Washington Post*. https://www.washingtonpost.com/news/worldviews/wp/2014/12/16/was-kony2012-a-failure/

Townsend, M. (2018). UK towns 'polarised' by rise of far right *The Guardian*. https://www.theguardian.com/uk-news/2018/oct/27/uk-towns-polarised-by-far-right-sara-khan-counter-extremism-commissioner

Townsend, M. (2019). Rise in UK use of far-right online forums as anti-Muslim hate increases. *The Guardian*. https://www.theguardian.com/world/2019/mar/16/rise-far-right-online-forums-anti-muslim-hate-wave

Watts, J., & Vidal, J. (2017). Environmental defenders being killed in record numbers globally, new research reveals *The Guardian*. https://www.theguardian.com/environment/2017/jul/13/environmental-defenders-being-killed-in-record-numbers-globally-new-research-reveals

5

Taking a Position Within Powerful Systems

James Randall, Sarah Gunn, Steven Coles, and With thanks to Gary H.

Diagnostic practice within psychiatry is the dominant paradigm for understanding human distress, both in and beyond the health service. However, this practice is increasingly contested both ethically and in terms of its evidence base by mental health professionals, survivor activist groups, service users and other interested groups, who claim that diagnostic labelling of mental 'ill-being' is either unhelpful or actively harmful (Kinderman et al., 2013; Pemberton & Wainwright, 2014). Although transdiagnostic practices (which apply the same treatment principles fitted to needs, rather than by diagnostic label) are slowly gathering steam, both clinically and in research, the predominance of the biomedical approach to diagnosis makes it difficult for psychologists to freely follow alternative approaches in clinical practice. Consequently, clinicians who are disenchanted with the diagnostic approach on ethical or evidence-based grounds adopt a range of stances to manage the conflict with working practically within the diagnostically driven system in the UK.

With thanks to Gary H.

J. Randall (✉)
University of Hertfordshire, Hatfield, UK

S. Gunn
University of Leicester, Leicester, UK

S. Coles
Nottinghamshire Healthcare Foundation Trust, West Bridgford, UK

C. Walker et al. (eds.), *The Palgrave Handbook of Innovative Community and Clinical Psychologies*, https://doi.org/10.1007/978-3-030-71190-0_5

In this chapter, we discuss the issues surrounding diagnostic labelling in clinical practice and the wider community in the UK. We then examine the stances adopted by practising clinicians in their attempts to integrate approaches critical of diagnosis within a resistant system. We argue that these fall on a spectrum, from clinicians who assimilate diagnosis into their practice (but risk complicity with a system they feel is unethical), through those who openly question the diagnostic approach and promote alternatives, to scientist-activists who directly act against diagnostic models in conjunction with community protest groups. We consider the risks and benefits of each position to clinicians and the wider community, and end with discussion of how alternatives to diagnosis can best be taken forward.

Understanding Distress

Problems with Diagnosis

Psychiatric diagnoses fail to adequately conceptualise distress, experience and troubled or troubling behaviour, predominantly because they often rely on biological conceptualisations that disregard or underplay essential cultural and other contextual factors.

Under the diagnostic model, poor mental wellbeing in many forms has often been attributed to a 'chemical imbalance of the brain', for example for depression and 'schizophrenia', effectively reducing misery to biological determinants. This has the potential to disregard sources of trauma and misery which are highly relevant to personal and collective distress, such as social exclusion, loss of income, impoverished or absent support networks, bereavement, stress, housing insecurity and otherwise unstable environments (including threatening, unsafe and abusive contexts). Diagnostic labels mask such contextual factors and reduce the ability of individuals to voice the sources of their distress (H, 2018). For example, Gary, a long-term user of psychiatric services, published an account explaining his experience of powerful others as removing his control and choice. He described the sense of an externally imposed narrative which subjugated his own understanding of his distress:

> *My very being and story had been told to me by others and…I didn't exist at all.* (H, 2018, p. 73)

In Gary's published account, he describes how he felt disempowered by being given a 'borderline personality disorder' diagnosis—which he saw as a medicalising of his distress, rather than an attempt to understand that his presenting struggles were very much rooted in his past experience of childhood trauma. It was this experience that motivated him to seek out others with similar experiences—gaining a sense of validation through connecting with others who could accept his personal narrative of psychological distress. Through building these links with others, who similarly shared their own related stories, Gary and his community of peers began to publish creative and non-fictional pieces of work on the subject of psychiatric care and survival. Gary described feeling 'awakened' through this alternative approach; noting it was as if he were beginning to speak with his own voice, rather than the voice of the diagnostic narrative imposed upon him. Gary's published account makes for powerful reading, particularly when he talks about his ongoing struggles with psychiatric services—whom he describes are less accepting of his trauma-focused understanding of himself. In personal communication, Gary elaborated on how a continued lack of safety within services entraps him in a psychiatric gaze—whereby his anger is understood solely in terms of diagnoses, whilst he continues to need some sort of diagnosis for ongoing psychological support and for the best chance of obtaining welfare benefits:

> *The mental health system (including the professionals who work within it), the welfare benefits system, and society in general, have made my threat responses much worse. One of the emotions I have identified is anger. I am furious all the time which can lead to me being more 'unsafe' and which are pathologised as a 'symptoms' of 'Borderline Personality Disorder' by most mental health professionals.* (Gary H, personal communication, 14 April 2019)

Within these restraining contexts, the benefits of individuals who also resist and attempt to ally with service users were clear, with Gary emphasising the importance of the sustained comradeship of his psychiatric nurse who has resisted the diagnostic scripts about Gary and supported this preferred narrative for over nine years. Gary's account is a striking example of the potential for harm if psychiatric discourses and related practices are allowed to prevail without questioning.

The 'export' of diagnoses cross-culturally further diminishes the value of personal understanding of trauma and mental health. Westernised and Eurocentric constructs of disorder are imposed across the world, in Foucault's "universal reign of the normative" (1977, p. 304). This reflects imposing Western and Eurocentric understandings on cultures which understand health and wellbeing in very different ways, which deviate from the predominant

Western psychiatric discourses and resonate more meaningfully for their members. For example, Loue and Sajatovic (2008) confronted cross-cultural ways of understanding voice-hearing in the context of spirituality, exemplified by a Puerto Rican woman diagnosed with 'bipolar disorder' who remarked that "psychologists don't believe in God, only medication" (2008, p. 604). Other examples include the interpretation of mental health in cultures such as India where this may be attributed to spirits (Singh, 2017) or Nigeria where it is commonly taken as a sign of God's disapproval (Kabir et al., 2004). In fact (according to a meta-synthesis by Choudhry et al., 2016), spiritual and supernatural causes are the second-highest attributed cause of poor mental health worldwide.

Clearly, these differences in interpretation present problems when attempting to impose a Western understanding and diagnoses upon cultures for whom it conflicts directly with local sense-making and established explanatory ideas. Many academics and mental health activists consider this process to reflect a discursive 'colonisation' of sorts. "Cultures are viewed as becoming more 'literate' about mental illness…[And] in the process of doing this we not only imply that those cultures that are slow to take up these ideas are in some way 'backward', but we also export disease categories and ways of thinking about mental distress that were previously uncommon in many parts of the world" (Timimi, 2014, p. 212). However, this is also a drastic problem for groups from different cultural backgrounds who live in or have moved to the UK. For example, a high proportion of refugees who have experienced significant trauma and face continued social exclusion and discrimination are diagnosed with a range of psychiatric conditions including anxiety, depression, post-traumatic stress disorder and psychosis (e.g. Robjant et al., 2009). Likewise, members of the Black Power Movement have historically been disproportionately diagnosed with schizophrenia—which arguably has more to do with the socio-political than biomedical (Metzl, 2011). Campaigns such as *the Inquiry into the 'Schizophrenia' Label* (ISL releases preliminary findings, n.d.) have identified serious problems with the labelling of Black, Asian and Minority Ethnic (BAME) individuals; with significant misunderstandings during the process of diagnosis, as demonstrated below:

> *The doctor at the hospital kept asking me if I heard voices. I didn't know what she meant by this. Was she checking my hearing, my awareness? Was she using a metaphor? I didn't know. I said yes as I could hear the voices of nurses and patients on the ward down the corridor. That sealed my fate.*

Sixty per cent of ISL survey respondents felt that race and ethnicity had played a part in their diagnosis, which some authors suggest may be attributable to a structural racism within diagnostic practices and criteria. For example, Wangari-Jones (2016) suggests that traits such as gesticulating or talking loudly may be identified as symptomatic of threatening, or possibly mentally unwell behaviour, whereas in other cultures this behaviour might be interpreted as excited or enthusiastic. Members of minority communities can therefore feel alienated from Westernised medical services, reducing their likelihood of seeking support. Diagnostic models consequently contribute to this ongoing culturally biased state of mental health services (see position statement by RAWOrg (2011) for a summary).

Although reductionist diagnostic accounts of distress have been disputed on the above grounds, explanations centring on biological imbalances and individual deficits, remain at the heart of the mental health professions; this is not least due to the traditional central role of psychiatry in mental healthcare, which keeps the biomedical model very much alive (Coles & Mannion, 2017). At the same time, this understanding permeates public socio-cultural discourse within Western culture. The dominance of biological perceptions across public and professional realms feeds into an overwhelmingly large market of 'self-help' literature in which the individual is exhorted to identify and 'repair' their perceived flaws. The parallel with diagnostic labelling is evident.

Efforts to reduce the dominance of individualistic, biological-deficit models of distress in psychology led to the generation of the biopsychosocial model, which incorporated supporting roles for psychological and social factors in models of mental health (Boyle, 2011). However, these psychosocial components remained very much supplementary to biological factors, leading critics to relabel the approach the 'bio-bio-bio' model (Read, 2005; Read et al., 2009). Overall, it does not go far enough to address the neglect of wider community and social factors in mental distress.

Table 5.1 summarises the two core issues with psychiatric diagnoses from the research literature and service user consultation, as published in a series of documents by the Division of Clinical Psychology (2013, 2015, 2016).

As demonstrated by the second core issue with diagnostic practices in Table 5.1, being labelled with a diagnosis can carry with it several costs to the person and society. These costs truly demonstrate that 'the personal *is* the political' (Dillon, 2011). Newnes (2016) described the discursive process of diagnosis, and the meaning it holds for those affected, as 'inscription' (the connotation of permanent etching in stone is no accident). In being inscribed with a diagnosis, it is implied that (a) there is something pathological within or about the individual themselves; (b) there is a powerful other with the right

Table 5.1 The two core issues with diagnostic classification as identified in the Position Statement (DCP, 2013)

Core issue 1: Concepts and models	Core issue 2: Impact on service users
Interpretation presented as fact	Discrimination towards those diagnosed
Limitations to validity and reliability	Stigmatisation and negative impact on identity
Restrictions in clinical utility and functions	Marginalising knowledge from lived experience
Biological emphasis	Decision-making impeded
De-contextualisation	Disempowerment
Ethnocentric bias: Specifically, Westernised and Eurocentric cultural biases in conceptualisation	Over-reliance on medication, underplays physical and psychological effects

and ability to inscribe this upon the individual; and (c) there is a permanence about the diagnosis—once inscribed, a diagnosis is difficult to shake off, can be associated with therapeutic pessimism (e.g. in the case of 'personality disorders') and remains engraved on the person's medical record throughout their life and indeed beyond.

Diagnoses decontextualise and can become stigmatising for the recipients. A significant example is the diagnosis of 'borderline personality disorder'. In practice, when personalities are diagnosed with 'disorder', further exclusion and discrimination are near-inevitable, and the impacts on self-esteem, well-being and prospects are critical (Shaw & Proctor, 2004). Such labelling can also be linked to therapeutic expectations of non-improvement, with the diagnosis overshadowing and 'clouding everything' (Cross, 2016). For example, in the case of 'emerging personality disorder', labelling/diagnosing in a sense excuses the clinician from any culpability or failure to help, if the condition worsens. An alternative approach comprises acknowledging the possible existence of unknown, ongoing or unvoiced trauma or adversities in a person's life, engendering the responsibility of knowing that the 'disorder' is fluid, not fixed and *could* (possibly) be moderated by looking outside the person at improving social/community/environmental factors, rather than diagnosing (or 'inscribing') the person and abdicating responsibility. As such, the lack of consideration of context in psychiatric diagnoses has the potential to distance practitioners from broader contextual issues in potentially harmful ways. For example, Gary H. creatively made a poster to demonstrate the ways in which for him, psychiatric diagnosis represents a political issue with deeply personal and agonising costs—as seen below (Fig. 5.1):

Clinicians can become complicit with these powerful acts of inscription through their own diagnostic practices, and consequently accept the concept

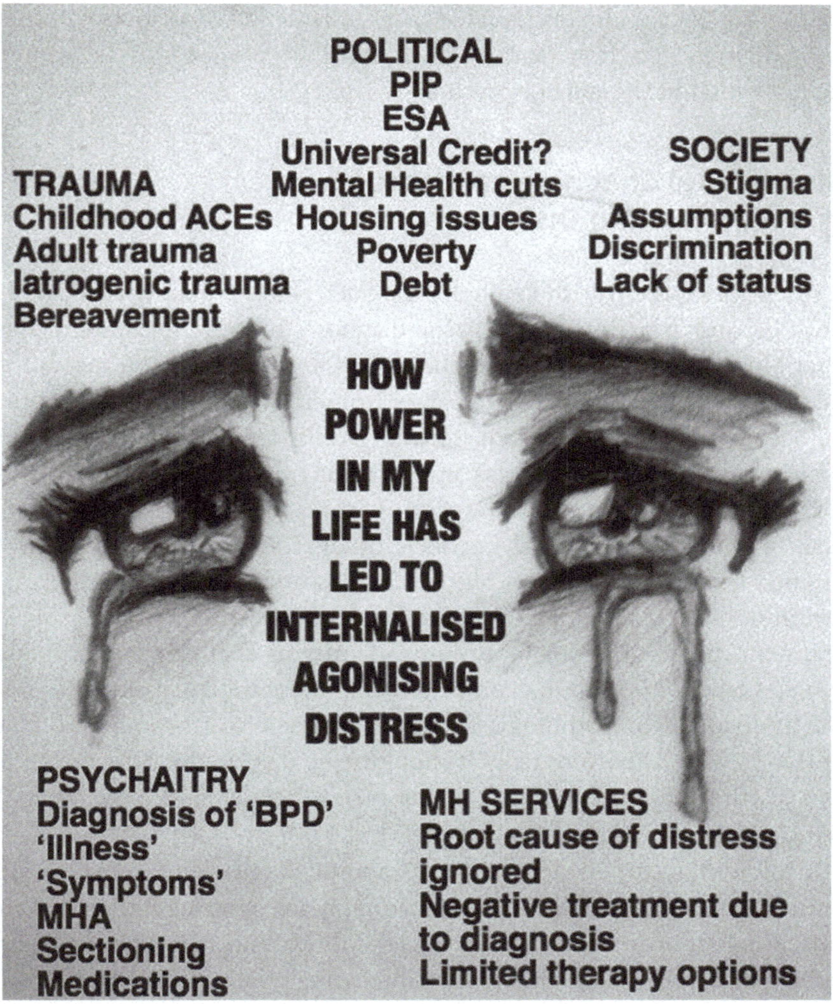

Fig. 5.1 The poster

of distress as an internalised disorder. Within services and society in general, individuals are encouraged to 'take control' of their despair, to change their responses to the world and to ultimately change *themselves*. David Smail describes this as a 'magical voluntarism' that independent of available resources, implies that if people cannot 'change themselves' successfully, it is some failing on their part (Lee, 2014; Smail, 2005). Once again, the blame falls on the somehow 'deficient' individual. However, Smail (2005) argues that magical voluntarism is "though highly plausible, doomed to impotence" (p. 28) due to its disregard of the disempowering dynamics involved in diagnosis, agency and choice; once again, deep-seated and fundamental contributing factors are ignored. Itten and Roberts (2014) colourfully describe this as "something [being] rotten in the state of psychology" (p. 223).

The (Slowly) Changing Landscape of Understanding Distress

In recent years, the British Psychological Society has explicitly advocated for a move beyond 'functional' psychiatric diagnoses to more meaningful ways of describing issues with mental wellbeing (DCP, 2013). With leadership from the professional body, small shifts away from an entirely diagnostic approach are becoming evident. 'Transdiagnostic' factors are beginning to emerge in some research agendas, such as investigations of the role of perfectionism across diagnostic constructs categorising eating-related difficulties, where the focus was on shared underlying foci for distress rather than on the label assigned to it (e.g. Shafran et al., 2002). Research into interventions is also beginning to explore shared 'process' factors between diagnostic groups and treatment modalities, moving towards identifying shared changes in adaptation and reaction to trauma and prioritising these in management of distress over individualised pathological 'disease markers' (e.g. Lambert & Barley, 2001). As Martín-Baró noted, "it shouldn't be theories that define the problems of our situation, but rather the problems that demand…their own theorisation" (cited in Burton, 2004, p. 587).

In addition to the changes in understanding distress which are emerging in research, shifts away from the diagnostic approach are emerging in the clinical conceptualisation of distress. The social context and material conditions of individual psychological distress are increasingly being identified as important. For example, significant links between early childhood trauma/adverse environmental factors and poor psychological wellbeing in later life have been identified and are the subject of ongoing research (see Felitti et al., 1998; Johnstone et al., 2018).

Evidence relating to the social-material origins of diagnoses is increasing; for a summary, see the Midlands Psychology Group (2012) manifesto for a social-materialist understanding of distress, which discusses the influence of social relations on the individual, the role of distress as a product of external trauma and subsequent invalidation of emotional responses, and that while biology may play an enabling role in mental distress, it does not take primary place. Trauma in particular significantly increases the risk of experiencing psychological distress, with retrospective studies often linking current presentations with historical traumatic events. Of those admitted in psychiatric inpatient settings, for example, 50–75% report physical and sexual assault in their childhood (McGregor, 2000)—statistics which quite frankly make the link between early trauma and later distress very clear. Non-diagnostic approaches rooted in contextualised understandings of distress are therefore sorely needed. Steps in this direction have arguably been made in terms of trauma-informed care which seeks to avoid re-traumatising, disempowering or further distressing those who have already experienced traumatic events, but much work is still required in this area (Sweeney et al., 2016) and in terms of other models of distress than trauma specifically, such as the aforementioned social-materialist understandings (Midlands Psychology Group, 2012). Trauma-informed approaches have also been critiqued ideologically and on a pragmatic level. First, the approach has been argued to reflect a political agenda, in which psychiatry can be dismantled through the 'awakening' of individuals who had not seen themselves as oppressed before (Vatel, 2015). Others have noted how trauma-informed approaches have galvanised organisational policies and structures in advance of evidencing that specific trauma-informed care practices can change people's lives for the better (Berliner & Kolko, 2016). The appropriateness of trauma-informed care at this early stage in its development is therefore by no means assured. Gary, whose experiences with diagnosis we shared earlier, described similar concerns about trauma-informed care:

> *I am increasingly concerned about the move by mental health services towards trauma-informed care. I see this as perhaps a buzzword. I worry that the more people that disclose trauma, the more people will be diagnosed with 'Borderline Personality Disorder'. I realise that stating "what happened to me" by disclosing childhood trauma all those years ago got me the sticky 'BPD' label in the first place. I think it is time to move on from 'What's happened to you?' to 'What are we going to do about it?'.* (Gary H, personal communication, 14 April 2019)

Additionally, we must consider the wider context of distress, that is the afflictions and adversities faced by communities and groups, which may have far greater impact on mental wellbeing than any counteraction the individual can undertake alone (Smail, 2005). A recent United Nations report, by Special Rapporteur and psychiatrist Dainius Pūras, argued that societal power imbalances must be addressed in order to improve health and wellbeing and that chemical imbalances have little relationship to psychological distress (Puras, 2017). Potential alternative conceptualisations integrating all of the above are being developed which focus on utilising relational, economic and socio-materialist resources within communities (e.g. Johnstone et al., 2018). The need for change across society to improve mental wellbeing for all was noted in context of Martín-Baró's (1996) 'liberation psychology', which sought to restore social justice through developing and applying psychological theory beyond the privileged—seeking transformative and collective change through raising consciousness with those most oppressed. It is also important to consider the influence of societal norms/values on what is considered a 'disorder'; Bentall (1992) for example, makes the argument that happiness meets many of the criteria, but of course is not considered an emotional disorder in need of diagnosis and treatment. These recent trends towards more relational and meta-level conceptualisations of distress introduce some sorely needed distance from the systemic inscription of disorder onto individuals.

Clinical Realities of Working with Distress

> *We cannot, I think, escape the clinic.... It would be a callous society indeed that stood back and offered [individuals] nothing just because nothing much is likely to provide any real 'cure' at the personal level. It is incumbent on us to do what we can, even if we cannot do much.* (Smail, 2005, p. 80)

Although diagnostic practices are thought of by many clinical psychologists and associated professionals as unethical, conceptually questionable and evidentially flawed, clinicians still report making decisions and choices in line with the diagnostic status quo. Randall and Coles (2018) reported clinicians "playing the diagnostic game", or participating overtly in use of diagnostic labels while more discreetly drawing on other methods of working with distress, in response to various factors in their working environments. Examples of factors which affected their likelihood of using diagnostic labels included the degree of experienced conflict between belief and practice, maintaining versus damaging relationships with colleagues, and dilemmas of position and power. Attempts to question the diagnostic model may be met with hostility or confusion from colleagues, which can be particularly intimidating for those early in their careers or in relatively junior positions. This is particularly true for those who lack confidence in their beliefs and capabilities, and are unwilling to risk their status and position to pursue change which they do not necessarily fully believe is necessary. Those who do risk their position and their relationships with colleagues by promoting non-diagnostic approaches are few, and the negative consequences can be high. In addition to these deterrents, the system rewards adherence to diagnostic models; diagnoses are required to access resources such as state benefits, clinical trials, therapies and medication. Rejecting diagnoses, therefore, may have negative consequences for the very people the clinician is attempting to support. In this way, the biomedical diagnosis-focused context of the majority of health services perpetuates itself; professionals who enter the service 'fall into line' with the established approach.

Some clinicians find ways to integrate diagnostic and alternative approaches, without directly challenging diagnostic practices, arguably to reduce anxieties and threat to themselves over the short term. However, over the long term, this integrative stance limits opportunities for concerted questioning of the overall diagnostic approach and contributes to maintaining the existing framework of individualising pathology. Arguably, successfully integrating diagnostic approaches with a more context-driven understanding of distress reduces the impetus to further decrease the influence of these biomedical constructions.

As well as external pressures to adhere to the diagnostic model, clinical psychologists may experience pressures from within the profession. Boyle (2011) describes clinical psychology as fearful of being accused of social and political bias, leading clinicians to cling onto sources of 'objectivity'. Diagnostic models offer a concreteness which is not necessarily available through more individualised process/trauma-focused models, and offers validation in this sense.

Until alternatives to diagnostic approaches become implemented at organisational levels, clinicians are faced with endless decisions as to continue to work with or within rigid diagnosis-orientated systems, or to choose to challenge these systems. For those looking to change their practice, there remains a need to adopt trauma-focused and contextualised understandings of distress, in order to provide flexible and non-judgemental support, that can continue to operate meaningfully and successfully within interdisciplinary teams who still predominantly think and work within the medical model.

In the remainder of this chapter, we explore a range of potential positions relating to integrative approaches, questioning and challenging approaches, and protest approaches to diagnostic practices, and how psychological practitioners may choose to work with these systems. We consider how these positions can be implemented in the workplace and beyond in practical, achievable ways and discuss some of the risks inherent in doing so, as well as how clinicians may seek to mitigate the perceived threat associated with challenging the status quo.

Positions on Diagnosis

A clinician's relationship to diagnosis is context-dependent, and it is important for clinicians to be aware of the changes in pressures across different working environments. In particular, some clinicians (despite acknowledging the problems with diagnosis-driven practice) struggle to act in accordance with their principles and values when faced with service-wide use of diagnosis, described by a participant in Randall and Coles (2018) as having to "still swim against the psychiatric tide". The second step after identification of the pressures on clinicians is adaptation to these pressures, in ways which enable effective co-working while allowing professionals to act in accordance with their values, beliefs and professional standards. Research by Randall and Coles (2018) explored how individual clinicians adapt their behaviours to the relational and social demands perceived as placed upon them, when working within services based around the diagnostic framework (as many or most health services still are). Typically, clinicians with concerns regarding the diagnostic approach fell somewhere between integrating diagnostic elements with other approaches and outright rejecting and campaigning against the diagnostic model.

What follows in this chapter, therefore, is examination of an evolving 'spectrum' of diagnosis-questioning positions adopted by mental health clinicians, with key examples of protest groups from the community. Towards one end of this spectrum, clinicians work with diagnosis (to varying degrees) alongside alternatives—integrating diagnostic and trauma/distress-focused approaches. Towards the other end of the spectrum are positions which directly criticise diagnosis and actively seek to promote alternatives. Some clinicians extend this further to explicit protest, often operating in conjunction with or sharing the values of survivor groups, and identifying themselves as community psychologists, scientist-activists, activist-practitioners. As noted, however, a person's adoption of a position may be fluid across contexts, dependent on the identified requests and needs of the people seeking their support, and the practitioner's perceived power, resources, support within the team and interests. For example, a clinician might choose to challenge the diagnostic approach only in cases where they feel they have sufficient social capital or a good relationship with other professionals, but might hold back when their position feels weaker. Such individuals oscillate between questioning diagnoses and pursuing an integrative approach, based on their judgement of when it may succeed, to pursue incremental change over time.

Integrating, questioning and protesting diagnosis carry differing degrees of trade-off between accepting diagnostic labels for their utility in service access and team working, and rejecting them to achieve better understanding and support for those in distress. Integrative approaches may therefore engender ethical/conceptual dissonance and guilt, while questioning or protesting may risk instability, threat and loss of inter-professional congeniality from challenging the status quo. We now discuss these three positions in detail, including potential risks of adopting each approach, and consider potential methods for mitigating such risks.

Integrating Diagnosis and Trauma/Distress Approaches

It would be disingenuous to propose that perspectives questioning or critical of diagnosis can only be adopted outside of services driven by this approach. While less constrained environments may be more conducive to free development of less traditional approaches (the Soteria project being a particularly good example—detailed later in this chapter), many psychologists and colleagues participate in scrutinising and seeking to work within and/or improve diagnostic services. However, as discussed above, such professionals are not always free to express or act upon their ethical convictions. Compromise between conviction and pragmatism often becomes necessary, with practitioners finding ways to integrate diagnostic practices with more ethical approaches without openly critiquing or challenging. For some, this is arguably a survival strategy and a means to maintain power and interests within professional practices (Randall & Coles, 2018). At the same time, there are clear examples of where diagnosis is used as capital to advocate on behalf of service users in accessing resources—which again, presents dilemmas in what can be considered most useful in the short and longer term.

Within their broader researcher, Randall and Coles (2018) explored how clinicians attempt to remain consistent with their ethical principles, while mitigating the risks associated with questioning diagnosis. Such strategies may include (though this list is not exhaustive):

- Using formulation alongside diagnosis within teams, to include contextual information to complement diagnostic labels.
- Emphasising social, historical and other contextual information.
- Engaging in research which challenges the reliability/validity of diagnostic constructs, or promoting transdiagnostic/process-based approaches in research.
- Supporting development of NICE guidelines regarding disorder-specific treatment pathways.

- Working 'around' diagnosis to address underlying causes. For example, this can include social-materialist causes of distress, such as poverty and/or social housing provisions. Likewise, clinicians can look to address contextual factors that are irrevocably linked to health inequalities, such as institutional sexism and racism, stigma and discrimination. This is represented in community psychology approaches in NHS services, where clinicians attempt to address the whole picture of a person's life and environment; it becomes less about what is wrong with the person, and more about what is not helpful about the person's relationships and environment—that is looking at their whole world, not just their internal 'disorder'.

Integrating diagnostic and trauma/distress-focused models arguably fits well within current services and 'the established order' (Diamond, 2008) and can be deployed without engendering significant conflict; for example, using psychometric research to question and challenge diagnoses through tests of reliability and validity can be promoted as exploratory work relating to evidence-based practice. Integrative approaches are, effectively, a compromise allowing professionals to operate within a system opposed to their own beliefs, as best they can.

However, there is a hidden risk; integrative approaches may inadvertently uphold harmful systemic and structural practices, while neglecting important contributing factors (explored further in Table 5.2). Positivistic acceptance of diagnostic truths is required to participate in such stances; clinicians including diagnostic models as part of their practice are still subscribing to the categorisations that demarcate people with 'disorders' as somehow 'different'. For instance, such a clinician may propose that 'personality disorder' exists on a spectrum with diagnosable 'degrees' and cut-off points of 'disordered personality' (e.g. Arbisi, 2014). This still, however, requires acceptance that there is such a construct as a 'disordered personality', with consequent stigmatising implications of the 'fragmentation' of the individual. Take, for example, the experience of Gary, whose psychiatric nurse worked with him to create a shared formulation but his psychiatrist and others persisted in applying the diagnostic construct of 'borderline personality disorder':

> *My Psychiatric Nurse wrote my Care Plan using a Formulation Approach. We wrote it together and this didn't mention diagnosis or disorder. However, this made little difference and I am still treated as someone with "BPD". I began to try to tell my psychiatrist that I didn't have "BPD" but I was told that I was lacking insight into my "illness".* (H, 2018, p. 73)

Table 5.2 Advantages and disadvantages to clinicians of attempting to integrate diagnostic stances with other approaches

Personal and professional implications of integrative approaches	
Advantages	Disadvantages
• Working within systems: Less resistance from structures and others, as practice is adapted to match service design • A pragmatism rooted in congeniality, familiarity and contested utility/evidence-base • Diagnostic practices have international reach and can provide a springboard for further elaboration, deconstruction and revision • Collaboration with colleagues that is based on established practices • Aligned to established practices of scrutiny and accountability based on outcome measures, electronic medical records and research grants • Arguably communicates with a greater ease across disciplines & teams • Adaptable to needs: Practice can look very different depending on the diagnosis in question • Potentially allows incremental changes via maintenance of positive working relationships with other professions	• Arguably perpetuates notion that distress is an internal pathology, decontextualising and masking societal causes of misery • Integrative practices could be argued to reify notion of 'abnormality'—leading to a thickening of an 'us and them' dichotomy (increasing stigma) • Practice may be incongruent with counter-evidence and survivor accounts relating to the psychological harm of diagnosis • Epistemological fragility: Concepts that underlie integrated practices are often contradictory or incompatible with one another, thus becoming misleading in their presentation as coherent approaches to working with distress

This highlights the difficulties of one practitioner alone pursuing integrative or non-diagnostic approaches; without a coherent approach from an entire team, the person is likely to experience conflicting interpretations of their experience and behaviour, which may increase distress further.

A significant example of integrating diagnostic and trauma/distress-focused approaches in clinical practice is the championing of psychological formulation; this is often touted as a means to collaboratively move beyond diagnosis without disposing of the approach entirely. Formulation is a core competency among clinical psychologists and comprises incorporation of interpersonal, biological, social and cultural factors in generating an individual model summarising psychological distress (DCP, 2011). Formulations are (supposed to be, although in practice not always) developed jointly with service users and focus on how their past and present experiences generate and maintain their current distress; these models are then used to produce plans to adapt to or change elements of the individual's situation, and are constantly open to review and reformulation (Johnstone & Dallos, 2013). It is often well received by individuals, who express a sense of collaboration rather than being 'inscribed upon'. One ISL survey respondent said:

> I am in favour of formulating a co-constructed narrative of the service user's problems and their personal meaning in the context of their life experiences. No diagnosis needed! (ISL releases preliminary findings, n.d.)

Within teams, clinical psychologists are often sought for their input in high-risk, complex cases, that is using formulation as a bolt-on rather than a self-sufficient alternative to diagnosis (Mohtashemi et al., 2016). This offers an integrative, practical route to changing practice by increments, encouraging the incorporation of psychological perspectives into the existing diagnostic system; it, therefore, manages some of the tensions between an awareness of the shortcomings of diagnosis and the sense of threat that challenging practices may engender. However, it carries the aforementioned problem of colluding with diagnostic practices while promoting distress/trauma-driven approaches. Additionally, the validity and reliability of formulation-based diagnoses have not been extensively researched (compromising their credibility within teams focused on evidence-based practice), although there is limited evidence that structured formulation remains highly reliable even in individuals with highly complex presentations (e.g. Critchfield et al., 2015).

Overall, integrating elements of distress/trauma-focused work into existing diagnostic frameworks minimises threat to the practitioner, but avoids challenge to the established system and maintains ethical discrepancies. We next examine the position of overtly questioning diagnostic practices.

Questioning Diagnosis

In questioning positions, clinicians explicitly emphasise problems with diagnosis and promote alternatives. Questioning perspectives highlight perceived inadequacies of the diagnostic approach, which typically leads to psychotropic medication being considered the primary or only treatment even in complex situations of adversity and human distress, such as loss, mistreatment and abuse. Rather than attempting to integrate diagnostic and trauma/distress-focused models, whereby practices appear improved at face value but remain relatively intact, many clinicians choose to confront and challenge diagnostic practices. This may be on an individual level or collectively with others; Box 5.1 details one such group-based approach, which seeks to reframe the conceptual underpinning of prescriptive practices.

Box 5.1 An Example of Questioning Diagnosis Beyond the Clinic Room

The Drop the Disorder Group

This highly inclusive group focuses on "critical questions of the day around the biomedical model in mental health" (A Disorder for Everyone, n.d.) challenging established approaches to distress, diagnosis, medicalisation and psychopharmacology. Originally inspired by the predominance of biomedical discourse in UK media and health campaigns (Watson, 2017), it attempts to engage healthcare professionals, service users and anyone with lived experience or engagement with psychological services in any context. While the core team comprise mental health professionals (a mental health nurse, psychotherapist and clinical psychologist), people strongly associated with the group include those with lived experience, academics, writers, poets and activists. It provides an important interface between various healthcare groups, service users and academics in relevant areas, allowing for exchange of knowledge and experience. Drop the Disorder also has positive links and shares associates, with Mad in America—a group with similar aims based in the USA (Watson, 2017). It should be considered, though, to what extent this represents another form of colonisation from Western culture; following the imposition of Western models of mental ill-being, this could be construed as the Western model of resistance. Arguably, supporting other modes of resistance from marginalised non-Western cultures and understandings would be more in line with the values the resistance hope to espouse.

There is a focus on public engagement via social media, including an active Facebook group (with almost 9000 members at the time of writing) and Twitter feed (with almost 28,000 followers) which encourage exploration of lived experience and how this relates to diagnoses, medicalisation of distress and associated language. Drop the Disorder has arranged multiple one-day 'A Disorder for Everyone' events in cities across the UK since October 2016. Events are intended to be accessible for people from all backgrounds and include workshops and creative presentations. The social media and events emphasise alternatives to "colluding with the message that people are "ill"", with an emphasis on relationships, attachment and distress/trauma as explanatory and maintaining components in poor mental health (Watson, 2017). Common themes on the social media forums include discussion of personality disorder diagnoses, electroconvulsive therapy and medication. The 'A Disorder for Everyone' (n.d.) website also carries related resources.

Drop the Disorder has been criticised at times for being overly biased against the biomedical model of mental health rather than presenting an even-handed appraisal, although the organisers contend that given the dominance of the biomedical model, their focus on alternatives is proportionate. In particular, the social media groups provide a source of support for those experiencing distress which they do not feel is well-explained by themes of sickness and medication and provides a forum for professionals to discuss working with different understandings of mental health difficulties within systems perceived as highly biomedical in approach. It can perhaps best be conceptualised as a group supporting the liaison between professionals and those with lived experience of distress (groups which of course may overlap). Future aims include development of a 'Mad in the UK' sites with resources and blogs supporting the group's aims and membership and continuing to build international networks with other organisations with related goals (Watson, 2017).

Questioning approaches are difficult to adopt for those early in their careers, who may be dissuaded from acting in accordance with their values due to the perceived risk of rejection from peers/superiors (detailed and explored further in Table 5.3). As part of their broader research, Randall and Coles (2018) note the following quote from a focus group of assistant psychologists:

Table 5.3 Advantages and disadvantages to clinicians of attempting to question diagnostic stances

Personal and professional implications of questioning diagnosis	
Advantages	Disadvantages
• A greater sense of adhering to values and ethics that reduces sense of incongruity and compromise. • Greater partnership with service users, with a greater tolerance for uncertainty in practice, to facilitate a greater degree of choice/control over one's journey through services. • Offers service users and colleagues different ways of understanding distress. This can include the biological and medical ways of understanding distress, but as contextualised to a broad range of factors. • Creates space for alternative theories of change and psychological models for consideration in the evidence-base (e.g. using, critiquing and replacing dominant practices). • Opens up the potential for pluralistic approaches, particularly in context of multidisciplinary team working. • Can contribute towards a gradual revision of professional and public conceptualisations of mental health difficulties—highlighting the multiplicity of contributing factors to psychological distress.	• Questioning humility: A potential to be seen as a 'lone wolf ' or troublemaker (e.g. seen as reluctant/contentious rather than curious), with little conceptual understanding of underlying values in questioning. • Position often based on different epistemological positions rooted in critical theory/social constructivism—creating a complexity and nuance to debate (e.g. complicating proposals to services/managers in culture of 'evidence-based' practice solely contingent on positivist approaches). • Services contexts increasingly faced with increasing demand, dwindling capacity and prospective cuts; leading to greater reliance on more mechanistic approaches above those that tolerate/accept uncertainty (i.e. categorisation over psychological formulation). • Questioning power: Diagnosis dominates public discourse, commissioning agendas, governmental policy and mental health service designs, meaning that those who take alternative positions will be occupying positions facing a great deal of opposing interests and power. • Individuals are often 'othered' by those critical of questioning approaches—being positioned into binary and dichotomous thinking (e.g. described as anti-psychiatry, anti-positivist, anti-pluralist).

> *It feels almost as if you are questioning [your supervisor's] experience and knowledge. I guess, in something competitive like training in clinical psychology, these people may be potentially writing you off.... And it's probably not conscious, but it is in the back of your mind that you know if I make too much trouble this could hinder my career path.*

Within this, they noted the negative connotations of being perceived as 'lone wolves' or 'troublemakers'—which were reminiscent of statements expressed by qualified clinicians within the broader study. Such considerations of power and interest are inherently linked to clinicians' decisions in practice and affect their ability to challenge diagnostic models.

Those who seek to integrate ways of working with diagnosis often make attempts to practise in line with their underlying ethical position, whilst at the same time managing perceived and actual risks of questioning diagnosis. In similar light, practitioners who explicitly question diagnosis also adopt a range of strategies and approaches to aid progress, whilst at the same time mitigating the risks and costs of doing so. Individuals and groups may question and critically challenge diagnostic practices in various ways and such strategies may include (though this list is not exhaustive):

- Fostering 'safe uncertainty' with service users (encouraging the mindset that it is acceptable not to have a concrete diagnosis and that this is not essential to achieving change/improvement). Safe uncertainty was conceptualised by systemic psychotherapist Barry Mason (1993), whose ideas are similar to efforts to improve informed decision-making through the development of accessible literature for service users on understanding formulation and diagnosis (DCP, 2016).
- Within teams, clinicians may directly challenge and offer alternatives during multidisciplinary work and during supervision.
- Working in partnership with service users through the design and delivery—working towards making co-production at the core of clinical practice.
- Further options for those later in their careers include becoming editors and peer-reviewers, to support diagnosis-questioning approaches in literature and research.
- Individuals and groups may go on to conduct their own studies and research around non-diagnostic-based practices.
- Collaborations with groups such as Drop the Disorder to offer training/teaching in alternative approaches (e.g. trauma-informed or formulation-based work).

- Efforts at integrating these questioning approaches into training should consider professional and disciplinary training pathways in order to include more critical and community psychology approaches and evidence into relevant curriculums and competency frameworks (from psychology undergraduate degree teaching through to clinical psychology doctorate training). Peacock-Brennan and colleagues have researched such provisions (Peacock-Brennan & Harper, 2018) and explored the feasibility of establishing policy-based placement provisions (Peacock-Brennan et al., 2018). However, it is important to note that these approaches are not specifically directed to reduce the influence of diagnostic approaches and could as easily encourage their use as discourage it.
- Designing self-help resources fitted to these approaches also help to improve awareness and relevant skills in the professional and broader communities. For example, clinicians developing self-help resources which focus on an awareness of trauma, power and distress in a person's relationships and environment may increase the likelihood of them using these techniques in their own practice or encouraging such formulations within their teams.
- Proactively seeking representation from marginalised groups and those with lived experience in investigations of mental health services and provisions, such as the aforementioned Inquiry into the 'Schizophrenia' Label campaign which specifically sought BAME experiences of being diagnosed with schizophrenia.

These approaches carry more risk than approaches integrating diagnosis and trauma/distress-focused stances. The challenge to the existing model is greater, and therefore there is more threat to multidisciplinary collaboration and professional relationships. There is also threat to perceived competence/expertise, and the clinician's ethical objections may be dismissed as preference or personal style, reducing their authority within the team. Finally, there may be service-level implications, such as reductions in diagnoses having financial implication (e.g. 'Payment by Results' within the UK) and more complex models making it more difficult to assess progress on routine or available outcome measures. There may therefore be resistance on an operational level, in addition to multidisciplinary reluctance to shift paradigms.

The potential for critically challenging diagnosis is far-reaching, particularly as groups such as Drop the Disorder have started to push for not only clinical but broader social change. However, the risks are off-putting to some. Following discussion of the last position (protesting diagnosis), we then provide some further strategies for mitigating the perceived personal and professional risks of such practices.

Protesting and Activism

The final of the three presenting approaches is for individuals to protest or seek to actively change diagnostic practices, usually by finding allies across disciplines and within public arenas. The development of the DSM-5 (American Psychiatric Association, 2013) saw a collaboration of professionals, service users, the public and mainstream media to contest a range of planned extensions to the diagnostic manual, in a protest which far overstepped merely questioning diagnosis (Kinderman et al., 2017). However, stances which overtly protest diagnosis are rare (but increasing). Other examples of protest/activist approaches include groups of professionals and service users who share their experiences and work to disseminate arguments further, for example, the Hearing Voices Network. Other collaborations go further, such as the Soteria network (see Box 5.2) which campaigns to provide drug-free, non-psychiatric alternatives to inpatient support for people experiencing 'psychosis'. Importantly, groups dedicated to ending racial inequality in mental health systems are also on the rise, such as Rights and Wellbeing of Racialised Groups (RAWOrg, 2011), who have the support of Mind and the Afiya Trust (another organisation working to reduce inequalities in healthcare provision for people from BAME backgrounds). The service user–led group Kindred Minds also offers peer support to BAME people who are experiencing mental distress, and additionally are involved in consultations and lobbying for social change to promote mental health service needs and wider societal issues for BAME communities. Their extensive manifesto by Griffiths (n.d.) was released in 2018. Often it is not professionals who organise such groups, with grassroots movements being initiated by service users and survivor groups—where like-minded practitioners may be welcomed into the group itself or invited to join particular activities and projects (rather than become group members themselves). An example of this is the Recovery in the Bin (RITB) group who are a self-defined critical theorist and activist collective. RITB exclaim that the recovery movement reflects an ideological stance grounded in neoliberal practices—operating on the denial of disability, coercive practices, victim blaming and continued removal of support services (see https://recoveryinthebin.org/ for further information). Advocating for 'unrecovered' status as a valid self-definition within what is considered wider class struggle, RITB calls upon professionals to protect service users from damaging and harmful governmental policies, and encourage dissidence and whistle-blowing in order to seek sustained systemic change.

As groups active against diagnosis develop in the community, activist-scientist groups are also emerging in clinical bodies—key examples are the Psychologist for Social Change and Psychologists Against Austerity groups (see McGrath et al.,

Box 5.2 An Example of Networks Set up Through and for Protest and Activism

The Soteria Network

Soteria (Soteria Network, n.d.) is a UK-based network committed to development of drug-free or minimum-medication therapeutic environments for people experiencing symptoms of 'psychosis' (i.e. having different experiences of reality to those around them). The network comprises service users, activists, professionals and carers, determined to promote the Soteria philosophy in UK mental health and to support the development of non-medical alternatives to 'traditional' UK psychiatry.

The Soteria approach emphasises the need for humane, non-coercive mental health support, arguing in support of the ability of people with psychotic experiences to recover without psychiatric/biomedical interventions. Psychosis is seen not as an illness or symptom, but as a sign of personal crisis arising from stressors such as traumatic experience, psychological/physiological harm, social distress or environmental instability. These are not biomedical conditions which can or should be remediated with medication, or certainly not medication alone. While Soteria warns of side-effects, inappropriate use of medication and unnecessarily prevalence of biomedical models in 'treating' psychosis, the network explicitly describes itself as not being 'anti-medication', simply as seeing medication as one option among many. The aim of treatment is not recovery, so much as change and transformation through the experience of psychosis, supporting people positively to make sense of and come through their experiences. The overarching drive is hope and autonomy, intended as a contrast to the pessimism inherent in psychiatric services, where people with psychosis are often expected to be on lifelong medication without opportunity for return to a healthy, fulfilling and meaningful life.

The network campaigns for Soteria-type mental health services, emphasising the need for patient-led decisions in mental healthcare, redressing the balance of power between patient and psychiatrist, and mechanisms to support those who wish to withdraw from psychotropic medication. Soteria-style projects emphasise home-like, non-professional, safe-feeling environments which offer minimum medication and maximum support. A review of evidence (Mosher, 1999) from the initial Soteria project and its successors indicate that 85–90% of acute and long-term people with psychosis could return to the community without conventional hospital treatment; Soteria-style environments reduced psychotic symptoms as effectively as antipsychotic medication over the first six weeks. It is argued by the network that such environments enable both short-term improvement in symptoms and long-term avoidance of institutionalisation, with better social adjustment, in contrast to medication which only offers the former.

The network's long-term aims include establishment of Soteria-style houses in the UK, for working with both people experiencing first-episode psychosis and those with longer-term psychotic experiences. The network also wishes to develop support networks for people living in the community, for example, by home visits from survivor support groups and offering support for withdrawal from psychotropic medication. Soteria sees its long-term aims as additional to NHS services, offering supportive resources in a manner and philosophy not currently available through UK mental health services.

2016) and the development of the Power Threat Meaning framework (Johnstone et al., 2018). However, protesting positions are even harder to enact in practice than challenging positions, with similar risks to questioning but exacerbated, such as risking outright adversarial dynamics with colleagues who adhere to medical/biological conceptualisations of distress. Overtly taking such positions can put individuals in direct conflict with the interests and priorities of their employers (see Cecchin et al., 1992; Diamond, 2008; Smail, 2005). Although collectives acting anonymously avoid this deterrent, any powers associated with professional status, which can be used helpfully to give some clout to activist groups, is lost. Such groups are also often viewed with suspicion. Some of the potential advantages and disadvantages to clinicians of assuming positions of protest and direct activism are listed in Table 5.4 below.

Table 5.4 Advantages and disadvantages to clinicians of assuming protesting or activist stances

Personal and professional implications of protesting diagnosis	
Advantages	Disadvantages
• Practising in-line with your values: A greater sense of adhering ethical standpoints & reducing incongruity and unhelpful compromise • Grassroots collaboration: Greater partnership with service users and survivor groups • Changing ideas about what constitutes help/ intervention, opens-up access to novel resources and establishes new approaches to support • May contribute towards establishing alternative conceptual frameworks and practice, or progress those already developing • Models approaches rooted in ethical values and practice which can be integrated into teams and service structures (e.g. demonstrating a different practice for those early-on in their careers) • Challenging and learning from one another: Supporting inter-agencies and cross-disciplinary working that embraces a whole body of perspectives • Dismantles 'us and them' discourses	• Requiring personal commitment to practice 'beyond' (e.g. working long hours) • Requiring persistence (e.g. meeting lots of resistance or barriers to progression) • Impact of activism and protests (e.g. systemic change) not always immediately realised or obviously visible; opening position to critique and dismissal from others • Significant responsibility: Objectives often linked with countering dangerous practices for others, so the costs of not succeeding can be hugely detrimental to one's own wellbeing • Extremely rare for protected time for activism; limited access to resources for this • Pushing against power: Requires challenging more established and powerful people and systems—with structural disadvantages (e.g. neoliberal structures bureaucratising and individualising) • Possible restrictions on career: Risking personal criticism, challenges to professionalism and loss of status within teams aligned to more medicalised discourses • Social media and 'trolling': Those who move away from the status quo risk being subjected to sustained 'attacks' from those who invest heavily in the established order of services—from persecutory, personal remarks (sometimes leading to 'trolling') to discursively oppressive tactics (e.g. labelling actions as 'virtue-signalling' or individuals as 'snowflakes')

What Then Can We Do?

Promoting non-diagnostic ways to understand distress requires three changes: (1) increasing general knowledge/awareness of alternative approaches, (2) reducing risks associated with adopting non-diagnostic conceptualisations where possible and (3) improving resources of clinicians to manage and mitigate remaining risks. This will require widespread national change, both within and beyond the health service, and consideration of practical means to achieve this is key.

Envisioning change is easier than achieving it, given the weight of tradition and biomedical predominance (Smail, 2005). As such, systems change is required to achieve overarching, longstanding improvement. Rather than simply looking at individuals and their immediate environments, systems change looks at the broader socio-political context and seeks to make appropriate changes to benefit wellbeing within this wider arena, consulting with and building cooperative relationships between involved individuals or groups to seek solutions. It also emphasises the interdependency between components; the aim is to create change by generalising attitudinal change across society, rather than by focusing on changing one element (Behrens & Foster-Fishman, 2007; Checkland, 1981). While there are many forms of systems change theory, they typically seek to address real-world messy problems in a holistic manner (Checkland & Holwell, 2005). Behrens and Foster-Fishman (2007) propose five key principles for implementing systems change: (1) to clarify its purpose, including the nature and boundaries of the current system and what resources are available to support change; (2) to identify whether a new system is required or if the existing system can be amended; (3) to conceptualise the work as systems change from its initiation and plan appropriately; (4) to use an integrative, eclectic approach; and (5) to identify leverage points and take advantage of arising opportunities. Essentially, the authors go a step beyond the reactionary responses to diagnosis (although they are writing about community change in general, not non-diagnostic approaches in particular) and argue for structured, planned change which is still responsive and flexible. In terms of generating a shift towards non-diagnostic approaches to mental wellbeing, this clarifies what is presently lacking; (1) the problems may have been identified, but their boundaries are not clearly drawn in terms of who is most affected and who should participate in solutions; (2) as outlined in this chapter, there is ongoing uncertainty as to whether a new system is required or whether diagnosis can or should be integrated with different understandings of distress; (3) certainly there is not currently a clear systems-change model for the shift, and cannot be until the former criteria are met; and (4) and (5) also rely upon clarification of the problem and what kind of solution is being sought. Initially, therefore, purposeful and inclusive collaboration between individuals using, providing, funding and directing mental health services is required to establish what systems change is appropriate and helpful.

For establishment of non-diagnostic practices, debate alone is insufficient (Smail, 2005); collaborative, sustained and collective action is necessary, across disciplinary groups and between mental health professionals and wider communities/society—in particular those with most political power. Practical changes clinicians can make to move towards this include:

- Engagement with policy and national consultations, in order to encourage overall change in models of conceptualising distress beyond the therapy room/multidisciplinary team. Indeed, Browne explored how applied psychologists can work towards influencing macro-level policies (Browne, 2017), highlighting a broad range of possible exits from inaction.
- Structured systems change approaches, following Behrens and Foster-Fishman's (2007) criteria for successful social change. This could initially be informed by systematic analysis of the structures, relationships and environment which maintain and reinforce the status quo. Griffith et al. (2007), for example, used three analytical tools to examine factors influencing race-related disparities in health provision and outcomes. Maintaining watchfulness for leverage points such as leadership changes or new funding is also important; as Behrens and Foster-Fishman (2007) note, systems change is often a matter of opportunistic seizing the day as much as planned, intentional change.
- Building relationships with the media and working confidently towards a change in discourse, influencing the communicative actions that follow. This could include writing original/accessible reports and letters, responding quickly to coverage of mental health issues in the media, recruiting allies to co-sign letters and co-write articles and offering interviews to local and national media.
- Running consciousness-raising groups regarding the underlying common experiences to presenting psychiatric diagnoses (e.g. social-materialist factors), for those accessing services and those supporting them (Fisher, 2017). Arguably, consciousness-raising groups should also be made accessible for many other groups, for example at policy and governance levels.
- Participating in research, seeking funding and adding to existing proposals to examine underlying causes and contributory factors in distress, rather

than adhering to diagnostic models when producing research. These efforts would suit action research methods and need to be democratic in process, participatory, and co-produced. A key focus might include further research into the reliability and validity of formulation-based diagnoses.

- Using research/audit to explore how local and social issues (e.g. suicide rates, poverty, high unemployment) relate to presenting levels of mental distress within services. Such small-scale research can enable services to innovate and accommodate to actual community needs—which may mean prioritising socio-materialist, political and governmental interventions to address mental health issues before or alongside offering the therapy chair.
- Finding allies in order to encourage meaningful action in the context of social injustices—leading to change and improvements in community experiences (Reynolds, 2010). Likewise, individuals should seek to become allies for those with least resources to move beyond adversities and difficult contexts—which can include disempowering contexts within the profession, alongside advocating for those accessing services or deciding to disengage from the established order.
- Supporting and linking in with groups who seek wider social change, such as RAWOrg, Kindred Minds and the Afiya Trust which attempt to address racial inequalities in mental health support in both formal services and wider society.
- In terms of decolonising mental health services (but also in broader community psychology), patient empowerment, education to improve social capital, reducing isolation and stress through building community connections, have all been shown to be helpful in support work with immigrants (Michael et al., 2008). Similarly, social network interventions have been used to encourage behavioural change and promote wellbeing (Valente, 2012). Both approaches take a wider view of mental distress, seeking to strengthen the resources and support available to individuals, rather than assigning a diagnosis and treating the person as somehow 'defective'.

There should be an awareness that change comes slowly and is more likely to be achieved through incremental steps and small acts of resistance and by aiming carefully/thinking small (Newnes et al., 1999). Importantly, this would mean not only seeking to change the socio-political and health service approaches to mental health, but to influence wider community lives for the better and re-align governmental practices towards a more humanistic and socially orientated understanding of distress and trauma. If we are to truly consider new ideas for new times, we must apply a concerted effort to building non-diagnostic approaches to psychological distress which give appropriate credence to contextual factors such as the availability and accessibility of social resources, and the origins of individual and collective traumas within and across societies. In doing so, we may well disentangle the inwardly looking gaze of diagnosis not from our bodies, but from the notion that our bodies are the cause or solution to distress. To look outside at a world that is causing significant and widespread mental distress is an important step in working more effectively in clinical practice and ultimately more ethical in working beyond psychiatric diagnoses.

Acknowledgements We would like to thank Gary H. for his comments and critical questioning. Importantly, he has helped us to critically engage with our own arguments and embed our observations in the lived experience of psychiatric services.

References

A Disorder for Everyone. (n.d.). Retrieved April 3, 2019, from http://www.adisorder4everyone.com/links/#useful-links

American Psychiatric Association. (2013). *Diagnostic and statistical manual of mental disorders*. American Psychiatric Association.

Arbisi, P. A. (2014). Introduction to the special section on the Personality Psychopathology Five (PSY-5) and DSM-5 trait dimensional diagnostic systems for personality disorders: Emerging convergence. *Journal of Personality Assessment, 96*(2), 117–120. https://doi.org/10.1080/00223891.2013.866571

Behrens, T. R., & Foster-Fishman, P. G. (2007). Developing operating principles for systems change. *American Journal of Community Psychology, 39*(3–4), 411–414. https://doi.org/10.1007/s10464-007-9106-3

Bentall, R. P. (1992). A proposal to classify happiness as a psychiatric disorder. *Journal of Medical Ethics, 18*(2), 94–98.

Berliner, L., & Kolko, D. J. (2016). Trauma informed care: A commentary and critique. *Child Maltreatment, 21*(2), 168–172. https://doi.org/10.1177/1077559516643785

Boyle, M. (2011). Making the world go away, and how psychology and psychiatry benefit. In M. Rapley, J. Moncrieff, & J. Dillon (Eds.), *De medicalizing misery*. Palgrave Macmillan.

Browne, N. (2017). Practice to policy: Clinical psychologists' experiences of macro-level work. Unpublished thesis.

Burton, M. (2004). Viva Nacho! Liberating psychology in Latin America. *Psychologist, 17*(10), 584–587.

Cecchin, G., Lane, G., & Ray, W. A. (1992). *Irreverence: A strategy for therapists' survival*. Karnac Books.

Checkland, P. (1981). *Systems thinking: Systems practice*. Wiley.

Checkland, P., & Holwell, S. (2005). *Information, systems and information systems.* John Wiley.
Choudhry, F. R., Mani, V., Ming, L. C., & Khan, T. M. (2016). Beliefs and perception about mental health issues: A meta-synthesis. *Neuropsychiatric Disease and Treatment, 12,* 2807–2818. https://doi.org/10.2147/NDT.S111543
Coles, S., & Mannion, A. (2017). Critical clinical psychology. In *The Palgrave handbook of critical social psychology* (pp. 557–578). Palgrave Macmillan.
Critchfield, K. L., Smith Benjamin, L., & Levenick, K. (2015). Reliability, sensitivity, and specificity of case formulations for comorbid profiles in interpersonal reconstructive therapy: Addressing mechanisms of psychopathology. *Journal of Personality Disorders, 29*(4), 547–573. https://doi.org/10.1521/pedi.2015.29.4.547
Cross, S. (2016). An exploration of the experiences of CAMHS nurses who work with adolescents with the label emerging personality disorder. Unpublished thesis.
Diamond, B. (2008). Opening up space for dissension: A questioning psychology. In A. Morgan (Ed.), *Being human: Reflections on mental distress in society*. PCCS Books.
Dillon, J. (2011). The personal is the political. In M. Rapley, J. Moncrieff, & J. Dillon (Eds.), *De-medicalizing misery: Psychiatry, psychology and the human condition* (pp. 141–157). Palgrave Macmillan.
Division of Clinical Psychology. (2011). *Good practice guidelines on the use of psychological formulation.* Leicester: The British Psychological Society.
Division of Clinical Psychology. (2013). *Classification of behaviour and experience in relation to functional psychiatric diagnoses: time for a paradigm shift. A position statement.*
Division of Clinical Psychology. (2015). *Guidelines on language in relation to functional psychiatric diagnosis.*
Division of Clinical Psychology. (2016). *Understanding psychiatric diagnosis in adult mental health.*
Felitti, V. J., Anda, R. F., Nordenberg, D., Williamson, D. F., Spitz, A. M., Edwards, V., … Marks, J. S. (1998). Relationship of childhood abuse and household dysfunction to many of the leading causes of death in adults: The adverse childhood experiences (ACE) study. *American Journal of Preventive Medicine, 14*(4), 245–258.
Fisher, M. (2017). 'It's not your fault': Consciousness-raising as a reversal of magical voluntarism. *Clinical Psychology Forum, 297*(9), 4–7.
Foucault, M. (1977). *Discipline and Punish: The birth of the prison.* New York: Random House.
Griffith, D. M., Mason, M., Yonas, M., Eng, E., Jeffries, V., Plihcik, S., & Parks, B. (2007). Dismantling institutional racism: Theory and action. *American Journal of Community Psychology*. https://doi.org/10.1007/s10464-007-9117-0
Griffiths, R. (n.d.). A call for social justice. Retrieved August 19, 2018, from https://www.nsun.org.uk/Handlers/Download.ashx?IDMF=c75197d7-824c-43ef-9a83-27ff33284147
H, G. (2018). A diagnosis of "Borderline Personality Disorder" Who Am I? Who could I have been? Who can I become? *Psychosis, 10*(1), 70–75.

ISL Releases Preliminary Findings. (n.d.). In *inquiry into the 'Schizophrenia' label.* Retrieved August 19, 2018, from http://www.schizophreniainquiry.org/news/isl-releases-preliminary-findings

Itten, T., & Roberts, R. (2014). *The new politics of experience and the bitter herbs.* PCCS Books.

Johnstone, L. & Boyle, M. with Cromby, J., Dillon, J., Harper, D., Kinderman, P., Longden, E., Pilgrim, D., & Read, J. (2018). *The power threat meaning framework: Towards the identification of patterns in emotional distress, unusual experiences and troubled or troubling behaviour, as an alternative to functional psychiatric diagnosis.* : British Psychological Society.

Johnstone, L., & Dallos, R. (2013). *Formulation in psychology and psychotherapy: Making sense of people's problems.* Routledge.

Kabir, M., Iliyasu, Z., Abubakar, I. S., & Aliyu, M. H. (2004). Perception and beliefs about mental illness among adults in Karfi Village, Northern Nigeria. *BMC International Health and Human Rights, 4*(3) (e-pub). https://doi.org/10.1186/1472-698X-4-3.

Kinderman, P., Allsopp, K., & Cooke, A. (2017). Responses to the publication of the American Psychiatric Association's DSM-5. *Journal of Humanistic Psychology, 57*(6), 625–649.

Kinderman, P., Read, J., Moncrieff, J., & Bentall, R. P. (2013). Drop the language of disorder. *Evidence Based Mental Health, 16*(1), 2–3.

Lambert, M. J., & Barley, D. E. (2001). Research summary on the therapeutic relationship and psychotherapy outcome. *Psychotherapy: Theory/Research/Practice/Training, 38*(4), 357–361.

Lee, J. (2014). Nine rather disconnected paragraphs: on Mental health, capitalism, creative education and the politics of friendship. *37 Pieces of Flair*, 6–8.

Loue, S., & Sajatovic, M. (2008). Auditory and visual hallucinations in a sample of severely mentally ill puerto rican women: An examination of the cultural context. *Mental Health, Religion and Culture, 11*(6), 597–608.

Martín-Baró, I. (1996). The role of the psychologist. In A. Aron & S. Corne (Eds.), *Writings for a liberation psychology* (pp. 33–46). Harvard University Press.

Mason, B. (1993). Towards positions of safe uncertainty. *Human Systems: The Journal of Systemic Consultation & Management, 4*(1), 189–200.

McGrath, L., Walker, C., & Jones, C. (2016). Psychologists against austerity: Mobilising psychology for social change. *Critical and Radical Social Work, 4*(3), 409–413.

McGregor, K. (2000). *Abuse-focused therapy for adult survivors of child sexual abuse: A review of the literature.* Unpublished thesis. Retrieved August 19, 2018, from https://www.researchgate.net/profile/Kim_Mcgregor/publication/238766469_Abuse-focused_therapy_for_adult_survivors_of_child_sexual_abuse_A_review_of_the_literature/links/0c96052c7c8e643b02000000/Abuse-focused-therapy-for-adult-survivors-of-child-sexual-abuse-A-review-of-the-literature.pdf

Metzl, J. M. (2011). *The protest psychosis: How Schizophrenia became a black disease.* Beacon Press.

Michael, Y. L., Farquhar, S., Wiggins, N., & Green, M. (2008). Findings from a community-based participatory prevention research intervention designed to increase social capital in Latin African American communities. *Journal of Immigrant and Minority Health, 10*, 281–289.

Midlands Psychology Group. (2012). Draft manifesto for a social materialist psychology of distress. *Journal of Critical Psychology, Counselling and Psychotherapy, 12*(2), 93–107.

Mohtashemi, R., Stevens, J., Jackson, P. G., & Weatherhead, S. (2016). Psychiatrists' understanding and use of psychological formulation: A qualitative exploration. *British Journal of Psychiatry Bulletin, 40*, 212–216.

Mosher, L. R. (1999). Soteria and other alternatives to acute psychiatric hospitalization: A personal and professional review. *The Journal of Nervous and Mental Disease, 187*(3), 142–149.

Newnes, C. (2016). *Inscription, diagnosis, deception and the mental health industry: How Psy governs us all.* Springer.

Newnes, C., Holmes, G., & Dunn, C. (1999). *This is madness: A critical look at psychiatry and the future of mental health services.* PCCS Books.

Peacock-Brennan, S., & Harper, D. (2018). How do clinical psychology programmes approach classification and diagnosis? Report of a brief survey. *Clinical Psychology Forum, 302*, 14–18.

Peacock-Brennan, S., Harper, D., & Patel, M. (2018). Developing policy-relevant skills in clinical psychology training. *Clinical Psychology Forum, 301*, 9–14.

Pemberton, R., & Wainwright, T. (2014). The end of mental illness thinking? *International Journal of Clinical and Health Psychology, 14*(3), 216–220. https://doi.org/10.1016/j.ijchp.2014.05.003

Puras, D. (2017, April 6). World health day: Power imbalances and inequalities big part of poor mental health. *Health and Human Rights Journal.*

Randall, J., & Coles, S. (2018). Questioning diagnoses in clinical practice: A thematic analysis of clinical psychologists' accounts of working beyond diagnosis in the United Kingdom. *Journal of Mental Health*, 1–7. https://doi.org/10.1080/09638237.2018.1437599

RAWOrg. (2011). In *Mind.* Retrieved August 19, 2018, from https://www.mind.org.uk/media/273467/the-end-of-delivering-race-equality.pdf

Read, J. (2005). The Bio-bio-bio model of madness. *The Psychologist, 18*(10), 596.

Read, J., Bentall, R. P., & Fosse, R. (2009). Time to abandon the Bio-bio-bio model of psychosis: Exploring the epigenetic and psychological mechanisms by which adverse life events lead to psychotic symptoms. *Epidemiology and Psychiatric Sciences, 18*(4), 299–310.

Reynolds, V. (2010). *Doing justice as a path to sustainability in community work.* Unpublished thesis.

Robjant, K., Hassan, R., & Katona, C. (2009). Mental health implications of detaining asylum seekers: Systematic review. *The British Journal of Psychiatry, 194*, 306–312. https://doi.org/10.1192/bjp.bp.108.053223

Shafran, R., Cooper, Z., & Fairburn, C. G. (2002). Clinical perfectionism: A cognitive–behavioural analysis. *Behaviour Research and Therapy, 40*(7), 773–791. https://doi.org/10.1016/S0005-7967(01)00059-6

Shaw, C., & Proctor, G. (2004). Suzi's story. *Asylum (Special Edition: Women at the Margins), 14*(3), 11–13.

Singh, S. (2017). 'I chained him to protect him from the spirits.' What are the challenges for psychiatrists in India? *BJPsych International, 14*(4), 100–102.

Smail, D. J. (2005). *Power, interest and psychology: Elements of a social materialist understanding of distress*. PCCS Books.

Soteria Network. (n.d.). *Soteria network*. Retrieved April 3, 2019, from http://www.soterianetwork.org.uk/resources/files/Soteria-Network-Booklet.pdf

Sweeney, A., Clement, S., Filson, B., & Kennedy, A. (2016). Trauma-informed mental healthcare in the UK: What is it and how can we further its development? *Mental Health Review Journal, 21*(3), 174–192.

Timimi, S. (2014). No more psychiatric labels: Why formal psychiatric diagnostic systems should be abolished. *International Journal of Clinical and Health Psychology, 14*(3), 208–215. https://doi.org/10.1016/j.ijchp.2014.03.004

Valente, T. W. (2012). Network interventions. *Science, 337*(6090), 49–53. https://doi.org/10.1126/science.1217330

Vatel, B. (2015, October). Unmasking trauma-informed care. *Clinical Psychiatry News*. Retrieved January 29, 2018, from https://www.mdedge.com/psychiatry/article/103429/unmasking-trauma-informed-care

Wangari-Jones, P. (2016, April 5). *How to decolonise mental health services*. Retrieved August 19, 2018, from https://www.opendemocracy.net/transformation/penny-wangari-jones/how-to-decolonise-mental-health-services

Watson, J. (2017, January 3). Time to 'drop the disorder' [blog post]. Retrieved April 3, 2019, from https://www.madinamerica.com/2017/01/time-drop-disorder/

6

Supporting Activists and Progressive Social Movements

Tod Sloan and John Brush

People with training in the psychosocial disciplines have neglected an important sphere of engagement: activism within social movements. While psychotherapists, counselors, social workers, and academic psychologists can and do participate in grassroots organizing, direct actions, and the non-profit sector, this participation generally happens *in parallel* with professional work. Such activity is rarely either the focus of, or particularly informed by, the repertoire of theory and practice associated with the field of psychology. Moreover, we are not aware of any coherent body of writing on actionable aspects of psychology designed for activists themselves (with the exception, to some extent, of the literature on working with burnout).

Over the last fifteen years, the authors have collaborated in a variety of practices putting psychology (and those psychologically trained) to work for

(Tod Sloan died in December 2018 while in the final stages of editing this chapter. It is dedicated to his memory.)

T. Sloan (Deceased)

J. Brush (✉)
Tryon Life Community Farm, Portland, OR, USA
e-mail: brush@tryonfarm.org

C. Walker et al. (eds.), *The Palgrave Handbook of Innovative Community and Clinical Psychologies*, https://doi.org/10.1007/978-3-030-71190-0_6

social change. One effort has been organizing networks of professionals offering *free, relevant therapy* for those on the frontlines of political action—and though we don't discuss it further here, we encourage others to do likewise. In this chapter, we report on our more experimental set of principles and practices that we and others have used in direct engagement with groups, collectives, and organizations (rather than individuals) to adjust *how they function* to be both more therapeutic for participants, and more effective in their actions. May it serve as a tool for those bringing about social change!

By the term "activist," we are referring to a person consciously and regularly acting with the intention to change an aspect of society. Such activism may involve physical proximity and ongoing collaboration with others, or it may be purely Internet-based, which limits the kinds and intensities of interpersonal relation that are possible. Moreover, activists come in all forms, spanning diverse demographic categories. This chapter is rooted in our experience supporting those advocating peace and social/environmental justice, specifically through left-leaning grassroots political organizing in European settler societies in the Americas. Nevertheless, we hope that the following recommendations can be useful for many sorts of activist groups, collectives, and organizations, considered both in terms of their explicit goals and in terms of the implicit well-being of the group.

Psychology *for* Activists

There is already, of course, an ample literature in social psychology that bears on understanding social issues, and attitude and behavior change. Important strands of this work are represented in the three-volume *Praeger Handbook of Psychology and Social Justice* (Johnson & Friedman, 2014). These works *analyze the problems* and describe professional tools for working with *special populations* most impacted by them. It is striking, however, that researchers rarely state the implications of their analyses: that we need to change the fundamental social structures that reproduce oppression. If they did, there would be a richer opportunity for psychological methods to inform the challenge of *how* to most effectively engage such change. As is, those in the psychological professions that *do* engage in political work do so largely without the benefit of directly relevant research in their field.

The disconnect is symbolized neatly, for example, by the existence in the USA of two separate organizations: the research-oriented Society for the Psychological Study of Social Issues (Division 9 of the American Psychological Association [APA]) and the action-oriented Psychologists for Social

Responsibility (see www.psysr.org). This division between science and practice merely reflects the longstanding divide between academic work and action in the "real world," despite (laudable) recent attempts to establish university-community partnerships and "engaged scholarship."

Why is it so hard to find a psychology *for* activists and their groups? In part, this is due to the myth of "scientific neutrality" historically adopted by professional psychology, which only vaguely refers to social betterment as one of its goals as a profession (Fox et al., 2009). It is also due to the emphasis most psychological theory and practice places on the individual level of behavior and experience. These two traits of the field have been repeatedly indicted by critical psychology as serving an *ideological* function—naturalizing and maintaining an unjust status quo by hiding the societal causes of injustice and personal suffering (cf. Fox et al., 2009; Parker, 2015; Sloan, 2000; Teo, 2014).

Building on their critique of scientistic and individualistic psychologies, critical psychologists and their allies have been developing engaged community-based psychologies for liberation and critical therapeutics (Parker, 2007; Watkins & Shulman, 2008; Loewenthal, 2015), to which this chapter contributes. Also useful for our purposes is a small body of literature on the psychology *of* activists, militants, revolutionaries, and transformational leaders (e.g., Anderson, 2009; Dobles & Zúñiga, 2005; Keniston, 1970; Lasswell, 1960; Moane, 2010). Much of this work can inform us, at least indirectly, about the factors that raise awareness, engage, and sustain activists, as well as about common obstacles that plague activists and their groups. However, much still needs to be done to forge links between the subdisciplines of psychology and the realms of action connected to progressive and radical social movements.

Social Movements

In this chapter, we emphasize working with social movements rather than with political parties or non-governmental organizations. If all levels of work are important, as Moyer's (2001) model of the stages and cycles of social movements suggests, why focus on the phase of change rooted in widespread, grassroots, nonprofessionalized "activism"? First, many existing approaches to organizational psychology or other fields can be adapted to formal structures and motivational mechanisms typical of parties and NGOs. They already are more visible to psychologists and have more resources to leverage. Second, we make the assessment that the most important social changes to come will originate in social movements that are nascent today, or tomorrow. Drawing inspiration from the movements to end slavery, for women's suffrage, for decolonization of the Global South, for gay rights, against corporate globalization, and to address climate change, we see the vitality and dynamism of bottom-up organizing as a key element in making deep change, and a level where the energies of the psychosocial professions are especially needed (Giugni et al., 1999).

Typical Challenges Activists Face

When North American activists were asked about their challenges (Sloan, 2013), the themes that emerged reflected two clusters: patterns of group dynamics and individual feelings.

Patterns of Group Dynamics

- Reproduction of structural oppression in and between activist groups: patriarchy, racism, homophobia, ageism, and so on.
- Privileging of identity political silos over intergroup solidarity and alliance-building.
- Lack of unity about the nature of the problem and the outcomes to pursue, leading to divisive debates over strategy and tactics, such as how radical a group's actions should be.
- Distracting interpersonal, subcultural, and procedural issues in groups and committees that exhaust participants.
- Difficulty maintaining a balance of work, organizing, and personal life, often leading to exhaustion and burnout.

Feelings

- **Feelings** associated with activism are often **intense** and **unpleasant**: fear, anxiety, passions, despair.
- Conversely, too much intellectualizing leading to a disconnect from passion and action.
- Overwhelm by the magnitude of the task, and frustration about slow progress and setbacks, leading to pessimism and paralysis.
- Feelings that much of their work is unseen and unappreciated.
- Sense of isolation from friends and family who do not understand their passion.

- Past traumatic experiences triggered by current actions and interactions, disrupting individual and group effectiveness.

There are additional, perhaps more extreme, challenges faced by many activists: complete ostracism by family; physical harm during protests; arrest and police maltreatment; loss of livelihood; long-term imprisonment; and disappearance, torture, and death by government or paramilitary. But even when activists do not face these heightened responses, most causes are daunting and progress is slow. As noted above, pessimism and despair can be rampant. This is an obvious place where psychological understandings and practices are relevant.

Although the practices of activists and their groups vary, activism in general can be seen as a form of "community of practice" (Lave & Wenger, 1991). For example, within a subculture of activism there are established ways of training new members, running meetings, making decisions, dealing with conflict or with "difficult people," planning for actions, and even socializing. In the next section, we look at principles and practices that can support activist groups to be at once more effective and enjoyable.

Framework: A Social Ecology of Activist Groups

A few years ago, we worked with a dozen US activists from different sectors and backgrounds who met as a collective, the Cascadia Center for Social Ecology, to develop training workshops for new activists during the Occupy movement in Portland, Oregon, USA. (Similar efforts can be found in many regions, e.g., the New Economy Organisers Movement Building Training in the UK and Training for Change in the USA.) In our workshops, we distilled principles and practices we had seen foster group effectiveness as well as participant retention and well-being. We understand that effectiveness and group well-being may not be among the primary goals of activists in some regions of the world, but we argue that good relations with comrades can be essential to momentum and solidarity.

The following framework and suggestions for practice are offered here as a starting point for thinking about the psychosocial dimensions of activism, where people with psychological training might make a special contribution. How psychosocial training or insight is shared with groups may range widely depending on the situation. Sometimes distrust of "professionalization," or other dynamics, may make explicit interventions rare and unobtrusive. Other times, there may be an opportunity to directly suggest shifts to the group's practices for psychosocial reasons. Indeed, in some cases trusted participants (or invited outsiders) may conduct workshops, organize dialogues, or lead exercises that strengthen the group on psychosocial dimensions.

In all such engagements, our fundamental principle is to shift our therapeutic attention away from a primary focus either on isolated individuals or on large-scale societal forces. Rather, we emphasize the *ecology of the small activist group*, be it a collective, an affinity group, a temporary project, a committee or chapter of a larger organization, or an intentional community.

Small groups are important for a variety of reasons:

- Individuals can relatively easily change them, and be changed by them, in a dynamic positive feedback cycle. For example, one or a few people can move the group to pursue their mission in ways that also support individual healing and development for their members, as well as engaging complicated intragroup processes focused on anti-oppression and decolonization (challenging white privilege, racism, patriarchy, etc.).
- Agile groups can more quickly adopt new practices that address common problems (such as those suggested below). Change can be faster because fewer people are involved, agreement can be easier to reach, and everyone can know each other and build trust directly. Furthermore, when multiple small groups are working on an issue or in a role, even major change involves less risk for the larger movement.
- Effective small groups can leverage their particular strengths in collaborating with other groups and making use of intergroup differences wisely. Such networks can realign these linkages in response to changing circumstances more rapidly than large organizations can either evolve or be superseded.

When this perspective on the small group informs our work, we can better support activists in persevering, enjoying, learning, and creating connection and community—at the same time as they are being effective in their immediate political aims. In our experience, as well as that of others (e.g., Starhawk, 2011), these outcomes can be attained by attending to matters at several different levels. One of the handouts we developed in the Cascadia Center summarizes practical suggestions for small groups functioning according to such levels, listed below. These are not a recipe for the perfect group; rather, they give a sense of the sorts of practices that groups are experimenting with and that might be encouraged by those with psychosocial training.

Individual Level of Participation in Activist Groups

- The group offers opportunities for members to **reflect with others** to develop a clear **personal mission**, vision, and values to support and direct their work.
- Meetings allow for regular processing with trusted others of the **emotional dimensions** of the work and the issues being addressed (frustration, despair, overwhelm, anger, grief, etc.).
- Members continue to learn because they are invited to **study together** and discuss puzzling aspects of the issues at hand.
- Ample time is devoted to **socializing** (share food, play music, etc.) both with others who share their values and with people who are not fellow travelers.
- **Embodiment** is fully acknowledged in the group's activities by taking time for creativity, exercise, experiencing the rest of nature, and slowing down together.
- Members have regular chances to examine **personal skills** and interests and consider how they may **dovetail with the group'**s current priorities and overall strategy (Rettig, 2006).

Group/Organizational Level

- The organization has **clear and wise processes** for holding its members **accountable** for unacceptable actions (e.g., racist speech, sexual assault, etc.).
- Meetings are **well facilitated** to ensure that **everyone** is able to contribute and **participate** in deliberation and decision-making (Bens, 2005).
- The group or organization has a **basic strategy** and plan that all members understand and have **opportunities to revise** in light of experience.
- Strategic goals are connected to **shared understandings** and expectations of member **commitment** and **behavior**.
- The group encourages **creative thinking**, especially by newcomers, as part of its planning and actions.
- The group integrates **non-verbal and embodied** modes of communication into its work—arts, dance, spirituality according to the wishes of members.
- The organization's **culture** supports **openness**, **trust**, acceptance of **diverse** perspectives.

Cultural/Societal/Political/Economic and Strategic Levels

- The group's internal and external actions **prefigure** the social arrangements they desire.
- Many **allied or linked groups** are also working actively to cultivate living alternatives to the dominant practices that the group is attempting to adjust or abolish.
- The group acts in ways appropriate to its **contexts** within larger struggles. It actively **cultivates direct links** with other groups as much as possible, and beyond that, maintains the sense that it is **part of a vast movement** of movements (Dixon, 2014; Derber, 2017).
- The group tries to **build bridges** with groups it does not usually work with in order to **find common ground** around shared goals (Smucker, 2017).
- Leaders directly represent group members in these relationships through internal **deep democracy** and regular reviews of vision, goals, and strategy.

Imagine: Psychosocial Understandings in Practice

What can all this mean for an activist who also happens to be psychology student, counselor, therapist, academic psychologist, community psychologist, social worker, or related professional? How can psychological insights into motivation, affect, identity, group dynamics, attitudes, personality, and all the other familiar topics in the field contribute to the functioning of activist groups?

Imagine you have been a member of an activist group or committee for a couple of months. Despite your role as a general member, your psychology "radar" has often been activated by the group or individual members. Imagine you have wanted to intervene directly given your observations and your psychosocial understandings, but this is not your role in the group (as you have not been appointed as "vibes-watcher"). You decide it would probably not go over well if you intervene explicitly, so you continue to observe and reflect. Over time, as a responsible member of the group, you find yourself bringing psychological understanding to bear on the sorts of issues listed below. You do this in an effort to help make the work of your group more effective and/or enjoyable. You recognize that these understandings are not the sole property of people trained in psychology, but that those with such training may be more likely to perceive problems and have insights or skills for addressing them.

The following are problems you may encounter and approaches you may consider.

Groupthink

Your observation: Your group often makes decisions without sufficient consideration of pros and cons or related concerns after a persuasive person argues for a certain course of action.

Possible approach: Social psychologists recommend various remedies for this foreclosed decision-making, including having someone play the devil's advocate. You may encourage your group to explicitly seek dissenting voices, especially for important decisions, and build in more time (multiple meetings, periods of silence) to ensure space for them to arise. Facilitated consensus decision-making may provide tools to ensure full participation and buy-in—various established procedures fit the needs of different sizes and types of groups (Bressen, 2019; Butler & Rothstein, 1987; Starhawk, 2011).

Group Bogged Down in Process Issues

Your observation: Your group gets stuck in long discussions about how they are going to go about their work. These may center on how decisions will be made, how authority/leadership will be organized, how the group mission should be worded, what gets on the agenda, and so on. These matters can be very important and necessary, but at some point, these deliberations can interfere in actually getting to "the work."

Possible approach: It is important to strive for a balance of process and action, because unresolved process level issues can seriously interfere with the success of the work. This points to the possibility of designating a psychologically minded facilitator who understands the agenda and can help the group attend to process issues effectively without stalling the work. Process issues tend to come up when unconscious group dynamics are active. These issues could reflect questions such as "Do we really trust each other enough to go ahead with this bold action?" or "Is the leader on a power trip that we need to interrupt?" Obviously, unconscious dynamics cannot be addressed in the way they might in a group therapy setting. However, simple interventions such as creating and periodically revisiting group expectations and norms, making time for personal check-ins at the beginning of meetings, taking a break when things get tense and members are tired, checking in with group about members' feelings, and reviewing the group's purpose can help dissipate anxieties. Vanucci and Singer (2010) offer interesting case studies of common group dynamics in non-hierarchical activist collectives.

Intellectualizing and Divisive Debates over Minor Issues

Your observation: Progressives and leftists are famous for seemingly endless debates about tactics and strategy. This is not necessarily a bad thing as it can develop a better analysis of challenges and bring about better results, but sometimes gets in the way of basic work.

Possible approach: When do activists tend to intellectualize and argue incessantly—and feel upset about it? This often happens when sufficient relationship-building has not occurred. Group members may sense differences and magnify them in debates, forgetting their common purpose. Anxiety or fear about other members, about the direction the group may take, about differences in opinions about strategy, disconnection from the issue or the community affected by the issue, subconscious biases, and other dynamics can appear in debates that seem to go on without resolution. With this dynamic, it can be helpful to facilitate group processes that encourage members to speak more personally with each other about hopes and worries to get at the root of the disagreements. Alternatively, sometimes it's helpful to take a break to relax and get perspective.

Tensions About How Meeting Time Is Used

Your observation: Group members express frustration with the meetings, attendance at meetings dissipates, or members report meetings are not addressing the most important issues.

Possible approaches: It is helpful for members to sense that they have a say in what happens at meetings. To address this, many groups have a process for collectively creating the agenda. Psychologically trained facilitators can help this process and observe group interactions to make sure members feel that appropriate emphasis is given to the most important items as well as help the negotiation process when there are discrepancies between priorities.

Racist, Sexist, Homophobic, Ageist, or Ableist Remarks and Actions

Your observation: Often, members of dominant cultural groups have not done the work to be aware of their privilege or their oppressive attitudes and behaviors. This makes the group less welcoming for members of frontline communities and interferes with healthy links of solidarity between your group and others.

Possible approaches: Require members to attend anti-oppression trainings (Crass, 2013). At the beginning of each meeting, repeat the agreement that all will work to reduce microaggressions, and share constructive ways to deal with them seriously when they occur, without becoming disrupted. Often this is just a matter of acknowledging a microaggression, apologizing and moving on. As needed, set aside specific time later to address further. (Resources for anti-oppression training can be found at https://organizingforpower.org/anti-oppression-resources-exercises/.)

Frequent "Calling Out" of Members for Oppressive Behaviors

Your observation: Well-meaning attempts to interrupt oppressive behaviors in the group can lead to a "call-out culture" in which quickly ostracizing scapegoats severs relationships, breaks group trust, and limits real transformation.

Possible approaches: Interrupting oppression is important. But sometimes "calling out" groups and individuals is not the most effective way of doing it. "Call outs" can be a tool for people who are insecure about their own privilege to prove themselves, or call attention to someone else to cover their own mistakes. When more nuanced tools aren't available, it can be a go-to for people triggered over and over by microaggressions, sometimes unfairly putting the burden on them. An alternate approach, especially useful inside a group where people have long-term relationships, is "call-in culture" in which trust and care are the foundation for calling attention to behavior that needs to change, along with ongoing support for change (Trần, 2013).

Disruptive Behavior

Your observation: Someone in the group frequently interrupts, sidetracks, blocks, gets upset, acts out, or otherwise interferes with the functioning of the group.

Possible approaches: This is a tricky one because the reason for the disruptive behavior is often not clear. Is it an appropriate reaction to group processes? Or is the behavior a function of the individual? Careful observation of group dynamics, expectations, and other points described in this section can allow for exploration of the relationship between the group functioning and individual member's behavior.

If the situation suggests individual issues, such as neurodivergence or other mental health needs, there may be a need for a different approach. Because the group is not a clinical setting, even those with professional training are not in a position to diagnose and treat. Instead, it may be helpful to facilitate the group in practicing compassion while acknowledging the necessity of getting the group's work done and identifying external resources that may better support the member's needs. Depending on the size and relationships within the group, you might ask to pause and address the relational and task issues that have become disrupted. Further, it may be helpful to facilitate a process to make explicit the challenges the group is having as well as revisit shared agreements and expectations. Perhaps the disruptive person feels excluded and simply needs an extra chance to feel heard or feels frustrated because they are unhappy with the way other members receive their ideas. In such cases, there may be simple solutions.

Revisiting shared goals and practices, as well as re-establishing agreements, can help re-calibrate the group. Staying on track with shared goals may eventually require interrupting the member. If, after group processing, the behavior continues to disrupt progress in the group, one-on-one intervention may be helpful. If the disrupting is done intentionally or repeatedly, it may be necessary to invite the person to a separate conversation to establish parameters for future participation, or to engage agreed protocols for removing a member (see Starhawk, 2011).

New Group Members Have Trouble Understanding What's Going On

Your observation: Activist groups are often so eager to move ahead with their work that they do not take the time to orient or explain complexities to new members. The new members may feel lost, find it hard to engage, and sometimes drift away.

Possible approach: Movements need to bring in new members who can share insights, energy, and new approaches. There are a number of ways to effectively integrate them. Leaders in the group can hold orientation sessions, both to educate about the group and to get to know new members, learn about skills they may bring, and let them know they're appreciated. Further, the group can discuss how they will welcome new members, and periodically revisit group goals and norms, either to integrate the ideas of new members or clarify existing rationales.

These scenarios are intended to stimulate thinking about how people with psychological training can help group function. Underlying these suggestions is a focus on the emotional, relational, often invisible currents beneath the group's surface, oft neglected by groups that focus primarily on tasks and action. Attending to the whole being of activists—physical, artistic, spiritual—can enliven meetings and retain participants. As a reminder of this theme, we suggest beginning holistically: reading a poem, doing art together, allowing time for silence (to accommodate different forms of spirituality), or singing a song.

Counseling, Therapy, and Support Groups

In addition to encouraging healthier groups, therapists and counselors can support activists directly in individual or group counseling or therapy. While it is rare for individuals to seek therapy to work on their activism per se, the need for spaces to address burnout, despair, pessimism, and trauma is increasingly recognized. There are a number of structured ways this may happen beyond self-referred individual psychotherapy or counseling. Some examples include: self-care groups designed for activists, process groups focused on specific social justice issues, counseling first aid teams during social action events, as well as wilderness experiences like those designed by eco-psychologist Bill Plotkin (2013), or deep emotional work in response to ecological destruction like Joanna Macy's *Work that Reconnects* (see Macy & Brown, 2014).

Hope and despair can be significant challenges in connection with activism. Fortunately, an extensive literature exists on the psychology of these experiences, including tools useful for activists (e.g., Doetsch-Kidder, 2012; Hoggett & Randall, 2016; Macy & Johnstone, 2012; Solnit, 2016; Zimmerman & Quiroz, 2016). Some recommendations include expressing and working through feelings of grief and despair in dialogue with others;

keeping a generational historical perspective on social change, since multiple setbacks are typical in processes that can last decades; and attending to multiple dimensions of our being as we struggle—the spiritual, the aesthetic, the interpersonal, the intergenerational, and so on.

In addition to books and Internet resources providing encouragement and insight, some communities offer opportunities for in-person events, like structured group workshops on hope and despair, often organized and conducted by people with counseling training. Another very promising reframing of psychosocial work in connection with social movements is Watkins' (2015) careful analyses of the ethics of "psychosocial accompaniment." Watkins describes various ways of witnessing, accompanying, and supporting those who suffer, all of which are relevant to social movements that confront injustice.

Changing the (Life)World: A Paradigm Shift

Much of the above is fairly straightforward and perhaps even obvious to those with some experience in grassroots activism. Hopefully, this invites people with psychosocial understandings to get involved. Now, we take the next step and look at ways psychological perspectives may inform and respond to a broader reconfiguration of activism.

Activists are continuously searching for more effective ways of bringing about desired changes. This is happening especially now, in the face of discouragement, as the globalization of capitalist economic relations continues, wars drag on for decades producing ongoing refugee crises, racism is reignited in many "liberal" societies, and at least some effects of climate emergency are now irreversible. Many committed activists feel they have failed and are doing a great deal of soul searching about what activism means and how it can achieve its goals.

To us, it seems a redefinition of activism may be emerging. Perhaps what we've called "activism" points further than what we do to bring about change in our spare time after paid work, family, friends, leisure, and community involvement. Beyond changing individual lifestyle and consumer habits (although this is a first step we all can do), perhaps it involves deeper questions of *who we are,* and who we are *to become*, if we are to live ethically. Radical social change is not the change of just ourselves, and it is not the change of social systems "out there," outside ourselves. It is something else, requiring participation in a collective social being between and beyond "self and society."

We have focused on small groups in this chapter, in part because imagining an ecosystem of such groups is a way to envision this social being as capable of creating the change we need. Systems—ecosystems, family systems, personality systems—can change rapidly and profoundly not by demolishing what exists and starting over, but by reconfiguring the parts into a new pattern. Perhaps small groups can be some of the parts that make new patterns if we help them function effectively. Through this intermediate scale, we may cultivate great personal realignments linked with broader social-scale shifts in shared life projects, a process in which individual and community *being* and *becoming* are transformed profoundly through inspiration, insight, and love.

In this final section, we suggest several aspects of this emergence for which existing fields of research related to psychology may be repurposed for radical ends. It will take the edgy creativity of all of us to expand to the scale of the challenges we face; perhaps these suggest ways for the psychologically trained to offer humane visions for a living future.

Decoloniality

Decolonial approaches remind us that most oppression in the world today is rooted in (historical and ongoing) violent conquest by a global empire-complex with roots in Europe (Mignolo, 2008). This challenges us to work not only to redistribute power and resources within a continuing (colonizing) social body, but for decolonialization (Bacchetta et al., 2019), decomposing the empire and ending the "white man's world" (Schwarz, 2011). As we see it, this entails:

- Interrupting ongoing processes of assimilating partially colonized peoples;
- Supporting movements to restore political-economic and psychosocial autonomy among partially colonized peoples; and
- Seeking formation of new peoples (ethnogenesis) from among those fully assimilated by the empire, to contest it from within its core demographics, becoming responsible accomplices of those fighting to remain relatively free of it.

These political challenges can seem unfamiliar. It can be hard to see beyond the horizon of the colonizing empire, the psychosocial fabric we've been born into. It's common to imagine colonization (or its euphemism, modernization) as a one-way street. To assume that once begun, it leads inevitably to assimilation, that only fighting for "rights" within the "real" power structure is worthwhile; that indigenous or "nationalist" struggles are merely local and secondary. And to see "ethnogenesis" as a countercultural pipedream to be recuperated by advertising execs. We need to build the psychological lenses to see beyond these narrow confines.

To this end, insights from the intersection between history, anthropology, and psychology may help. The range of human behaviors and social structures is immense, the emergence of new peoples through amalgamation or splitting is quite common and these movements have not been one-way. Indeed, it may be that one of the most common reasons for ethnogenesis is the political imperative to resist or escape oppressive states. For example, Scott (2009) shares a rich ethnographic and historical argument describing the hill peoples of Southeast Asia and elsewhere. (For a brief review, including references to other scholars of premodern examples that may inform post-postmodern strategies, see Friedman, 2010.)

In that context, what is it like to be a human person acted on by forces of colonial assimilation, yet also striving decolonially? What are the psychosocial tools that may help us resist the one and support the other? For example, what ties us emotionally to one mode of political economy, and makes us fearful of another, even if it is "objectively" in our interests? What are ways that spirituality and ritual practices can galvanize courage to help us make such hard changes, to link us to each other in ways that are new to us?

Perhaps a first step is to recognize that what social scientists ambivalently call "cultures," or "peoples," or "nations" are complex collective systems reproduced through all parts of us—psychology, politics, spirituality, economics, kinship—to result in profoundly different ways of being human. Western liberalism tends to implicitly universalize one version of human individualism, obscuring the structural integrity of other ways of being people and peoples—especially those disrupted by colonization. In this regard, the academy can be an echo chamber. A tool for growing beyond these blinkered biases is cultural translation written by indigenous people who know clearly who they are (Wahpimaskwasis, 2008).

Understanding that reproducing a lifeworld involves the whole of a social system, we can see why attempts to cure the ills of assimilation often fail when addressing economics alone, childhood formation alone, trauma alone, electoral politics alone. Since the cultural system is self-regulating and complex, all aspects need to be engaged together, often through a conscious political project. (For an exploration of the nuanced example of the Métis, see Anderson, 2014. For a review focusing on the value of such scholarship from an "insider," see Sawchuk, 2015.)

Much the same can be said of most attempts to create "new culture" by radical activists—too often, only a small subset of cultural aspects are addressed, making it just a "subculture." To move toward anticolonial ethnogenesis requires a much more integrated approach. An example that points in this direction is that of the "hoopwalkers" of western N. America—who are attempting to create new lifeways rooted in cycles of tending wild gardens, gaining most of their physical and psychosocial needs in the process (Saine, 2013). It also illustrates how such work is fraught with the risk of carrying settler baggage when insufficiently grounded in tangible relations of solidarity with decolonizing indigenous peoples (Seraphin, 2016).

Indeed, this is also true for psychology professionals. There is a great deal of work to do, whether supporting communities healing from generational traumas, confronting the mental health field to make radically more space for indigenous and decolonial worldviews and therapies, or accompanying small activist groups as they transform the social and psychic patterns of activism itself as part of decolonializing the revolution. But to do so effectively, such professionals must be in ongoing, deep interrogation of their own participation in colonization. Uncritical psychology, as an academic discipline and through its related professions, selects for assimilated people and reinforces coloniality. Culture change starts at home.

Conclusion: A Call for Therapeutic Contagion

At this tumultuous moment, what activists, liberation psychologists, and ultimately all humans are faced with, is a profound remaking of the fabric of the empire's human being. Activists moving beyond simply opposing the most recent outrage must learn to design new patterns of material and social existence, because *everything has to change* (Escobar, 2018). Psychologists and social workers willing to look beyond the familiar boundaries of the profession may be particularly well placed to support willing activist groups. Such groups, woven through relationships, may become the very body of transformative new social beings. For them, their process—how they help people work together, feel differently, and imagine change—must become at least as important as any short-term product. Indeed, in the words of a profoundly influential Italian activist:

> In the days to come, politics and therapy will be one and the same. The people will feel hopeless and depressed and panicked, because they can't deal with the post-growth economy and they will miss our dissolving modern identity. Our

cultural task will be to attend to these people and to take care of their trauma showing them the way to pursue the happy adaptation at hand. Our task will be the creation of social zones of human resistance, zones of therapeutic contagion. (Berardi, 2009, p. 220)

References

Anderson, A. (2009). On being an activist. *Journal for Social Action in Counseling and Psychology, 2*(1), 44–50.

Anderson, C. (2014). *'Métis': Race, recognition, and the struggle for indigenous peoplehood.* University of British Columbia Press.

Bacchetta, P., Maira, S., & Winant, H. (Eds.). (2019). *Global raciality: Empire, postcoloniality, decoloniality.* Routledge, Taylor & Francis Group.

Bens, I. (2005). *Facilitating with ease.* Jossey-Bass.

Berardi, F. 'Bifo'. (2009). *The soul at work: From alienation to autonomy.* Los Angeles: Semiotext(e). Retrieved from https://libcom.org/files/Franco%20"Bifo"%20Berardi%20-%20The%20Soul%20at%20Work%20From%20Alienation%20to%20Autonomy.pdf

Bressen, T. (2019). Tree Bressen's Group Facilitation Site. Retrieved from https://treegroup.info/

Butler, C. T., & Rothstein, A. (1987). *On conflict and consensus: A handbook on formal consensus decision making.* Portland, ME: Food Not Bombs Publishing. Retrieved from https://theanarchistlibrary.org/library/c-t-butler-and-amy-rothstein-on-conflict-and-consensus-a-handbook-on-formal-consensus-decisionm

Crass, C. (2013). *Toward collective liberation: Anti-racist organizing, feminist praxis, and movement building strategy.* PM Press.

Derber, C. (2017). *Welcome to the revolution: Universalizing resistance for social justice and democracy in perilous times.* Routledge.

Dixon, C. (2014). *Another politics: Talking across today's transformative movements.* University of California Press.

Dobles, I., & Zúñiga, V. (2005). *Militantes: La vivencia de lo político en la segunda ola del Marxismo en Costa Rica.* University of Costa Rica Press.

Doetsch-Kidder, S. (2012). *Social change and intersectional activism: The spirit of social movement.* Palgrave Macmillan.

Escobar, A. (2018). *Designs for the pluriverse: Radical interdependence, autonomy, and the making of worlds.* Duke University Press.

Fox, D., Prilleltensky, I., & Austin, S. (Eds.). (2009). *Critical psychology: An introduction* (2nd ed.). Sage.

Friedman, P. K. (2010, November 9). *Ethnogenesis: A radical constructionist case.* Retrieved from https://savageminds.org/2010/11/09/ethnogenesis-a-radical-constructionist-case/

Giugni, M., McAdam, D., & Tilly, C. (1999). *How social movements matter.* University of Minnesota Press.

Hoggett, P., & Randall, R. (2016). Sustainable activism: Managing hope and despair in social movements. Retrieved from https://www.opendemocracy.net/transformation/paul-hoggett-rosemary-randall/sustainable-activism-managing-hope-and-despair-in-socia

Johnson, C. & Friedman, H. (eds.). (2014). *The Praeger handbook of social justice and psychology.* 3 vols. Santa Barbara, CA: Praeger.

Keniston, K. (1970). Student activism, moral development, and morality. *American Journal of Orthopsychiatry, 40*(4), 577–592. https://doi.org/10.1111/j.1939-0025.1970.tb00716.x

Lasswell, H. D. (1960). *Psychopathology and politics.* Viking Press.

Lave, J., & Wenger, E. (1991). *Situated learning.* Cambridge University Press.

Loewenthal, D. (Ed.). (2015). *Critical psychotherapy, psychoanalysis, and counselling: Implications for practice.* Palgrave.

Macy, J., & Brown, M. Y. (2014). *Coming back to life.* New Society.

Macy, J., & Johnstone, C. (2012). *Active hope.* New World Library.

Mignolo, W. (2008). *I am where I think: Globalization and the de-colonial option.* Duke University Press.

Moane, G. (2010). Sociopolitical development and political activism: Synergies between feminist and liberation psychology. *Psychology of Women Quarterly, 34*, 521–529.

Moyer, B. (2001). *Doing democracy.* New Society.

Parker, I. (2007). *Revolution in psychology: Alienation to emancipation.* Pluto.

Parker, I. (Ed.). (2015). *Handbook of critical psychology.* Routledge Press.

Plotkin, B. (2013). *Wild mind: A field guide to the human psyche.* New World Library. http://animas.org

Rettig, H. (2006). *The lifelong activist.* Lantern Press.

Saine, S. J. (2013). *Toward a theory of rewilding psychology.* Gaia University. Retrieved from http://portfolios.gaiauniversity.org/view/view.php?t=0jpWnoKPxtmUYJ6FOQXf

Sawchuk, J. (2015). 'Métis': Race, recognition, and the struggle for indigenous peoplehood. *Labour/Le Travail* 76, 231–233. The Canadian Committee on Labour History.

Schwarz, B. (2011). *Memories of empire, volume 1: A white man's world.* Oxford University Press.

Scott, J. C. (2009). *The art of not being governed: An anarchist history of upland Southeast Asia.* Yale University Press.

Seraphin, B. (2016). Rewilding, 'the hoop,' and settler apocalypse. *The Trumpeter, 32*(2), 126–146. https://doi.org/10.7202/1042989ar

Sloan, T. (Ed.). (2000). *Critical psychology: Voices for change*. Macmillan Press.
Sloan, T. S. (2013). Activist support as a form of critical psychology praxis. *Annual Review of Critical Psychology, 10*, 952–963.
Smucker, J. (2017). *Hegemony how-to: A roadmap for radicals*. AK Press.
Solnit, R. (2016). *Hope in the dark*. Haymarket.
Starhawk. (2011). *The empowerment manual: A guide for collaborative groups*. New Society.
Teo, T. (Ed.). (2014). *Encyclopedia of critical psychology*. Springer-Verlag.
Trần, N. L. (2013, December 18). Calling IN: A less disposable way of holding each other accountable. *Black Girl Dangerous*. Retrieved January 1, 2014, from http://www.blackgirldangerous.org/2013/12/calling-less-disposable-way-holding-accountable/
Vanucci, D., & Singer, R. (2010). *Come hell or high water: A handbook on collective process gone awry*. AK Press.
Wahpimaskwasis Little White Bear/Makokis, J (2008). Nehiyaw iskwew kiskinowâtasinahikewina—paminisowin namôya tipeyimisowin: Learning self determination through the Sacred. *Canadian Woman Studies = Les Cahiers de la Femme, 26*(3, 4), 39–51.
Watkins, M. (2015). Psychosocial accompaniment. *Journal of Social and Political Psychology, 3*(1), 324–341. https://doi.org/10.5964/jspp.v3i1.103
Watkins, M., & Shulman, H. (2008). *Toward psychologies of liberation*. Palgrave.
Zimmerman, K., & Quiroz, J. (2016). Love with power: Practicing transformation for social justice. Oakland, CA: Movement Strategy Center. Retrieved from https://movementstrategy.org/b/wp-content/uploads/2016/07/MSC-Love_With_Power.pdf

7

Statactivism and Critical Community Psychology: Using Statistical Activism to Resist Injustice in the NHS and Higher Education

Carl Walker and Anna Zoli

Introduction

Social justice is a complex and largely elusive concept when analysed from a theoretical perspective. Nonetheless, a good deal of research has been generated by scholars making claims to social justice activities. In the discipline of critical community psychology, social justice has been defined by Kagan et al. (2011) as the possibility for people to live in peace and freedom, and to receive a fair share of collective resources. Moreover, social justice has been articulated as one of the values driving the discipline, together with community and stewardship.

In the UK in 2021, we are witnessing a mobilisation of the tactics of accumulation through the aggressive corporate takeover of key public services and such accumulation is routinely legitimated by questionable practices of evidence collection and public consultation (Fine, 2016). What form social justice should take against the backdrop of the recent hollowing out and colonising of public institutions, often supported by peculiarly neoliberal processes of consultation, participation, and user empowerment, is not straightforward. Invoking practices of stewardship oriented towards a version of social justice in a context marked by persistent, often hidden, circuits of dispossession is challenging, and possibly the reason why so much critical community

C. Walker (✉) • A. Zoli
School of Applied Social Science, University of Brighton, Brighton, UK
e-mail: c.j.walker@brighton.ac.uk; a.zoli@brighton.ac.uk

C. Walker et al. (eds.), *The Palgrave Handbook of Innovative Community and Clinical Psychologies*, https://doi.org/10.1007/978-3-030-71190-0_7

psychology work has been critiqued as accommodationist and politically conservative (Fryer & Fox, 2015).

We are currently confronted with novel and inordinately complex configurations of how power operates, penetrates, and legitimises the conditions for the disposability of previously valued public services (Fine, 2016), and this is no more obvious than in the English National Health Service (NHS) and Higher Education (HE). In this piece of work, we draw on two case studies in these domains where we consider a form of critical community psychology praxis designed to expose and ultimately disrupt some of the hidden relays of dispossession mandated by recent health and HE policy and practice.

In our experience of attempting to tackle social inequalities with the tools of critical community psychology, we often find ourselves void of effective means to counter attack the overwhelming dominion of numbers and statistics (Zellini, 2018) that are problematically mobilised to justify what we consider to be little more than state-sponsored economic violence masquerading as public service modernisation. Power (2000) describes how New Performance Management techniques have contributed to an audit 'explosion' across the public services with untested and uncritically implemented regulating systems applied to discipline and control doctors, teachers, university lecturers and other professionals. This flood of social measures that Power describes are quantifiable bureaucratic audits that have been justified as the necessary tools to ensure accountability, transparency, and efficiency (Espeland & Saunder, 2007).

However, while absorbing specific accountability recipes may be crucial for political and managerialist regimes to legitimise behaviour, they do not necessarily bear positively on either standards or democratic answerability (Gulbrandsen, 2008). Instead, audit cultures tend to construct a vocabulary of knowledge that legitimises state and managerial power at the expense of the many professionals working in, and service users who use, public services (Craig et al., 2014).

Montero (2009) suggests that the mode of community and critical psychologies developed in many countries have openly manifested social transformation as their ultimate goal. However, what is abundantly unclear is the way in which that goal is to be obtained in so far as there are few methods explicitly formulated with that task in mind. In this chapter, we introduce statactivism as a potential critical community psychology tool, applied to two projects co-ordinated by Brighton scholars and students—the Brighton Citizens' Health Services Surveys (BCHSSs) in the domain of healthcare provision and the National Senior Management Survey (SMS) in the domain of higher education.

Statistical Activism

Statactivism is a consolidated movement seeking to challenge the dominion of quantification set by neoliberal hegemonic discourses and realities that they privilege (Bruno et al., 2014). Quantification is not a neutral tool to enhance efficiency, rather it is a force that creates new streams of power; shapes social and political action; and informs and transforms institutional, collective, and community practices (Didier, 2018). The proponents of statactivism claim that it contrasts the blind faith in the truth of numbers by exposing the intrinsic paradoxes, the unethical behaviours, and controversial consequences of adopting a doctrine of measurement in the provision of essential services, such as security (Didier, 2018), healthcare (Zoli, 2017), and higher education (Walker et al., 2019).

Statactivism has been articulated as a militant use of figures (Baudot, 2014) whereby previous representations of reality can be challenged and contested (Bruno et al., 2014). And although statistics, and the metrics through which they are produced, have long been associated with the regressive social accounting practices of the neoliberal state (Bruno et al., 2014), forms of collective action that use numbers, measurements, and indicators as means of denunciation and criticism allow the capacity of previous indicators to be brought into doubt (Lury & Gross, 2014). A major aim of those who use statactivism is to subvert problematic models of social accountability (Walker et al., 2019).

Drawing upon this ethos, the authors of this chapter, together with other scholars, students, and community groups, felt compelled to collect data in order to challenge two sets of practices. The first was the commissioning of privatised healthcare services in Brighton and Hove, United Kingdom (UK). The second was the invisibilisation of senior management in UK Universities who at the time had been characterised as a 'mercenary army of professional administrators' (Halffman & Radder, 2015, p. 165) maintaining a UK HE sector being eaten alive by corporate logic and a pedagogy of debt.

Statactivism and Critical Community Psychology

The concept of statactivism arose with the worker movement fighting-class inequalities (Desrosières, 2008) and has been applied to an increasing number of topics focusing on social disparities (Desrosières, 2014). Recent writings on statistical activism in France and more distant Liberation Psychology from Latin America have provided an impulse for the research contained herein.

There is resonance with the principles of statactivism and liberation psychology. Montero and Sonn (2009) discuss the need to produce a science which is constructed by praxis, which they define as 'practice that produces knowledge and knowledge that turns into action' (p.). Jiminez-Dominguez (2009) points to the value of Ignacio Martín-Baró's effective use of surveys as deideologisation tools against the military dictatorship in El Salvador in the 1980s. Martín-Baró believed that such tools could be mobilised to give voice to dissent. For Martín-Baró, neo-positivist methods could be very useful once separated from their epistemological assumptions, allowing the practices of quantifying people's experiences can also help to reveal injustice (Samuel, 2014).

Where statactivism is oriented to producing calculative infrastructures that can be organised to make surfaces or planes for action and resistance (Lury & Gross, 2014), liberation psychology can be made manifest by using surveys to enable social ruptures that contribute to the transformation of the institutions and practices enabling oppression. Both approaches entail political practices that involve the conscientisation of participants while seeking to strengthen democracy (Montero & Sonn, 2009). Such activities resist and subvert the understandings of reality mediated by what schemata designed in other worlds can capture (Burton & Gomez Ordonez, 2009, p. 349). Martín-Baró (1994) suggested that survey tools could be used as deideoligising instruments and constituted a valid approach by psychologists seeking to introduce into the collective consciousness elements and schemata that can help dismantle the dominant ideological discourse.

We took as a start point the notion that surveys could be used to interrogate and interrupt the circuits of dispossession that had been legitimised by previous mobilisations of evidence to reform public institutions (Fine, 2016). We were interested in the role of knowledge in shaping political activities and in exploring whether statactivism, as a militant use of figures (Baudot, 2014), could be a valuable tool to disrupt the previous 'dominant schemata' in health commissioning and higher education that had tended to be limited to documenting 'safe events' (Smith, 2010). We were interested in using surveys to challenge dominant contemporary ways of knowing localised health commissioning and national HE practices and to challenge forms of consultation whereby the more public participation was mobilised, the more the power relations of local and national communities were masked (Miraftab, 2004).

We have sympathy with Fryer and Fox (2015) who question the versions of 'critical' and 'liberation' that are invoked in many pieces of community psychology praxis where, despite provocative and radical injunctions to action, much of the praxis itself is politically conservative and largely acritical. The following project sought to use statactivism as a means to engage in work that was disruptive, confrontational, and challenging of the manifestations of regressive neoliberally informed policy in higher education and health commissioning. In this work, we tested out statactivism as a methodological approach for critical community psychology in order to produce forms of evidence and participatory practices which, rather than feed into mainstream normative policy making and practice, dislocated and challenged the ways in which injustice was being visited, not through a distant tyrannical power, but through the everyday practices of well-intentioned liberal society (Iris Marion Young, 1988, p. 272). Our approach to statactivism included projects with explicit aims of unsettling dominant logics that boost the narratives of those in power and silence the voice of those who are excluded, and of enacting transformative social change by having marginalised voices heard by decision makers.

The two projects, the Brighton Citizens' Health Services Survey (BCHSS) and Senior Management Survey (SMS), stem from a reflection on existing power dynamics within two UK public institutions, NHS and HE, and take a clear stand in designing actions with the transformative potential to promote political participation and increase political action.

Statactivism in Action—Two Cases

NHS Privatisation in Brighton

Through the UK 2012 Health and Social Care Act (HSCA), £80bn of UK health commissioning budget was controversially entrusted to newly formed Clinical Commissioning Groups (CCGs) (DoH, 2013). One of the key concerns during this period was whether this act of parliament mandated for the mass privatisation of the British National Health Service. Recent research suggests that healthcare professionals, including GPs, do not feel that their CCG policies reflect their own views and that they have very little chance to impact CCG's policy decisions (Murphy, 2015). Moreover, there have been suggestions that cost-efficiency appears to be overriding service quality during the dysfunctional CCG tendering processes (Checkland et al., 2013; 350:h149), and problems of transparency have been considered to routinely arise due to the institutionalised secrecy through which these contracts are procured, awarded, and performed (Deith, 2013).

Moreover, there have been suggestions that the engagement and accountability practices that have emerged post-HASC have suffered from many of the previous limitations that have befallen their predecessors (Hudson, 2015; Tritter & Koivusalo, 2013). That is, increasingly prescriptive and centrally driven set of performance metrics such as waiting times (Currie & Suhomlinova, 2006; Speed & Gabe, 2013), audit regimes working in combination with central command structures and vertical control (Dommett et al., 2016) and very few examples where citizen participation has actually led to tangible improvements in services or changes in policy (Smith, 2006).

Following several instances of public contracts being transferred or awarded to private health providers in the city of Brighton, South East England, academics and students at the University of Brighton conceived an action research project to create a provisional space to explore, extend, and challenge the knowledge and practices mobilised in post-HSCA healthcare public engagement and commissioning. This work was based on the premise that people do not only have a consumer-oriented relationship to health services. Health services, and hospitals in particular, are important to peoples' ideas about local identity and sense of place (Jones, 2016; Brown, 2003). In the UK, hospitals play an important symbolic role; they are more than just buildings where healthcare is delivered and it was our contention that members of the public would have legitimate opinions on local NHS privatisations although until this point no organisations had sought these opinions.

The Brighton Citizens' Health Services Survey

In response to a perceived need for greater public say in local healthcare commissioning, the first Brighton Citizens' Health Services Survey (BCHSS) was conceived by academics and students at the University of Brighton. The project was initially designed to hold regular six monthly public consultations with a substantial number of citizens from Brighton and Hove. Within the BCHSS the intention was to use survey methods to identify and 'map' moments of commissioning controversy and, through the process of collecting data and reporting the survey results, to provide the basis for a disruption or slowing down of the practices that function to stabilise and legitimise current healthcare commissioning and the limited forms of democracy that they make possible.

The BCHSS was developed as an 'engagement technology' to explore the conditions for developing a form of evidence-based healthcare activism that foregrounded many of the commissioning and budgetary activities that were operating beyond public knowledge and consent (Desrosières, 2014). In so doing, the project team hoped that the findings could be used to start a local conversation where disparities between commissioning decisions and public needs and values can be made clear and acted upon. In this context, citizen information was used as a legitimate counter point to 'official' information.

Through the creation of an 'animating set of questions' (Espeland & Saunder, 2007), the BCHSS sought to open up a space through which to make visible some of the ways of knowing and valuing the NHS and health services that had been erstwhile minimised through the consumer-oriented commensuration practices of post-2012 public engagement. In this way, there was a clear agenda to explore and broaden previously consumer-oriented engagement opportunities.

The project developed surveys that were designed to move beyond the post-HASC (2012) accountability dominance of recording consumer experience with the health services they used. Rather they sought to capture unmeasured and excluded forms of knowledge representing the voices of the people of Brighton & Hove on important topical health issues like funding cuts, privatisation, and the broader tensions between local commissioning and national funding policy directives. These potentially controversial issues were not at the time of data collection any part of the suite of accountability and transparency practices employed across the city.

The project was established using a distinctive approach to survey design and involved developing a public engagement tool aligned to public consultation, participation, and deliberation rather than the production of a 'validated instrument'. The methodology that underpinned the project enabled the survey design to evolve as part of a participatory, consultative process.

The questions on current commissioning issues were drawn from the minutes of local Health and Wellbeing Board (HWB) and Clinical Commissioning Group discussions, with a focus on issues that were or had the potential to be controversial. For instance, the transfer of the contract for patient transport from a statutory to a commercial provider was the subject of considerable debate and press coverage. The list of currently tendered contracts and their end-dates were available on the CCG website. However, since upcoming commissioning intentions were unavailable on the public website, a Freedom of Information request was submitted for a list of services that will be subject to new tendering processes in the forthcoming calendar year. Given the claims that the post-reform English NHS was in the midst of privatisation by stealth programme, this tendering process was (potentially at least) very controversial.

The first survey was a two-page, multiple option questionnaire that took three to four minutes to complete. Online and paper versions of the survey were produced. It was disseminated by the survey teams through various forms of social media, including most prominently Twitter and Facebook. The project team sought to sample as broadly as possible and so for this reason the survey was circulated to organisations and groups who might be expected to display a broad political and demographic membership. This included all major local political parties, all resident's associations in the city, all church groups, two universities, and the three local trades unions. Moreover, several hundred surveys were complete by a convenience sample of passers-by in Brighton city centre over four consecutive Saturdays. In total, 1300 completed first surveys were collected and analysed, and 700 of the second survey.

When the survey was released, the survey team attempted to contact the local CCG, Healthwatch and the Health and Wellbeing Board. Despite numerous attempts at contact, no reply was received from either the CCG or Healthwatch. The lead councillor from the local Health and Wellbeing Board replied by email that they would be interested in viewing the findings.

Once the results had been collected, an initial report was produced (Brighton Citizens' Health Services Survey team, 2016), and a launch event of the initial report was held at the University of Brighton (BCHSS, 2016). A press release was issued to all local media outlets, including newspapers, radio stations, and online news sites. The launch event drew 40 local stakeholders, including local politicians, academics, NHS staff, and campaign groups. While the CCG did not attend the launch event, their lay representative did although it was not clear whether he was there in a personal capacity or representing the CCG.

The report concluded that the public in Brighton & Hove held clear and compelling views on the values that they felt should underpin the ways that they wanted their health services to be commissioned, and it restated Brighton and Hove CCG's (B&H CCG's) statutory remit to ensure that these views were appropriately reflected in their decision making. It stated that, in the city of Brighton and Hove, a vast majority of the public were against the use of private companies in the local health economy and very concerned about some of the recent decisions that had been made to commission private companies to undertake certain services. Finally, there was an acknowledgement that further work was needed on the part of B&H CCG to reflect the public needs and values in their commissioning decisions.

In terms of engaging with the CCG, a deputation to the local council Health and Wellbeing Board was arranged for July 2016. Formally, a deputation consists of a member of the public presenting a statement which is submitted to the board seven days in advance (selected members of the CCG are also members of the HWB). All board members see the pre-submitted statements and have a prearranged response at the ready. The deputation received a mixed reception by members of the Health and Wellbeing Board. Some of the members were in favour of the work, and some appeared to be challenged by the findings.

As the survey project developed over its first two iterations, numerous local media, (such as the local newspaper, *The Argus*, regional radio, BBC Sussex and Juice FM, and regional television, BBC South Today) started to pick up on the findings and use the data collected as a means through which to develop local healthcare stories and to check their information when writing their own stories.

There were several moments where the stakeholders with the most powerful interests in this context sought to directly challenge the veracity, ethics, and appropriateness of the survey project. These included emails and communications in personal and public meetings. The project was challenged by commissioners as potentially unethical, unrepresentative of the local population and methodologically flawed. It was suggested that the survey addressed national policy issues that were beyond local commissioner control. Moreover, a knock-on effect was that several of the key stakeholders in the city who had been criticised in the results of the survey made it clear that they were not willing to work with the lead investigator or anyone working with the investigator. This was communicated indirectly via a number of sources.

HE Marketisation in England

Recent literature documenting the current state of UK higher education appears to point to a sector beset by a range of disparate but related issues. Gill (2014) describes an increasing reliance upon corporate management techniques, the expansion of student numbers without an associated expansion of staff, workforce casualisation, increasingly unmanageable workloads and a proliferation of audit regimes oriented towards problematic notions of accountability as central to recent changes in the sector. Outside of higher education a sense of disinterest and bewilderment is matched by a growing and pervasive sense of crisis from within and Gill (2014) describes forms of exploitation that have largely been protected by the seemingly privileged spaces of the university.

Ball (2012) suggests that in such regimes of performativity, experience is nothing and productivity is everything—an ever intensifying upward spiral of standards where last year's efforts are a benchmark for improvement. There is little evidence that this metric explosion in higher education improves educational performance, with the Research Excellence Framework (REF) having been described as 'hallucinatorily wasteful' (Gill, 2009).

Senior management teams now appoint self-selecting and self-reproducing boards of governors which allow senior management teams to exercise largely unlimited powers that are endorsed by governing boards, usually after faux exercises in consultation (Holmwood et al., 2016). There has been a relative dearth of literature on university senior management leadership (Perry & Miller, 2017). However, that which has been published has tended to be unequivocal in representing university management as sociopathic leaders befuddled by a caustic combination of narcissism, psychopathy, and Machiavellianism (Perry & Miller, 2017). Craig et al. (2014) characterise university senior management regimes as supporting courts of conformers and colluders who are selfish, ambitious, and openly supportive of toxic tyrants where universities, bedevilled by audit culture, are characterised as psychotic.

The National Senior Management Survey

The UK Senior Management Survey represents the first nationwide attempt to understand the realities of UK higher education through schemata designed within the sector. A group of lecturers in the UK started this action research project to explore the direction of higher education management and evaluate different accountability measures. The survey sought to move the gaze from the narrow metrics of staff performance to the senior management teams who set the conditions through which staff performance becomes possible so that senior managers could be opened to much-needed scrutiny. The survey mirrored the NSS process and set up a national league table of senior management teams. It focussed on:

- senior management impact on students
- senior management performance
- work pressure and wellbeing
- treatment of staff

Six thousand academics from across the UK completed the survey from 80 universities.

The very top-scoring university had 37% of staff satisfied with management, the average across the sector was 11% of staff satisfied with senior management and several universities at the foot of the table didn't have a single member of staff satisfied with management. Key findings showed

- 70% of academics said their SM didn't give them enough hours to support their students
- Only 21% of academics believed their SM positively impacts how they can support students
- 67% of academics believe that NSS and module feedback scores are not being ethically used to encourage staff performance
- Only 8.8% of academics believe their managers deserve the salaries they are paid
- Only 12.6% of academics believe their senior management favour holding down tuition fees
- 15% of staff feel respected and valued by their senior management
- 80% of staff work evenings and/or weekends to fulfil their roles

Preliminary findings and the final table were published in the Times Higher Education magazine; the findings were presented to an audience of UK HE senior managers (see Fig. 7.1) at a Westminster Policy Forum Conference on the REF, and a motion presented to the Union UCU which was passed agreeing to continue a biannual version of the survey.

A forthcoming paper (Walker et al., forthcoming) details a qualitative account of the 4000 comments provided by academic staff on senior management. This paper provides a scathing critique of a sector beset by continuous revolution, the crushing of institutional memory, change fetishism, expensive vanity projects and shocking incompetence that has created impossible and toxic conditions for staff where a cohort of powerful and governance-free managerialists have a decreasing understanding of the teaching, research, and administration of a university.

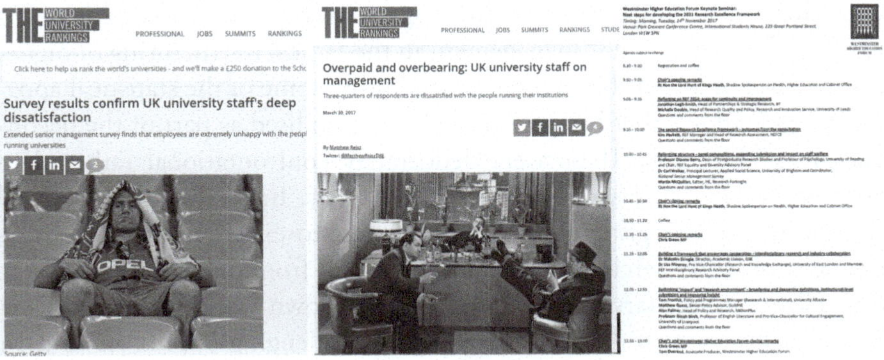

Fig. 7.1 Publicity for the survey

Concluding Thoughts on Statactivism and Critical Community Psychology

Martín-Baró (1994) said that our role as psychologists should not be to understand the world but to change it. In these projects we have sought locally, and nationally, to challenge dominant ideologies that provide the invisible scaffolding for acts of oppression organised through the prism of 'austerity'. The two examples drawn upon here, the marketisation of higher education and NHS privatisation and defunding, are two examples of economic and social violence that have been positioned as progressive social policy through the legitimising policy discourses of austerity.

The cases outlined above represent attempts to incorporate statactivist practices into critical community psychology praxis as a way of introducing into the collective consciousness elements and schemata that can help dismantle the dominant ideological discourse and practice in Higher Education in England/UK and Health Commissioning in Brighton. We mobilised statistics in order to bring about a disruption in the tactics of aggressive corporate accumulation in public health and higher education that have been normatively legitimated by the mainstream politics of evidence (Fine, 2016). We sought to counter the ways in which evidence and public consultation have been deployed to legitimate land grab, and hollow out public institutions (Fine, 2016). Critical community psychology praxis influenced by Liberation Psychology and Theology demands a more 'action-oriented', less 'academic' critical psychology where praxis is developed to make violence and its perpetrators visible (Burton & Gomez Ordonez, 2009). These two statactivist projects were influenced by such demands.

In the BCHSS, forms of privatisation and NHS cuts, which had been largely invisible to the public, were made visible, and the reactions of the public drawn back into the deliberative spaces of powerful stakeholders. For the SMS, the role of senior management in the radical restructuring of higher education was made visible and challenged using some of the statistical apparatus (league tables) that has previously been mobilised as part of the deconstruction of UK HE. These were deliberately confrontational rather than reformist projects that sought to engage publicly. In so doing, the critical community psychologists involved were subject to experiences of intimidation, control, and coercion both from inside and from outside their institutions. However, as Martín-Baró noted about his own work, 'these attacks at the university confirm that our activities are challenging oppressors to their very core' (in Jiminez-Dominguez, 2009, p. 46). While one must be careful about drawing insensitive parallels between the military junta in El Salvador and neoliberal 'briefcase wars' of capitalist England, it is and should be the case that such work as this invokes consequences when the disrupted institutions seek to resteady their trajectories. Any critical community psychologist embarking on such a statactivist project should keep in mind the potential consequences of such actions. We don't say this to dissuade scholar activists from such activities, just to ensure that people don't embark on romanticised notions of praxis free of potential retaliations.

Unlike many versions of community psychology which have been characterised as acritical, politically conservative, and inherently accommodationist (Fryer & Fox, 2015), these projects used statactivism in a more confrontational and militant manner in order to bring into being figures, statistics, and ways of knowing practices that previously did not appear, to make these ways of knowing policy and commissioning available publicly and to directly challenge dominant stakeholders in a variety of deliberative spaces. The current fascination of community psychologists with participation and empowerment fails to attest to the ways in which these concepts have been depoliticised and indeed mobilised in order to mask power relations locally and nationally. These projects sought to reveal and challenge these power relations, not to empower a mythical consumer of health and education but to challenge some of the entrenched silences of neoliberal governance (Miraftab, 2004).

The mode of community psychology and of critical psychology developed in many countries have openly manifested social transformation as their ultimate goal but what is not clear is the way in which that goal is to be obtained, for in so far there are few methods explicitly formulated with that task in mind (Montero, 2009). This work constitutes an attempt to formulate and implement potential methods. Rethinking the role of universities in supporting communities should become a priority for our discipline, particularly when they have the latitude to challenge oppressing forces to their very core (Jiminez-Dominguez, 2009). Universities can (sometimes) act as protected spaces in which thoughts and idea of this kind can be pursued to the highest level, and should be a privileged vehicle to convey such knowledge to citizens. For critical community psychology to play a meaningful role in deliberative governance and social change, its practitioners must be increasingly prepared to step outside the safety of the accommodationist reformism which enables much of the violence against our public services to continue undisturbed.

References

Ball, S. J. (2012). Performativity, commodification and commitment: An I-spy guide of the neoliberal university. *British Journal of Educational Studies, 60*(1), 17–28.

Baudot, P. Y. (2014). Who's counting? Institutional autonomy and the production of activity data for disability policy in France (2006–2014). *Partecipazione e Conflitto, 7*(2), 294–313.

Brown, T. (2003). Towards an understanding of local protest: Hospital closure and community resistance. *Social & Cultural Geography, 4*(4), 489–506. https://doi.org/10.1080/1464936032000137920

Bruno, I., Didier, E., & Vitale, T. (2014). Statactivism—Forms of action between disclosure and affirmation. *PACo, 7*(2), 198–220.

Burton, M., & Gomez Ordonez, L. H. (2009). Liberation psychology—Another kind of critical psychology. In M. Montero & C. Sonn (Eds.), *Psychology of liberation—Theory and applications*. Springer.

Checkland, K., Allen, P., Coleman, A., Segar, J., McDermott, I., Harrison, S., & Peckham, S. (2013). Accountable to whom, for what? An exploration of the early development of clinical commissioning groups in the English NHS. *BMJ Open, 3*(12). https://doi.org/10.1136/bmjopen-2013-003769

Craig, R., Amernic, J., & Tourish, D. (2014). Perverse audit culture and accountability in the modern public university. *Financial Accountability & Management, 30*(1), 0267–4424.

Currie, G., & Suhomlinova, O. (2006). The impact of institutional forces upon knowledge sharing in the UK NHS: The triumph of professional power and the inconsistency of policy. *Public Administration, 84*(1), 1–30. https://doi.org/10.1111/j.0033-3298.2006.00491.x

Deith, J. (2013). A healthy market? Lack of transparency raises doubts about NHS commissioning. *BMJ, 347*, Article f7115. https://doi.org/10.1136/bmj.f7115

Department of Health. (2013). The mandate: A mandate from the Government to the NHS Commissioning Board: April 2013 to March 2015 (Presented to Parliament pursuant to section 13B(5)(b) of the National Health Service Act 2006). Retrieved from https://www.gov.uk/government/uploads/system/uploads/attachment_data/file/256497/13-15_mandate.pdf

Desrosieres, A. (2014). Statistics and social critique. *Partecipazione e Conflitto, 7*(2), 348–359.

Didier, E. (2018). Globalization of quantitative policing: Between management and statactivism. *Annual Review of Sociology*. https://doi.org/10.1146/annurev-soc-060116-053308

Dommett, K., MacCarthaigh, M., & Hardiman, N. (2016). Reforming the Westminster model of agency governance: Britain and Ireland after the crisis. *Governance: An International Journal of Policy, Administration and Institutions, 29*(4), 535–552. https://doi.org/10.1111/gove.12227

Espeland, W. N., & Saunder, M. (2007). Rankings and reactivity: How public measures recreate social worlds. *AJS, 113*(1), 1–40.

Fine, M. (2016). Chapter 5—accumulation and its dis'(sed) contents: The politics of evidence in the struggle for public education. In M. Spooner & J. McNinch (Eds.), *Dissident knowledge in higher education*. University of Regina Press.

Fryer, D., & Fox, R. (2015). Community psychology—subjectivity, power, collectivity. In I. Parker (Ed.), *Handbook of critical psychology*. Routledge.

Gill, R. (2009). Breaking the silence: The hidden injuries of the neoliberal academia. In R. Flood & R. Gill (Eds.), *Secrecy and silence in the research process: Feminist reflections*. Routledge.

Gill, R. (2014). Academics, cultural workers and critical labour studies. *Journal of Cultural Economy, 7*, 1.

Gulbrandsen, L. H. (2008). Accountability arrangements in non-state standards organisations: Instrumental design and imitation. *The Organ, 15*(4), 563–583.

Halffman, W., & Radder, H. (2015). The academic manifesto: From an occupied to a public university. *Minerva, 53*, 165–187.

Holmwood, J., Hickey, T., Cohen, R., & Wallis, S. (2016). *In defence of public higher education: Knowledge for a successful society*. Convention for Higher Education.

Hudson, B. (2015). Public and patient engagement in commissioning in the English NHS. *Public Management Review, 17*(1), 1–16. https://doi.org/10.1080/14719037.2014.881534

Jiminez-Dominguez, B. (2009). Ignacio Martin Baro's social psychology of liberation. In M. Montero & C. Sonn (Eds.), *Psychology of liberation—Theory and applications*. Springer.

Jones, L. (2016). Policy as discursive practice: An ethnographic study of hospital planning in England (Doctoral dissertation, London School of Hygiene andTropical medicine, London, United Kingdom). https://doi.org/10.17037/pubs.02997234

Kagan, C., Burton, M., Duckett, P., Lawthom, R., & Siddiquee, A. (2011). *Critical community psychology*. Wiley.

Lury, C., & Gross, A. (2014). The downs and ups of the consumer price index in Argentina—From national statistics to big data. *Partecipazione e Conflitto, 7*(2), 258–277.

Martín-Baró, I. (1994). *Writings for a liberation psychology*. Harvard University Press.

Miraftab, F. (2004). Making neoliberal governance: The disempowering work of empowerment. *International Planning Studies, 9*(4), 239–259.

Montero, M. (2009). Methods for liberation: Critical consciousness in action. In M. Montero & C. Sonn (Eds.), *In psychology of liberation—Theory and applications*. Springer.

Montero, M., & Sonn, C. (2009). About liberation and psychology: An introduction. In M. Montero & C. Sonn (Eds.), *Psychology of liberation—Theory and applications*. Springer.

Murphy, E. (2015). Primary concerns 2015. Retrieved from Cogora website: http://www.cogora.com/wp-content/uploads/2016/11/primary-concerns-2015.pdf

Perry, C., & Miller, P. J. (2017). *Dysfunctional leadership in Universities: Identifying and dealing with sociopaths*. Management, Leadership and Marketing in Universities and Colleges of Higher Education.

Power, M. (2000). The audit society—Second thoughts. *International Journal of Auditing, 4*, 111–119.

Samuel, B. (2014). Statistics and political violence-reflections on the social conflict in 2009 in Guadeloupe. *Partecipazione e Conflitto, 7*(2), 237–257.

Smith, G. (2006). Studying democratic innovations: An analytic framework. In *Democratic Innovations: Institutions for citizen participation* (pp. 8–29). Cambridge, United Kingdom: Cambridge University Press.

Smith, G. (2010). *Studying democratic innovations. An analytic framework. In democratic innovations*. Cambridge University Press.

Speed, E., & Gabe, J. (2013). The health and social care act for England 2012: The extension of 'new professionalism'. *Critical Social Policy, 33*, 564–574. https://doi.org/10.1177/0261018313479010

Tritter, J. Q., & Koivusalo, M. (2013). Undermining patient and public engagement and limiting its impact: The consequences of the Health and Social Care Act2012 on collective patient and public involvement. *Health Expectations, 16*, 115–118. https://doi.org/10.1111/hex.12069

Walker, C., Artaraz, K., Darking, M., Davies, C., Fleischer, S., Graber, R., Mwale, S., Speed, E., Terry, J., & Zoli, A. (2019). Building spaces for controversial public engagement – Exploring and challenging democratic deficits in NHS marketization. *Journal of Social and Political Psychology*, 2195–3335.

Walker, C., Erickson, M., Hanna, P., et al. (forthcoming). Change fetishism, incompetence and governance free zones—A statactivist confrontation of contemporary UK higher education. *Journal of Community and Applied Social Psychology*.

Zellini, P. (2018). *La dittatura del calcolo*. Adelphi.

Zoli, A. (2017, October). Community well-being in the era of health care privatisation. In S. Di Martino (chair), *Community Well-being: Theories, Indicators, and Strategies of Intervention*. Symposium conducted at the ECPA 10th European Congress of Community Psychology. Newcastle.

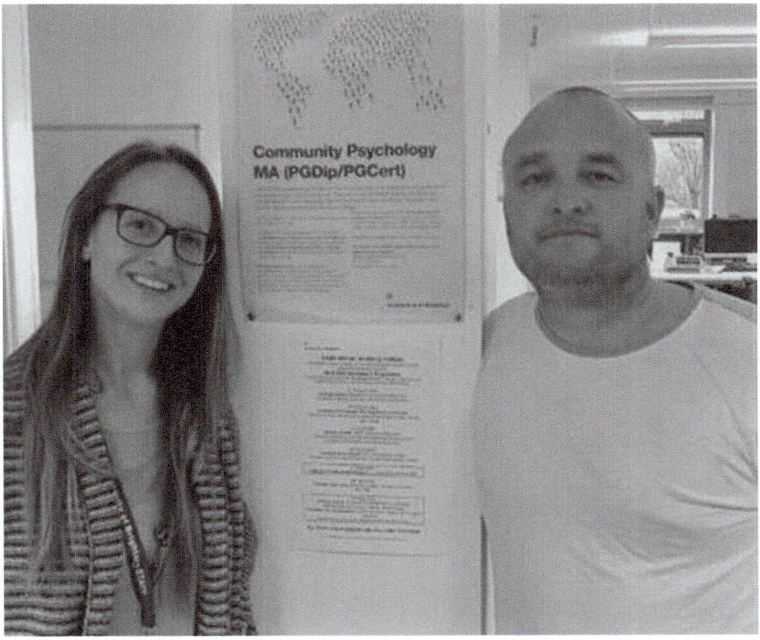

Carl and Anna try hard to do, as well as teach and research, community psychology. Carl is an academic, community activist, council member, and stand-up comedian—not necessarily in this order—and his enthusiasm is deemed contagious by many, but not (yet) alarming by the authorities. Anna is a transdisciplinary scholar, erratic soul, and human rights advocate; she loves laughing but sometimes struggles to understand jokes. Carl and Anna run the only Master's degree in Community Psychology in the UK, hoping to inspire many and not to enrage too many with their bold, epistemologically value-driven, and methodologically heretic work, and programme. With the ongoing thirst for a science that serves the marginalised, for a collective knowledge that subverts privileges, and for an education that inspires learners as well as teachers, they hope to provide a chapter which meets these ambitious goals.

Part II

Working in Radical and Disruptive Spaces

> And I bid you this, go there, where wagons do not pass; do not drive your chariot along the same ways as others, nor along the broad path, but the untrodden roads, although you will drive a narrower route. (Callimachus, Aetia)

This section presents a number of works that challenge the conventionally accepted notions of therapeutic spaces and practices. These projects are theoretically underpinned by the increasing understanding that there is not (and most likely never will be) a unifying framework to standardise care and mental health provision. This is due to the "magnificent overabundance of reality" (Bagemihl, 1999) and the unpredictable forms of human realities (Arendt, 1978) which daily overturn the presumptuous assumption of a universal expert-driven truth (Chomsky, 2002).

In Chap. 8, Malherbe, Suffla, and Seedat provide an example of community-driven epistemic disobedience as an invitation to reflect on decolonial practices even in critically oriented contexts. With a similar emphasis on reflexivity, in Chap. 9 Denton et al. present their experience with 'Options', an alternative model for therapeutic intervention where practitioners from different backgrounds and service users co-create unpredictable insights on mental distress, a process which, the authors argue, requires the actors involved to dismiss the asymmetries based on expert-driven truth models.

In Chap. 10 Vavvos and Triliva offer an application of Action Research to tackle the structural sources of mental distress working with a network of evicted and indebted citizens in the distinctive context of Greek austerity measures, showing how psychological research can serve people's interests in their strive for social justice. Looking at how community has the power to self-organise and create inclusive spaces, in Chap. 11 Wilcox and Graber explore a queer community pub as a healing, informal, and radical place in Brighton, UK. The transformative power of language and space is also conveyed through the events under which scientific knowledge is branded, and shared. In Chap. 12, Hadjiosif and Desai discuss how the British Psychological Society (BPS) Community Psychology Festival was born and became an annual flagship event for like-minded people, and how this new format sets an accessible, inclusive alternative to an academic conference.

Further exploring 'untrodden roads' through co-production and creativity, in Chap. 13 Taggart et al. present and discuss the 'Define Normal Project', an experiential training for mental health staff to learn about psychiatric care provision from the eyes of young service users. Similarly, in Chap. 14 Anderson et al. present 'Converge', a project radically challenging the roles and spaces of university and mental healthcare, where service users are offered art-based education (rather than therapy), within the same university structures of all other students (rather than in segregated spaces such as hospitals or centres). In Chap. 15, the last one of this section, Arshad argues how cyberspace can provide a safe healing space for British-Pakistani women of Muslim faith to collaboratively bridge the hiatus between their Islamic spirituality and Western understanding of the suffering through the metaphor of 'The Jannah Tree'.

All the chapters in this section are joined in the urge to abandon the 'broad path' of ineffective, patronising, and dehumanising spaces of Western-global-North centric mainstream psychology in favour of value and users' driven modes of participation and healing. Upon an academically informed critique, they also take up the challenge to describe and reflectively analyse new routes which can create such needed epistemological and methodological ruptures.

References

Arendt, H. (1978). *The life of the mind.* New York: Harcourt Brace Jovanovich.

Bagemihl, B. (1999). *Biological exuberance: Animal homosexuality and natural diversity*. New York: St. Martin's Press.

Chomsky, N. in Mitchell, P., & Schoeffel, J. (eds.). (2002). *Understanding power: The indispensable Chomsky*. New York: The New Press.

8

Reflexively Interrogating (De)colonial Praxes in Critical Community Psychologies

Nick Malherbe, Shahnaaz Suffla, and Mohamed Seedat

The destruction and distortion of particular knowledges, and their construction (see Fanon, 1963), casts colonised subjects as Other and ascribes to them dehumanising modes of being. Certainly, colonised peoples and their knowledge systems are rarely, if ever, able to sufficiently meet the 'requirements of respectability'—or what is sometimes referred to as the master codes (Mbembe, 2001)—of a colonial world that is made largely in the image of wealthy, white, cisgendered, heterosexual, male able bodies. In this way, epistemic violence—the manner by which particular knowledge systems are arranged for the purposes of marginalising and subjugating particular groups (Spivak, 1988; Teo, 2018)—seeks to drain colonised subjects of autonomy and historical agency for purposes of control. Colonised peoples, subsuming all rendered as Other through historical and contemporary colonising forces, then become defined along colonial coordinates that afford them only partial humanism (see Said, 1978). However, the global history of popular resistance on the part of dominated peoples, which includes constructing alternative, liberatory knowledge-praxes, has demonstrated that systems of oppression, such as colonialism, are

N. Malherbe • S. Suffla (✉) • M. Seedat
Institute for Social and Health Sciences & Masculinity and Health Research Unit, University of South Africa & South African Medical Research Council, Cape Town, Western Cape, South Africa
e-mail: malhenr@unisa.ac.za; suffls@unisa.ac.za; Shahnaaz.Suffla@mrc.ac.za; seedama@unisa.ac.za

C. Walker et al. (eds.), *The Palgrave Handbook of Innovative Community and Clinical Psychologies*, https://doi.org/10.1007/978-3-030-71190-0_8

always incomplete *attempts* at full domination (Gordon, 2017). Through various politicised forms of resistance to foreclosed ways of knowing and being, understood as epistemic disobedience (see Mignolo, 2009), people can and have overcome seemingly omnipotent structures of domination.

Epistemic disobedience must be considered with respect to hegemonic knowledge-making spaces, such as the academy. In psychology, the discipline within which we are most dominantly situated, the revolutionary work of Martinican psychiatrist Frantz Fanon (1963, 1967) ushered in what has been referred to as a decolonial turn (see Maldonado-Torres, 2017). Fanon's work has been especially influential in the conceptualisations and enactments of certain psychologies, typically critical in orientation. Yet, mainstream psychology remains characterised by Euro-American-centrism, conservative individualism, false claims to an apolitical orientation, and a neoliberal agenda (Seedat & Suffla, 2017). Dominant psychologies thus remain tethered to coloniality, that is, existing systems of power that act to maintain colonial relations of exploitation and domination well after the period of 'classic colonialism' (see Maldonado-Torres, 2017). Even (critical) community psychologies—themselves a response to oppressive mainstream psychologies—have, in recent years, been increasingly institutionalised and largely denuded of their liberatory impulse (see Yen, 2008).

By examining a particular moment of community-driven epistemic disobedience, it is the purpose of this chapter to explore reflexively some of the tensions, regressions, contradictions and unevenness, as well as the creativities and imaginations, that are inherent to the ways in which critical community psychologies, and their numerous institutional restraints, approach decoloniality. Certainly, decolonising iterations of critical community psychologies, which attempt to remain vigilant to currents of epistemic violence in the field, do not discredit their own existence, but instead strive to constantly resist their disciplinary predispositions towards coloniality. We, therefore, propose that critical community psychologies commit to a relevant, historically sensitive mode of decoloniality that connects to other sites of civil, ideological, political and social struggle. Simultaneously, critical community psychologies are obliged to engage in the difficult, yet crucial, task of considering reflexively their liberatory ambiguities, which frequently act to reinscribe coloniality in different ways. Following this, we might begin to imagine critical community psychologies that are aware of and resist their disciplinary complicity in the coloniality of knowledge, power and being. These psychologies may also facilitate innovative and democratic means of envisioning, articulating and—most importantly—deploying decolonising knowledges for the purposes of psychosocial liberation (Fanon, 1967), and challenging colonial conceptualisations of justice (see Gordon, 2017).

Psychologies and the Decolonial Turn

In his book *Black Skin, White Masks*, Fanon (1967) demonstrates that the foundations of colonised peoples' collective psychological anguish are not to be located exclusively in individual psyches. Rather, such anguish is to be expected when one lives in a world structured by coloniality, wherein one's very being is perceived as a kind of anti-social violence towards normative colonial structures and conceptions of respectability (Gordon, 2017). Fanon (1967) thus asserts that a decolonising psychology will support colonised subjects in uncovering the societal connections to their psychological well-being and foster among them the decolonial attitude imperative to remaking a world in which their humanity is recognised and cherished (Maldonado-Torres, 2017). Through the fostering of a decolonial attitude, psychology's decolonial turn therefore strives to unhinge various available modes of being, power and knowledge from systems of coloniality. In this way, if we are to consider coloniality as the dismemberment of a colonised people from their consciousness, history, land, memory, being, the body, and fellow colonised subjects (see Ngũgĩ wa, 2009), then a decolonising psychology must look to establishing a collective re-memberment in the service of psychosocial emancipation.

Underscoring this conception of a decolonising psychology is an awareness that coloniality is not a conclusive or closed system and can be, as has been the case throughout history, resisted by movements that seek to critique and transform. It would then appear that the decolonial attitude is always alert to the fact that colonialism is only an *attempted* erasure of people's agency and humanity (see Gordon, 2017), through, for example, imposing closed systems of organised knowledge—such as fixed identity categories—on to people in order to predetermine their ways of being and knowing (see Fanon, 1963; Oyěwùmí, 1997).

While community psychologies, specifically, are a response to some of the inadequacies of mainstream psychologies, not all forms of community psychology are critical and those that are, are not by definition also decolonising. We contend that a decolonising community psychology is one that is marked by a sharp criticality, characterised by emancipatory consciousness, knowledges and praxes.

In May 1965, the *Boston Conference on the Education of Psychologists for Community Mental Health*, held in Swampscott, Massachusetts (United States) advocated a proactive, prevention and strengths-orientated approach to extending psychological services to vulnerable and disenfranchised populations (Viola & Glantsman, 2017). Today, this conference, usually referred to as the Swampscott Conference, is widely understood as having disciplinarily officiated community psychology in the United States. However, there have been numerous criticisms levelled at the Swampscott Conference (e.g., Fryer, 2008; Seedat & Suffla, 2017) for instituting an apolitical, unreflexive and somewhat myopic conception of community psychology, wholly uncritical of the very construct of 'community', the capitalist system in which communities are forged (Coimbra et al., 2012), as well as the unequal power relations intrinsic to enactments of community psychology. Furthermore, early iterations of community psychology in the US tended to overlook more radical, anti-capitalist articulations of community psychology throughout Latin America (see Gokani, 2011). During the 1970s, however, community psychology work began employing an increasingly critical approach than that envisioned at Swampscott, referencing itself against political repression, bourgeois government policy, complacent mainstream psychologies, and the globalised exclusion of vulnerable populations from apparatuses and systems of power (Fryer, 2008; Yen, 2008).

With specific reference to South Africa, the location from which we offer this contribution, critical community psychologies emerged in the late 1980s, forming part of the popular resistance to the turbulent psychosocial landscape instituted and maintained by the oppressive apartheid State. Today, South African critical community psychologies have accrued institutional recognition and legitimacy. Notwithstanding, they have also had much of their liberatory impulse subdued (Yen, 2008), recast to suit or—at best—antagonise only minimally, the arrangements of a neoliberal capitalist global ordering (Seedat & Suffla, 2017).

Decolonising Critical Community Psychologies

The fostering of decolonial attitudes is not requisite of even the most committedly critical enactments of community psychology. In this way, critical community psychology is certainly not impervious to the shifting ebb and flow of coloniality and may in fact, contradictorily, even serve to acclimatise people to particular social norms, rather than promote the conditions by which to resist and remake these norms and their governing master codes. For example, community psychologists played a role in pacifying resistance to both neoliberal austerity in 1970s Britain and the second Intifada in Palestine during the early 2000s (Coimbra et al., 2012). We would, therefore, do well to heed Gordon's (2017) insistence that conceptions and applications of justice are not exempt from the urgency of decolonisation. Critical community psychologists who seek to decolonise their work, along with the forms of justice that they endeavour to promote, must engage with a range of social actors, as well as reflect on and trouble their own collusion with the coloniality of being, power and knowledge.

There is an increasing scholarly focus on the revitalisation of the decolonial turn in psychology, including, in many instances, critical community psychologies. Specifically, in the introduction to the Special Issue of the *Journal of Social and Political Psychology*, Adams et al. (2015) outline three central approaches to decolonising psychological praxis: indigenisation, denaturalisation and accompaniment. Expanding on each of these praxes in a subsequent article, contained in the Special Issue of the *South African Journal of Psychology*, Adams et al. (2017) argue that although they conceptualise each of these approaches as discrete, they typically do not manifest as such in one's decolonising engagements. Further, these approaches are not absolutely or immanently decolonising in and of themselves. Instead, it is how they connect to wider struggles and forms of resistance that exemplify their decolonising aspirations. We would also add that the three approaches do not speak comprehensively to the complexities and messiness of community engagement and decolonising work, both of which call for critical forms of compassionate and sustained activism. Below, we provide a brief outline of these three approaches.

Indigenisation

Indigenisation is concerned primarily with dominant epistemic arrangements. It sees researchers and practitioners attempt to (re)claim indigenous wisdom in order to produce knowledge forms that are more suited to particular communities' realities, thereby serving them better than the kinds of Euro-American-centric knowledges that are frequently imposed by mainstream psychologies. It follows then that in taking seriously and normalising indigenous knowledges, indigenisation highlights the inability of apparently universal mainstream psychologies to serve all people. Yet, indigenisation remains highly community-specific in its scope and risks essentialising cultural knowledges by collapsing into an attempt to identify and romanticise 'authentic' indigenous knowledges, without problematising these knowledges (Adams et al., 2015).

Denaturalisation

Denaturalisation encompasses a contextually sensitive re-thinking of that which is posited as natural—including the coloniality of being, power and knowledge—by mainstream psychologies and broader hegemonic formulations of social science, as well as numerous master codes. Denaturalisation does, however, risk ignoring issues of direct and/or structural violence by focusing predominantly on epistemic violence (Adams et al., 2015). Further, there lies the danger of not connecting denaturalisation processes to other political struggles for social justice, thereby limiting its change-making capacities (see Gordon, 2017).

Accompaniment

In seeking to acknowledge the experiences of others and make possible new forms of interaction (Sacipa et al., 2007), accompaniment is defined, broadly, as an encounter between people from a given community and community psychologists—who are, generally, outsiders to the community—with the ultimate goal of constructing liberatory knowledges and praxes (Rodríguez et al., 2009). In rearranging the conventional relationship between researcher/therapist and participant/patient, accompaniment fosters a mutual being and sharing, which concludes only once a predetermined task has been completed, irrespective of whether such completion takes place within the confines of a specific project. In this way, researchers lend what expertise they can to those fighting coloniality so that, in standing alongside others, feeling and action occur together in the service of social action (Adams et al., 2015; Sacipa et al., 2007). There are, of course, myriad limitations to accompaniment. For instance, beyond a somewhat hollow acknowledgement, it is difficult to navigate the fact that the accompaniers are usually privileged outsiders who set the terms of accompaniment, its duration, as well as when it is to be initiated and concluded (Watkins, 2015). Accompaniers may also fall into the 'saviour' trope that characterises so much community work, wherein power imbalances are used for self-gratifying purposes (Adams et al., 2015).

Considering these three approaches and their stated limitations, we argue that one of the central imperatives for decolonising critical community psychologies is the fostering of a reflexive stance towards the compound pursuit of the social justice ideals to which critical community psychologies commits. As Fanon's (1963, 1967) work reminds us, this includes a consciousness about colonial and colonising designations of humanness. Maldonado-Torres (2016) elaborates that living in the zone of being (see Fanon, 1967) implies recognition of "one's status as a full human being with a broad range of potentials and possibilities" (p. 13), whereas living in the zone of non-being denotes "not only that one is not meant to have easy access to basic means of existence, but also that it is normal for everything and everyone, including oneself, to questions [*sic*] one's humanity" (p. 13). Community psychology, with its ability to construct that which constitutes 'normativity', the 'pathological' and even 'community' (Coimbra et al., 2012), holds the potential to signify that which is superior, human and socially respectable (see Grosfoguel et al., 2015), and therefore must at all times be considered in relation to zones of being and non-being.

Here, it is important to be cognisant of the positionalities of community psychologists themselves. Indeed, it the case that certainly, black community psychologists, for example, are positioned within zones of non-being. However, most psychologists, by virtue of their proximity to the discipline of psychology and its institutional embeddedness, are enmeshed within a practice that has historically configured, constituted and supported zones of being and non-being. Community psychologists who seek to interrogate critically the coloniality of knowledge and society therefore do so incompletely if they do not at the same time consider the discipline as well as themselves in relation to zones of being and non-being. It is thus through a continuous, critical and reflexive interrogation that we may begin to imagine liberating being, epistemologies and humanism from predetermined colonial zones.

The Ebb and Flow of (De)coloniality: A Reflexive Analysis

As a means of demonstrating the complexity inherent to the fostering of decolonial attitudes within critical community psychologies, we offer in this section an instance of community-driven epistemic disobedience that exemplifies the uneven terrain within which we find ourselves.

Context

For approximately two decades, residents from a South African township, located in the southern region of Johannesburg, have worked on numerous intervention projects with critical community psychologists from the research institute to which we are affiliated, the Institute for Social and Health Sciences (ISHS) at the University of South Africa and its Masculinity and Health Research Unit, co-directed by the South African Medical Research Council. Established in the 1980s, this particular community constitutes predominantly shack dwellings that are inhabited by South Africans as well as foreign nationals, most of whom identify as black. Although the community registers relatively high rates of crime, violence and unemployment (Statistics South Africa, 2011), residents have expressed dissatisfaction at being characterised within media reports and popular discourses by these descriptors exclusively, recalling colonial constructions of an Other who is to be managed and read solely on the terms set by these constructions (see Said, 1978). The community also has a rich history of social activism, such as petitioning and protest action, which has, at times, been met with violence from State actors.

Rather than episodic, brief and/or resource-dependent interventions, much of the critical community psychology work that takes place in this community strives for a sustained engagement that fosters a culture of safety and just peace within the community. Frequently drawing on innovative methodologies that, at different moments and to varying degrees, move between denaturalisation, indigenisation and accompaniment, much of our work in this community focuses on violence and injury prevention, safety and peace promotion, the privileging of subaltern voices, speaking back to dominant metanarratives and epistemic violence, structural resistances and community cohesion. In practice, this sees community members drawing on a host of creative methodological and distributive procedures that strive towards collective mobilisation, speaking back to dominant State actors and the collective articulation of desired systemic changes. Although the work endeavours to intersect with and inform existing modes of grassroots activism, it must be conceded that institutional constraints, such as funding preclusions to address directly the immediate material conditions of the community, have limited our own capacities to support community-led activist efforts. It is, therefore, essential that the work is continuously evaluated and reconstituted through dialogical community feedback.

Scope

In attempting to complicate the simplistic, reductionist manner by which violence is frequently understood by mainstream community psychologies, our current interventions include several projects that cohere to facilitate social change at multiple levels. Taken as a whole, the work seeks to address three central dimensions of violence, each of which interlocks with the other in complex ways. First, direct violence—on which many mainstream community psychologies are usually focused—is understood against Galtung's (1990) well-known conception, where it is defined as the physical and/or psychological violence that occurs between individuals or groups. Second, structural violence is contained within numerous intersecting systems that sustain disadvantage over certain communities and population groups (Galtung, 1969). Finally, epistemic violence, which forms the focus of this chapter, and as indicated earlier, refers to the marginalising capabilities of dominant knowledge systems (Spivak, 1988; Teo, 2018).

Although the scope of this work undoubtedly renders it a form of critical community psychology, we accept that it is only a partial signification of our decolonising praxis. By conceptualising the various ways by which the interlocking manifestations of direct, structural and epistemic violence sustain and legitimise structures of coloniality, and how such coloniality can be resisted, we are continually challenged to centre the Fanonian decolonial turn in our work. Below, we offer our interpretation of a moment of community-driven epistemic disobedience that was enacted at an event hosted by the ISHS for the community. We focus on this exemplar in order to demonstrate: how critical community psychology work can reinscribe the coloniality of knowledge, power and being; the importance of our own reflexive engagement throughout decolonising work; and the complex decolonising potentialities and regressions inherent to epistemic disobedience and its interpretation.

Community-Driven Epistemic Disobedience

On 6 December 2016, an annual event was held at the ISHS office in Johannesburg to acknowledge the community with which we collaborate, review the research activities for that year and jointly assess the year's successes and challenges. Furthermore, several community-based groups were invited to discuss activities in which they had been involved that year. The event, therefore, harnessed the university's discursive and material resources to officiate a formal, ceremonial and institutionally sanctioned interaction with the community. Importantly, the event was conceptualised as an enactment of relational accountability, which represents meaningful and ethical engagements with community partners in research (see Reich et al., 2017). This also entails a critical stance that is attentive to the relational dynamics inherent to the research encounter and the respective accountabilities of the actors concerned.

With staff members seated at the front of the room and community members and representatives at the back, the Head of the ISHS (the third author of this chapter) began his address, which was intended to inaugurate the event. However, as he began to speak, he was interrupted by a well-known member of the community, who is also recognised as a key community leader. It soon became clear that the interruption was not to be a brief remark, but a premeditated counter-inauguration of sorts. After greeting both staff and community members in his—and much of the community's—first language (thereby symbolically and literally ushering in the very 'community voice' that the event acknowledged, but did not accommodate sufficiently), the community member presented the Head with a small clay pot, or calabash, known as an *ukhamba*. The community leader explained that the *ukhamba* represented an acknowledgement of the ISHS on behalf of the community and that it was to be received by the Head on behalf of the Institute on the basis that he is both its leader and a male-bodied individual. Despite the Head's insistence that the ISHS as a collective should accept the *ukhamba*, the community leader asserted repeatedly that it was to be given to the male Head.

Retrospectively, considering the event's initial constitution from a critical standpoint, it may be said that the event sought to consciously mobilise the university's status, as well as its cultural, social and financial capital so that the event was established, self-referentially, as 'important' and to be taken seriously by both university staff and community members (the latter presumed as guests). The presentation of the *ukhamba* disturbed this particular arrangement of power between the researchers and the community, instituting a form of epistemic disobedience. When elaborating and building on understandings of the complicated and uneven contours along which decolonising praxes lie, such moments of epistemic disobedience that emerge from outside zones of being cannot be overlooked by researchers.

First, the presentation of the *ukhamba* at this moment must be located both culturally and temporally. In traditional isiZulu cultural practice, the *ukhamba*—a vertical, oval-shaped vessel, approximately 20–25 cm in height with a flat base and wide mouth (Fowler, 2006)—is utilised for serving, drinking, preparing, transporting and/or storing homemade beer as well as, albeit less frequently, medicine (Jolles, 2005). Although commercialised to an extent (it is sold as a decorative item to consumers outside of its cultural base), the *ukhamba* is an artefact that represents everyday or ceremonial cultural practice. In this way, it is inscribed with a plethora of meanings which become especially charged as we engage with this moment of epistemic disobedience.

In reading critically this moment, we also consider the ontological position of the disruptive subject, that is, the community member who presented the *ukhamba*, functioning here as a disruptive object. Throughout his time working with the ISHS, this particular community member has been open in his critique of many of our community intervention projects. Although we are not always in agreement with the form and content of his resistance, and given that limited work has been undertaken on community resistances to community psychology work, his dissenting voice is always encouraged and, where possible, provided with the requisite communicative platform. His frequent embodiment of the 'disruptive actor' role moves between centring the community and a centring of the self, and disturbing binaries between the two to problematic and progressive effects. However, in this particular instance, although he—as a single subject—handed over the *ukhamba*, he was insistent that the community, and not himself, be acknowledged in its display. In this way, he ensured that the legacy that the *ukhamba* signified was to be one characterised by an insurgence of community-driven voice, rather than individualised disruption.

As mentioned previously, in attempting to reify the perceived successes of numerous community projects, many of which were framed theoretically as both critical and decolonising, the event drew on the status and the resources of the university, an institution characterised by coloniality and, increasingly, a neoliberal agenda. Certainly, university spaces have been shown to subscribe to a regime of hegemonic knowledge-making and epistemic violence (see Campbell, 2011), much of which mimics dictums of coloniality that distort, disfigure and destroy the representations of colonised peoples (see Fanon, 1963). Indeed, for their participation in different projects, various community members were scheduled to receive certificates of acknowledgement which, in themselves, signify a kind of neoliberal metric of excellence within the university. By setting the terms of engagement within this space that sought to acknowledge what is clearly an incomplete conception of community members, we, as representatives of the university, may very well have limited the range of channels of agency and autonomy available to community members. The disruptive introduction of the *ukhamba* therefore came to insert and centre community voice within the university space—a re-memberment of sorts (see Ngũgĩ wa, 2009). Introducing the *ukhamba* into this moment shifted focus away from certificates and neoliberal metrics, towards regard, respect and—as was revealed to the Head in subsequent conversations with this community member—a form of epistemic justice that was located in African cultural practice. In this way, the community members did not simply introduce their voices temporarily within zones of being; rather, their interruption disturbed the very logic by which the existence of these zones is predicated, destabilising as well as exposing colonialities of power which, to function effectively, must take on symbolic, hidden formulations. This visibilising and partial reconstitution of the discursive contours of coloniality inscribed on to this space served to remind us that our decolonising work must push back against the very structures in which it is located and through which it finds expression. In short, this brief moment of epistemic disobedience demonstrates that decoloniality must challenge the coloniality written into the content, process and social actors pertinent to the spatio-discursive positions occupied by critical community psychologists.

In subjecting our work to a form of reflexive, decolonising critique, we examine this disruptive moment with reference to Adams et al.'s (2015) three modalities of decolonising psychological science. While we recognise that Adams et al. (2015) offered their conceptualisation with specific reference to approaches to decolonisation in psychological science, we find their contribution to be nonetheless a useful framework for analysing the micro-level elements of decolonising praxis, as encapsulated within a single moment of epistemic disobedience. Importantly, in our analysis, we understand that this framework does not sufficiently capture the complexities inherent to decolonising practice, but is nonetheless useful when interpreted as an interacting, shifting and disordered hermeneutic lens to interrogate (de)colonial praxes in critical community psychologies.

In considering indigenisation, the presentation of the *ukhamba*, its cultural signification and its spatio-temporal meaning within this setting centred—or indigenised—marginalised knowledge forms within the university's hegemonic, epistemically violent and Euro-American-centric knowledge-making space. The space was then reconstructed to acknowledge 'alternative' knowledge forms which are typically muted or distorted under the university's subscription to the coloniality of knowledge.

The spatial arrangement of the event and the manner by which it configured the knowledge-making and agentic capabilities of community members is particularly germane to considerations of denaturalisation. The room in which the event was held was arranged in a manner that situated most of the university staff at the front, a position from where they were able to address the audience. By interrupting the proceedings, the presentation of the *ukhamba* dislocated the geographies of power implicit to the ceremony's spatial arrangement. In this way, the interjection of community voice denaturalised the functioning of particular master codes by exposing concealed dynamics of power, rendering their very constitution arbitrary, that is, not *normal* or *natural*.

In addition to exposing the event's imbedded hierarchical structure, the interposition from the community member acted to undermine somewhat this unequal spatio-discursive arrangement. A levelling of this sort may be read as a kind of accompaniment, whereby the dominant meta-narrative was remade along lines of mutuality and inclusion. Indeed, the event's aim of acknowledging the community was not wholly rejected; rather, the coordinates by which it attempted to do this were recast along engagement lines characterised by more of a dialogical exchange than was communicated through the opening of the event. In moving between each mode of decolonisation, participants enacted a kind of epistemic disobedience that did not wholly disregard our knowledge-making projects, but inserted their agency within it, thus transforming and partially decolonising it. While perhaps not a complete or full enactment of accompaniment, the presentation of the *ukhamba* allowed community members to momentarily move alongside researchers.

Finally, in appreciating the complexities of decolonising praxes, we may turn our attentions to the community member's insistence that the Head as a leader and as a male-bodied subject was to receive the *ukhamba*. Decolonising conceptions of justice (see Gordon, 2017) entail nuanced, contextually sensitive discussions that endeavour to conscientise all parties, rather than impose the hermeneutic lens of, for example, an imperial feminism (see Amos & Parmar, 1984) on to the knowledge, power and being of one party. Therefore, although we attempted to implement a flat, 'gender neutral' structure in our receiving of the *ukhamba*, it became clear that it was to be the male leader that was to receive it on behalf of the ISHS. Our terms of engagement were resisted in this sense. Rather than assuming an essentialised interpretation of gendered performances, common to many Western bourgeois feminisms, we remain mindful that African feminisms resist monolithic representations of gendered enactments that tend to yield static and often oppressive readings of sociocultural relations of the Other. As such, we continue to engage with undoubtedly gendered moments such as these through ongoing conversations with community members, who both critique and support community social justice efforts that are explicitly and implicitly undergirded by patriarchal assumptions and practices. It is through situated and participatory analyses that we may then develop gender equitable praxes that are sensitive to the "myriad gender relations, practices and identities in Africa" (Lewis, 2001

p. 4), while at the same time remain critical of patriarchal practice. All of this serves to remind that decolonisation is a project as much about race, as it is about gender, as it is about everyday enactments, and as it is about a host of organised knowledge systems. Accordingly, decoloniality must assume expansive approaches to liberation.

Concluding Remarks

Almost 60 years after Frantz Fanon's death, the decolonial turn in psychology remains as urgent and relevant as ever. In this chapter, we grapple with the complexities of revitalising the decolonial turn in critical community psychology by reflecting on a moment of community-driven epistemic disobedience within the university, a setting that has traditionally been typified by coloniality and epistemic violence. We examine this moment not as a means of positing reflexivity as a decolonising end in and of itself, but rather to present the insidiousness of coloniality even within work that strives towards decoloniality. In this way, we also pronounce the importance that epistemic disobedience serves within the project of decolonisation.

Following our reflexive analysis, albeit a single moment interpreted through a decolonising lens, we suggest that our reading is instructive for the contributions of critical community psychologists whose liberatory praxes seek to transform knowledge arrangements and institutionalised practices, expose the ubiquity of coloniality and uncover the imprints of power that characterise our disciplinary and ontological positions. While it is not our intention here to offer formulaic recommendations, we encourage critical community psychologists to undertake what Teo (2018) refers to as meta-reflexivity. In our context, meta-reflexivity functions to problematise the social and epistemological order and entails reflecting on and assessing how, or if, community-engaged work appreciates the project of decoloniality. While meta-reflexivity requires that critical community psychologists continually challenge themselves and one another, we argue that the transformatory potential of the meta-reflexive process is enhanced considerably in and through the interpersonal and inter-subjective context inherent to our engagements with communities.

In this chapter, we examine a particular event, as well as the manner by which it was disrupted—neither of which was entirely decolonising in its constitution. Yet, considered together, both demonstrate the deep-seated complexities of decolonisation, which are not always identified by actors of decolonisation themselves. Instead of dismissing or revering in absolute terms moments such as these, we argue that they should be placed under dialectical scrutiny; that is, we should perceive them as moving between decoloniality and coloniality, sometimes simultaneously. In heeding these moments, we may gain greater insights into how better to enhance the decolonising potentialities of our work. The presentation of the *ukhamba* as a decolonising insurgence of community voice should not be interpreted as a pure or perfect kind of decolonising praxis. Rather, it may be considered as a means of understanding the uneven grounds of decolonisation, and as a platform through which to explore the role of epistemic disobedience—as well as (meta-)reflexivity—in challenging, reformulating and dismantling zones of being and non-being within and beyond critical community psychologies.

References

Adams, G., Dobles, I., Gómez, L. H., Kurtiş, T., & Molina, L. E. (2015). Decolonizing psychological science: Introduction to the special thematic section. *Journal of Social and Political Psychology, 3*(1), 213–238.

Adams, G., Gómez, L. H., Kurtiş, T., Molina, L. E., & Dobles, I. (2017). Notes on decolonizing psychology: From one special issue to another. *South Africa Journal of Psychology, 47*(4), 531–541.

Amos, V., & Parmar, P. (1984). Challenging imperial feminism. *Feminist Review, 17*, 3–19.

Campbell, J. (2011). *Today's university: Mimicry versus creativity, presented at Decolonising our universities*. Paper presented at the fourth Multiversity Conference.

Coimbra, J. L., Duckett, P., Fryer, D., Makkawi, I., Menezes, I., Seedat, M., & Walker, C. (2012). Rethinking community psychology: Critical insights. *The Australian Community Psychologist, 24*(2), 135–142.

Fanon, F. (1963). *The wretched of the earth*. Grove Press.

Fanon, F. (1967). *Black skin, white masks*. Grove Press.

Fowler, K. D. (2006). Classification and collapse: The ethnohistory of Zulu ceramic use. *South African Humanities, 18*, 93–117.

Fryer, D. (2008). Some questions about "the history of community psychology". *Journal of Community Psychology, 36*, 572–586.

Galtung, J. (1969). Violence, peace, and peace research. *Journal of Peace Research, 6*(3), 167–191.

Galtung, J. (1990). Cultural violence. *Journal of Peace Research, 27*(3), 291–305.

Gokani, R. (2011). Marxian currents in Latin and North American community psychology. *Annual Review of Critical Psychology, 9*, 110–117.
Gordon, L. R. (2017). When justice is not enough: Toward the decolonization of normative life. In F. F. Bragato & L. R. Gordon (Eds.), *Geopolitics and decolonization: Perspectives from the global south* (pp. 39–48). Rowman & Littlefield.
Grosfoguel, R., Oso, L., & Christou, A. (2015). 'Racism', intersectionality and migration studies: Some theoretical reflections. *Identities, 22*(6), 635–652.
Jolles, F. (2005). The origins of the twentieth century Zulu beer vessel styles. *South African Humanities, 17*, 101–151.
Lewis, D. (2001). African feminisms. *Agenda, 16*(50), 4–10.
Maldonado-Torres, N. (2016). *Outline of ten theses on coloniality and decoloniality.* Fondation Frantz Fanon. http://frantzfanonfoundation-fondationfrantzfanon.com/IMG/pdf/maldonado-torres_outline_of_ten_theses-10.23.16_.pdf
Maldonado-Torres, N. (2017). Frantz Fanon and the decolonial turn in psychology: From modern/colonial methods to the decolonial attitude. *South Africa Journal of Psychology, 47*(4), 432–441.
Mbembe, A. (2001). *On the postcolony*. University of California Press.
Mignolo, W. D. (2009). Epistemic disobedience, independent thought and decolonial freedom. *Theory, Culture & Society, 26*(7–8), 159–181.
Ngũgĩ wa, T.'o. (2009). *Something torn and new: An African renaissance.* Basic Civitas Books.
Oyěwùmí, O. (1997). *The invention of women: Making an African sense of western gender discourses.* University of Minnesota Press.
Reich, J., Liebenberg, L., Denny, M., Battiste, H., Bernard, A., Christmas, K., Dennis, R., Denny, D., Knockwood, I., Nicholas, R., & Paul, H. (2017). In this together: Relational accountability and meaningful research and dissemination with youth. *International Journal of Qualitative Methods, 16*(1), 1–12.
Rodríguez, S. S., Guerra, C. T., Villarreal, L. F. G., & Bohórquez, R. V. (2009). Psychological accompaniment: Construction of cultures of peace among a community affected by war. In M. Montero & C. C. Sonn (Eds.), *Psychology of liberation* (pp. 221–235). Springer.
Sacipa, S., Vidales, R., Galindo, L., & Tovar, C. (2007). Psychosocial accompaniment to liberate the suffering associated with the experience of forced displacement. *Universitas Psychologica, 6*(3), 589–600.
Said, E. W. (1978). *Orientalism*. Pantheon Books.
Seedat, M., & Suffla, S. (2017). Community psychology and its (dis)contents, archival legacies and decolonisation. *South Africa Journal of Psychology, 47*(4), 421–431.
Spivak, G. C. (1988). Can the subaltern speak? In L. Grossberg & C. Nelson (Eds.), *Marxism and the interpretation of culture* (pp. 271–313). University of Illinois Press.
Statistics South Africa. (2011). *Community profile databases.* https://census2011.adrianfrith.com/
Teo, T. (2018). *Outline of theoretical psychology: Critical investigations.* Palgrave Macmillan.

Viola, J. J., & Glantsman, O. (2017). Introduction. In J. J. Viola & O. Glantsman (Eds.), *Diverse careers in community psychology* (pp. xxv–xxxi). Oxford University Press.

Watkins, M. (2015). Psychosocial accompaniment. *Journal of Social and Political Psychology, 3*(1), 324–341.

Yen, J. (2008). A history of community psychology in South Africa. In C. van Ommen & D. Painter (Eds.), *Interiors: A history of psychology in South Africa* (pp. 385–412). Unisa Press.

9

Options: Conversation in Collaboration

Hannah Denton, Mark Haydon-Laurelut, Duncan Moss, Angela Paterson Foster, and Jan Shepherd

In this chapter we hope to convey our experience of using the 'Options' model: a brief consultation approach originally developed in an Adult Mental Health setting. This collaborative and non-pathologising way of working draws on a hybrid of ideas and practices from Community Psychology and Social Constructionist therapy.

Prologue

> *Where do we start when we want to give an account of our experience? How do we honour the complexity and 'polyvocality' of life?* (Gergen, 1999)

H. Denton (✉) • A. Paterson Foster
Sussex Partnership Trust, East Sussex, UK
e-mail: Hannah.Denton@sussexpartnership.nhs.uk

M. Haydon-Laurelut
Department of Psychology, University of Portsmouth/Sussex Partnership NHS Foundation Trust, West Sussex, UK

D. Moss
Department of Clinical Psychology, Plymouth University, Devon, UK

J. Shepherd
Health in Mind, East Sussex, UK

C. Walker et al. (eds.), *The Palgrave Handbook of Innovative Community and Clinical Psychologies*, https://doi.org/10.1007/978-3-030-71190-0_9

As four authors we want to honour our differing 'voices', rather than homogenise into a single narrative. We hope, in doing this, to achieve two things. One is to keep alive something we each hold true (in our own way) conceptually: there is danger in reduction, in creating accounts that hide multiplicity, uncertainty, contradiction and—yes—even confusion. In doing so, we draw from the Social Constructionist tradition where:

> *constructionism invites a collaborative and polyvocal orientation toward inquiry. There is less demand for hierarchy—and solid ground to distinguish between good and bad.* (Mattes & Schraube, 2004, para. 18)

Secondly, we would like to offer in the process of writing this chapter some kind of mirroring—in process—of the 'Options' Service that we are here to describe. So we want to start (as perhaps someone using our Service might start) with going back into the past. From there each narrative takes a different tack, but in our wandering and wondering, we hope we have given at least a flavour of some of the philosophy, ethos, practices, procedures and most importantly 'the feel' for each of us, of working within this quietly radical model.

And, as with an Options session we will at the end offer a 'reflecting team'—a further commentary, through conversation, of what we have heard in reading each other's accounts, and where for each, this may leave us, at the end of the session and the end of the chapter.

Duncan's Story

I want to reflect on how I wondered into Options.

The threads to this go back to multiple places. Some I can place from undergraduate encounters.

I had the great good fortune of studying as an undergraduate with two radical psychological thinkers—John Shotter (see Shotter, 2012) and David Smail (see Smail, 2005). There is no space here of course to do much other than 'name check' these prolific writers or do even remote justice to their perspective. In brief though, they had established for many a huge question mark over the 'project' of therapy. In John Shotter's case what I most recall is that he introduced for me the idea of the 'hermeneutic circle', a circle where we can never interpret the world free from social constructed values and assumptions.

The hermeneutic circle seems to interfere with, if not absolutely preclude the possibility of, objective knowledge. This is so because our reasoning would seem to be circular. For example, a description of circular interpretation or hermeneutics of emotion given by the philosopher Charles Taylor regarding the emotion 'shame':

> *'Shame' can only be explained by reference to other concepts which in turn cannot be understood without reference to shame. To understand these concepts we have to be in on a certain experience, we have to understand a certain language, not just of words, but also a certain language of mutual action and communication, by which we blame, exhort, admire, esteem each other* (Taylor, 1973: 58).

Exploring the hermeneutic circle at that time was one of these 'defining moments', where we don't quite see the world the same afterwards. If, put simply, the circle shows that we can only perceive and understand through 'lenses' laden and shaped by personal, family and cultural values and assumptions, what—to cut to the chase—is happening when a therapist suggests to a client what is wrong with them?

In David Smail's case, he actively (and explicitly) questioned the potency of therapy from my very first encounter with him. His first teaching session with us undergraduates involved him playing tapes of his sessions as a therapist, to highlight how therapy doesn't work (or at least doesn't work 'magically' beyond the modest gains of comfort, encouragement and a little illumination).

In a nutshell David Smail's perspective, and in his own words, is this:-

> *Hardly any of the 'symptoms' of psychological distress may correctly be seen as medical matters. The so-called psychiatric 'disorders' are nothing to do with faulty biology, nor indeed are they the outcome of individual moral weakness or other personal failing. They are the creation of the social world in which we live, and that world is structured by power. … One cannot hope to understand the phenomena of psychological distress, nor begin to think what can be done about them, without an analysis of how power is distributed and exercised within society* (Cited in Tweedy, 2016: 208).

This perspective did not arrive via a defining moment but was more almost as a reluctant and gradual process of dis-illusion as I gradually let go of my own dreams of therapeutic magic (and that letting go came through both receiving and offering therapy).

So, coming to train and practice as a Clinical Psychologist, both deeply sceptical of the claims to objectivity and potency of Therapy, was not a comfortable ride. But the final encounter I want to share here, crucially, helped scaffold a space that could honour such uncomfortable truths and yet still carry on offering a tentatively helpful conversational space.

And it was on my first placement with a busy London Psychological Therapies Service for Adults, steeped in individual-focused Psychodynamic Psychotherapy. By chance I was introduced to a psychologist in the team called Karen Partridge. Karen, as it turned out, was at the forefront of attempts by brave practitioners influenced by the thinking current at the time in family therapy, to bring such ideas into this less obviously welcoming realm of individual Psychotherapy (see Partridge et al., 1985).

Many of these ideas can be distilled down to a practice—the practice of the 'reflecting team', but really for me at that time it boiled down to an invitation, in the midst of a therapy session with an individual, for Karen and I to pause, and to start to speak about what we might be 'up to'—in other words to publicly walk around our hermeneutic circle. With this I noticed came a giving up of mystique and power, but also a strange kind of solidarity between the three of us, that I felt David Smail would approve of. This was a therapeutic space made visible for what it was—a tentative, collaborative, space of 'Safe Uncertainty' (Mason, 1993). Overall, it's hard to overestimate how this first 'reflecting team' experience just broke a 'frame'—somewhat like breaking the 'fourth wall' (the pretence to not 'see' the audience) in acting. So many things flowed through that breached wall, and one of them was Options.

Jan's Story

The first sparks of Options began in the mid-1990s with the government's expectation that the Community Mental Health Teams (CMHTs) should focus attention on clients with severe and enduring mental health difficulties. Suddenly many people with less severe mental health problems that had routinely been referred to the CMHTs by their GPs, no longer had a service. In response to this dilemma, a local group of managers, clinicians and primary healthcare staff, of which Duncan and I were a part, gathered to find a way of addressing the problem. The goal was to develop a way of offering a brief mental health intervention to primary care patients with little or no specified funding and taking advantage of the mental health skills and experience found throughout the healthcare system—both statutory and community/voluntary. In the room were people interested and skilled in a variety of approaches: drawing on ideas from narrative therapy (e.g. Epston & White, 1990; Freedman & Combs, 1996), social constructionism (e.g. Gergen, 1999), systemic approaches (e.g. Andersen, 1987; Anderson, 1997) and community psychology (e.g. Kagan et al., 2011) as well as brief, single session and solution-focused ways of working (e.g. De Shazer & Berg, 1997; Hoyt, 2000). The question was: how could we develop a brief, effective, mental health and well-being intervention that made the most of the range of experience, knowledge and perspectives available in community mental health services?

After a phase of exploration, and building on ideas already being used locally (Jones et al., 1997), the model of 'Options' was conceived.

Part of the model was to ensure that the service was as accessible as possible and that the decision to access the service was handed over to the client—this meant that the GP sent in a referral and also gave the client information about the service. It was then up to the client to contact the service and book an appointment (Seager, 1991). Clients were offered between one and three sessions with a *single session* expectation, that is that one session could well be all that was needed to enable the client to find a way forward. Each session involved two practitioners. One, whom we called the 'interviewer', started the conversation by inviting the client to share their story, difficulties or what brought them to the service. The other, whom we called the 'reflector', would 'sit back' and listen. At the point in the conversation where there was a pause in their account, when it seemed that enough of the story had been told to grasp the issues, the 'interviewer' would invite the client to 'sit back' and listen whilst the two practitioners had a conversation where they shared any thoughts or ideas that they had. These might include the impact of the story, any themes, strengths and resources (that sometimes the client might not have recognised), dilemmas and ideas about ways forward. After this short conversation, the 'interviewer' would return to the client and ask them to comment on what they found helpful or unhelpful in listening to this conversation, explicitly asking them to comment on what did not fit with them. The 'interviewer' would follow what the client had picked up on so the client was in charge of the direction of the ensuing conversation. This *reflecting team* approach allowed clients to take a step back from the problems they had brought to the session, and to listen to their own story from an alternative perspective along with the different thoughts and ideas discussed by the two practitioners. In addition to the therapeutic element of this intervention, there was also a wide range of information and contact details for local community and support organisations that would be shared with the client if appropriate.

The service was offered in GP surgeries and community venues and staffed by a range of practitioners including mental health nurses, health visitors, volunteers from local community services, counsellors and psychologists. During any Options appointment we paid attention to the mix of practitioners, ensuring that every session was led or supported by a practitioner experienced in the way of working. At the end of each session there was time for a short debrief or supervision. A local group of GPs supported an initial pilot of the service and the evaluation showed that the service model offered good outcomes for clients as well as reducing GP attendance (Shepherd, 2000, unpublished MSc Dissertation). As support and enthusiasm for the service grew, it attracted a small amount of funding from local National Health Service (NHS) commissioners, and developed to cover most of the county. Apart from some local GP counsellors, Options was the only primary care mental health service for several years. Unfortunately during the commissioning process for the Improving Access to Psychological Therapies (IAPT) programme the funding for Options ended.

Hannah's Story

I first started working in the Options service when I was a newly qualified counsellor. I was immediately drawn to the approach. Initially this was the warmth and openness of the therapists involved but as I learned more I also valued the rejection of the expert position in favour of genuine curiosity in understanding another person's life world, focusing on whatever the client wanted to rather than driven by prior assumptions or the demands of the organisation, and offering ideas and tentative suggestions but without any expectations about which direction the client might choose to go. I also enjoyed the breadth of what might be considered helpful, rather than assuming a 'traditional' therapy was optimal, suggestions might range from sports and community groups to political activism depending on the client's story. These values have ended up influencing the way I have worked throughout my career.

As a counsellor you rarely get the opportunity to do therapeutic work with another therapist. As an inexperienced practitioner I initially took on the role of 'reflector'. This gave me the chance to watch another person engage a client in a therapeutic conversation. It felt both a privilege and a great opportunity to learn from practitioners with more experience than myself. It was fascinating to see the different stories about the person develop as the 'interviewing' therapist asked gently inquiring questions. I always enjoyed being in the reflecting role. It was an opportunity to 'sit back' and allow my mind to be free to wonder as I did not have the task of generating questions or deciding in which direction to go. It was a chance to be in a different space whilst still being in the conversation, with both the information provided by the client and a sense of how they interacted with another: to have the time to really try to understand the experience of the client and how they see their world and themselves within in.

The moment when the person taking the 'interviewer position' turned to me to ask whether I had any thoughts was always a nerve-wracking moment. As a newly qualified counsellor having an experienced practitioner being interested in any ideas I had was always quite surprising. The attitude of openness offered to the client was also brought to the reflecting conversation and as long as I also participated with same degree of curiosity, tentativeness and acceptance that my view was mine then there was a freedom to share any thoughts or ideas however unformed they may be. The fact that each therapist and the client would all have slightly different understanding and ideas was celebrated rather than one version was seen as the truth. It was an interesting experience to invite the client to observe us, our conversation and any ideas we had. Like laying your cards on the table and saying what do you think? Is any of this any use? Or do you have other ideas that we can explore together?

As I became more experienced I started to more often take the lead role in sessions. Although it could be exposing, having another practitioner watching me as I worked, it could also be incredibly supportive. If it was a practitioner I knew well then I was confident that they had 'my back' and that if I did not have any useful ideas then they would. And it was always interesting to see what they were curious about and what I might have totally missed. As I was still fairly inexperienced it also challenged my belief that I was not very good as I was being observed working clinically by people I respected and no one came out of sessions saying 'you cannot do this!'. Now that I have been working as a psychologist for many years I really value having had this experience as I feel very comfortable having other practitioners join me for assessment and review sessions without an anxious need to always be getting it 'right' and appearing the 'expert'.

Even after many Options sessions I still felt a moment of discomfort when telling the client that this was going to be the time that I was going to talk to the other practitioner. Was this going to be the time that the client would hate it, it is after all breaking rules of conversation. This rarely happened however and most often when you returned to the client their first statement was about feeling really heard. And heard by two people who were interested and thinking about their story not just one. When it worked well the sessions felt engaged, supportive, creative, opening and warm. A particular kind of relationship seemed to develop and most clients seemed to find just the one session helpful.

I ended up in a service development role for Options and a part of this was training and working with people with little experience in the model. I also undertook a qualitative evaluation of the service (Denton & Michie, 2006). This gave me a chance to see what did not work so well. Joining together with another worker who did not share the same values, in particular not wanting to reflect and be tentative, would also feel at odds with what we were trying to do. Although there was some space for a range of professionals, including those that preferred to work from an expert model, this only worked if they owned their position and reflected on there being other just as valid ideas. There is a danger that this way of working could be disempowering if the practitioners shared their ideas in a dismissing way or with a fixed agenda or pre-established plan: no one wants two 'experts' in a room telling them what to do.

Mark's Story

Theories, Feelings and Practices

I joined Options in 2000 already having an interest in systemic and social constructionist ideas through my work with people with learning disabilities. I was drawn to the theoretical influences of the service, chiefly social constructionism (Gergen, 1999), which considers the importance of language in creating shared realities—post-modernism (Lyotard, 1984), with its focus on the importance of local knowledges, and the Co-ordinated Management of Meaning (CMM) (Pearce, 2007) with its attention to the multi-contextual ways in which communication processes make our social worlds. Important as these ideas are they do not capture the experience of working with the service. Below I will describe in session practices.

Having a Conversation

Options is a place where three (or more) people *come together to have a conversation*. The sessions most often involved two practitioners and one client. The word *'conversation'* is important and is, unlike *'assessment'* or *'intervention'*, implicitly reciprocal. This give-and-take form of interaction implies that we cannot know before or outside of a particular talk with a client what will or should occur. In the Options model one person volunteers to *'begin the conversation'*. They are not the lead therapist and they may or may not be the most experienced person in the room. They are the person who begins to talk first. The conversations I have participated in might appear by turns quite chatty, serious and sometimes involving humour. This is perhaps not what 'therapy' would be assumed to consist of.

Community in Mind

A part of this approach concerns consideration about who and what the conversation might include. Communities are persons in language, ideas, practices and ways of making sense. They are epistemological (they have ideas about what counts as knowledge) and ontological (they have ideas about what exists). Communities are therefore much more than the physical spaces we inhabit. Knowledge of self and world is constructed in community. We may inhabit them but they also inhabit us. An Options session doesn't have an entire physical community in the room but has community in mind. In addition to the wealth of local resources clients would be introduced to (see Jan and Hannah's Story), in considering the metaphor of *'practising from a park bench'* (Moss, 2002), the three-person conversations look out towards the contexts within which the difficulties that brought people to their General Practitioners and Options are co-created. How to practise this? Relational questions support this approach that, in common with systemic practice more generally, seek to go beyond individualisation, psychologisation and medicalisation of difficult experiences. These questions can take the following kind of forms:

> *What ideas did you have about coming here today?*
> *If we finished our hour here together and you felt this had been a worthwhile talk, what kinds of things would we have discussed?*
> *Who else might have a view about this? What would they say if they heard what I had just heard?*
> *What kinds of ideas about 'X' (gender, age, race, disability, religion, sexuality, feeling anxious, becoming unemployed …) have you encountered?*
> *Which ideas might be useful/not useful to you right now?*

These kinds of questions support the client to lead the direction of the talk, offer the possibility for opening up and developing new stories and reframe the issues across multiple contexts beyond the self.

Warming the Context

Unusual forms of practice are not useful if the client is unable to connect with and make sense of them. This kind of practice (in particular the reflecting conversation between practitioners) was (and remains) somewhat unusual. Warm ideas according to Burnham (2005) are more likely to survive than 'cold' ones and so in order to warm the context in an Options session the issue of seeing two practitioners might be addressed by using non-technical language to explain that *'three heads can be better than two'.* We also explained using non-jargon filled language, as Hannah noted earlier, that one person will *'sit back and listen'* to the conversation (importantly their role was not to observe the person called 'client' but to observe the exchange itself) and that once we have heard what the listener has to say we can comment upon it together if we wish.

> ***We think you should think like this.*** (Shotter, 2007: 22)

Let us consider the reflecting team (RT) model a little further. Family therapy had prior to the RT adopted a model wherein a therapist and client(s) would have a conversation whilst another team of therapists (often students and a supervisor) would sit behind a one-way mirror. The team behind the mirror would have conversations unheard by client and therapist and would at some point in the session often deliver a therapeutic message to the family. Tom Andersen turned the practice on its head. He switched on the lights and the audio in the team room and asked them to speak so that the family could hear and subsequently have an opportunity to respond. This became known as the reflecting team and latterly, to highlight the important processes of dialogue and reflection rather than the structure of this particular practice, reflecting processes. For Shotter (2007) writing about Andersen's work, Tom had a feeling—not a theoretical insight—not the implementation of a piece of decontextualised 'evidence' rather a sense, a moral intuition that he did not want to continue to tell people how to live, to tell people:

> *'we think you should think like this', they (Tom Andersen and his team), felt the unpleasantness of it. For in effect they were saying, you should stop thinking like you do, and start thinking like us; it was about telling other people how they should live their lives. They could not continue with it.* (Shotter, 2007: 22)

My experience of Options was very much a three-way collaborative conversation where we looked out onto the world together and thought about how a person might go on in their lives. We might offer ideas but not blueprints for how we thought people should live.

Witnessing, Uncertainty and Dialogue

Uncertainty and the witnessing of a person's story are key aspects of an Options conversation. People are asked to say more as they elaborate their stories. If a person brought a story they were struggling to live with connections were made with key points, questions asked about alternative views and meanings. I characterise my Options experiences with words such as dialogue, conversation, reflection and not-knowing (Anderson & Goolishian, 1992). An Options session was (and I understand is) not a place for diagnosing, inducting people into (or out of) the language of the mental health profession, focusing only on the 'deficits' a person brings or indeed refusing to talk about difficulties and problems in favour of talking only of solutions.

The conversations I had were dialogical. What I said felt like an unfinished offering subsequently shaped by the contributions of the two others. These conversations are alive to in-the-moment possibilities, responsive and in my experience of being an Options practitioner often very useful conversations for those who took part in them.

Angie's Story

I had been in the mental health system for many years and, despite receiving a range of interventions and treatments, was still in a place where my mental health was not improving and my medication was continually being raised. When the situation came to a head, with near fatal consequences, I was referred for an Options session, in Adult Mental Health Services, to try a different form of therapy.

From the first session it felt more of an equal environment to previous experiences in mental health services. I was taken aback by being able to witness the counsellors actually processing the information I had relayed. It was affirming to hear that the counsellors had listened to what I had been saying. It can be difficult to get perspective when you are feeling very angry and overwhelmed. Listening to them talk helped me to rationalise what had felt messy in my head. The experience felt calming and gave a space to think and to think differently, with moments when the penny dropped when I could see things from different angles. I had heard my story from my perspective for many years but to hear other people tell my story allowed me to be interested again and this was engaging and refreshing. I started to work harder as a result. Although I was the 'patient' with two 'professionals' it felt like three people in the room so I did not feel intimidated and was able to share whatever I wanted. It also seemed effective and productive for the counsellors as they processed the information by talking with each other. I had left previous one-to-one counselling sessions feeling anxious, and had gone back to dysfunctional behaviour, because of having no idea about how the counsellor viewed what I had just said. Hearing the ideas of the counsellors allowed a sense of closure. The experience was a revelation as I left feeling empowered and validated.

I feel I came into my first Options sessions as a whirlwind of anxiety and angst, that was all consuming, and by the last session I felt I had the tools to be able to deal a lot more constructively with the issues that had brought me to the therapy in the first place. I felt sad to leave but did not feel abandoned as I had done at the end of previous therapies. Options felt like a catalyst to getting on the road to recovery, to being able to live a functional, successful and happy life. It was important to know that I could always get back in touch if I needed another session.

I look back with fondness on Options as it seems like that was when my life started to change. In this therapy I did not feel like a sick person. I was no longer a label or a statistic. I felt like a respected individual. During the 5 years since my last Options session I have conquered my eating disorder having struggled for 25 years, come off all medication, climbed Kilimanjaro, am happily married in a functional and healthy relationship and am about to sell my very successful business.

Reflections

Duncan

So I guess we can just tune into how we feel right now and how it felt writing that section? In some ways it flowed quite easily and that in itself was a surprise because I thought it would be too remote or hard to dredge up but actually it felt very fresh.

Hannah

I found it surprisingly easy to write, and it is has been a real pleasure to meet up again. And one of the things that struck me was how much those ideas, even though it might not be 'Options' exactly any more, have been significant throughout what I have done since.

Mark

I also have found that although I have not worked for Options for some time now the ideas and experiences have stayed with me.

Angie

It has been really positive for me to share my story and show that you can recover with the right help and support. After having years of counselling, and going round in circles, I feel passionate about this way of doing therapy. It feels a shame it wasn't available to me sooner as I could have avoided some of the turmoil.

Jan

It has actually been really nice to have a reason to sit down and tell a bit of the story of Options. That actually felt quite a special thing to do. Because I think Options is quite a unique service and, although we have kind of all stepped away from it in different ways, it is kind of, in the service I have something to do with, it has kept going. It has enough strength of itself. So it has been really nice to have a reason to acknowledge that this is a unique model, that can be really helpful. It is quite a powerful model, both with how staff respond to it as well as clients. And to have a reason to write that down and map that out.

H

I always enjoy revisiting and reconnecting to the ideas because they, well there is that sort of interesting paradox, they are quite subversive ideas, you know, they don't fit in the medical model, they don't really fit in the NHS, and yet somehow they persist. People keep wanting to come back to them. So it keeps going despite the fact … and I love that it is a bit subversive and challenging and different. And that makes it surprising that it somehow survives.

D

Just in the spirit of talking about the impact personally of doing this process, I remember now that I felt quite sad writing it thinking about the people I mention as having been influences on me, as they have all recently died and there was almost a kind of panic connected to that. A sense that these ideas could disappear and I felt both a little sad and anxious about that. The order of things in general do not support these ideas

H

No, if anything we are moving further and further away from them.

J

Absolutely, we definitely are.

H

And there is not … fundamental to Options is having that space to think isn't it, like the reflecting conversation is thinking out loud, it is really forcing a thinking space into the session and most of the services now seem to be built on not having time to think. That is a privilege that we don't have any more. And there is another paradox isn't there because maybe there would only be one session. And yet there would be space. Whereas now you have got more sessions and yet no space.

D

I remember I used to use this metaphor in Options training that if you have only got a very short time with someone you have got to act as if you have all the time in the world.

J

In the middle of writing this I had to go and do some teaching on Options for another service that was possibly interested in the model and one of the things that I find, when I do some teaching, people always start of being skeptical. And what I say is what you need to do to learn it, is to do it. And that spaciousness of doing it helps people to connect. Because there is a lot of spaciousness around this particular way of working, it is not pressured, it is not 'have to do this' or 'have to do this', there is a framework and within that framework there is a lot of space for people to sit back, think and listen. And people really value that.

A

I totally agree with this. It was really important for me to have space to sit and think whilst the counsellors were talking. In one-to-one counselling you are doing all the talking so you do not have time to process. It also seemed that the counsellors were able to use the space to process their ideas. And that this created a way of us all being able to think and work together on problems in a very equal way.

D

I think for me that is one of the things I was most struck by reading Mark's account because although Mark does draw on some philosophical or theoretical ideas actually for me the thread of his account is about the human level, it is about for example Tom Anderson just feeling that it didn't feel right to have a reflecting that was out of ear shot. And I think that the thing about these ideas, that although they can be esoteric, there is, I think, a way that we were inspired at a very human level by their implications of how we can just be as human beings together in a space and that is anything but esoteric or philosophical. About human beings valuing conversations where power is shared and named and where there is an honouring of the sense of multiplicity and inconsistency and dilemmas and not wrapping things up in a tidy way. And yet the very act of being heard powerfully can have a validating, encouraging, and comforting impact which is actually one of the things that David Smail wrote about. What we can offer is that sense of solidarity, sense of collective encouragement and validation, which are human things which are not magic and they are not technical.

H

They just require a kind of stance don't they.

D

They require a stance that allows, like a door that opens to just to let that in, and be contained in a slightly scaffolded way.

H

And maybe there is … because I think in Options there are all these paradoxes, all these things that sit alongside each other that maybe don't obviously don't sit alongside each other, and that is why so difficult for people to understand it until they do it, until they have that felt experience of doing it and then it makes sense.

M

I am glad you raised this Duncan, Jan and Hannah as I was initially attracted by the ideas and then as I began to work in the service with all three of you in different sessions and with different clients it was in that space of practice that I experienced both common themes (of witnessing, sharing, opening up possibilities) and also how the conversations were unique.

J

One of the things that I really liked about doing this chapter was reading each other's accounts because they are so different. There are different perspectives and they have paid attention to different things and brought different things alive in a way that was really kind of helpful and interesting. It reminded me of the way that the model works that we have each brought a different voice to make this work.

D

I suppose I am just thinking about the future, about all of this, for me I am distinguishing between these ideas being held by a service and these ideas being held almost in private and that they come out implicitly. And I think there are advantages and disadvantages to both. For me that has been my journey into just holding these more implicitly. But there are some advantages to that because you haven't got the weight of trying to maintain an organisation and an articulation of that. And the dangers that we did often experience in Options of it getting eroded. And it is almost like, again paradoxically, the bigger it got the more likely it was to get eroded and there were drivers that were increasingly coming into Options like well 'couldn't you get by with just one of you', or we wouldn't have as much time for training or reflective practice etc.

H

Measuring, risk assessments ….

J

And those things, certainly trying to negotiate a way for Options to have the space to be as it is within a context where there is constant push of targets, and just being allowed to trust, have that space to be open and just see what comes up and what happens without having to dictate what it is or to make it something and it is, to hold that space, in the midst of a very tight framework or a service is actually a real challenge.

D

Because that is one thing we haven't really talked about, or we haven't also had here, I guess that the spirit of the Options Manager and other people who managerially for many years, the best years of Options, held a kind of gap that was almost like an invisible gap between the edges of the Options service and the pressures and the demands of the general management of mental health services. If that gap hadn't been there for a while I don't think we could ever really have created the container in the way that we did. And I think the Manager, and others, did a lot of work behind the scenes to just hold at bay, and I think that is another context of the spaciousness that we are talking about in the sessions was also mirrored in a certain kind of spaciousness allowed to us for a while and as that space began to collapse I think it then did begin to be in danger of eroding Options even if Options had then been recommissioned. In a way that might have been the worst outcome, that it could have remained in name only, recommissioned but lost its teeth because that space had collapsed in. For me it worked best as a kind of cottage industry. If you try to host an innovative idea in a very un-innovative way and that you make it party to all the usual scaffolding and pressures then it actually loses essentially what it is. In a nutshell that is what could have happened to Options if it had become integrated into IAPT.

J

I hear what you are saying, about how can you hold that space as it should be in the midst of a targeted service. It is not … it just takes a lot of work. But it feels to me like, without those spaces, what would the service be like. Without any of those spaces. For the staff as well.

D

And what we haven't written so much into our accounts is if we just talk about the experience of being part of the options, Hannah you talked about this in yours, about the experience of your own wellbeing as a practitioner, and there is a whole other story on a human level of stressed mental health workers being able to sit in a room with another colleague sharing, and really sharing, the human experience of trying to offer help.

J

So one of the interesting things is that in some of the places where Options works, some of the practitioners would say that having that space and working with other colleagues in this way is one of the things that enables them to cope with a stressful work environment.

H

I am aware of the time, any final thoughts before we end.

D

For me I would like to hold again the contradictory and paradoxical range of emotions we have expressed thinking about the future, or the past of Options, is that sense of both optimism, a sense of hope and possibility but also a sense of melancholy, sadness, anger, dissolution, and I kind of wouldn't like to narrow it down to any one of those emotions and hold them all. And I don't really have a strong allegiance to any one of those emotions in relation to this. I feel that mix.

J

Yes, I think I would second that.

Final Thoughts

Although we have not written a conventional chapter or how-to manual we hope we have managed to convey a sense of Options by describing our personal experience of being involved in the service. It is an approach based on a number of different influences and so we would encourage you to follow up on the references if you want to explore these ideas further. Although in Options the ideas were formed into a service, with a particular framework that provided a scaffolding, they can also be used more implicitly as an individual therapist, practitioner or even manager. They underpin a stance, a way of having a conversation with another, rather than a particular model, and a stance that perhaps sits at the edge, or in the gaps of other large-scale and more dominant services and ideas. In our experience, this is where Options often fits, with clients whose presentations are more complicated or who may not be in a position to make the most of a longer focused therapy intervention. They may have current life problems and more complex issues, have had several therapeutic interventions that have not been helpful or simply not have the time and space for a longer therapy intervention. For staff there is also a lot to offer in this model: an opportunity to work with colleagues, to learn from each other and to receive live feedback and affirmation—a rare spacious and innovative therapeutic window in a frequently pressured context.

References

Andersen, T. (1987). The reflecting team: Dialogue and meta-dialogue in clinical work. *Family Process, 26*(4), 415–428.

Anderson, H. (1997). *Conversation, language and possibilities. A postmodern approach to therapy*. Basic Books.

Anderson, H., & Goolishian, H. (1992). The client is the expert: A not knowing approach to therapy. In S. McNamee & K. Gergen (Eds.), *Therapy as social construction*. Sage.

Burnham, J. (2005). Relational reflexivity: A tool for socially constructing therapeutic relationships. In C. Flaskas, B. Mason, & A. Perlesz (Eds.), *The space between: Experience, context, and process in the therapeutic relationship*. Karnac Books.

De Shazer, S., & Berg, I. K. (1997). 'What works?' Remarks on research aspects of solution-focused brief therapy. *Journal of Family Therapy, 19*(2), 121–124.

Denton, H., & Michie, F. (2006). Users' experience of an innovative primary care service: An in-depth exploration. *Primary Care Mental Health, 4*(4), 235.

Epston, D., & White, M. (1990). *Narrative means to therapeutic ends*. W.W. Norton.

Freedman, J., & Combs, G. (1996). *Narrative therapy. The social construction of preferred realities*. Norton & Company.

Gergen, K. J. (1999). *An invitation to social construction*. Sage.

Hoyt, M. F. (2000). Some stories are better that others. Doing what works best in brief therapy and managed care. *Clinical Psychology Forum, 23*, 21–26.

Jones, S., Moss, D., & Holtom, R. (1997). A consultation service to adults referred as having mental health problems. *Clinical Psychology Forum, 105*, 21–26.

Kagan, C., Burton, M., Duckett, P., Lawthom, R., & Siddiquee, A. (2011). *Critical community psychology*. Wiley.

Lyotard, J. F. (1984). *The postmodern condition: A report on knowledge* (Vol. 10). University of Minnesota Press.

Mason, B. (1993). *Human Systems: The Journal of Systemic Consultation & Management, 4*, 189–200.

Mattes, P., & Schraube, E. (2004). "'Old-stream' psychology will disappear with the dinosaurs!" Kenneth Gergen in conversation with Peter Mattes and Ernst Schraube [39 paragraphs]. *Forum Qualitative Sozialforschung / Forum: Qualitative Social Research, 5*(3), Art. 27. Retrieved from http://nbn-resolving.de/urn:nbn:de:0114-fqs0403275

Moss, D. (2002). Practising from a Park Bench. *Mental Health Today*, August.

Partridge, K., Bennett, E., Webster, A., & Ekdawi, I. (1985). Consultation with clients: An alternative way of working in adult mental health. *Clinical Psychology Forum, 83*, 26–28.

Pearce, W. B. (2007). *Making social worlds: A communication perspective*. Blackwell Publishing Ltd.

Seager, M. (1991). Waiting lists are not the only problem: Changing a referral system. *Clinical Psychology Forum, 36*, 20–26.

Shepherd, J. (2000). Evolution of a Brief Therapy Service. Unpublished MSc Dissertation.

Shotter, J. (2007). Not to forget Tom Andersen's way of being Tom Andersen: The importance of what 'just happens' to us. *Human Systems, 18*, 15–28.

Shotter, J. (2012). More than cool reason: "Withness-thinking" or "systemic-thinking" and "thinking about systems". *International Journal of Collaborative Practices, 3*(1), 1–13.

Smail, D. (2005). *Power, interest and psychology: Elements of a social materialist understanding of distress*. PCCS Books.

Taylor, C. (1973). Interpretation and the sciences of man. In D. Carr & E. S. Casey (Eds.), *Explorations in phenomenology. Selected studies in phenomenology and existential philosophy* (Vol. 4). Springer.

Tweedy, R. (2016). *The political self: Understanding the social context for mental illness*. Routledge.

10

Protesting Against Property Foreclosures in a Fragmentized Socio-Political Sphere: An Action-Oriented Model

Andreas Vavvos and Sofia Triliva

Introduction

From the late nineteenth century up until contemporary times, the issue of "the crisis of psychology" has generated long-lasting and intense controversies (Sturm & Mülberger, 2012). Recently, a large body of academic literature has supported that this crisis-ridden discipline has played a key role in the solidification of the neoliberal model of governance and uncritically reflected and reproduced the sort of atomistic individualism associated with it (Burton, 2015; Mentinis, 2013; Walker et al., 2014). Along these lines, deconstructing the role of the psy-complex in the neoliberal workings of personal debt and the debt industry constitutes a task of vital importance. The institutions of mainstream psychological science and the psy-experts have reinforced the propagation of debt as a matter of "cognitive delinquency" and "financial illiteracy" and enabled the sole attribution of indebtedness to the moral deficits and the internal pathologies of the "irresponsible" and "deceptive" indebted citizens (Burton, 2015; Walker, 2012; Walker et al., 2014). Ignoring and concealing the structural dimensions of personal debt (widespread precariousness, unemployment, recession, stagnation of wages, etc.),

A. Vavvos (✉) • S. Triliva
Department of Psychology, Faculty of Social Sciences, University of Crete, Crete, Greece
e-mail: psy2921@psy.soc.uoc.gr

C. Walker et al. (eds.), *The Palgrave Handbook of Innovative Community and Clinical Psychologies*, https://doi.org/10.1007/978-3-030-71190-0_10

psychological science has remained solely restricted in helping indebted and evicted individuals to adapt to the new conditions and function better in an unjust system (Ballester et al., 2015).

This chapter challenges these conservative understandings of psychological science and offers insights from an action-oriented project that focuses on a network of evicted and indebted citizens in Greece's austerity context. The research initiative is informed by the community psychology principles of giving voice and empowering the most oppressed and vulnerable social groups and critically analyzing hegemonic practices and discourses. In Greece, community psychology as an integrated academic and professional practice has not yet been fully developed (Triliva & Marvakis, 2007). However, vis-à-vis the neoliberal transformations and conceptualizations within Greek society, many psychologists and mental health professionals are taking a critical and reflective stance toward the individualized and psychologizing approaches applied by social scientists in understanding or intervening in people's lifeworld. They are more skeptical of the decontextualized conceptual tools of mainstream psychological science and are moving toward alternative forms of interventions (Mentinis, 2013; Triliva et al., 2013).

The Fragmented Socio-Political Sphere in Crisis-Ridden Greece

Greek society has been subjected to destructive neoliberal adjustments and to the painful austerity policies that were implemented as a remedy to the Greek sovereign debt crisis. The austerity packages imposed by European Central Bank, the European Commission, and the International Monetary Fund (IMF) included unpopular measures, such as widespread privatizations and massive cuts in social welfare spending, wages, and pensions (Blyth, 2015; Williams & Maruthappu, 2013). A large body of academic literature has already outlined the lack of empirical support for the narratives of austerity policies and sovereign debt crises that have imbued public space (Blyth, 2015; Burton, 2015). The pernicious psychosocial effects of the neoliberal management of the "Greek" crisis have also been documented (Triliva et al., 2013; Vavvos & Triliva, 2018; Williams & Maruthappu, 2013). The socio-political and economic landscape in Greece was and is replete of crises, including a healthconomic crisis (Williams & Maruthappu, 2013) and the unprecedented global refugee crisis (Kousoulis et al., 2016). According to Public Issue's data for 2012, four in 10 households (41%) have taken out a bank loan (Public

Issue, 2013), while Sapounakis and Katapidi (2017) report that 4501 court decisions on evictions from primary residences had taken place in the Country Court (Eirinodikeio) of Athens in 2013.

Likewise, within the political landscape, confusion and complexity have abounded, including the rise of Golden Dawn, a neo-Nazi political party (Zartaloudis, 2013), and the results of two elections (January and September 2015) where a historically uncommon coalition government between the radical right-wing party of Independent Greeks and the radical left-wing party of Syriza was formed. The political parties that coalesced were voted to usher in "the politics of hope" and a counter-neoliberal policy agenda (Katsambekis, 2016). Just a few months after taking on the realms of governing, Prime Minister Alexis Tsipras called for a referendum vote and the 61.3% of those casting a ballot in the so-called Greferendum—the Greek austerity referendum of 5 July 2015—voted "no" to the harsh third bailout package proposed by creditors. Despite these results, the government broke its anti-memorandum promises and implemented another round of brutal austerity measures (Giannacopoulos, 2016). This added to the political muddling, people's bemusement, and political identity confusion. The latter is an important component in cultivating a common identity which is an integral part of mobilizing and collective action. Given the conflictual context, forging and upholding unity and common action is not a facile task for solidarity coalitions.

The Local Context and the Emergence of SAOR

During the crisis years, thousands of citizens in many European countries have been expelled from their homes and evicted from their residences due to their inability to pay their rent or make mortgage payments (Ballester et al., 2015; Ordóñez et al., 2015). Following this collapse of a failing Euroatlantic social and political system, many anti-debt and anti-foreclosure coalitions such as Plataforma de Afectados por la Hipoteca (PAH) in Spain and Bündnis Zwangsräumung Verhindern (BZV) in Berlin have taken direct action addressing crucial issues regarding debt and housing through grassroots activism (Ordóñez et al., 2015).

A paradigmatic case of the "foreclosure protestors" is SAOR (Network for the Mutual Assistance of Debtors), an anti-foreclosure network established in 2013 in a Cretan city. The network's charter and members' praxis include an agenda of actions planned and implemented in order to transverse a crisis-ridden economic and political arena. In a socioeconomic sphere where crises prevail, have taken hold, and ravaged Greece, the SAOR coalition can be dubbed a populist social movement, which according to Aslanidis (2016) is a

> non-institutional collective mobilization expressing a catch-all political platform of grievances that divides society between an overwhelming majority of pure people and a corrupt elite, and that claims to speak on behalf of the people in demanding restoration of political authority into their hands as rightful sovereigns. (pp. 304–305)

The aim of the coalition is to protect, inform, and empower debtors so that they can reclaim and redeem their lives. According to the members of the coalition, they have disrupted and prevented more than 1000 planned court foreclosure proceedings during the past seven years. The arsenal of their collective action praxes includes physically averting the serving of eviction notices and impeding court officials from completing the legal processes involved in foreclosures, creating a human wall to protect the threatened home from foreclosure, and protesting against the existing housing legislation. Due to their "unlawful praxes," many members of the coalition have been arrested for trying to disrupt and impede the eviction procedures which were regularly scheduled in the town's courts. Table 10.1 provides the information for the trajectory of the coalition, the stages of the intervention, and the key events in Greek politics.

The aim of this chapter is to inquire into how qualitative research can be used as practical knowledge. After a brief review of the first phase of this project which contained a qualitative study conducted with members of SAOR in 2014, the chapter presents the second one which included a public presentation of the results of this qualitative study and a focus group with members of the coalition. The scope of these research activities was to stimulate critical conscientization processes regarding the hegemonic and ethnocentric undertones of coalition's praxis and discourse and to investigate how initial findings could have resonance and relevance for the participants' daily struggles (see also Baldwin, 2001). In the third and last phase of the research we endeavored to work collaboratively with members of SAOR and use media and documentary film to bring public awareness to the mental health challenges of debtors and to engender community dialogue on the complexities involved when the political is equated with the personal sphere, especially in contested and conflictual public spaces.

Table 10.1 Key events in this research initiative and in Greek politics

Timeline	The trajectory of the coalition and the stages of the intervention	Key events in Greek politics
October 2009		Newly elected Prime Minister George Papandreou from the socialist party of PASOK reveals the country's large budget deficit. Greece's borrowing costs skyrocket and its credit rating is downgraded to "junk status."
May 2010		First bailout of Greece in a context of political and social upheaval, including demonstrations and riots against austerity.
October 2011		Prime Minister Papandreou proposes a referendum vote focusing on the second bailout agreement. Prime Minister Papandreou resigns and a unity coalition government headed by economist Lucas Papademos takes over and implements more stringent austerity measures.
February 2012		Second IMF–EU bailout is approved, including a restructuring of debt.
November 2013	The charter of the coalition is written by its members. On a weekly basis, members of the network will meet in or outside of courtrooms in order to disrupt the scheduled foreclosure processes.	
October–December 2014	Implementation of the first stage of research: 11 interviews and one focus group with members of the coalition are conducted.	Prime Minister Antonis Samaras does not enter negations for another bailout agreement.
25 January 2015		Elections and formation of a coalition government between Independent Greeks and Syriza: showdown with creditors, amid discourses of default and Grexit.

(*continued*)

Table 10.1 (continued)

Timeline	The trajectory of the coalition and the stages of the intervention	Key events in Greek politics
5 July 2015		The Greek bailout referendum takes place, in a context of "capital controls." A "NO" vote overwhelmingly rejected the new bailout terms.
14 August 2015		With 222 voting in favor, the Greek parliament approves the third bailout program and the harsh austerity reforms. The Syriza Party splits into two.
21 September 2015		The Greek legislative election was held following Prime Minister Alexis Tsipras' announced resignation on 20th August.
28 September 2016	The coalition is blamed by the antifascist network of Rethymno for being xenophobic and for participating in the campaign against hosting refugees in Crete.	
5 February 2017	SAOR and other coalitions in Crete merge into a larger anti-foreclosure network, the PanCretan Network of Forces of Resistance and Mutual Help.	
2 October 2017	Three members of the administrative council of SAOR are arrested for alleged crimes they committed. The coalition's actions receive a great deal of media attention.	
21 October 2017	Presentation of the research in the conference and conduct of the focus group.	
October 2017–February 2018	Publication of the interview articles in the local newspapers.	

(*continued*)

Table 10.1 (continued)

Timeline	The trajectory of the coalition and the stages of the intervention	Key events in Greek politics
24 October 2017	The first author and two members of the coalition speak about the research project in a local radio channel.	
04 November 2017–31 December 2017		Greek notaries decide to abstain from all auctions due to safety concerns.
29 November 2017		Greek government launches the platform for online auctions, a prerequisite of the third bailout program. The launch of online auctions was a means of keeping the protestors away from courtroom proceedings and brought the auction procedures in public courtrooms to a halt. Violent clashes of protesters with riot police in Athens and Thessaloniki take place.
02 December 2018	Presentation of the documentary *SAOR: A Reflection of the Crisis?* in an academic conference.	

The Neoliberal Myth of Austerity: Indebted Personhood in a Bankrupt Nation

In May 2015, members of SAOR turned to the Department of Psychology at the University of Crete, requesting psychological help for debtors in their coalition, who were confronting mental health challenges connected to socio-economic difficulties. As they requested, a qualitative inquiry was conducted to clarify their needs and contextualize their stories and collective struggles. During the period from October through December 2014, 11 semi-structured interviews and one focus group (six participants) were conducted and analyzed using phenomenologically informed thematic analysis (Braun & Clarke, 2006). Three superordinate themes comprised an analytic narrative under the title: "The neoliberal myth of austerity: Indebted personhood in a bankrupt nation" (see Vavvos & Triliva, 2018).

In this study, participants described the collapse of their dignity and the feelings of shame and guilt they experienced as indebted citizens during the austerity era. They explained how SAOR had constituted a sociospatial topos where they could grasp the commonality of their suffering and question the individualizing narrative of indebtedness. The emancipatory (saving homes, redefining the narrative of debt, producing solidarity discourses, etc.) and the ambiguous (ethnocentric and individualized focus, the demands for the return of neoliberal pre-crisis conditions, lack of critical reflection on the neoliberal growth-oriented lifestyle, etc.) aspects of their struggles were also critically discussed. A second phase of research could ultimately aid in the exposure of these socio-political contradictions. Conscientization of the ways in which psychic functions and processes and social circumstances constitute each other and co-produce SAOR's members' realities and activities was necessary.

The Step from "Research on" to "Action-Oriented Research"

The findings of this qualitative research were presented in a local scientific conference focusing on solidarity economy. After informing the coalitions' stakeholders about the conference, eight members participated in the discussion that ensued the presentation. All in all, rather than imposing our "expert" perspective on the data and overshadowing participants' voices, the democratic process of a public presentation ensured equal participation in the co-construction of knowledge and constituted a space to critique, provoke, and challenge the participants' and our own interpretations and perspectives. That process was a necessary step for this project and forced us to move into more intricate discursive positions and call into question the dominant positivist conceptualizations of data ownership and validity (see Baldwin, 2001).

The presentation was audiotaped and transcribed verbatim. Participants in the conference discussion provided informed consent after the study's aims, benefits, and procedures were explained to them. Participants' names were replaced with pseudonyms and all recordings were deleted once the anonymized transcripts were completed. Given that populist movements claim to express the will of the people (Katsambekis, 2016), we focused the analysis on how researchers, SAOR members, and activists present in the conference had constructed the concept of "the people" and how these constructions were promoting social justice. The systematic procedures and data analysis processes described by Braun and Clarke (2006) provided a framework for coding the data. The thematic analysis included familiarization with the data, data reduction via coding, searching, and deriving themes, and producing condensed data in conceptually grouped analytical units. From this process, two overriding themes were identified: (1) the dispute between a pragmatist and an ideological discourse and (2) crossing the blurred lines of politics: a first-person reflection. Thematic analysis will be drawn on to critically examine the hegemonic undertones of coalition's praxis and discourse and the researcher's positionality.

The Dispute Between an Ethnocentric and a Left-wing Discourse

Academics and activists, present at the conference, expressed their animosity toward SAOR's aims, tactics, and members. The "class" issue dominated the discussion and there were persistent questions about the class position of SAOR's members. Promoting a cross-class unification of Greek people against austerity measures and elites, SAOR members were criticized for reproducing an ethnocentric rhetoric and protecting the rights and interests of the beneficiaries of the neoliberal order. Zizis, an academic, pointed out: "Behind these, a discourse about the Greek people surfaces. ... Greek populace is not one populace, there are classes etc." and Christos, an activist, added: "How do you decide ... which business or which houses are you going to help, by stopping its foreclosure?"

The people present at the conference were members of grassroots economic initiatives, representatives of the social solidarity economy, and strong supporters of a radical social and economic restructuring of society. Hence, they were critical of SAOR's reformist and pragmatist demands (return of normal market conditions, urgent requests for dignified existence, finding jobs, canceling debts, etc.). Furthermore, apart from the appeals for a cross-class alliance against corrupt elites and foreign economic institutions, SAOR, similar to other anti-eviction groups, aimed to unite and include ideologically diverse actors and heterogeneous groups under the umbrella of a common objective—stopping foreclosures.

In the discussion, the inclusion of members and voters of a neo-fascist party in the coalition was the focal point of the discord. The articulatory links between austerity, Euroscepticism, and nationalism and the rise of neo-fascism galvanized the political atmosphere. Hence, there was a disputable and controversial issue at stake for solidarity initiatives: should a "solidarity" coalition include members or voters of neo-fascist communities and parties? Iakovos, a member of SAOR, declared: "People, who are in the coalition, support different parties. … I have seen people from Communist Party of Greece, I have seen people from neo-fascist groups, from New Democracy." And Vasilis, an activist, responded regarding supporters of fascist ideologies: "The existence of these people in SAOR's circles is a very serious matter … because we are talking about dangerous people … if we do not do something tomorrow or the day after tomorrow, we are going to mourn victims."

In the local community, there was much discord and condemnation for the reproduction of a "right-wing" populist rhetoric by, at least, some members of SAOR; namely, a rigid conceptualization of the people as a homogeneous ethnic group (the "Greek" people). This framing of the movement in patriotic terms accompanied by inclusion of all classes (among others, those who strategically do not pay their debts and elite debtors) and ideologies (among others, members of neo-fascist groups) created a hodgepodge with regard to the common identity of the collectivity. The process of public presentation made apparent these ambiguities and contradictions in the coalition's members' political stance. They were besieged to adopt a more critical and reflective stance.

Crossing the Blurred Lines of Politics: A First-Person Reflection

Taking into consideration what Paulo Freire has ironically described as the academic "air of messianism" (see Freire, 1994, p. 79), we attempted to be, also, "conscientized" by the conference dialogue and exchange and question our own political assumptions and ethical stances. As researchers we were not neutral in that the ethnocentric rhetoric that was very evident in the first phase of the research brought up lots of critical analysis regarding the political ramifications of such narrations and our positionality as researchers. This issue captured the ideological complexity of the research project and became the focal point of the discord between participants. Dimitris, an activist, stated:

> I believe that we have to overcome … this neutrality about the values, which, let's say, Weber, has established … if there was here someone from a neo-fascist party … what should we do? And what should you do as a researcher when you face those people or even the choice of this subject matter.

Panagiotis, an activist, said addressing Dimitris: "I will disagree with my friend … of course, reality includes people who belong to neo-fascist groups. What can we do? It is perspicuous that when you do research, obviously there are fascists." The discussion generated a heated debate and revolved around the researchers' positionality and constraints of SAOR's struggles in generating a social justice agenda. On the one hand, the coalition had offered a socio-spatial space where debtors, who had been gravely oppressed by destructive neoliberal adjustments, could express their growing indignation and grievances. On the other hand, the SAOR coalition, similar to other anti-eviction networks such as PAH and BZV (Ordóñez et al., 2015), had not shaped an explicit political agenda to frame the issues of personal debt and affordable housing. As a result, their unstated ethnocentric rhetoric provided a fertile ground for the oppression of other social groups (refugees, migrants, etc.) and for the tolerance and indifference toward neo-fascist groups' actions.

We attempted to address this difficult impasse denouncing the intolerance espoused by neo-fascist groups and while showing respect to the personal stories participants had shared with us and our collaborative relationships with the coalitions' members. As qualitative researchers and psychologists influenced by principles of community psychology, we rejected a value-neutral stance and endeavored to make the tolerance toward neo-fascist parties a matter of public and rational argumentation. Given the rise of right-wing populist parties and movements in the European context (Katsambekis, 2016), we propose that it is crucial for community psychologists to critically highlight and analyze activists' tacit political assumptions and "claim, in the name of tolerance, the right not to tolerate the intolerant" (Popper, 2003, p. 293).

Focus Group: The Aftermath of the Tumultuous Conference Discussion

Immediately after the conference presentation, a focus group was conducted in the Center of Research and Studies of the University of Crete. The focus group lasted one hour and, apart from the researchers, six male members of the coalition participated: Iakovos (53 y/o), Stelios (64 y/o), Panagiotis (51 y/o), Lefteris (59 y/o), Vasilis (48 y/o), and Nikos (58 y/o). Based on the researchers' and participants' concerns and on the feedback from the presentation and discussion, the focus group was based on five thematic axes.

1. The relevance of the qualitative research and the discussion that ensued for their daily struggles.
2. The arrest of coalition members for being involved in criminal activities and the episodes of violence and fierce clashes of SAOR members with the police.
3. The challenge of the electronic foreclosures.
4. The need for common dialogical rules and how they interface with the lack of mobilization of a large sector of those that "belong" to the coalition.
5. The presence of people supporting a neo-fascist ideology in the coalition and the racist and ethnocentric rhetoric of some members of the coalition. The discussion was focused on this issue and caused a critical debate between participants. Most of the members of the group expressed their stance on these issues. Lefteris declared:

> Because in our circles there was expression of an unprocessed rage and indignation, many tried to invest on this. This member of the neo-fascist group … had said "the Muslims are threatening us" and I told him "I am a Muslim" [laughter] … or against homosexuals … or Nikos [pseudonym] was coming and saying "no immigrant in Crete." I told him "no racist in Crete."

The focus group discussion led to the decision to make a documentary film and to publicize in local media channels (radio, newspapers) the participants' silenced stories of indebtedness in order to bring under public scrutiny the hardships, the problems, and the socio-political perceptions and actions of SAOR's members. The scope was to engender public conversation and awareness regarding the complexities that were forging SAOR's praxis with regard to the debt and foreclosures.

Using Interviews as a Tool for Self-Reflection: Debtor's Stories in the Public Space

During the third phase of this research, SAOR members' interviews conducted in 2014 were published in two newspapers and in their electronic sites, Kritiki Epitheorisi (Cretan Inspection) in Rethymno and Agonas Kritis (Cretan Fight) in Chania. The general public of this intervention included Greek-speaking citizens that had access either to the printed or to the online edition of the newspaper. As stated in the introductory article in Agonas

Kritis, "the aim of this cooperation is to open a fertile channel of communication and dialogue between the university, society and the 'stop' foreclosures movement" (Aggelakis, 2017, p. 3). The journalist from Kritiki Epitheorisi declared that "a research like that, which does not stop with the data of 2014, but follows the developments, has an unquestionable interest and concurrently proves the quality of collaboration that university can have with the local community" (Vilara, 2017, p. 6).

Initially, we came in contact with all the interviewees, explaining the aim and the scope of this intervention. Eight SAOR members responded positively. Furthermore, they each selected the parts of the interview that would be publicized in the newspaper article. Additionally, we jointly re-read, reflected, and critically commented on the transcript of the interview based on two thematic questions: (a) what emotions and thoughts did the reading of the transcript trigger and (b) how had their lives changed since the interview was conducted (three years later). All the final articles were approximately 800 words and were published from October 2017 to February 2018. Table 10.2 provides the following information: the pseudonym of the interviewee, the title and meaning of the title of the newspaper article, and interviewee's comments on his/her interview in 2014.

SAOR members reported that it was redempting and empowering to critically reflect on their biographical trajectories and make the public aware of their suffering. Most of them stressed that it was valuable to actively engage in an intervention that aimed to document how the crisis had impacted theirs' and others' lifeworlds. In a nutshell, the use of a newspaper article as a tool for community intervention provided a way to avoid circumscribing and limiting the research endeavor opening it up to a community-wide audience.

The Psychology of Indebted Man and the Shortcomings of the Anti-foreclosure Movement

The media coverage phase of the research continued with the participation of the first author in a local radio channel on 24 October 2017. The first author was invited to speak about this research project and the discussion had the title: "The Psychology of Indebted Man and the Shortcomings of the 'Stop' Foreclosure Movement."[1] Apart from the researcher, two members of the

[1] For the radio broadcast see [in Greek]: https://soundcloud.com/andreas-vavvos/25-10-2017a

Table 10.2 Debtor's stories in the public space

Name	Title	Meaning	Comments
Michalis	In a cell	The fear that police would arrest and imprison him because of his debts.	Financially, I'm in a worse situation, but for some reason I continue to hope for something better. Reading the transcript I smiled, reflecting on how my life was three years ago and where I am now. For me, the coalition still inspires hope for human power and will, even after the tragic events.
Vasilis	No you do not pass five, you pass ten	A debtor living in the austerity era is like a student, who despite the fact s/he was initially told that s/he needs to pass five, s/he is finally forced to pass ten courses.	Today I am free. I have accepted that I cannot save anything. The trap was well positioned. I fell in. I gathered all my psychic strength with my family and some good friends and we are trying to get our lives back.
Aristotelis	When you hear the bell tolling, do not ask for whom it is tolling, know that it is for you	Using Ernest Hemingway's famous quote, in order to highlight the importance of getting informed and taking action.	I found interesting the idea of cooperating with the Department of Psychology. I was glad that this discussion took place, because I think that the well-documented presentation of conclusions helps in knowledge construction and informs society regarding the debt problem.
Ioanna	The "cheapskate" Character from the book *Christ Recrucified*	Parallelizing her daily life with the character "cheapskate," scrooge from the book *Christ Recrucified*.	It was very pleasant to re-read the interview. It is almost 3 years ago. I mocked myself about the innocent answers that I gave then and I thought "Was this me? Who was saying these things?" I have no contact with the coalition and its members anymore.

(*continued*)

Table 10.2 (continued)

Name	Title	Meaning	Comments
Themistoklis	Finding equilibrium in a descending elevator	Giving voice to precarity and insecurity.	In general, the situation remains stable. Only with a bank I had a major improvement. Seeing my interview three years later, I am realizing how stagnated the financial situation continues to be. Psychological malaise continues unchanged. Eventually the elevator's belt may break.
Iakovos	Wherever you look, you see walls	Describing his life as a trap where he feels hemmed in and cannot find a way out.	Personally, nothing has changed since the interview. The state has closed the doors to us. What the University of Crete did was a good praxis, following what SAOR requested. From that process one sees what every citizen feels.
Stelios	They are the same like you	Expressing feelings of solidarity between SAOR's members.	My life has no improvement, the opposite is true. I do not stop hoping, since SAOR is in a developing process.
Despoina	Debt as a recourse	Depicting debt as systemic necessity in order to deal with daily financial problems.	My life has changed a lot. My health is not good. Cancer treatment brings many complications and I am unable to work. Regarding the interview, my emotions are mixed. On the one hand, I feel relieved because I shared with someone my problem, but on the other hand I feel shame.

In the Greek educational context, a student is obliged to pass a specific amount of courses each semester. Vasilis uses this analogy in order to depict how he was finally forced to pay over the odds and describe the false promises that governments and creditors gave to debtors.

coalition participated in the discussion. The discussion lasted almost 17 minutes and was focused on the following themes:

1. Description of the nature, the aims, the results, and the methodology of the research and a brief literature review.
2. A critical evaluation of the differences and similarities of creditors' and debtors' discourses, as presented in the specific research, and the blame-game around the Greek crisis.
3. A discussion about the limitations, contradictions, political aims, and future of the "stop" foreclosures movement.
4. The relationship of university with the local community and the collaboration of university members with local actors.

SAOR: A Reflection of the Crisis?

The audiovisual part of the project took the form of a documentary[2] entitled *SAOR: A Reflection of the Crisis?* and added useful insights as compared to other documentaries, such as *Mietrebellen* and *La Plataforma*, that refer to anti-foreclosure coalitions (Ordóñez et al., 2015). The final version of the documentary was a result of an in-depth collaboration between SAOR members, a journalistic working group, and members of the Department of Psychology, who had been working on interviewing the coalition's members in the first phase of the research process in 2014. The researchers and the interviewees commonly chose the interview excerpts that would be included in the documentary. The excerpts chosen highlighted best the essence of the participants' narrations and stories and were befitting with the documentary's aim.

The documentary was initially inspired by the growing insecurity and precariousness that the crisis brought to peoples' lives. Its aim was to highlight the psychosocial effects of the economic crisis in the specific region, from 2015 to 2017. The focus was directed on SAOR as a reflection of the crisis in the region, since this anti-foreclosure network was first founded in Greece and the subject of "foreclosures" received national publicity at that time. This interlacing of discourses, media broadcasts, and information brought to the surface the connection between the facts in a more cogent, complete, and

[2] This part was co-written with Matthaios Kapetanakis, journalist, main director, and producer of the documentary. For the documentary, see: https://filmfreeway.com/SAORacrisisreflection

valid way. This form of triangulation revealed that there was a climax in coalition's protest events that finally led to arrests, but also in the hidden criminal activity of some people who took advantage of the SAOR network's members' recognition, acceptance, and friendship, so as to hide their clandestine and illicit activities. Another significant issue that arose was the hidden facts and information in the course of some of the collectivity's praxes. Using multiple sources, unapparent or only circulated as rumors events, what came to light was a climax that had provided an unofficial safe environment for illegal activities.

An initial version of this documentary was presented in the conference "Crete in the 21st Century: Problems, Challenges and Perspectives in the Cretan Society, Economy, Politics and Health."[3] After the viewing, a fruitful discussion followed between SAOR members, researchers, academics, and members of other coalition groups. This revealed the impact of the incidents to the main actors, the members of the community, who had the chance to reflect on how the political economy of debt had contextualized human suffering and on the political narrations of the "stop" foreclosures movement.

Conclusions

In the first phase of this research project, participants likened their realities to a "fairy tale." Their stories highlighted that austerity is a "fairy tale" narrated by those yielding power in order to portray "a happy ever after" for "elites" and, to concurrently be applied, "as a made-up story" designed to hoodwink and mislead the populace. This simile resembles what Martín-Baró depicted as the Social Lie, which "consists in constructing a reality that is ideologically compatible with the interests of the dominant class" (Martín-Baró, 1994, p. 188). We hope that this research has contributed to bringing a more critical awareness of what SAOR members had described as a "fairy tale" and helped to bolster SAOR's members' critical reflection on how bringing about political change is complex. Collective action proved to be tricky and, although the austerity regimes continue to be enforced, the SAOR coalition is struggling to find a cohesive political identity and to fight the foreclosures in what proved to be shifting and highly contested socio-political spaces.

Our long and reflexive engagement with the coalition, the community, and the multifaceted literature emanating from different fields of study kept us aware and actively involved with the complexities of doing the research and

[3] For the conference see [in Greek]: http://30years.soc.uoc.gr/

also in recognizing, examining, and understanding our own assumptions and positioning throughout the process. We learned a great deal both personally and professionally, since it was demanding to deconstruct the political, personal, and economic forces and their confluence. Endeavoring into the community and assuming the role of intermediaries between the tainted identity of the coalition, other collectivities, public condemnation regarding the criminal activity of three of SAOR's members, and the fragmented political space was and continues to be an arduous task for us and all involved. Furthermore, conducting action research at a time of constant change and debate about the roles of those governing, people's responsibilities, and the nation's future placed all involved in the process in precarious positioning. Working with people within the same community, who concomitantly espouse diverse and antithetical values was laborious, yet crucial. In doing this, we focused on community psychology's critical agenda, bringing to the forefront and underscoring the many contradictions that pervade neoliberal practices and the political subjects it produces.

In terms of practice, we propose that future community psychologists should engage in community-based art initiatives such as the documentary produced in this research initiative. Community-based theater (theater of oppressed, documentary theater, etc.) is also an alternative medium of disseminating research findings. Theatrical activities, apart from being a means of self-expression and self-growth, can be a tool for a "gentler" and "softer" social activism for adults with psychiatric experiences (Faigin & Stein, 2015, pp. 157). In particular, documentary theater, a performance style which cites real documents such as interview transcripts, can be a useful tool for community psychologists and qualitative researchers engaging in conversation with communities where discord and divisiveness exist. The use of reflexivity throughout the research process from the outset until the end can also be a catalyst for an innovative research practice. Creating a manuscript open to criticism and comments from academics, activists, journalists, members of community groups, and local citizens is an eye-opening process where different filters offer perspectives that are valuable. This community collaboration creates a participative framework that highlights complexity and the many different aspects of social issues. Stretching and blurring these technical boundaries between researchers and researched and engaging in the anxiety-producing process of venturing out of the "ivory tower" of academia is the task at hand for psychologists interested in political activism and social change.

References

Aggelakis, I. (2017, December 12). "Το παραμύθι της λιτότητας": Μεγάλη έρευνα για το κίνημα ενάντια στους πλειστηριασμούς στην Κρήτη ["The fairy tale of austerity": A big research about the anti-foreclosure movement in Crete]. *Agonas Kritis,* pp. 3-5. Available in: http://agonaskritis.gr/το-παραμύθι-της-λιτότητας-μεγάλη-έρευ/

Aslanidis, P. (2016). Populist social movements of the Great Recession. *Mobilization: An International Quarterly, 21*(3), 301–321. https://doi.org/10.17813/1086-671x-20-3-301

Baldwin, M. (2001). Working together, learning together: Co-operative inquiry in the development of complex practice by teams of social workers. In P. Reason & H. Bradbury (Eds.), *Handbook of action research: Participative inquiry and practice* (pp. 287–293). Sage.

Ballester, A., Carmona, M., Fernández, R. D., González, A., Jiménez, J., Martínez, E., ... Viano, C. (2015). The consequences of evictions in Spain. In S. M. Değirmencioğlu & C. Walker (Eds.), *Social and psychological dimensions of personal debt and the debt industry* (pp. 84–100). Palgrave Macmillan.

Braun, V., & Clarke, V. (2006). Using thematic analysis in psychology. *Qualitative Research in Psychology, 3*(2), 77–101. Retrieved from: http://eprints.uwe.ac.uk/11735/2/thematic_analysis_revised

Blyth, M. (2015). *Austerity: The history of a dangerous idea.* Oxford University Press.

Burton, M. (2015). Debt dynamics in the UK and beyond: How propaganda impedes effective political action. In S. M. Değirmencioğlu & C. Walker (Eds.), *Social and psychological dimensions of personal debt and the debt industry* (pp. 123–137). Palgrave Macmillan.

Faigin, D. A., & Stein, C. H. (2015). Community-based theater and adults with psychiatric disabilities: Social activism, performance and community engagement. *American Journal of Community Psychology, 55,* 148–163. https://doi.org/10.1007/s10464-014-9695-6

Freire, P. (with notes by Freire, A.M.A.). (1994). *Pedagogy of hope: Reliving pedagogy of the oppressed* (R. R. Barr, Trans.). New York, NY: Continuum (Original work published 1992).

Giannacopoulos, M. (2016). Sovereign debt crises, referendums and the changing face of colonial power. *Continuum: Journal of Media and Cultural Studies, 31*(1), 33–42. https://doi.org/10.1080/10304312.2016.1262098

Katsambekis, G. (2016). The populist surge in post-democratic times: Theoretical and political challenges. *The Political Quarterly, 88*(2), 202–210. https://doi.org/10.1111/1467-923X.12317

Kousoulis, A. A., Ioakeim-Ioannidou, M., & Economopoulos, K. P. (2016). Refugee crisis: Not a one-country job. *International Journal of Public Health, 62*(1), 1–2. https://doi.org/10.1007/s00038-016-0890-0

Martín-Baró, I. (1994). Public opinion research as a de-ideologizing instrument (J. Caroll & A. Aron, Trans.). In A. Aron & S. Corne (Eds.), *Writings for a liberation psychology* (pp. 186-197). Cambridge, MA: Harvard University Press.

Mentinis, M. (2013). The entrepreneurial ethic and the spirit of psychotherapy: Depoliticisation, atomisation and social selection in the therapeutic culture of the 'crisis'. *European Journal of Psychotherapy & Counselling, 15*(4), 361–374. https://doi.org/10.1080/13642537.2013.855248

Ordóñez, R. V., Feenstra, R. A., & Tormey, S. (2015). Citizens against austerity: A comparative reflection on Plataforma de Afectados por la Hipoteca (PAH) and Bündnis Zwangsräumung Verhindern (BZV). *Araucaria. Revista Iberoamericana de Filosofía, Política & Humanidades, 17*(34), 133–154. https://doi.org/10.12795/araucaria.2015.i34.07

Popper, K. R. (2003). *The open society and its enemies: The spell of Plato* (Vol. 1). Routledge.

Public Issue. (2013). *Greek social issues 3–2013: Loans to Greek households, 2012.* Retrieved from: http://www.publicissue.gr/en/1731/loans-2012

Sapounakis, A., & Katapidi, I. (2017). Evictions from primary residences in Greece: Methodological concerns regarding the collection of data from Civil Courts' records for tenancies. *European Journal of Homelessness, 11*(2), 149–162.

Sturm, T., & Mülberger, A. (2012). Crisis discussions in psychology: New historical and philosophical perspectives. *Studies in History and Philosophy of Biological and Biomedical Sciences, 43*(2), 425–433. https://doi.org/10.1016/j.shpsc.2011.11.001

Triliva, S., & Marvakis, A. (2007). Community psychology initiatives in Greece. In S. M. Reich, M. Riemer, I. Prilleltensky, & M. Montero (Eds.), *International Community Psychology: History and Theories* (pp. 363–374). Springer.

Triliva, S., Fragkiadaki, E., & Balamoutsou, S. (2013). Forging partnerships for mental health: The case of a prefecture in crisis ravaged Greece. *European Journal of Psychotherapy & Counselling, 15*(4), 375–390. https://doi.org/10.1080/13642537.2013.849275

Vavvos, A., & Triliva, S. (2018). The neoliberal myth of austerity: Debt and solidarity in the forefront of public space. *Journal of Social and Political Psychology, 6*(2), 315–330. https://doi.org/10.5964/jspp.v6i2.740

Vilara, X. (2017, October 26). Έρευνα του Τμήματος Ψυχολογίας του Πανεπιστημίου Κρήτης για τις ψυχολογικές επιπτώσεις της κρίσης στους δανειολήπτες και για το κίνημα κατά των πλειστηριασμών [Research of Department of Psychology of University of Crete about the psychological consequences of crisis in debtors and the 'stop' foreclosures movement]. *Kritiki Epitheorisi*, pp. 6-7.

Walker, C. (2012). Personal debt, cognitive delinquency and techniques of governmentality: Neoliberal constructions of financial inadequacy in the UK. *Journal of Community & Applied Social Psychology, 22*(6), 533–538. https://doi.org/10.1002/casp.1127

Walker, C., Burton, M., Akhurst, J., & Değirmencioğlu, S. M. (2014). Locked into the system? Critical community psychology approaches to personal debt in the context of crises of capital accumulation. *Journal of Community & Applied Social Psychology, 25*(3), 264–275. https://doi.org/10.1002/casp.2209

Williams, C., & Maruthappu, M. (2013). "Healthconomic crises": Public health and neoliberal economic crises. *American Journal of Public Health, 103*(1), 7–9. https://doi.org/10.2105/AJPH.2012.300956

Zartaloudis, S. (2013). Greece and the recent financial crisis: Meltdown or configuration? In F. Panizza & G. Philip (Eds.), *Moments of truth: The politics of financial crises in comparative perspective* (pp. 158–176). Routledge.

11

'We the Marlborough': Elucidating Users' Experience of Radical, Informal Therapeutic Practices Within a Queer Community Pub

Charlotte Wilcox and Rebecca Graber

Charlotte Wilcox became interested in working radically after working in community psychiatry, witnessing how the mental health system can be functionally anti-therapeutic in its creation of resistance, otherness, and disempowerment, especially for those who are already marginalised. She became aware of the implications of this lack of containment, particularly in traumatic distress. While training in psychotherapy, she began thinking about trauma as a relational phenomenon. At the same time, over a period of a few months, she and her partner lived in the queer community in rooms above the Marlborough pub. Living within the queer community, she was heartened to experience the ways in which people were supporting each other emotionally, demonstrating in these informal practices a sophisticated engagement with the relational nature of trauma. She was astonished at how community members were doing this healing work for each other apparently spontaneously, drawing on shared experience and tacit knowledge about containing distress. She and co-author Rebecca Graber bonded over a shared belief that given the right conditions and space, people will do this healing work for each other. Rebecca's research is driven by a belief that psychology often overlooks the healing power of people's existing relationships. By contrast, together Charlotte and Rebecca are interested in the I-Thou dynamic in which kindness can permeate knowledge, policy and therapeutic practice. They choose to use phenomenology because this method valorises experience and

C. Wilcox • R. Graber (✉)
School of Humanities and Social Science, University of Brighton, Falmer, East Sussex, UK
e-mail: C.Wilcox@brighton.ac.uk; r.graber@brighton.ac.uk

C. Walker et al. (eds.), *The Palgrave Handbook of Innovative Community and Clinical Psychologies*, https://doi.org/10.1007/978-3-030-71190-0_11

provides the tools for seeing, and understanding, another person's lifeworld. They believe that human connection not only is a therapeutic precursor to recognition, but should form the foundation of psychological practice and knowledge-making.

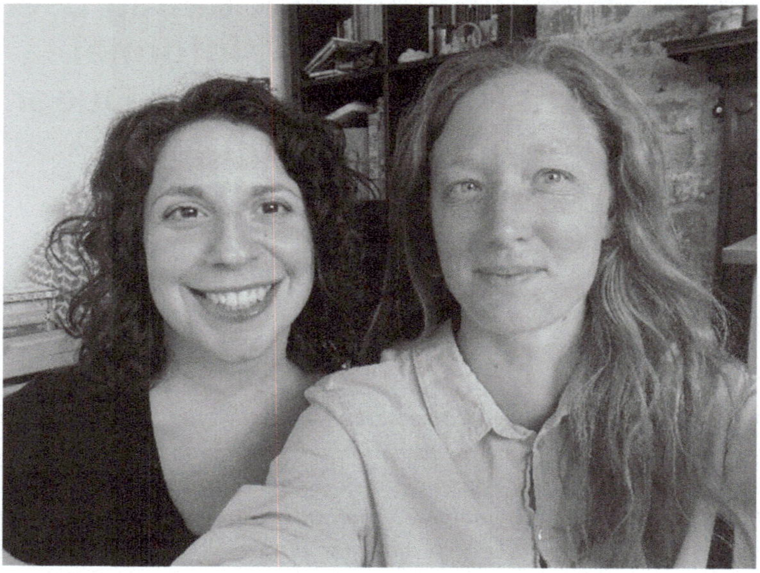

Introduction

In 2016, the Marlborough Pub received an award for Best Community Resource from MindOut, a Brighton-based queer mental health charity. The Marlborough has been associated with the LGBTQIA+[1] community since the 1970s when a queer theatre organisation set up in the upstairs theatre. In the last five years or so the pub has become a focal point for the Brighton queer scene and specifically for the increasingly visible trans and nonbinary community. The centrality of a pub in functioning as a radical space for a marginalised community is not new. But the MindOut award recognised that something happens in *this* pub community that supports people's mental health.

[1] In this chapter, we interchangeably use the terms queer (reclaimed and in popular use since the late 1980s) and LGBTQIA+ (Lesbian, Gay, Bisexual, Queer/Questioning, Intersex and Asexual and others). These acronyms are currently in wide use and are understood to hold maximum inclusivity for what are increasingly referred to within the mental health field as GSRD (gender, sexuality and relationship diversity) communities. Terms were used synonymously by all participants, although P10, aged 53, said they found 'queer' difficult as they remember when its only use was as a homophobic slur.

Prompted by public recognition of this pub's value and by the first researcher's own lived experience as a Marlborough community member, this chapter aims to describe and theorise existing radical informal therapeutic and peer support practices within the queer community, situated within the 'space and place' of the pub itself. We suggest that, here in the pub, a form of relationality emerges which resists the oppression of 'psychologising' elsewhere in LGBTQIA+ people's lives, it is radical and disruptive. This is particularly compelling given the paradoxical situation in which many community members find themselves: both desiring mental health support but disincentivised from accessing it, for example from experiences of ignorance and discrimination by service providers or controversies over the diagnostic status of gender variance (Drescher, 2010; Stonewall Scotland, 2014; LaSala, 2013).

Perceived social support from embedded social relationships (i.e. naturally occurring social relationships such as friendships) has been consistently linked with various indicators of well-being, happiness and resilience (Graber et al., 2016). More broadly, such relationships address needs for belonging, mutuality and inclusion (Jordan, 2013; La Guardia, 2008). Not everyone has access to supportive embedded relationships, nor desires to use those relationships to deal with specific challenges. Peer support is an alternative to formal care often used within health promotion, disease prevention and chronic care frameworks to share experiential knowledge and emotional support, addressing stigma reduction, social connectedness and instrumental support (Dennis, 2003; Graber, in press).

The Marlborough is generally recognised as a cohesive community in which emotional support is given and received, beyond narrow categories of formal care, peer support or even friendship. What happens at the Marlborough is organic and attests to the healing significance and 'richness of everyday relationships' (Postle, 2013). The community can be understood as a place where informal relationships of care happen. This has a double significance. Firstly, it is increasingly understood that social networks and identities have a profound protective impact on mental and physical health (Jettan et al., 2012). Social identities, and factors associated with them (such as social support and a sense of community), can promote coping, and well-being for individuals dealing with a range of illnesses, injuries, trauma and stressors. Secondly, the role of informal community-based and socially oriented approaches in alleviating mental distress is now recognised (Walker et al., 2017). 'Social recovery' is understood to be recovery from distress through nurturance via the richness of informal relationships rather than any cure dispensed from formal healthcare.

In recent times queer people have critically engaged with the negative impact of heteronormativity on mental health theorisation and mental health treatment of LGBTQIA+ people. Moon (2010) confront the heteronormativity of predominant counselling ideologies. Moon draws our attention to the struggle for recognition within mainstream therapeutic practice, identifying an ongoing impasse arising from complicit subordination to the dominant group. She argues that a form of epistemic violence—a 'gentle violence'—is perpetuated which legitimates oppression, resists radical shifts in power and has implications for emotional citizenship and sociality. Queer theory provides an alternative reading which can complicate the terrain and offer a way out of this impasse (Butler, 1990; Moon, 2011). It not only allows us to interrogate the Marlborough as a 'space and place' in which informal therapeutic practice happens as a response to gaps in existing services, but encourages us to question how the Marlborough exists as a radical community on its own terms, forging its own practices and conceptualisations of 'well-being' that are created outside of heteronorm and the normative structures of psychiatry. This complements recent moves to bring queer experience, knowledge and theory to therapeutic contexts (Carroll & Gilroy, 2001; Giammattei, 2015).

Such practices encourage us to follow Sedgewick (1990) in thinking phenomenologically about political action in what has become known as 'affective activism' (Johnson, 2015). Affective activism 'transforms queer subjectivities' via 'new forms of relating across identity difference, producing a vitalist politics that sustains people through their everyday lives' (Johnson, 2015, p15). These forms of relating create potential for affective solidarity, connecting beyond identity differences through shared affective experience, and the '(sometimes unexpected) process of being moved' (Johnson, 2015, p. 173). This way of thinking demands greater attention to the affective component of queer lived experience.

Together, an orientation towards affective lived experience, desire to undermine heteronormative readings of mental health and interest in how social relationships can provide a crucial alternative or challenge to statutory care form a theoretical landscape from which to ask: What are users' experiences of radical informal therapeutic practices and peer support situated within a queer community pub?

We intend to contribute to the radical critique countering both anti-therapeutic neo-liberal psychiatric structures and the heteronormative assumptions that impact LGBTQIA+ people in two key ways. First, we aim to generate novel understanding of the lived experience of radical informal therapeutic and peer support practices in the queer community. Second, we aim to provide inspiration for new ways to undertake psychotherapeutic and community psychological practice, within queer and other communities engaging in informal care practices.

Method

Research design and data generation

Understanding and richly describing the lived experience of people in this 'space and place' is necessary to give name to what is happening in this radical space. We use Husserlian descriptive phenomenology of qualitative interview data to allow radical immersion in the lifeworld of participants (Wertz, 2011). An explicitly relational and reflexive phenomenological stance calls on 'fragments of being' such as sociality, self, space and embodiment, as analytical ways in to understanding experience (Finlay & Dawsonera, 2011; Ashworth, 2003). A descriptive phenomenological approach is consonant with therapeutic practice since it aims to describe rather than interpret, honouring the participants' expertise as the ultimate arbiters of their subjective experience (Wertz, 2011). Descriptive phenomenological analysis (Wertz, 2011) was applied to semi-structured individual interviews eliciting LGBTQIA+ users' experience of informal radical therapeutic practices. We used photo elicitation at the start of interviewing to stimulate emotional memory responses and allow participants to share and define their phenomenological experience, although in practice participants referred to the images infrequently (Bates et al., 2017). Photo elicitation did not feature in the analysis as participants did not particularly engage with the stimuli. We suspect that their strong affective connection to the pub means that they did not need any visual stimuli to prompt discussion, but future research might use photo elicitation more strictly to guide verbal data generation. Visual artefacts were drawn from community-based social media (Instagram: #TheMarlborough), a rich source of user-led data. After a prompt to explain what the Instagram images meant to them, participants were asked questions, including a description of times they used the pub community for support with their mental and emotional health, how their experience of support in the Marlborough may have differed from their experiences receiving services, how the Marlborough may differ from other queer spaces and how the provision of support in the community could be improved.

Ethics. Ethical approval was obtained from the University of Brighton Tier 2 Ethics Committee. Participants were considered vulnerable since as a group they experience more frequent mental and/or emotional distress, and/or symptoms of a mental illness as defined by the DSM-5 (APA, 2015; Stonewall Scotland 2014). Potential participants were excluded who were in *active* state of mental crisis at time of potentially giving consent, although pre-existing and ongoing emotional and mental distress were not an exclusion criterion because of the research topic. Charlotte Wilcox (CW) exercised clinical judgement in discussion with the participant as to whether current mental state would impact capacity to give informed consent to participate, or if taking part might even potentially exacerbate distress. This was re-assessed regularly. Participants could not be intoxicated at consent and/or interview. A single drink was not considered to amount to intoxication, in recognition of the fact that interviews were held at the pub, and that users may order a drink in the ordinary course of being on site. No ethical concerns arose during recruitment or data generation. Gatekeeper permission was secured from the pub managers and directors of the queer theatre company Pink Fringe/The Marlborough Theatre Company, based upstairs from the pub. Written consent was obtained prior to the interview and reiterated prior to commencement.

Participants and recruitment

Participants were ten regular users of the Marlborough Pub who self-identify as queer and/or as a member of 'the Marly community' (see Table 11.1). Recruitment was via word of mouth and via a poster displayed in the main pub to facilitate widespread awareness of the research study.

Analytical procedure

We followed standard procedures for descriptive phenomenological analysis (Wertz, 2011). CW coded meaning units within each transcript. Two transcripts were double-coded by Rebecca Graber (RG) and discrepancies were

Table 11.1 Participant demographics

Participant no	Age	Gender/sexuality expression	Relationship to Marly
1	33	Queer man	Managerial
2	32	Queer man	Resident artist
3	38	Queer woman	Regular
4	31	Queer woman	Regular/ex-staff
5	26	Queer woman	Regular/ex-staff
6	30	Queer nonbinary	Resident artist
7	44	Queer nonbinary	Regular
8	25	Bisexual trans woman	Regular
9	30	Trans man	Staff/regular
10	53	Two spirit	Regular

discussed. Summaries of phenomenological themes were written for each participant. These were collated across accounts to identify initial themes, which were finalised through ongoing discussion, imaginative variation and iterative movement between themes and codes, to arrive at our final six-theme structure. We engaged with critical reflexivity through a diary (CW) and ongoing discussion in recognition of the intersecting relationships held between personal and professional ways of being, grounded in the communities in which this work is situated. We addressed rigour by self-assessing whether the analysis faithfully conveyed lived experience, addressed phenomenological essences and typicalities, noted variations in experience according to meaningful demographics and conveyed accounts with empathy, openness and naivety (Elliott et al., 1999; Wertz, 2011).

Analysis

Analysis revealed six themes delineating forms of support experienced by Marlborough community members (see Table 11.2). These themes were: feeling recognised as you are; feeling safe to express the true self; experiencing intimacies of 'queer family'; engaging in queer listening; choosing community for humanised/humanising support; and experiencing ongoing healing of the self. For brevity and with the aim of most effectively addressing the needs of clinical and community psychology practitioners, we present only the analyses of the first, second and fourth themes in full.

Theme 1: Feeling Recognised as You Really Are

Participants experienced a recognition of who they really are within the space of the pub. While this has some connotations of 'acceptance', 'recognition' goes beyond 'acceptance' to involve a sense of being seen, known and celebrated, not merely tolerated or made to fit into, or being assessed against, an existing mould. This involved a felt sense of loosening norms, welcoming difference and embracing the weird.

Participants experienced the Marlborough as a place those who don't feel welcome or who might feel marginalised elsewhere could be recognised for who they are, as expressed simply by P5: 'I can be me here. There's no pretence' (48). This absence of 'pretence' appears crucial for countering the sense of heteronormative gaze that participants experience in other spaces, allowing participants to feel 'known' as they are. Said P10: 'It's just good to walk in,

Table 11.2 Theme descriptions and exemplar quotes

Theme name	Description	Exemplar quotes
Feeling recognised as you really are	Recognition of who participants really are within the space of the pub Involves sense of being seen, known and celebrated, not merely tolerated or made to fit into, or being assessed against, an existing mould Felt sense of loosening norms, welcoming difference and embracing the weird	*It's just good to walk in, and be known…they are just treating you as the person next to you, they are not treating you like the animal in the zoo, and just looking.* (P10) *There's such an openness—it not just about identity. It's about way more than that—people who come here are open-minded in all the ways.* (P9)
Feeling safe to express the true self	Pub as a sanctuary: a place of safety, where they could just 'be' Feelings of embodied safety tied up with feelings of belonging and inclusion, such that the body feels no pressure to perform but can be a comfortable vehicle for the self	*I don't feel nervous coming here. Which I might feel if it was just a random pub. I would be always looking a bit over my shoulder a little bit I guess. While here it's not like that.* (P8) *To be really crude, this is the only place other than my house where I can take a poo. This is the only place because it's literally like there's no defence….I don't know it feels like my personal space.* (P5)
Experiencing intimacies of the queer family	Consistent experience of the pub as both a symbolic 'family home' for living out close-knit relationships and reliably accessing experiences of intimacy unavailable elsewhere Particularly valuable for trans/nonbinary participants and those whose home lives have been disrupted, who seek a place to ground and be welcomed	*It's even more home than home. It's been the one constant since I've been in Brighton.* (P9) *Loads of pubs would be like, yeah, we're family. But this is actually family….I think it's the politics of it really. And the genuine caring thing. People are genuinely looking out for each other. And are aware.* (P4) *I've got a lot of siblings at the Marlborough. And parents. And children…the roles just pop about all over the place…but it works, and it's ok.* (P3)

Engaging in queer listening	Experience of specifically queer style of relating, characterised by sensitivity to the emotional life of self and others within this community Reciprocity in tacit commitment to support others in their expression of emotions, refusal to shame people for their feelings and keen sense of responsibility Question over skill as learnable or innate.	*I practice actual—you can call it queer—listening, when you don't hear anything else in your head. It's like you're really listening to another human being instead of thinking about your own shit.* (P6) *I just think queer people are especially magic [giggles] and just really caring and looking out for each other...not many other people look out for us. And I guess kind of a greater understanding of respect, consent, love, the different types of love and different types of relationships, and different understandings and a lot of emotional intelligence.* (P3)
Choosing community for humanised/ humanising support	Frequent experience of formalised services as instrumental, unaccommodating or unavailable in contrast to 'human-ness' of pub encounters Avoiding collapse into unhelpful binary of happiness/wellness and mental ill-health/sickness Community embrace of complexity of mental health to enable such feelings as 'radical joy'	*The DIY is always so much better than the institution because the institution has no room for joy because it only has room for numbers and results and feedback and data....It needs to feel enjoyable because actually to enjoy something, to be joyous is radical, it's as radical as being angry.* (P6) *This is my place I come to if I feel anxious...outside was one of my friends and I was like 'can I have a hug?'...five people all came out just to check on me....They were like, 'no, this is mental health, you do what you need to be doing to make yourself feel better'....I was like, 'well they're not judging me, and it's nice.'* (P4)
Experiencing ongoing healing of the self	Transformative healing and growth with lasting repercussions outside of the pub walls Detoxing of shame, promotion of self-worth, becoming of self, practice of compassion	*The amount of self-expression and the common sense of identity that it's given me, or the new kind of tools to re-contextualise my identity....Shame and guilt, you know it's the kind of queer building blocks of identity....It's given me some other things to feel proud about which are not rooted in shame and guilt.* (P2) *It gives me permission and validity you know to then go to other places and feel that I don't need to conform to you now!* (P1)

and be known…they are just treating you as the person next to you, they are not treating you like the animal in the zoo, and just looking' (368–369). For P10, being 'known' provides affirmation of personhood, in contrast to a reductionistic, entrapping categorisation to type ('like an animal in a zoo'). Friendships based in the pub were therefore experienced as pivotal in recognising the self and bringing it to a public expression, as P9 expressed about his gender transition: 'They have literally made me who I am now' (14–15). For P9, recognition was intertwined with presenting a new self in his own mould.

This sense of being recognised created a welcoming atmosphere that was experienced as a genuine integration of difference, as P3 expressed: 'There were people from all…different parts of the LGBTQIA+ community and really really integrating, and nobody felt that they were on edge.…I can be quite sensitive to atmospheres in places, and I didn't pick up on anybody being worried about being there, and the door was open, and people just floating in and out' (133–37). P3 acknowledges the difficulty in creating a genuinely integrated space in [their] sensitivity to 'atmospheres'. The fluidity of movement between spaces is felt to echo the freedom to be wherever, and whoever, one feels called to be.

This open-mindedness transcends gender or sexuality and was experienced as encompassing an overall loosening of norms: 'There's such an openness—it not just about identity. It's about way more than that—people who come here are open-minded in all the ways' (P9, 11). For P9, being part of this community comes part and parcel with an expansiveness that moves beyond identity concerns. Consequently, a new norm of the 'weird' emerges in which the non-normative is accepted, paving the way for recognition. P9's account goes on to exemplify a tension between acceptance and recognition that is at play in loosening norms to create a new norm of what might be called 'weird' elsewhere: '[People who] behave in ways that are not [neuro-]typical, or might be seen as "weird" but that's totally accepted here. Those things are not seen as weird, they're totally accepted' (P9 126–128). Here, that which brushes up against 'weird' is recast. A sense of difference ('they') and observation ('are not seen') are maintained, but norms are recast to envelop those who might otherwise be cast without.

While in P9's example of interpretation of neurotypical behaviours, a sense of acceptance is maintained, in most other contexts the 'weird', aka the different, was also celebrated. The distal presence of the theatre space often featured in accounts to emphasise this celebration. P5 imagines a 'nonbinary kid', on their inaugural trip to Brighton, stumbling up to the theatre and 'seeing a bad-ass non-binary person stripping their clothes off, singing a song, you'd be like, "Holy Shit! It's not just me!" You know, it's like family' (P5, 417–419).

P5's example invokes a felt sense of being brought in from the cold into the fold of family—through a perspective shift from seeking to recognition ('it's not just me!'), and within a celebration of the body, to be included in the community as one really is.

Theme 2: Feeling Safe to Express the True Self

Participants experienced the Marlborough as a sanctuary: a place of safety, where they could just 'be'. While 'recognition' has an existential cast, feeling safe involves feelings of embodied safety that are tied up with feelings of belonging and inclusion that allow for a physical de-armouring, such that the body feels no pressure to perform but can instead be a comfortable vehicle for the self.

Running through multiple accounts was a somatic experience of safety within the pub. Feelings of belonging and inclusion were expressed in an embodied fashion (e.g. 'there's just some sort of warmth about the Marly' [P8 354–355]). Safety was then localised within the body:

> It's just that I don't feel nervous coming here. Which I might feel if it was just a random pub. I would be always looking a bit over my shoulder a little bit I guess. While here it's not like that. It's just kind of normal. (P8, 111–113)
>
> You can kind of slightly unclench. And go ahhhh right, ok, there's lots of problems here, but being attacked isn't one of them. (P2)

These extracts point to the existential burden of the omnipresent threat of implied or actual violence in the straight world, with participants experienced heightened vigilance in monitoring their environment and holding physical tension. By contrast, the Marlborough is experienced as a place to physically relax ('ahhh'), in freedom from bodily threat. P2, a manager of the pub, is clear that things are not perfect here and that management of the space brings 'problems' of its own. This emphasis merely serves to underline the weight of the pressure that is relieved when this gay cis man steps into a phenomenological world that is not defined by straight masculinity.

Other participants noted that even within LGBTQIA+ community spaces, threats can stem from performative expectations. For example, 'gay' places can make P6, who identifies as nonbinary, feel like they're 'not enough, not lesbian enough. But the Marlborough never makes me feel like that. I just am, and that's enough' (P6, 53–54). For P6, there is a perceived threat to self in feeling pressured to contort themselves into ill-fitting labels even within other queer spaces. Interestingly, multiple accounts conflate the people of the Marlborough with the place itself, suggesting just how deeply this security is embedded within their sense of the space.

Other accounts suggest that this felt sense of safety is related to a felt sense of support prevailing within the community. Feeling safe is experienced as a permitted de-armouring as vigilance checks are abandoned, bodies are unclenched and unhelpful personas are dismantled. Said P1, a cis gay man, the Marlborough 'allows for you to take down some guards and some borders and some boundaries that you put on yourself because you thought that's what's expected of you'. Even while P1 acknowledges the normative and, perhaps, limited usefulness of being boundaried, such 'guards' and 'borders' (in militaristic metaphor) are ultimately untrue to the self. In the Marlborough, then, where bodily threats abate, the real self does not need to be hidden from view.

The embodied experience of sanctuary was most vividly expressed by P5: 'To be really crude, this is the only place other than my house where I can take a poo. This is the only place because it's literally like there's no defence.…I don't know it feels like my personal space' (49–50). For P5, in absence of the need for its constant defence, with the body permitted to meet the self ('my personal space'), the body could finally lay down its arms.

Theme 4: Engaging in Queer Listening

Participants engage in a specifically queer style of relating, characterised by sensitivity to the emotional life of self and others within this community. Relating was reciprocal—participants experienced a tacit commitment to support others in their expression of emotions, a refusal to shame people for their feelings and a keen sense of responsibility. Some felt this style of relating was learnable while others located it as innate.

The term 'queer listening' was used by P6, who explain their personal experience seeking support in the Marlborough during bereavement:

> I practice actual—you can call it queer—listening, when you don't hear anything else in your head. It's like you're really listening to another human being instead of thinking about your own shit. (P6 427–428)

For P6, being fully present to another person is experienced as fundamentally queer. They create a counterpoint to the relating offered by formal services and the straight world through their experience of being profoundly witnessed in their grief. To fully set aside 'your own shit' and bear witness to another soul is experienced as 'queer': a happening outside the norm, an authentic way of being, a movement outside of the self. Other participants experienced a contrast between queer listening and that experienced in the straight world. 'I don't have to hold myself in. No-one is going to come over to me and be like "I'm sorry, you're being a bit too much right now"' (P6 330–332). P3 often felt that her distress was too much in straight circles and compares with the Marly community: 'I didn't get any sense that people felt obligated to be nice, it was like a real love' (P3 114–115). Listening is experienced as an authentic expression of love, rather than performative; judgements about appropriateness and concerns about the listener's self are set aside in service to the support-seeker. The perceived intrinsic queerness of this love-imbued listening is reiterated by P3: 'I just think queer people are especially magic [giggles] and just really caring and looking out for each other…not many other people look out for us. And I guess kind of a greater understanding of respect, consent, love, the different types of love and different types of relationships, and different understandings and a lot of emotional intelligence' (233–236). This evokes the 'queer family' as bringing an emboldening unconditionality to queer friendships: 'People are very, very good at telling it straight, like it is. And not upsetting each other... I feel much more able in that space to say to my friends if I think they're being an idiot. And that be it' (P3 250–256). For P3, transparency and commitment to authenticity fosters intimacy, resulting in a deeper bond, but like most family relationships this may come alongside truth-telling, disputes and conflict.

While P3 suggests a sort of innate emotional intelligence for queer people, accounts also held the sense that queer listening is highly skilled. P9 talks about a special kind of attention required to meet others' experience, overladen with the responsibility to get this listening right: 'this is the one point of contact for a lot of people, they don't have friends (373–374). P9 said, 'there can be a scary amount of pressure to get this right, because if you fuck up there's that kid's first shot [at coming into the trans world] ruined' (265). Queer listening, in these accounts, necessitates making space for the person speaking, with all their attendant vulnerabilities and possibilities. This was underpinned by an understanding that those who support will also need to be supported. P6 said, 'it's like "you do you, and I'll do me". And that's it. And if you need anything, let me know, and if I can help, I will, and if I can't I won't, but I'm not going to say, "I'm sorry", you know, "you can't be sad, don't cry"' (336–338). Listening entailed a sense of responsibility for both parties, with individuals taking ownership for the management of their emotional selves-in-relationship—acknowledging the challenge and importance of being able to be fully present for another person, and demonstrating their own vulnerability without constricting the support-seeker. Crucially, this was a learnable skill: 'And also like teaching people how to respond to being called out' (P4 512–513).

The experienced effect of queer listening was that emotionality was fundamentally permitted:

> They're not gonna feel like they are overreacting, or being silly, or being too sensitive. It's just, these are your emotions and we accept that.... It's ok to be upset. (P4 505–516)

These extracts highlight that while queer listening entails presence and hearing, it does *not* entail a sense of gaze or judgement. Queer listening is experienced as meeting distress by another's presence: it is fundamentally an act of recognition. P4 knows that having expressed these feelings will not then lead to being rejected. They can be heard, without having their emotions labelled and judged in the moment of their being experienced. This allows for a release of unexpressed affect. While this permits an expansive release of emotionality, queer listening can also be experienced as containing those affective states that threaten to destabilise and destroy. For example, P9 noted that 'when it's all been too much for me to hold by myself, they've been there for me to help me hold it together it too' (86–87). For P9, queer listening is experienced as 'holding' the self, so that when he himself feels he is 'too much', others can maintain the disparate threads of his emotional state. Queer listening is, then, experienced as listening without monitoring, seeing without watching—holding with open hands.

Discussion

Analysis demonstrated ways in which queer people experienced the giving and receiving of emotional support in a queer community pub. Complex emotions and distress were welcomed, enabling the pub to operate as a relational matrix for support, with numerous types of relationships available for community members—including, but not limited to, close friends, acquaintances, lovers, 'queer family' members, staff. This community was experienced as characterised by reciprocity, interconnected relationships, embodiment and moves away from binary experiences of emotionality as indicative of either mental health or mental illness. In characterising some practices of fictive kinship—'queer family'—and empathetic listening as inherently queer, analysis speaks to the need to understand and celebrate the unique emotional support provided by and within this community. Johnson's (2015) psychosocial manifesto for sexuality invites us to attend to the transformative potential of queer forms of relating.

Within the relational matrix of the Marlborough is a space/place in which queer people can feel supported in their free expression of subjective experience, without having their being-in-the-world reduced to categorisations and/or performances of gender and sexuality. This evokes Heidegger's notion of a 'clearing' as an illuminated place where phenomenological expression—Gelassenheit ('letting beings be')—happens (Heidegger, 1993 p125). Given the contexts of heteronormativity, silencing, embodied threats, instability, fragmented familial relationships, social oppressions and even reductionism stemming from within other realms of the LGBTQIA+ community, the maintenance of this space and cultivation of a clearing in which to see and be seen becomes a fundamentally radical act.

A person's subjective experience is made up of 'selves-in-relationship', engaged in an ongoing and ultimately unrealisable process of 'being-in-becoming' (Atwood & Stolorow, 1996). In these accounts, selves-in-relationship are conducted in ways that are shame-healing, expressive, generative, creative and health-promoting. This conceptualisation, again, relies on an understanding of the self as inherently intersubjective, breaking a binary of self/other to understand subjectivity as relational. As suggested by ongoing experiences of healing and by experiences of 'queer listening' as involving a dance between maintaining the self and setting it aside, this allows participants to radically 'include' the self, others and all aspects of self-in-relationship, some of which may be painful and previously disowned, in ways that might not have been possible in other contexts and settings. Indeed, accounts speak not only to recognition (not acceptance) *between* individuals, but to the unfolding recognition and expression of multiplicities *within* the individual. This becomes a radical act in a wider context of oppression, categorisation and silencing. Undertaking this work within the informal, social sphere has a fundamentally humanising flavour. Although the Marlborough does not have the intensity of a formal psychotherapeutic dyad, it is, effectively, a dedicated informal therapeutic space. The powerful healing force of mutual recognition is readily available—on tap, as it were. It is experienced across accounts as a more phenomenologically resonant alternative to, complement to or substitute for formal service provision. Clinical psychologists are therefore invited to challenge the binary of therapeutic/non-therapeutic spaces, while community psychologists are invited to consider the necessity of cultivating and maintaining places to be *seen*, amongst wider discussions of empowerment.

This analysis adds to calls within clinical psychotherapy for two related shifts in perspective. First, we conceptualise some kinds of traumatic distress as a *relational* injury to 'self' to be healed, as inflicted, through the healing processes of relationship, as evidenced by the accounts (Van Der Kolk, 2009). Second, we reconceive trauma healing as a primarily phenomenological task, grounded in the principle of supporting somatic experience in the here-and-now (Levine, 2005). Shifting from the cognitive treatment paradigm to 'somatic experiencing' has been shown to be effective when working with gender-variant expressions (Briggs et al., 2018).

The analysis presents an invitation to community psychologists to integrate trauma-aware ways of working into our understanding of queer experience. A sense of existential permissibility—of being led by somatic experience, and of building trust in the body's capacity to restore equilibrium through unfettered expression—is key to trauma resolution treatments that understand trauma as living on residually in our nervous systems (Ogden 2012; Van der Kolk 2013). We suggest that participants are, informally and without clinical direction, engaging in some version of affect regulation process. Affect Regulation Theory suggests that individuals are in one of three affective states (threat/safety/drive) at any given time, which cycle in three distinct but dynamically interlinking systems (Gilbert, 2013). Threat, safety and drive/expression recur in participant accounts. By stilling fears of threat, promoting safety and encouraging full expression of emotionality and identity within the relational matrix, emotional support within the Marlborough may rise to loosening norms, unbuttoning the self and expressing feeling. Affect Regulation Theory links with the attachment paradigm to help clinicians think about processing of emotions, self-coherence and the role of the dyad (Benjamin, 2017). More than simply being seen and witnessed by another, intersubjectivity, mutual regulation and recognition describe processes at the implicit, co-created level of interpersonal exchange. This down-regulates hyperarousal, essentially making feelings easier to bear—as emotions are increasingly shared between partners, so can the *range* of feeling be shared, leading to co-regulation. Turning to the other can also be understood in attachment terms as a navigation towards subjective feelings of safety and security (Benjamin, 2017). Flexible affect regulation is associated with a well-engaged social engagement system, determining outward expressiveness and contact with others, with overall benefit to mental and physical health (Porges, 2014).

Indeed, for these queer participants, there is an embodied flavour to experience, particularly in managing feelings of shame and in the internalisation of long-standing physical threats. This is perhaps not unexpected when the body has been experienced as a site for battle, at worst, or negotiation, at best, and particularly for trans and nonbinary bodies (Johnson, 2015). Strong affects such as shame can be dysregulating—'too-muchness'—and can sometimes supersede the capacity of the other to absorb it, with the risk of becoming hyper-aroused themselves (Benjamin, 2017; De Young, 2015). Accounts speak to the complex intersubjective work done through emotional support within the Marlborough to contain and mitigate shame and other embodied threats. Analysis suggests that once the significant affective energy tied up in shame is affectively metabolised, it becomes available for expression of self (Finlay, personal communication, 2018).

This community, with its radically self-organising practices, constitutes a space/place for living out of queer lives, encompassing the full range of affective possibilities, from aspects of the joyful, the life-saving as well as the mundane. This itself is experienced as a resistance to the norm. The space further resists the erasure of queer experience threatened under hetero- and homonormativity (Duggan 2003), challenging the collapsed binaries that have frequently reified queer experience into stereotyped polarities of health and happiness/ill-health and mental illness, shame/pride, embodiment/performativity (Blackman, 2011). While the status of the Marlborough as a space/place for the 'indwelling' of complex queer lived experience is undoubtedly tied to the vision and activist practices of its management, our findings speak to a deep relational resonance that could not, be manufactured.

Participants' accounts attested to the experience of shared commitment to maintaining safety; inclusivity; acknowledging difference, welcoming diversity and celebrating expression. Literature on intergenerational and collective trauma suggests there is something profoundly reparative, indeed *vital*, about being part of a co-created culture that stands together to make and protect space—the 'clearing'—in which this unfettered expression of feeling-to-the self and to-the-other is welcome (Gobodo-Madikizela, 2016).

We can question why the Marlborough is experienced by these participants as a place for relationship, not 'just' for political activism—after all, shared values are commonly striven for throughout the community sector. We suggest the key here is the intersubjective underpinning of the lived experience of the Marlborough. This applied queer politics feels organic to participants because it is embedded within a complex relational matrix of support. The community, through both deliberate activism and spontaneous cultural practice, acknowledges and addresses the phenomenological needs of its members. Undoubtedly the Marly's queer community participates in affective activism in multiple ways, with its curated theatre programme, showcasing assertive celebrations of difference and emphatic practices of inclusion.

Queer theorists speak to the state of 'precarity' arising from neo-liberal economic conditions, which queers are disproportionately impacted by (Halberstam 2008; Munoz 2008). As we present our findings about the support undertaken in a 'queer local', we note with irony the disappearance of the neighbourhood 'boozer', as the privatisation of space gathers apace (CAMRA, 2017). This community came into being through the work of the theatre-makers in the company upstairs.

The current queer-led cooperative management structure exists in uneasy tension with the commercial interests of the large pub chain that owns the lease on the pub, and doubts for the financial viability of the pub surface regularly. The theatre company depends almost entirely on receding UK Arts Council funds, and has recently launched a crowdfunding appeal to raise £10,000 for basic running costs to mark its ten-year anniversary. The Marlborough is, unfortunately, typical of wider trends in which gentrification has led to a 'hostile environment' for queer community space: a review of LGBTQIA+ nightlife in London reports drastic closures of venues over the last five years (UCL Urban Academy, 2018). In richly describing the informal mental health support work being done here, this analysis provides evidence towards the essential benefits of creating and maintaining queer community places that allow for life-as-lived.

Implications for Community Psychologists

This unique pub community culture offers an exemplar for community psychologists interested in alternative models of distress and care. Here radical and self-organising 'informal care' practices function to mediate distress that otherwise is held by pathologised individuals, amplifying this distress. The valorisation of shared affective experience within a socially mediated framework is an important step in which community psychology can contribute by recognising this affective activist work.

Implications for Public Health Service Commissioners

The pub community is a significant resource for LGBTQIA+ community public health. Its precariousness should be of concern to those in local and central government who have a stake in maintaining public health in the city. The shift towards discourses of well-being that would recognise the impact of both community and a public art practice is reflected in the theatre's funding bids, which increasingly invoke mental health promotion as a key outcome. Mental health funders and providers would be similarly advised to widen their scope of what mental health services actually look like. Specifically this would involve allocating resources to strengthen institutional capacity within informal care providers. This could mean links with formal mental health providers, such as MindOut, in the form of training and support for Marlborough staff. Notably, bar staff frequently progress from working at the Marlborough to roles within formal care provision and/or therapeutic services.

Limitations

Since early 2017 the majority of Arts Council funds received by the Marlborough was allocated to working with Queer People of Colour (QPOC), with the dual strategy of improving representation in the arts, and engaging QPOC as audiences and as community members within the LGBTQIA+ community. This was not reflected within the sample since none of the participants identify as QPOC, although a number of participants alluded to this key strategy in their accounts.

Conclusions

A Husserlian phenomenological analysis of radical informal therapeutic practices in a vibrant queer community pub highlights varied and powerful forms of emotional support amidst experiences of shame and marginalisation. Queer listening emerges as a form of tacitly held knowledge and a learnable skill, transforming individually held distress into an experiential foundation for social bonds and points of resistance. Community psychologists are invited to work from within and/or in partnership with queer communities to recognise, develop and strengthen the practices of pre-existing affective communities through programme development and resource provision.

Acknowledgements We kindly thank Abby Butcher, Tarik Elmoutawakil and David Sheppeard, for access to the Marlborough Pub community, and our participants for sharing their experiences.

References

APA. (2015). The Diagnostic Statistical Manual.

Ashworth, P. (2003). An approach to phenomenological psychology: The contingencies of the lifeworld. *Journal of Phenomenological Psychology, 34*(2), 145–156. https://doi.org/10.1163/156916203322847119

Atwood G., & Stolorow, R. (1996). The Intersubjective Perspective. *Psychoanalytic Review, 83*, 181–194.

Bates, E. M. C., Kaye, L., & Taylor, J. (2017). "Beyond words": A researcher's guide to using photo elicitation in psychology. *Qualitative Research in Psychology, Vol, 4, 459–481.*

Benjamin, J. (2017). *Beyond Doer and Done To: Recognition Theory, Intersubjectivity and the Third*. Routledge.

Blackman, L. (2011). Affect, Performance and Queer Subjectivities. *Cultural Studies, 25*(2), 183–199.

Briggs, P., Hayes, S., & Changaris, M. (2018). Somatic Experiencing Informed Therapeutic Group for the Care and Treatment of Biopsychosocial Effects upon a Gender Diverse Identity. *Frontiers Psychiatry*, https://doi.org/10.3389/fpsyt.2018.00053

Butler, J. (1990). *Gender trouble: Feminism and the subversion of identity*. Routledge.

CAMRA (Campaign for Real Ale). (2017). Save Our Pubs campaign. https://www.camra.org.uk/pubs/campaigns/ (accessed 21/09/19).

Carroll, L., & Gilroy, P. J. (2001). Teaching "outside the box": Incorporating queer theory in counselor education. *Journal of Humanistic Counseling, Education and Development, 40*(1), 49.

Dennis, C-L. (2003). Peer support within a health care context: A concept analysis. *International Journal of Nursing Studies, 40*, 321–332.

De Young, P. (2015). *Understanding and Treating Chronic Shame: A Relational/Neurobiological Approach*. Routledge.

Drescher, J. (2010). Queer diagnoses: Parallels and contrasts in the history of homosexuality, gender variance, and the diagnostic and statistical manual. *Archives of Sexual Behavior, 39*(2), 427–460. https://doi.org/10.1007/s10508-009-9531-5

Duggan. (2003). *The Twilight of Equality? Neoliberalism, Cultural Politics, and the Attack on Democracy*. Beacon Press.

Elliott, R., Fischer, C. T., & Rennie, D. L. (1999). Evolving guidelines for publication of qualitative research studies in psychology and related fields. *British Journal of Clinical Psychology, 38*(3), 215–229. https://doi.org/10.1348/014466599162782

Finlay, L., & Dawsonera. (2011). *Phenomenology for therapists: Researching the lived world*. Wiley-Blackwell.

Giammattei, S. V. (2015). Beyond the binary: Trans-Negotiations in couple and family therapy. *Family Process, 54*(3), 418–434. https://doi.org/10.1111/famp.12167

Gobodo-Madikizela, P. (2016). *Breaking intergenerational cycles of repetition: A global dialogue on historical trauma and memory.* Opladen; Berlin: Barbara Budrich Publishers.

Graber, R. (in press). Peer support interventions. In *Cambridge Handbook of Psychology, Health and Medicine, 3rd Edition.* (Edited by Ayres, S., Llewellyn, C., Baum, A., McManus, C., Newman, S., Wallston, K., Weinman, W. & West, R.)

Graber, R., Turner, R., & Madill, A. (2016). Best friends and better coping: Facilitating psychological resilience through boys' and girls' closest friendships. *British Journal of Psychology, 107*(2), 338–358. https://doi.org/10.1111/bjop.12135

Graber, R., Madill, A., & Turner, R. (in press). You must be the place: the lived geography of resilience processes among British young people and their best friends in low-income communities.

Halberstam J. (2008). The Anti-Social Turn in Queer Studies. *Graduate Journal of Social Science, 5*(2).

Jettan, C., Haslam, J., & Haslam, S. A. (2012). *The Social Cure: Identity, Health and Well-Being.* Psychology Press.

Johnson, K. (2015). Sexuality: A psychosocial manifesto. Cambridge: Polity.

Jordan, J. V. (2013). Relational resilience in girls. In S. Goldstein & R. B. Brooks (Eds.), *Handbook of Resilience in Children* (2nd ed., pp. 73–86). Springer US. https://doi.org/10.1007/978-1-4614-3661-4_5

La Guardia, J. G. (2008). On the role of psychological needs in healthy functioning: Integrating a self-determination theory perspective with traditional relationship theories. In J. V. Wood, A. Tesser, & J. G. Holmes (Eds.), *The Self and Social Relationships* (pp. 27–48). Psychology Press.

LaSala, M. C. (2013). Out of the darkness: Three waves of family research and the emergence of family therapy for lesbian and gay people. *Clinical Social Work Journal, 41*(3), 267–276. https://doi.org/10.1007/s10615-012-0434-x

Levine P. (2010). *In an Unspoken Voice: How the Body Releases Trauma and Restores Goodness.* North Atlantic Books.

Moon, L. (2010). *Counselling ideologies: Queer challenges to heteronormativity.* Ashgate.

Moon, L. (2011). The gentle violence of therapists: Misrecognition and Dis-location of the other. *Psychotherapy and Politics International, 9*(3), 194–205. https://doi.org/10.1002/ppi.251

Munoz, J. E. (2008). *Cruising utopia: The Then and There of Queer Futurity.* New York University Press.

Ogden, P. (2015). *Sensorimotor Psychotherapy: Interventions for Trauma and Attachment.* Norton Series on Interpersonal Neurobiology.

Porges, S. W., & Carter, C. S. (2017). Polyvagal Theory and the Social Engagement System: Neurophysiological Bridge between Connectedness and Health. In P. Gerbarg and P. Muskin (eds.) *Complementary and Integrative Treatments in Psychiatric Practice* (pp. 291–310). Arlington, VA: American Psychiatric Association Publishing.

Postle, D. (2013). The richness of everyday relationships. *Therapy Today, 24*(3), 1.
Sedgwick, K. (1990). *Epistemology of the Closet*. University of California Press.
Stonewall Scotland. (2014). Your Services Your Say: LGBT people's experiences of public services in Scotland. https://www.stonewall.org.uk/resources/yourservices-your-say-lgbt-peoples-experiences-public-services-scotland-2014
Van der Kolk, Bessel A. (2015). T*he body keeps the score: Brain, mind, and body in the healing of trauma*. New York, New York: Penguin Books.
Walker, C., Hart, A., & Hanna, P. (2017). *Building a New Community Psychology of Mental Health: Spaces, Places, People and Activities*. Palgrave Macmillan.
Wertz, F. J. (2011). *Five ways of doing qualitative analysis: Phenomenological psychology, grounded theory, discourse analysis, narrative research, and intuitive inquiry*. Guilford.

12

The Evolution of the Community Psychology Festival

Miltos Hadjiosif and Meera Desai

Miltos Hadjiosif and Meera Desai met while organising the first ever Community Psychology Festival and also spent some time together on the BPS Community Psychology Section Committee, becoming two of the main people behind the Festival's many iterations. They both feel very grateful for the wonderful people they have met through these activities. Miltos is a Senior Lecturer in Counselling Psychology at UWE Bristol, an institution that enables him to teach psychology from a critical, reflexive angle and support his students to think of psychology as holding potential for liberation at a personal and collective level. Meera is a clinical psychologist who has always been inspired by systemic, narrative and community approaches in her work with children, young people and families. Miltos' main ambition in life is to have either PJ Harvey or Pearl Jam curate a Festival. Meera has no idea who either of these are, but judging by Miltos' excellent taste in Avril Lavigne albums, she can only assume that said Festival would be pretty great.

M. Hadjiosif (✉)
UWE Bristol, Bristol, UK

M. Desai
Ealing Council, London, UK

C. Walker et al. (eds.), *The Palgrave Handbook of Innovative Community and Clinical Psychologies*, https://doi.org/10.1007/978-3-030-71190-0_12

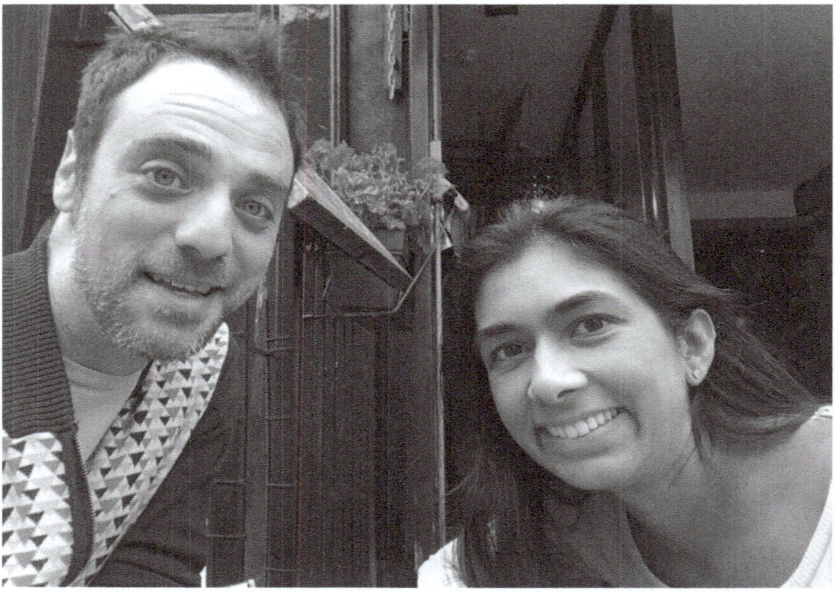

Festivals have been a staple of human culture since antiquity. They usually take place within a pre-specified time period, during which various activities such as music, theatre, and food feasts occur to attract and unite people in celebration of a particular cause. Many festivals have spiritual or religious ties, while others have been born out of trade and commercial interests. In contemporary popular Western culture, the word 'festival' brings to mind annual commercial music events such as Glastonbury in the UK and Coachella in the US. At the same time, scientific disciplines increasingly seek to engage the public by using this appealing format. It was against this backdrop of definitions, and exciting possibilities, that the idea of launching our very own festival as an alternative to an academic conference came about.

The concept of a Community Psychology Festival grew out of a discussion between members of the British Psychological Society (BPS) Community Psychology Section Committee. We asked ourselves what was unique about community psychology, how to bring our passion for it into our everyday work contexts, and how to be more inclusive within and beyond the narrow confines of our discipline. Parallel discussions noted that it tended to be the same people speaking at and attending the conferences and events that the Section put on, and that speakers at these events were typically preaching to the converted. We felt that we needed to do something more aligned with the values of community psychology, something distinctive, to attract people to the field and demonstrate its potential to do psychology differently. One committee member made a throwaway comment about how we should put on a festival instead of a conference. Instead of laughing and moving on, another asked, “Why not?!” and thus the Community Psychology Festival was born. This brief exchange foreshadowed the start of an ethos of dreaming big, making connections during informal moments, and trusting the process even when the details are far from being worked out, an ethos that has woven its way through each Festival.

November 2014 saw the inaugural (or ‘first ever’, as we liked to call it) Community Psychology Festival in London. What began as a vision for an accessible, inclusive alternative to an academic event culminated in a two-day festival of presentations, performances, and participatory learning. Subsequent years saw a second Festival in Manchester, a third in Bristol, and a fourth in Hertford. At the time of writing, preparations were underway for the fifth Festival in Brighton. In this chapter, we outline how the flagship event of the Community Psychology Section took shape, share our learnings from organising three such Festivals, and offer some thoughts regarding the future of the Community Psychology Festival in the hope of inspiring alternative ways of sharing knowledge and practice.

Combining Values from Critical Community Psychology and Festival Culture

Each Festival has been unique to time, space, and local context. It is important to stress that there is no set formula to be followed for each iteration of the Festival; thus it takes a lot of work on behalf of the organising team to create an event that strives to educate as well as entertain. The planning stages of the first Festival saw us spend much time considering our hopes and ambitions and laying down objectives that were aligned with Community Psychology. Much of our teleconference time was spent questioning taken-for-granted concepts, attempting to inspect each of our decisions with a critical eye, and challenging each other; it was perhaps our shared values that allowed us to do this relatively casually despite some of us having never met in person. We rallied around critical community psychology’s guiding principles of community, social justice, and stewardship (Kagan et al., 2011) and were clear that the creativity afforded by a Festival format needed to be capitalised to serve these values rather than simply becoming a marketing gimmick. We were also keen to attract the attention of potential contributors who might be put off by traditional conferences in order to showcase work that sat on the fringes of mainstream psychology.

Many of us were inspired by Paulo Freire's (1972) view of every 'learner' as an expert and educator with something to offer, and every 'expert' or 'educator' as having a lot to learn from those whom they purported to teach. Therefore, our aim was to create a learning community within the Festival, one in which the power dynamics that normally play out in academic events could be undermined. Our experiences suggested that these dynamics were often enacted between those who identified as psychologists and those who did not, between seasoned professionals and students, and between groups who held varying degrees of power in society, such as people of different genders, ethnic backgrounds, or abilities. For example, a common observation in mainstream conferences was that those who deliver talks and speak when delegates are invited to comment tend to be white, male, and with many decades of experience within a particular profession or discipline. This suggested that we had been losing out on some of the knowledge and experience held by those falling outside this privileged group. Another common critique of psychology is its historic exclusion of 'experts by experience' from the generation of knowledge, which is at odds with community psychology's preference for co-production of both knowledge and human services (Mayer & McKenzie, 2017). We believed that it was important to reach out to people with lived experience of mental distress, social injustice, and/or exclusion, as well as those in less professionalised roles who played a crucial part in helping people at a collective level, such as community organisers.

Although we acknowledged that we may not be able to wholly eradicate some of these power imbalances, we were determined to do our best, and learn from our mistakes for any future Festivals. By doing so, we hoped that we might be able to hear and learn from those who typically had less of a voice and whose wisdom was therefore obscured by more traditional knowledge-sharing events. We were confident that this would enrich any discussion, learning, and action which took place during and beyond the Festival. This required a shaking up of the rituals and 'taken-for-granteds' of traditional conferences, to prevent us from slipping into the ways of being and relating associated with them. It also required some subversion of the traditional expert versus learner roles, in accordance with Freire's idea of a 'learner-educator'.

An example of one of the early challenges we encountered was around how to signal that the Festival not only welcomed, but vitally relied on attendance by non-psychologists. We considered the benefits and drawbacks of a tagline that was half-jokingly suggested for our promotional material: '*Psychologists welcome, non-psychologists more welcome*'. There was a tricky balance to strike as we wanted to attract people who did not necessarily have a psychology background without alienating psychology colleagues who could become potential allies in our attempts to infuse a social justice agenda into the discipline.

We were also attracted to aspects of festival culture which we felt complemented critical community psychology values. Victor Turner (1966) coined the term 'communitas' and developed the concept of 'liminality', two ideas central in comprehending the nuanced group processes that take place during festivals. Communitas refers to the feeling brought about by a collective experience that happens when people come together. It can be thought of as 'inspired fellowship' or a sense felt by a group of people when their life together takes on full meaning (Turner, 2012, p. 1). Importantly, communitas occurs through the readiness of people to rid themselves of their concern for status and dependence on structure, and have an experience in each other's presence (Turner, 2012). Liminality is a state of 'in-betweenness', such as when one identity has been shed before another has been adopted (Turner, 1966, p. 94). It is a threshold often found in rituals, as well as natural daily phenomena when one state of being merges into another, for example, the hour of twilight. Fuelled by our own experiences of significant learning often taking place both within a collective and on the edge of boundaries, we hoped to make space for communitas and liminality as part of the Festival experience.

Themes, Rock Stars and Community Psychologists

Music festivals tend to rely on headliners, which receive top billing above less known names. This trend can similarly be discerned in many contemporary conferences listing keynote speakers who can be thought of as the heavyweights of each discipline at any given time. We were very clear that we did not want to have keynotes for the Festival as this would dilute the communitas we were aiming for and introduce an untoward hierarchy of significance in contributions that we consider of equal value. However, as with every movement, community psychology has its 'rock stars' and we paid homage to one of them, the late David Smail (cf. Cosway et al., 2017) who had passed away shortly before the first Festival, by naming one of the stages after him.

Academic conferences tend to cohere around one or more themes to give some focus to the content and publicity of the event, and in this case, we felt that it may be a useful structure to lean on. The theme of the Festival typically depended on where the organising committee's interests lay, as well as the socio-political zeitgeist of the time. The theme of the first Festival was 'Children and Young People'. We did not exclude any submissions on the basis of their relevance to this theme and ended up with some workshops and events which did not directly relate to it. However, holding children and young people in mind reminded us to foreground prevention and systems over intervention and individuals, and to give value to the resources of a group which holds much potential, but relatively little power in society (Burman, 2017). As part of this, we enjoyed talks, refreshments, and break-time performances provided by young people representing London-based social enterprises and community projects.

The second Festival had the theme of 'Creativity, Collaboration, and Community' and was promoted as an event open to anyone with an interest in social justice, wellbeing, and community cohesion. Beyond local and national third-sector organisations, we hosted participants and contributors from Spain, Greece, Italy, the Netherlands, and Israel. The spike in international interest presented us with the dilemma of how to maintain this appeal without contributing to an increase of the event's carbon footprint and we trialled some remote contributions using video links as well as streaming the Festival online.

The theme of the third Festival was 'Falling apart, pulling together: Collaboration in times of division'. This was a response to shifts in the contexts in which we were working, playing, learning, and living (Karanikolos et al., 2013; Feigenbaum & Iqani, 2015; Hirsch, 2013), and a call-out to groups who might be able to teach us about finding hope and shared meaning within this. It is probably not a coincidence that the theme was selected in the aftermath of the polarisation shaking the UK in 2017, following a highly controversial referendum on leaving the European Union (colloquially referred to as 'Brexit') and leadership instability across the political spectrum (Mance, 2017). In the call for contributions we additionally included some more 'concrete' sub-themes, for example, 'Housing and Mental Health', in order to signify the types of contributions that we were interested in receiving. These also helped with publicity by letting people unfamiliar with community psychology know what to expect from an event of this type.

Perhaps the most consistent piece of constructive feedback we received following the first Festival is that people would have benefitted from an early session on what community psychology is. Responding to this was somewhat tricky as definitions of community psychology inevitably fall short of capturing the ethos that we believe makes one a community psychologist. In addition, community psychology is an umbrella term that attracts psychologists working in different areas of research, training, and practice. As a result, we have refrained from including an orientation session in any of the Festivals and instead point those who want to find out more to resources such as the

Section flier and a collection of online articles which *The Psychologist* magazine has put together and typically updates prior to each Festival.[1]

Contributions

Interdisciplinary collaboration is a vital aspect of community psychology (Maton et al., 2006). Although we would have loved to have more members of the public attend our Festivals, we recognised the limitations on our budget and the amount of time we could spend on promotion. Actively seeking contributions from other disciplines felt like a more realistic first step towards an outward-facing Festival, and one which acknowledged the fact that psychologists certainly don't have all the answers.

Let us give an example of the interdisciplinary work that the event tried to foster, from the third Festival in Bristol. An economics lecturer who teaches large numbers of undergraduate students at a redbrick university came to deliver a participatory workshop. The session had the explicit dual function of introducing the economics of the housing market to the audience whilst also gathering their ideas on how to enrich the lecturer's material with insights that might sensitise her students to the effect of housing on mental health. A lively discussion followed, which illustrated the importance of allies, especially those from professions such as economics which risk being portrayed as villains in an all too simplistic manner.

The arts have been a strong thread running through the Festivals, and the reasons for our commitment to them were threefold. Firstly, we felt that the visual and performing arts have universal emancipatory and healing potential which is not amenable to conceptualisation within Western, euro-centric psychologies (Naidoo, 1996; Osei-Kofi, 2013; Rogers, 1993; Seedat & Suffla, 2017). Secondly, arts-based workshops can offer a participatory element, which we thought was crucial to the success of our Festivals. Serving the values of community, social justice, and stewardship often brings with it tensions and dilemmas; we believed that innovative solutions to some of these challenges would best be borne out of creative, participatory spaces, particularly those which encourage a sense of liminality. Thirdly, community psychology does not position itself as a science in which 'benefit' can be neatly measured; we wanted to resist austerity culture and its focus on an auditable surface by protecting and celebrating collectivist creative projects with real felt impact. Sessions ranged from arts-based community action projects to an experiential Biodanza workshop, in which even the most cynical festival goers seemed to

[1] To see these please go to https://thepsychologist.bps.org.uk/festival-community-psychology.

experience an embodied sense of community, connection, and positive affect through music and movement (Bateman, 2004).

Contributors for all sessions were encouraged to prioritise ongoing audience participation over structured slide show presentations ('participation over powerpoint') followed by a 'Q&A'. Continuous feedback was collected during the days of the Festival by encouraging festival goers to write on an 'Ideas Wall' and each day was structured so as to include sufficient time for connection whether during refreshment breaks or sessions which included higher levels of participation. However, every year feedback points to the fact that there is never enough time to do what mainstream conferences call 'network' and we prefer to think of as connecting with each other outside of sessions.

Making It Easier to Attend: Venues and Access

Each Festival aimed to organise itself in the heart of a local community, rather than take people out of the spaces in which they might typically live, work, play, and gather. We also wanted to avoid unnecessarily intimidating or elitist venues, thus accessibility is a key criterion for any potential Festival venue. Mindful of cuts to community centre funding, this meant choosing community and/or arts-based venues as far as possible within our budgetary and logistical constraints as a way of giving back to our host area.

We ended up with three very different venues across the first three Festivals. The first ever Festival took place in a spacious church in the heart of London. We were attracted to the venue due to its location, explicit commitment to accessibility, inclusivity (including an assertively inclusive stance on issues of gender identity and sexual orientation), political action, and non-conformity. However, although we would not rule the possibility of having a future Festival in a building of worship, we did receive feedback that some festival goers were less comfortable in such a venue. The second Festival was held in a refurbished mill in Manchester, a venue which prioritised sustainability in its purchasing, building, and catering practices, and provided low to no cost venue hire for community and activist groups. The third Festival was held in a publicly funded arts house on the Bristol harbourside which plays a central role in engaging under-represented communities with the arts.

We were aware that hosting a Festival which spanned one working day and one weekend day may prove to be a barrier to those with childcare responsibilities, so when we were asked whether children could be brought to the first Festival, we had an opportunity to put our organising principles to the test. Consciously putting aside our discomfort at breaking academic convention, and reminding ourselves that this was a festival and *not* a conference, we saw no reason to say no. Feedback following the Festival suggested that going back to our critical community psychology values in this instance had paid off:

> *I just wanted to say a huge thank you for the wonderful festival (please pass on my thanks to the other organisers, as I don't have their e-mails). It was absolutely one of the best things I've been to in years. It totally embodied the spirit of community psychology. I loved the way everyone was included in such a natural way, including children. if only more spaces were like that, then the problem Sue Holland named of mothering and activism wouldn't be so acute. Myself and my colleagues who took part absolutely loved it and I've been buzzing with the inspiration ever since.*
>
> *Email following the first Festival (included with festival goer's permission)*

Invigorated by this positive response, our dream for the third Festival was that our team of volunteers could use a spare room to create a family space with free childcare; however, our energy and commitment to inclusion were no match for UK Health and Safety policies. We welcomed several infants and young people to the Festival nonetheless and they played a key part in a place-building intergenerational workshop that took over the entire Auditorium for half a day. Perhaps it was the ice-cream show, courtesy of a local enterprise, but we would like to believe that the radiant smiles on the youngsters' faces indicated a growing interest in community engagement! We wanted festival attendees to mirror what an actual community might look like and saw it as a real strength that this crowd cut across generational, among many other, divides.

Venue permitting, the Festival uses independent, local caterers as far as possible. Sustainable produce, the reduction of waste, and the avoidance of plastics were other factors that were considered when planning the food and refreshments to sustain festival goers over the two days. For the first Festival, fruit and morning pastries were bought from an independent café, and a community-based children's charity agreed to bake cakes for us free of charge as part of one of their regular activities. We later decided to use some of our underspend to make a donation towards equipment as a thank you. We were delighted to contract Community Interest Company the Social Kitchen to provide lunch on both days as part of their *Mamas to Market* project, which supported a group of first-generation Vietnamese women towards running their own local market stall. Although it took some organising to transport hundreds of freshly cooked spring and summer rolls, aromatic stew, and dumplings across London, we ended up with some of the best food participants had ever experienced at a festival (or conference!).

Costs

Funded by some generous grants from the BPS Research Board's Section Initiative Fund, the BPS North West Branch, and the BPS Division of Clinical Psychology's Faculty for Children, Young People and their Families, we were able to keep registration fees relatively low for our first Festival. We were also able to offer a number of full bursaries, which meant that a large proportion of festival goers were from community organisations, activist networks, and service user/survivor groups. With each successive Festival attracting more and more interest from within as well as beyond psychology, culminating in a sold-out third Festival, we also grew in confidence and felt increasingly able to use pricing models which allowed us to fund a significant number of bursary places ourselves.

Critical psychology helps us see that language constructs as well as conveys (Potter & Wetherell, 1987) and we wanted to use words that created an inclusive festival ethos (hence the 'first ever' instead of the 'inaugural' Community Psychology Festival). Clearly, an event like the Festival is allergic to the term 'patient' but we found that making bursaries available to 'service users' was also linguistically problematic as it obscures those who had experienced other sorts of marginalisation. As a result, our bursaries were available to 'community members' who could not afford the price of the ticket.

A large team of volunteers from local undergraduate psychology courses ensured the smooth running of the third Festival, and allowed some of the exuberance to be contained with an invaluable operation involving lists, rotas, and timetables. This had the added benefit of allowing a group who might otherwise not have been able to afford the registration fees to immerse themselves in a branch of psychology which is largely absent from undergraduate curricula.

Keen to foster the sense of communitas which had developed over the two days at previous Festivals, and with the awareness that attendance fees were significantly lower than those of a typical academic conference, we also refrained from offering a single-day discount to registration fees for the third Festival in order to incentivise full participation over the two days. This had the unforeseen effect of helping to partially address the issue of there never being enough unstructured time for connection, as many festival goers spontaneously made use of the hours between the first and second days to continue their conversations. However, this pricing model is a point of debate amongst the organising team, as it effectively discourages people that can only attend one of the days from coming.

Having a university as an affiliate for the third Festival was advantageous for a number of reasons, including being able to use their press office and online payment facilities, as well as involving their talented students and staff in all aspects of organisation. The extent to which an academic institution with a more or less traditional psychology department will skew the Festival's focus towards mental health oriented content is something we often debate. On the one hand, attaching the Festival to a university means that we get a chance to probe the boundaries of psychology right at the root of its dissemination, while on the other it signals a compromise that future Festivals will try to rectify. Nonetheless, we are keen for the Festival to remain an independent entity and it is important for any partner organisation to appreciate that it is not a profit-making venture. After all costs have been covered, any remaining profit goes into the planning of the next one, mainly in the form of bursaries to increase accessibility.

The Finishing Touches

We were aware that the formality and structures of academic conferences were contributory factors to their inaccessibility by early career psychologists and members of the public. As many of our 'day jobs' were focused on the reduction of mental distress, we found the resultant exclusion of service user/survivor/lay groups particularly unhelpful. Therefore, we consciously attempted to foster a flexible, informal approach to hosting the Festival, one which acknowledged the necessity of play (Fig. 12.1). During the first Festival, organisers identified themselves by wearing welly boots; we also referred to glitches as 'Glastonbury rain' and rooms as 'stages'. By the time of the third Festival, we had given up any pretence of needing to be taken seriously, and went all out with our (optional) festival attire as organisers, including sequins, 'festival hair', and copious amounts of glitter. The feedback obtained would suggest that this stance was particularly well received and succeeded in its attempts to foster inclusivity. We experienced no negative effects of 'being human', or 'being ourselves' on our ability to tackle weighty topics or engage in academically rigorous debate, although we have yet to submit this to empirical testing. The signature object of the Community Psychology Festival is a wristband (Fig. 12.1 and 12.2), which acts both as an easy way to identify festival goers and a keepsake to remind ourselves of the festival magic long after the final curtain call.

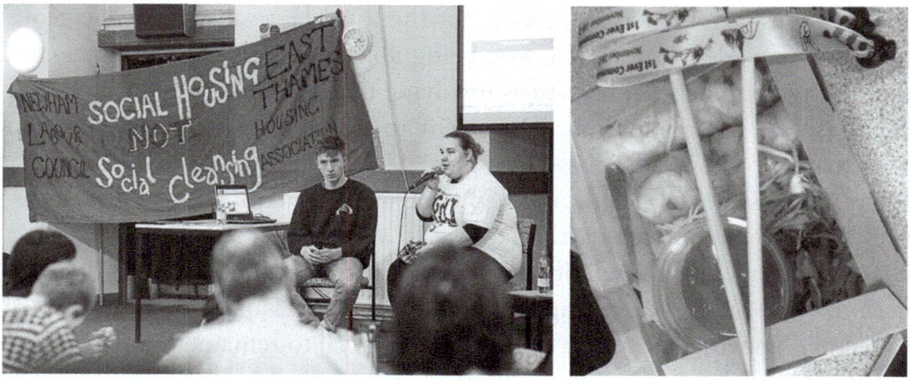

Fig. 12.1 Images from the festival

Fig. 12.2 Wristband from the third Community Psychology Festival

Looking Ahead

In a study of Edinburgh's Beltane Fire Festival, Matheson and Tinsley (2016) charted the festival's evolution as it progressed from the initial stages of revival, through development and regulation, to maturation. The carnivalesque early days offered greater participation for all and a lack of division between performers and audience, which was an important element in its communitas. However, as audience sizes increased, the event became increasingly professionalised, leading to, for example, the exploration of different event funding models, the involvement of external stakeholders, and the acquisition of charity status. Despite careful navigation, it was felt that the original communitas was eroded by these regulatory influences. As we look ahead, we are conscious to ensure that a similar fate does not befall the Community Psychology Festival. Everybody involved in the organisation of the Festival volunteers their time, enthusiasm, and skill-set as best they can, and it is this non-hierarchical ethos that will perhaps best protect the Festival from commercialisation. Our hope for the future is that community organisations will become more involved in each successive Festival; however, hope is perhaps not enough to ensure that we don't become complacent with the Festival's success only within the networks that are familiar to us. We are currently wondering what a more concerted effort to attract and engage with the local communities might look like. The Section is exploring a more strategic plan for the future of the Festival, which could culminate in some pre-specified roles relating to community outreach being put in place.

Another challenge pertains to how we can meaningfully capture and articulate the 'impact' of the Festival. Feedback consistently indicates that what people value the most are the intangible qualities, liminal experiences, thought-provoking conversations, and moments of connection. At the same time, it strongly hints at frustrations regarding how to translate all this into action and bring about much desired changes in the contexts where people live and work. This should not be an unfamiliar tension to community psychologists, yet it is one that the Festival seems to bring into focus each year. Perhaps one way of thinking about the Festival's role is as a physical forum where we can come together and 'fail better' (Prall, 2004) at bridging the proverbial 'talk-walk' divide. Figuring out how to sustain new collaborations and the following through of ideas is one area in which we have much further work to do.

We are aware of the dangers of being biased towards urban sites, particularly as the Festival was born right in the centre of London. Moving each Festival to another part of the country has brought its own challenges, as we have needed to balance responsivity to feedback from previous Festivals against responsivity to the needs of local communities. There have also been practical issues around needing to have at least a portion of each Festival's organising committee based in the region, which has meant that the art and science of hosting a Festival has had to be re-learnt to some extent each year. This links to our hope of each Festival inspiring attendees and giving rise to a new team that picks up the mantle of putting on the next one, as indeed was the case for the organising team of the fourth Festival in Hertford.

Personal Reflections

The rationale and theory behind the decisions we have taken when organising each Community Psychology Festival are important, as are the basic 'nuts and bolts' of how to run a Festival. However, it can be hard to convey in such concrete terms exactly how the Festival has managed to embody communitas and liminality, or the subtle ways in which it chips away at the barriers to community, social justice, and stewardship. Therefore, we would like to conclude with some reflections on what the Festival represents for the two of us.

We met during the planning stages of the first Festival, at a time when we had not yet joined the Community Psychology Section Committee. Our involvement with community psychology came at a particularly inspirational time, when many ideas were exchanged (some of them too wild to put to print) in the articulation of a shared vision of what this event might look like.

We were struck by the affinity we felt towards each other and the rest of the organising team with whom we held regular teleconferences. We knew each other's voices before we saw each other's faces, on the first day of the first ever Festival. It is no understatement that we were swept away by the enthusiasm and solidarity of the festival goers, and saw our anxieties about everything going according to plan give way to relief and a surrendering to the communitas of a psychology event that was truly different—people were standing shoulder to shoulder whether they were trainees, professors, activists, or their children.

We witnessed genuine reflexivity, an openness to new ideas, those with traditionally more power stepping back to encourage those who might not normally be allowed to speak, camaraderie, an appetite to contest the status quo, and invitations to be challenged. Most probably as a result, we also benefitted from attendees from a wide variety of backgrounds confidently participating and feeling connected to each other and to the elements that attracted us to community psychology in the first place. We were always amazed at how quickly the festival spirit took over and the line between organisers and attendees became blurred; people were very keen to help with the running of the event in a way that suggested that for most people, it was an event that they co-created and took ownership of, rather than attending in the expectation that they would be catered for. While we are certain that there were times when our community psychology values were less embodied, and where we could have done better, what we saw provided a stark contrast, for four successive Festivals, to many mainstream psychology events that we had attended.

Returning to the Festival each time brings us the joy of reconnecting with familiar faces and forging new connections alike. We believe that one of the Festival's most important functions is to energise those that attend it, and inspire those who follow it from afar, as it provides a galvanising experience which can be crucial in sustaining community psychology work. As with many 'continuing professional development' events, it also provides a pause for us to reflect on the ways in which we have, and have not, brought community psychology values into our work, and re-energise ourselves to continue this cycle of action, reflection, and dialogue over the coming months and years.

References

Bateman, C. (2004). Can we dance towards health? *South African Medical Journal, 94*(2), 76.

Burman, E. (2017). *Deconstructing developmental psychology*. Routledge. https://doi.org/10.4324/9780203946169

Cosway, R., Foley, J., Jones, J., Morgan, S., Priest, P., Richards, C., & Wainwright, T. (Eds.) (2017). Power, interest and psychology: Developing David Smail's ideas [Special Issue]. *Clinical Psychology Forum, 297*.

Feigenbaum, A., & Iqani, M. (2015). Quality after the cuts? Higher education practitioners' accounts of systemic challenges to teaching quality in times of 'Austerity'. *Journal of Further and Higher Education, 39*(1), 46–66. https://doi.org/10.1080/0309877X.2013.778961

Freire, P. (1972). *Pedagogy of the oppressed*. Penguin Books.

Hirsch, D. (2013). *A minimum income standard for the UK in 2013*. https://www.jrf.org.uk/sites/default/files/jrf/migrated/files/income-living-standards-full.pdf

Kagan, C. M., Burton, M., Duckett, P. S., Lawthom, R., & Siddiquee, A. (2011). *Critical community psychology*. Wiley-Blackwell.

Karanikolos, M., Mladovsky, P., Cylus, J., Thomson, S., Basu, S., Stuckler, D., … McKee, M. (2013). Financial crisis, austerity, and health in Europe. *The Lancet, 381*(9874), 1323–1331. https://doi.org/10.1016/s0140-6736(13)60102-6

Mance, H. (2017, December 30). British politics in 2017: Terror, tragedy, Theresa May and Brexit. *The Financial Times*. https://www.ft.com/content/861c1054-e57f-11e7-8b99-0191e45377ec

Matheson, C. M., & Tinsley, R. (2016). The Carnivalesque and event evolution: A study of the Beltane fire festival. *Leisure Studies, 35*(1), 1–27. https://doi.org/10.1080/02614367.2014.962591

Maton, K. I., Perkins, D. D., & Saegert, S. (2006). Community psychology at the crossroads: Prospects for interdisciplinary research. *American Journal of Community Psychology, 38*(1-2), 35–49. https://doi.org/10.1007/s10464-006-9062-3

Mayer, C., & McKenzie, K. (2017). '…it shows that there's no limits': the psychological impact of co-production for experts by experience working in youth mental health. *Health & Social Care in the Community, 25*(3), 1181–1189. https://doi.org/10.1111/hsc.12418

Naidoo, A. V. (1996). Challenging the hegemony of Eurocentric psychology. *Journal of Community and Health Sciences, 2*(2), 9–16.

Osei-Kofi, N. (2013). The emancipatory potential of arts-based research for social justice. *Equity & Excellence in Education, 46*(1), 135–149. https://doi.org/10.1080/10665684.2013.750202

Potter, J., & Wetherell, M. (1987). *Discourse and social psychology: Beyond attitudes and behaviour*. Sage.

Prall, W. (2004). Failing better: Integrative theory as work in progress. *British Journal of Psychotherapy Integration, 1*(1), 24–32.

Rogers, N. (1993). *The creative connection: Expressive arts as healing*. Science & Behavior Books.

Seedat, M., & Suffla, S. (2017). Community psychology and its (dis)contents, archival legacies and decolonisation. *South African Journal of Psychology, 47*(4), 421–431. https://doi.org/10.1177/0081246317741423

Turner, E. (2012). *Communitas: The anthropology of collective joy*. Palgrave Macmillan.

Turner, V. (1966). *The ritual process: Structure and anti-structure*. Cornell University Press.

13

The Define Normal Project

Danny Taggart, Cheryl Nye, Jessica Taylor, Jacob Solstice, Matthew Harrison, Rebecca Bryant, Stacey Clark, and Wendy Franks

The authors would like to dedicate this chapter to the memory of our colleagues and friends Oz Osborne (1972–2018) and Dr Wendy Lara May Franks (1969–2021). Oz was instrumental in the development of the Define Normal project and several other Community Psychology ventures in Great Yarmouth over many years. He was and continues to be an inspiration to us through his commitment to working for social justice and transformational change in the field of mental health. Wendy was a co-author of this paper and the project coordinator. Wendy was the central influence on the devlopment of Community Psychology praxis in Great Yarmouth, and her thinking, work and commitment continues to inpsire us all.

"I think that's what Define Normal is all about really…people get scared of the unknown and they like you to fit in a certain box. People don't like unpredictability, people feel comfortable…everyone's got a certain way they communicate, a certain way they behave and when people are different I think it worries people, it scares people and the only thing they can think to do is to try to fix it when maybe it doesn't necessarily need fixing." Cheryl

D. Taggart (✉) • C. Nye • J. Taylor • J. Solstice • M. Harrison • R. Bryant • S. Clark • W. Franks
Colchester, England
e-mail: dtaggart@essex.ac.uk

C. Walker et al. (eds.), *The Palgrave Handbook of Innovative Community and Clinical Psychologies*, https://doi.org/10.1007/978-3-030-71190-0_13

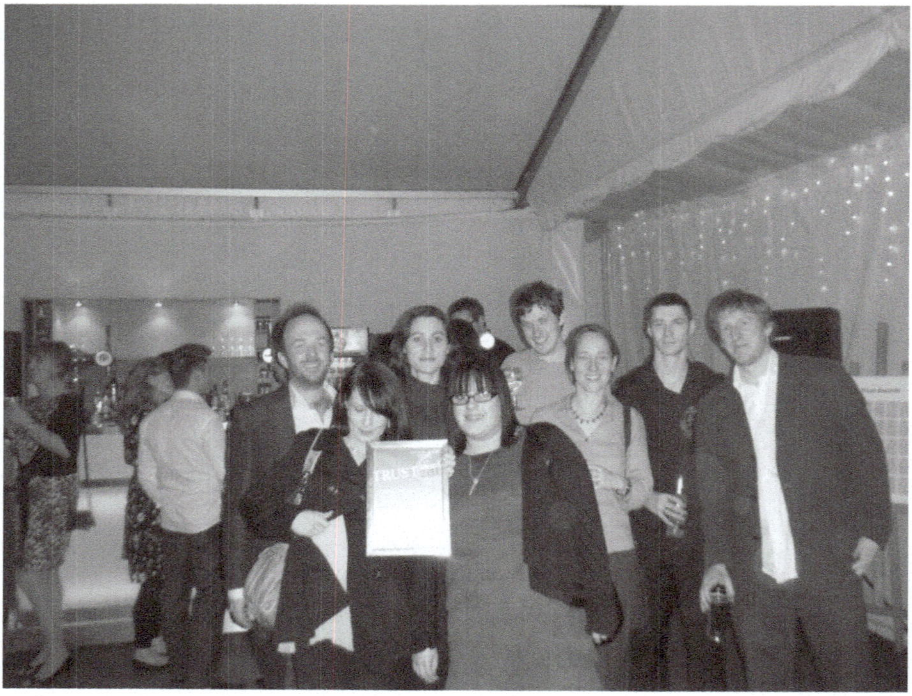

The chapter format draws on the work of Kagan et al. (2011) which loosely structures community psychology praxis along stages of action research—think, consult, act, reflect. Following some contextual scene setting, we divide the project into these four overlapping phases in order to illustrate how each stage of the work can be considered as part of an action research cycle. In actuality the project was more dynamic and circular than this, with cycles of theorising, consulting, acting and reflecting occurring at all stages throughout the project. This structure also largely reflects the theoretical concerns of the two clinical psychologists involved in the project (Danny & Wendy), as will be seen the young people and to a lesser extent the other staff involved were more task and process focused, with less concern for the community psychological orientation. From this perspective, therefore, community psychology praxis *enabled* the project by providing a framework, but it was the collaboration with the young people and their creative control that *drove it.*

Context

This project was undertaken in a seaside town in the Eastern Region of the United Kingdom, Great Yarmouth. The town experiences significant levels of socio-economic deprivation, including much higher than national average rates of child poverty, income deprivation and eligibility for free school meals. Health-related statistics show higher than national average rates for alcohol-related hospital admissions, child safeguarding referrals, instances of domestic abuse and teenage pregnancy. Social and economic statistics show higher than average rates of NEET (Not in Education, Employment or Training) among young adults, rising levels of youth homelessness and below national average educational achievement (Norfolk County Council, 2015).

On the other hand, Great Yarmouth is a historic fishing town and seaside resort dating back to the thirteenth century, which has been catering for Britain's tourists since the eighteenth century. It has higher than average levels of migration for the region and enjoyed something of a renaissance during the New Labour years with higher than average levels of investment, particularly into public services.

The funding for this project came from an under-spend from a regional commissioning body's training budget for professionals about 'emergent personality disorders' in young people. It was administered through the local NHS Mental Health Foundation Trust. At least some form of young person involvement was required for the use of the under-spend. This was based on feedback from participants who attended the original training. Two of the authors had experience of working with the local community in participatory ways (Franks, 2013; Taggart et al., 2013) and so were approached by Mental Health service management to develop the training with service user involvement. The project therefore began from a 'top-down' organisational directive, was initially professionally led and task-focused. In the context of the previous work from this funding, the use of diagnostic frameworks to describe young people's mental health was contested.

Think

This section will address the theoretical conceptualisation that informed the project's development.

Critical community psychology and the action research model (e.g. Reason, & Bradbury, H. (Eds.)., 2001) were the overarching approaches initially employed by the professionals to inform the strategies for engaging young people and steering the process of this project. As such, from the outset this project was clearly shaped and driven by professionals, held accountable within professional structures. Within this framework, the intention was to be as participatory *as possible* within the expectations and instructions of the funding and managing bodies. This tension between the emancipatory, critical praxis of community psychology and the instrumental, corporate culture within NHS Foundation Trusts defined aspects of the project with certain project members keen to push boundaries further and others needing to maintain organisational accountability. We suggest that this is likely to be a feature of many such projects and a key strategy early on was to ensure the *nature of participation* was spelt out clearly in all project documents. So on the Define Normal project participation meant that the young people could have complete editorial and creative control of all aspects of the training *content*, while professionals were responsible for making decisions about training *delivery*. This strategic planning mattered later on to the young people as Jacob points out, "It was complete freedom to express ourselves, no one ever said, 'Oh, don't know if that's a good idea'."

A further tension was that there were some differences between the commissioning directives and the involved professionals' recognition of user-based knowledge and critique of services, particularly the original training's emphasis on Emerging Personality Disorders, a diagnostic expansion that all the professionals involved had concerns about. We aimed to develop a respectful relationship that valued the expertise of both professionals and service users. One of the areas of commonality among professionals involved was a shared critical understanding of the dominant way of understanding and treatment of young people's mental health such as forced treatment, medicalisation and labelling. This interacted in a complementary way later with the young people who also had a radical and critical take on mental health services, in some ways even more so than the professionals. Managing this difference in the extent of critique between different project members was another feature of the process.

Previous community psychological work in the locality were underpinned using a UK-influenced community psychology approach (Kagan et al., 2011; Orford, 2008) and typically followed a structure of research or consultation with relevant key informants from within the community, followed by development of collaborative projects to build upon findings that could be beneficial for the community. Two earlier projects have been possible because of funding from a Neighbourhood Renewal Fund (Franks et al., 2007) and trainee time from a specialist clinical psychology training placement (Taggart et al., 2013). Both of these projects were made possible through supportive management within locality mental health services. Clinical psychologist relationships with mental health management demonstrated the value of permitting time and workforce resources to undertaking service development activity. It also reflected political priorities of the New Labour government at that time, which were still emphasising social inclusion, community capital and transformational initiatives aimed at empowering marginalised communities. While arguably, many of these constructs were little more than empty signifiers which could be twisted to suit prevailing neoliberal orthodoxy, the project was able to appropriate the discourses in order to pursue a community psychology agenda. For example, at that time empowerment was not only a psychological construct but a policy priority, so making this an aspect of the Define Normal project fitted with commissioner priorities. Once embedded in the project, we theorised empowerment to mean young people taking *actual power*, as opposed to a watered-down *psychological sense of empowerment*. It is without doubt more difficult to harness policy constructs to community psychology ends under conditions of austerity, but this formula of using contemporary ideas like resilience to justify clinical community psychology working may still have utility.

With the Define Normal project, a psychological formulation of the broad issues was initially generated from a professional's perspective (see Fig. 13.1), which would ultimately be superseded by a collaborative formulation, generated within the group. This collaborative formulation would shape the development of the training materials and strategy. Our hypothesis embedded in Fig. 13.1 was that young mental health service users had little claim to expertise within the system as it exists. Theoretically this represents both forms of what Miranda Fricker (2007) has helpfully theorised as Epistemic Injustice. It is a Testimonial Injustice in that the perspectives of the young people are not given the status of experts in relation to their mental health care by virtue of an 'irrationality' arising from their 'mental illness'. At the same time there is a Hermeneutical Injustice operating as in their isolation as patients the young people would struggle to form the social bonds and shared meanings that could enable them to forge new forms of knowledge where their expertise could be recognised. It was the projects intention to intervene in this cycle; if the young people developed a collective voice, then it was possible for them to be experts, albeit in the limited context of some training days. In speaking about her previous artwork Stacey articulates this sense of isolation: "I used to see the things I used to draw as personal and that people wouldn't understand them, so I kept them to myself. For myself, I feel invisible to the world, people see through me and don't see me as a person." This is in relation to a piece of

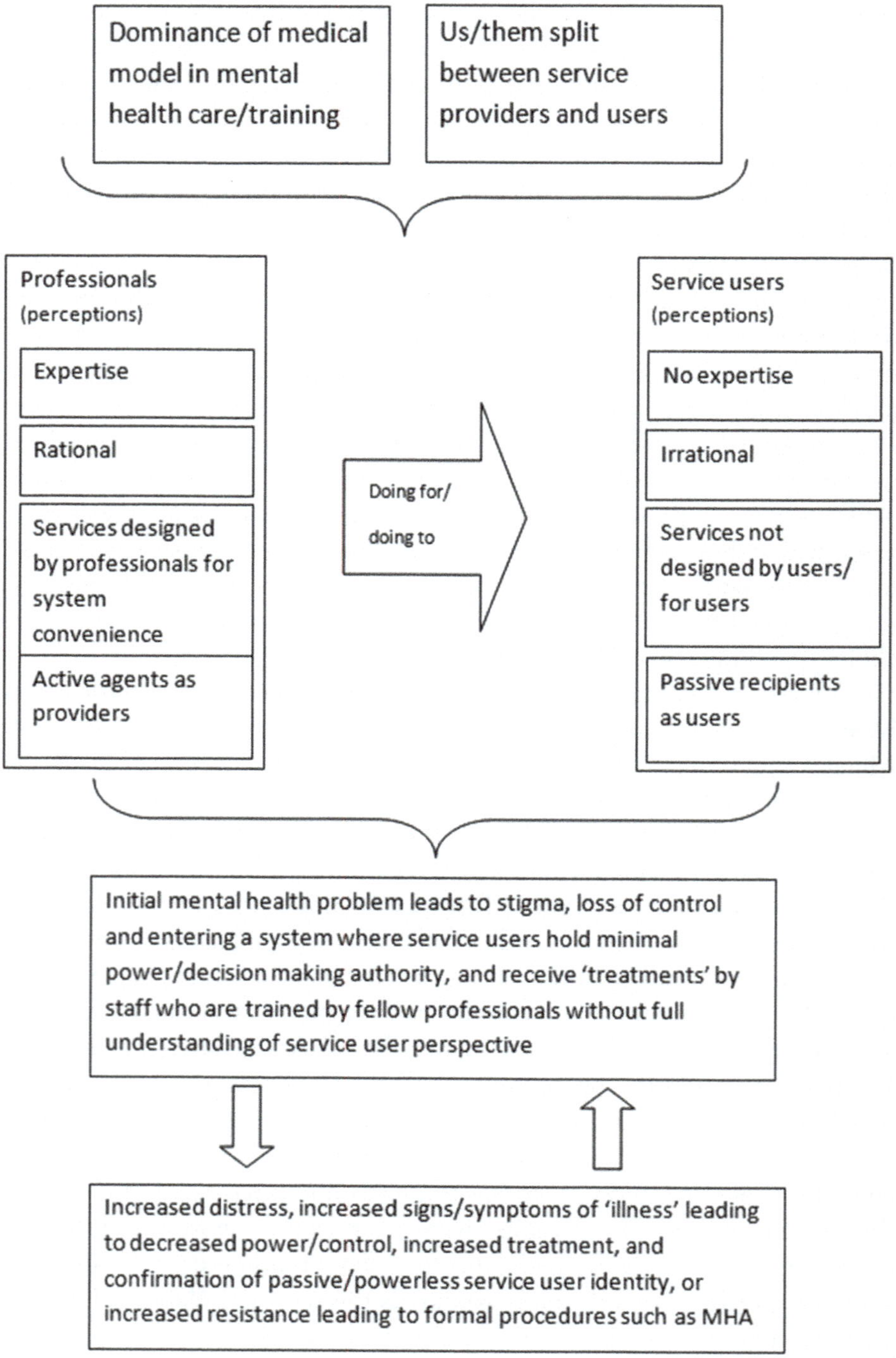

Fig. 13.1 Professional-generated formulation

artwork Stacey produced for the training, in the form of a short graphic novel. So in coming into the project, what had been personal and unseen could be put into the world as a training resource and shared with other people. Therefore our initial formulation recognised the need for the definition of who is an expert to be broadened to incorporate people with 'experiential knowledge' alongside creative potential. However, this statement of intent could only be realised once the young people brought into the project what had previously been silenced, with epistemic justice in this project meaning little theoretically in the absence of action.

Consult

This section outlines the development of the project as well as considering 'process' issues germane to its success.

The original aim was to work with a group of 6–8 young people (likely to be between 16 and 25 years of age) who had experiences of complex mental health needs, and who were interested in working together to develop a training package for service providers. Involvement was sought from young people within the age range on the basis of their experience and motivation rather than criteria such as diagnosis or other demographic characteristics.

The first points of contact came through the existing inter-agency networking group: the Youth Emotional Wellbeing Forum (YEWF), and local mental health services. A small group of staff across different agencies was originally engaged to support the development and delivery of the training. There was initially a considerable level of interest in involvement in this project from colleagues in the YEWF. The initial planning meetings included staff from different agencies including Young Minds, Rethink, Mental Health Services, Connexions and the local Further Education College. However, as the project developed, professionals from services outside of the Mental Health Trust found it difficult to prioritise this work and were unable to continue their involvement. The staff from the Mental Health Trust had time allocated within their roles for this project, and this is what enabled the project to continue. The young people were recruited from a range of sources: a local sixth form college, the local Early Intervention service and a local Young People's Mind. Seven young people attended the initial meetings, reducing to five core project members who were involved all the way through to delivery of the training days. The young people took on different roles depending on their expertise and interest, but the experiences of each of them contributed to the creative content of the training resources.

"We threw lots of ideas together…" (Zombie Dave). As Dave points out here the initial stages of the project were fairly free flowing. The professionals within the team worked together to provide a space for young people to explore their experiences of mental health and mental health services. The aim of this initial stage was to develop ideas about what the young people would like professionals to understand, so that this could inform professional practice in providing services. This process involved flexible group discussions and focused activities to generate a set of themes that would shape the training. The themes were integrated into a large collaborative formulation. There was initial anxiety from the young people about the relative lack of direction from the professionals involved; there was a task focus but they were needed to take control of the creative content and artistic direction of the training resources. Their initial uncertainty spoke to previous experiences of working with professionals; they did not expect to be allowed to take control.

The detail of the collaborative formulation was too large to include in this chapter and is summarised below.

The process of building the collaborative formulation began with asking the young people to come up with ideas that they would like professionals to understand about their experiences of mental health services. All of these single words or phrases were collected and arranged by the group into themes that fit together under overarching categories. The categories included 'What Happens When Put in a Box', 'Bad Experiences with Staff', 'What It Feels like', 'What Staff Should Understand', 'Communication Skills' and 'What We'd Like'. These categories were based on experiences young people had within psychiatric services, for example, being 'put in in a box' referred to several of them finding the process of diagnosis to be limiting, objectifying and invalidating of their own understandings of their subjective experience. Likewise 'bad experiences with staff' referred to all the young people having experienced coercion and several having coping strategies such as self-harm undermined as attention seeking, adolescent and demonstrating a lack of responsibility. Interestingly when one of the graphic novels showing a young person's struggle with self-harm was later shown to trainee clinical psychologists, one commented along similar lines that the person needed to take responsibility for their behaviour. This illustrates how these prejudicial views are not the preserve of other professions but embedded in our own responses to behaviour we find disturbing. 'Communication skills', 'what staff should understand' and 'what we would like' were linked ideas with the young people desiring a different type of relationship with staff, less paternalistic and more focused on collaboration and respect. As can be seen the young people as group were unhappy with the underlying psychiatric model that underpinned staff attitudes and rejected the invalidation that they encountered. They wanted a different relationship to their mental health and saw that this would require a shift in ethos. Therefore the different themes were collected under a high-level theme of 'Changing Staff Opinions' which drove the training.

As the project developed, the young people who were involved had creative ideas that took the project away from an adaptation of existing experiential knowledge generated in real-time training, into the development of a unique training package that incorporated new ideas. In essence as the creative process took hold and was given space, the young people made the project their own and developed training resources beyond the scope of what the professionals involved could have foreseen. The process of how this happened was inclusive as Jacob noted: "The training we came up with wasn't just based on one person's experience, it was a composite of everyone's experiences. People came from quite different backgrounds and experienced different things and so gave you a different perspective." Echoing this emphasis on pluralism and diversity of views Cheryl said: "If we had an opinion, if anyone had an opinion, it was listened to and considered."

The professionals working in this project aspired to genuine engagement between collaborators and questioned the success of this outcome throughout. On reflection, we considered that traditional quantitative measures of outcome would be inappropriate and fail to subvert the power imbalance between collaborators on the project. In our qualitative evaluation, we could see that a core group of young people remained involved, attended regularly, produced creative project work, delivered the training and went to a national community psychology conference to present the project. Feedback from the young people in the documentary about the project described their feeling valued, respected and heard. As Jacob said: "The fact that we were treated with respect, and that we had the opportunity to get our feelings and our opinions across for a whole day was really positive." Stacey described how her experience of the project changed her own original perception of mental health professionals: "Having past bad experiences, I painted (professionals) as like this monster, but professionals are not really monsters. They (the Define Normal project staff) answered a lot of questions and they basically gave me a better understanding of how professionals should work."

How was it possible to achieve this level of collaboration and engagement?

Time was flexible. The project did not work to organisational deadlines completely, although this did mean that the project over-ran. The staff time allocation to the project was not tightly managed or costed, so this 'inefficiency' was among the factors that enabled the project to succeed. While this flexibility was a symptom of a time that feels very far away today, we argue that there are still opportunities for clinical psychologists to carve space out for this type of community psychology work. As discussed above we utilised the policy discourse such as empowerment and inclusion so prevalent at that time. Today, much rhetorical discourse goes into emphasising the importance of 'co-production' and 'involvement'. While, much of this can be seen as a cynical attempt to take responsibility off services and onto communities, and points to the shift away from us being patients or service users and becoming consumers or customers, they also offer opportunities. It means that services need to be seen to be engaging in participatory activities and we would encourage community clinical psychologists to utilise this language in order to subvert traditional practice and to engage critically with communities such as this one in order to find out their priorities for change, as opposed to getting them to ratify ours. What undoubtedly also helped in the case of Define Normal was a collective of like-minded professionals of different grades supported by a clinical psychologist manager. This work is likely to be too difficult for us to do it alone; partnerships between different professionals and community members are crucial in sharing the load.

Staying 'under the radar' and out of the hospital. There was no micromanagement, enabling unstructured, unpressured sessions that could be fun and creative. It was possible to develop informal working relationships between professionals and young people. Professionals with close involvement with the young people during project sessions were skilled at maintaining engagement and given space and freedom to carry our project activities alongside the young people. Delegated project management was transparent and visible but not always present or directly observing the day-to-day activity of the project.

Engagement with young people was on their terms and with their needs in mind. The location of project activity was taken out of institutional mental health settings and located in a more neutral community college environment.

Inclusive of diverse mental states and mental health crises. One of the criticisms of service user involvement in mental health care is that participation can often involve service users who are 'recovered' and well enough to engage in 'professionalised' contexts. We have some sympathy with this position in desiring a diversity of involvement but also do not want to denigrate contributions wherever they come from. However, as it happened as the Define Normal project developed it became clear that there was considerable diversity among the group and that mental health crises could not only be managed within the project but actually contributed to the creative content of the training. For example, for a period some project members were under inpatient care and in coming off the ward to the project they were able to pour in their experiences that day into the animation. There are scenes in the

Transparent Joe animation that have a visceral quality because of the real-time, raw quality of the experiences that informed them. These sections are less imagined than described, which adds to the potency of the training while increasing the project's critique of the young people's mental health care and adds to the overarching pessimism surrounding the creative content developed. However, while this diversity of experiences and having young people involved who had ongoing mental health struggles enriched the content of the training, it was not without its complexity. The primary one was how hard it is to engage in project work while undergoing inpatient psychiatric treatment. From a professional point of view, there were organisational challenges that may be similar in other clinical community psychology projects. A particular challenge was the paradox of the young people's experiences being seen as evidence of mental illness in one context and legitimate experiences that can be used to generate creative context in another. This contradiction caused distress for both young people and staff in the project, concerns about the safety and trustworthiness of the project among some clinical staff and created ethical dilemmas for how we linked up the various systems. These contradictions were managed primarily by referring back to the contract of work which explicitly stated that the young people had creative control of all training materials and so their decision to portray mental health differently to the mainstream. The contradictions did however come to a head when one project staff member was reprimanded by senior clinical staff from the local Early Intervention Service who took issue with the portrayal of what they perceived to be psychotic phenomena as the young person's truth. We would recommend to colleagues that future projects should be careful around framing mental health differently from mainstream services and that doing so in a way that brings outside staff along with you is advisable rather than creating such a different viewpoint that it becomes incompatible and conflict ensues.

Welcoming of critical perspectives: Young people's views were met with alignment from professionals who also personally held critical perspectives on systemic failures in traditional mental health services. Professionals working within this project were permitted by senior management to have a relatively unsupervised oversight of the project as a result of previous performance and existing relationships of trust. The project's central emphasis on the young people being in creative control was what guided conversations with external clinical staff and privileging the truth of their experiences rather than aligning the project with 'clinical' reality as seen by other professionals was key in maintaining trust among young people and professionals as can be seen by Jacob's feedback; "*our views were still heard even when they were critical…how we were able to turn our negative stuff into positive.*"

Act

This section refers to the delivery of the training, its contents and reception.

The young people involved in the project were interested in using a range of creative media for sharing their knowledge and experiences within a training context. One of the professionals within the project team, Danny (Taggart et al., 2013), had previous experience of working with a film-maker, Matthew, on projects with young people who had mental health problems. The film-maker was invited to come and talk to the group, and following the initial meeting, was contracted to help make a stop-motion animation film about young people's experiences of a *composite* mental health journey. The young people in the project called this film *Transparent Joe*, based on how one person described her experience of feeling invisible and disregarded. The animation reflects the isolation and alienation the young people experienced going through a frightening and confusing psychiatric system. The principal character 'Joe' upon experiencing distress resulting from social factors is immediately picked up and placed in a box where he is tested, observed and buried in medication in an objectifying and dehumanising way. The scene where the character is literally buried under a wave of pills was particularly affecting for one training delegate: "The film was really powerful, the bit about the medication. I've got an image in my head of the medication just covering the whole of the character…the way it literally consumed the character." The denouement features a less obviously medicalised professional taking Joe out of the box and leaving him in a wasteland full of blank signs pointing nowhere. The overall tone of the animation is one of loneliness, fear and confusion with a disjointed soundtrack composed by Jacob.

Alongside the film-making, some of the young people also designed their own mini-graphic novels depicting elements of their individual experiences. These were deeply personal testimonies of individual young people's experiences of mental health problems turned into art through a graphic novel medium. Like the film, the graphic novels do not have positive stories to tell about help seeking and take a critical perspective on forced treatment and the medicalisation of idiosyncratic identities. They also address themes of loss of identity through conformity, suicide and self-harm.

Delivery of the Training

The project team delivered three full-day training sessions to local professionals from statutory and third-sector organisations. All sessions were delivered by the whole Define Normal team and involvement of the young people was flexible according to their preferences on the day. Young people's roles included introducing elements of the training, taking part in group discussions, answering questions from the audience, providing a spoken-word summary of the day and role-playing in the experiential elements of the training. The training sessions were structured to give trainers and delegates opportunities to watch, listen, experience, reflect and discuss. The morning involved group discussion of hopes for the day and brainstorming participants' understanding of factors that contribute to young people's mental health problems. Feedback from these activities was discussed. Before lunch, *Transparent Joe*, the Define Normal film, was shown. Participants had opportunities to discuss their responses to the film. The three graphic novels were made available to delegates to read and discuss.

After lunch, the group moved to the large hall in the building to take part in the experiential element of the day.

'Walk in My Shoes' involved experiencing a service user's journey through elements of the mental health services that young people had experienced and identified as difficult and unhelpful. These experiences included:

- Being spoken about, rather than spoken to, in a role-played meeting between a consultant psychiatrist (Jacob dressed in a suit) and junior doctor (Danny) with the participant seated in a small chair and not addressed directly during the 'ward round'. The interrupted and hurried conversation between these professionals included numerous unexplained acronyms, a dismissive language and tone relating to the 'patient' experience, behaviour, treatment adherence, engagement and prognosis. As one participant who worked on an inpatient ward reflected after undertaking this task that it was not so satirical as may have been assumed with those not familiar with the ward round culture: "Sadly I think it is really accurate and I think it is often like that, except that there should have been another eight people doing it as well."
- Having to tell your story repeatedly while being referred from one professional to another, none of whom appear able to offer any help or explain the confusing fictitious diagnosis that the person has been given. Professional roles were Mental Health Linkworker (Stacey), Psychiatrist (Jacob),

Psychologist (Wendy) and Receptionist (Rebecca). Participants were asked to complete questionnaires at each stage of the referral process, and frequently had to wait for long periods between brief and hurried 'appointments'. The final diagnosis of MTID (Multiple Transferential Iatrogenic Disorder) was a reflection of the symptoms delegates may develop as a result of journeying through a confusing and ultimately pointless system.

- Being asked to undertake a task while fitted with heavy weights (to represent the effects of psychiatric medications) and earphones playing voices. One participant found this "really, really good, really effective, really powerful…an insight into how hard it might be to concentrate, or remember, or even just move about when you are feeling so heavy and lethargic".

Reflect

This section considers some of our learning from the project, including what we could have done differently.

It was important to facilitate young people's involvement in the project by providing more support to attend meetings than was initially expected. Although this was not a service being provided to young people, it was necessary to offer support with transport to facilitate attendance. Some of the young people involved in the project were under the care of specialist mental health teams during the project. This has meant that professionals were involved in organising collection from and return to the inpatient unit during periods of admission.

In addition to practical issues relating to maintaining engagement in the project, the experience of working with young people who were experiencing mental health problems has meant that the professionals in the project team needed to be mindful of their mental health needs. For example, this meant that it was important to remain flexible about timescales for completion of the project, and required an extension of the staff time available to the project. It was difficult at times to maintain a task-focused approach during some of the sessions, and although the project in general was task-focused, there was a need to approach the sessions flexibly and for professionals to be responsive to the needs of the collaborators.

The professionals working on the project did not have regular clinical supervision in relation to this element of their work. In retrospect this was an oversight, and the smooth-running of the project relied on their professionalism, joint working and clinical skills. We would recommend a clear supervision structure where the process of project development can be thought about psychologically, with particular attention paid to boundary issues that might come up due to the different working relationships forged between young people and staff. In the event of a crisis, this would have been managed through existing lines of communication, although there were no acute crises during the project and this seems likely due to the respectful, transparent relationships between all project members. Often a 'flattened hierarchy' (Holmes, 2010) approach to relationships prevailed where project members took collective responsibility for the task focus. In feedback sessions the young people relayed that this type of relationship stood in stark contrast to their previous experience of contact with mental health professionals.

There were additional issues with some of the professionals working on the project who also worked in teams that provided services to some of the young people involved in the project. It was important for professionals to clarify within their team that their role with young people in this project was not a clinical role. It was therefore important to observe professional boundaries regarding the sharing of information within the services, due to potential role conflict. This proved challenging when issues central to the project, such as compulsion, entered into team discussions around the young people's mental health care. Having a first-hand perspective from young people on the traumatic nature of detention in a psychiatric hospital made it difficult to then be involved in discussions regarding that within mental health services. In short, seeing things from the young people's perspectives made it difficult to return to mainstream services. This may also have been the case for delegates, as the young people's perspectives as deployed through the training media were not reformative but rather calling for a complete overhaul of the system. A question remains as to whether it would have been better to sacrifice the critical edge and rawness of the project in the service of a more realistic message for change. The novelty of the project stood in its opposition to mainstream psychiatric practice as channelled through creative media by the young people. However, a more reformist position, focusing on achievable goals may have generated more immediate systemic change. Future clinical community psychology projects working with young mental health service users may want to consider the primary task of the project: to enable young people's empowerment or to reform services? In our case these two were partly incompatible and the former became the default priority.

Feedback from delegates who took part in the training was generally positive. People expressed admiration for the young people and their courage in developing this project. After the first day, some delegates expressed concerns that the training presented a negative picture of mental health services without detailing how they could be improved. The second training day incorporated a section at the end to provide opportunities for delegates to discuss what actions they could take to improve the services in which they work. It was emphasised that the training development was creatively led by young people with the intention of providing a platform for their voices to be heard. Therefore, the decisions about the content of the training were made by young people who were involved. This dimension of the project did present some challenges to the professionals who facilitated the process. When developing the 'Walk in My Shoes' experiential element of the training several of the young people wished to make this experience quite punishing for delegates. During this time the professionals in the project asked the young people to consider how to make the process as constructively educational as possible, bearing in mind that many of the delegates would not be individuals who had been directly involved in their own worst experiences. Many delegates expressed finding the experiential element of the training very uncomfortable through exposure to a first-hand example of young people's experiences in mental health services. However, as one delegate observed: "I think all of my colleagues should have to come and do it as well, it was a really good experience, a difficult one, but I think pretty accurate from what I see."

Implications for Future Clinical Community Psychology Work in NHS Settings

In addition to reflections for future work peppered throughout the text we would like in drawing our chapter to a close highlight four key points.

To reiterate a point made earlier on, for Define Normal it was crucial to work within and in accordance with NHS power structures for the project to be acceptable. This stands in contrast to other community psychology projects which take a more radical approach to critique and work hard to stand outside the mainstream. For us both approaches have value, although we accept a possible criticism of NHS-based clinical community psychology that it is so bound by institutional power structures as to not be truly community psychology at all. This debate can bedevil work in the field but we argue that the friction that can be caused by such discussions can lead to a creative dialectic whereby new forms of praxis can emerge. For example, while the work of our critical psychology colleague David Fryer stands in contrast to the Define Normal project by virtue of the extent of the critique and the level of engagement with mainstream institutions, we feel he and others have had a profound influence on the shaping of this project (see Fryer & McCormack, 2011, for an example of a more critical approach to community psychology and co-production). It was in relation to this type of community psychology praxis that the Define Normal project was conceptualised, while the actual construction and delivery of the project was constrained by organisational limits.

Co-production is the latest iteration of a commonly held trope in health and social care, that involving service users in policy, research, training and service development is *a good thing*. As we have outlined, this rhetoric can be harnessed by clinical community psychology projects to demand more meaningful engagement with communities but what then? The art of co-production on this project was largely process driven. That is to say that the project succeeded in so far as the relationships between project members enabled the tasks to be completed. In the absence of these relationships there would simply have been no project. The ingredients that make up successful co-productive relationship are as variable and difficult to define as any other human relationships. However, what we can say is that from the perspective of the Define Normal project, they take time to develop, cannot be based on professionalised models of co-working and require space to reflect on how they change over time. Suffice to say many project members have kept in touch intermittently since the project finished and we hope this is some indication of the strength of the connection we made with one another.

In undertaking clinical community psychology work in the NHS and other statutory settings, it seems crucial to us that critical perspectives are brought in under the guise of co-production. With service user involvement now a statutory responsibility for all health and social care providers in the UK, there is a risk that the transformational radical edge of the service user movement can be lost in procedurally based, consensus affirming tokenistic practices. This is a well-articulated concern already (see Beresford, 2016 for a discussion of tokenism in involvement), but for us community psychology with its adherence to social justice values and emancipatory praxis offers a grounding that can ensure involvement is meaningful and committed to change. The Define Normal project was modest in scale and achievement but deeply critical ideas about the violence of the psychiatric system were articulated through the use of subversive means. We think without having the inspiration of international community psychology to build upon, the project may have become more cautious.

A final reflection is on the importance of experiential knowledge forms and the significance of the young people's contribution to the project. To undertake a project like this as a professional carries risks. However, the risks the young people took in bearing their experience publicly and using personal traumas to inform a creative process that resulted in a training programme cannot be underestimated. It was not without its costs, as Cheryl puts it: "I felt a little bit, sort of, on parade. Like, I'm crazy and I'm here to show you what I think about it." We suggest this is an inherent risk in any project of this sort and it is worth noting that any benefits for community members have to be balanced against the risks of overexposure, entering into a potentially frightening professionalised world and also managing the disappointment of the inevitable limits of what can be achieved. However, the benefits of involvement for the Define Normal project are clear to see. Not only was the content of the training enhanced by the young people having creative control but the actual structure and fabric of the events were transformed beyond what could have been possible with a professionally led project. We suggest that this form of transformative, rather than additive, co-production work is best achieved by taking a community psychology approach and adapting appropriately for clinical settings. The results of this are probably best appreciated by watching the two Vimeo videos which show the *Transparent Joe* animation and feature a brief documentary of the project. Links can be found in the Abstract.

References

Beresford, P. (2016). *All our welfare: Towards participatory social policy*. Policy Press.

Franks, W. (2013). Turning 'Them' into 'Us': Reflecting on the regulation of participatory research in public health services. *Journal of Critical Psychology, Counselling and Psychotherapy, 13*(1), 9–17.

Franks, W., Gawn, N., & Bowden, G. (2007). Barriers to access to mental health services for migrant workers, refugees and asylum seekers. *Journal of Public Mental Health, 6*(1), 33–41.

Fricker, M. (2007). *Epistemic justice: Power and the ethics of knowing*. Oxford University Press.

Fryer, D., & McCormack, C. (2011). The war without bullets: Socio-structural violence from a critical standpoint. In E. Almeida (Ed.), *International community psychology: Community approaches to contemporary social problems* (Vol. 1, pp. 213–232). Universidad Iberoamericana.

Holmes, G. (2010). *Psychology in the real world: Community based groupwork*. PCCS Books.

Kagan, C., Burton, M., Duckett, P., Lawthom, R., & Siddiquee, A. (2011). *Critical community psychology*. Wiley.

Norfolk County Council, Supported by Business Intelligence & Performance Service and Public Health. (2015). *0-19 District Profile*. Great Yarmouth.

Orford, J. (2008). *Community psychology: Challenges, controversies and emerging consensus*. Wiley.

Reason, P., & Bradbury, H. (Eds.). (2001). *Handbook of action research: Participative inquiry and practice*. Sage.

Taggart, D., Franks, W., Osbourne, O., & Collins, S. (2013). 'We are the ones asking the questions'. The experiences of young mental health service users conducting research into stigma. *Educational and Child Psychology, 30*(1), 61–71.

14

Rewriting the Space Between a University and a Healthcare Provider: The Model of Converge

Emma Anderson, Adam Bell, Paul Birch, Lucy Coleman, Paul Gowland, Matt Harper-Hardcastle, Eloise Ingham, Bekhi Ostrowska, and Kev Paylor

From co-author, Lucy Coleman: It feels as if the majority of health and social care focuses on ensuring people have the right medication and means to survive. We need more than this to fulfil us as human beings, to help us be happy. Converge offers more. Working in this way doesn't feel radical—it's simply helping people feel confident and gain a sense of achievement through education and art, which is why I enjoy working there and why I started a music charity, Emerging Voices.

E. Anderson (✉)
School of Humanities and Social Science, University of Brighton, Brighton, UK
e-mail: e.anderson2@brighton.ac.uk

A. Bell • P. Birch • L. Coleman • P. Gowland • M. Harper-Hardcastle • B. Ostrowska • K. Paylor
York St John University, York, UK
e-mail: p.birch@yorksj.ac.uk; L.coleman@yorksj.ac.uk; p.gowland@yorksj.ac.uk; m.harperhardcastle@yorksj.ac.uk; rebecca.ostrowska@yorksj.ac.uk

E. Ingham
Independent researcher, UK

C. Walker et al. (eds.), *The Palgrave Handbook of Innovative Community and Clinical Psychologies*, https://doi.org/10.1007/978-3-030-71190-0_14

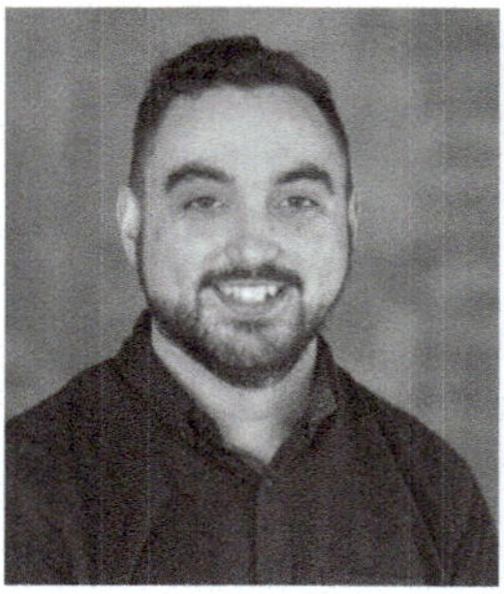 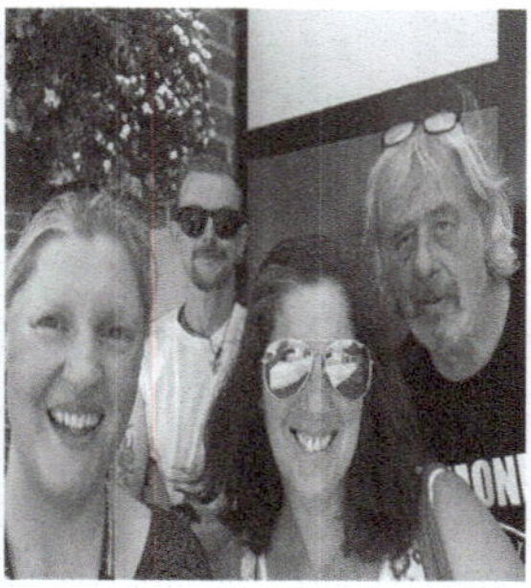 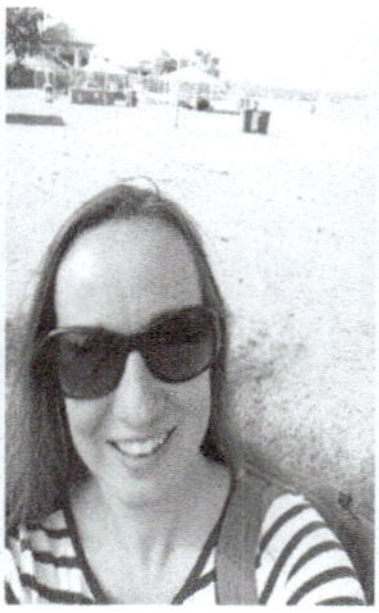 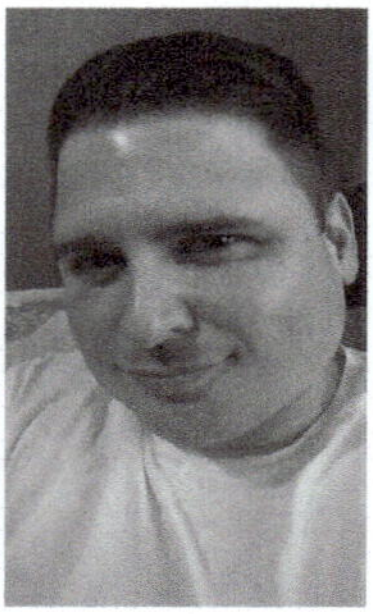

For the past 171 years, the buildings of Bootham Park Psychiatric Hospital and York St John University (YSJ) have stood opposite each other. It takes just five minutes to walk from one to the other, yet despite the geographical proximity, there has been a vast social, cultural and systemic distance between the two. Converge, a partnership between YSJ and Tees, Esk and Wear Valleys National Health Service Trust, aims to bridge that divide and challenge the social exclusion and stigmatisation surrounding mental distress by opening up the university and working with people who access mental health services as students.

Converge started in 2008 when Nick Rowe, an associate professor of theatre at YSJ, and one of his third-year students, Gemma Alldred, offered an eight-week introduction to theatre. Eight people completed this course, and their positive reaction and desire to continue sparked a commitment to run it again—and then to gradually expand Converge's offerings. There are now 19 different courses, in visual arts, theatre, dance, textiles, music (including a new gamelan group), storytelling and more. There is also a choir, Communitas; two theatre companies, Out of Character and In the Moment; and a band, 1/2/6. Recent developments include a publishing house to help distribute creative writing outputs, a film company and the Converge Evaluation and Research Team (CERT), a group composed of Converge students, staff and YSJ students who learn and develop research skills and bid for paid evaluation work. In the academic year 2016–2017, 318 people completed courses and 85 university students were involved in course delivery or support.

Running alongside Converge is the Discovery Hub, a sister organisation launched in 2015 that aims to act as a broker between mental health services and the community by supporting people to achieve their wider learning goals. Converge students can attend signposting sessions with Discovery Hub to find out about opportunities in the local area, doing things that are important to them, such as volunteer placements. Notably for a university-based mental health initiative, Converge grew out of, and remains rooted in, the University's Arts department. However, there are growing links between the psychology department, with the involvement of current and former community psychologists based at the university, and an increasing number of psychology students engaged in the service-learning opportunities that Converge offers.

In this chapter, written by a group composed of Converge students, support-workers, university students and academics, we outline the work of Converge, illustrating it with pieces of creative and reflexive writing. We will focus on three interlinked features of Converge that draw on community psychology praxis to rework the relationship between a university, healthcare provider and people with experience of mental ill health. First is the emphasis on education, not therapy, which helps us move beyond the disempowering and often oppressive psychiatric model of mental health (Cromby, Harper, & Reavey, 2013; McCubbin, 2009). Second is the opening up of the university—a traditionally privileged space—to resist the exclusion and 'othering' of people who have experience of mental distress. And third is the collaborative, exploratory approach of Converge as a community of learners, which we argue has led to some beneficial, yet unexpected developments. We also stress that the initiative has had reciprocal benefits for the university community too, and consider what Kagan, Burton, Duckett, Lawthom and Siddiquee (2011) and Prilleltensky (2003, 2012) argue is a fundamental component of community psychology praxis: a deeper understanding of how political and societal systems affect individuals' and communities' wellbeing.

Offering Education, Not Therapy

In Western countries, there has been a recent shift towards programmes and treatments for mental distress that emphasise self-management and patient expertise (Rimke, 2016; Scott & Wilson, 2011). However, Harper and Speed (2014) argue that the current emphasis on 'recovery' and 'resilience' in mental health practice and rhetoric can encourage a deficit model of mental health and an individualised understanding of distress, obscuring the structural factors, such as inequality and poverty, that contribute to it.

Converge does not offer 'therapy' or align itself with the recovery model. Instead, it is built around a framework of education and the idea of 'discovery'—open-ended, creative, dynamic and non-prescriptive. Whereas 'recovery' can imply getting back to a previous state, many people talk in terms of finding a new, richer identity as a result of engaging with Converge. Converge has students not 'patients', 'service users' or 'customers', and this in itself offers a more empowering and less-stigmatised identity, and changes the stories available to us to talk about ourselves and our lived experience (Rowe, 2015). The structure of Converge courses enables students to develop their creative ideas and abilities, working as part of a group to create something new under the guidance of tutors. Participants take ownership of the work they produce, motivating them to come back each week. This approach is grounded in the idea that it is better to tackle mental distress at a community level, rather than focusing on discrete individuals, as this is more likely to have positive effects on the wider collective, as well as the distressed individuals (Campbell & Jovchelovitch, 2000; Keating & Hertzman, 1999).

Indeed, there is evidence that the language of education and discovery employed at Converge may also work to alter wider perceptions about mental health, helping to work towards what Townley and Sylvestre (2014) call transformative change, which they describe as moving beyond change that happens *within* a system to altering the underlying values and assumptions of that system. Converge classes are taught by University staff, students and, increasingly, Converge students. York St John students also take part in courses and activities as buddies, working with Converge students who have requested extra support. A striking consequence of university students' contact with Converge students was a change from regarding people who use mental health services as ontologically different, highly vulnerable and in need of special treatment, to engaging with them as learners: a relationship and a purpose far more familiar to students (Rowe, Forshaw, & Alldred, 2013). Eloise Ingham, who graduated from York St John in 2017, wrote this reflection on her involvement with Converge.

> *Before I started working with Converge I had no idea what to expect from the students. Mental illness as a whole seems to receive so much bad publicity and still to this day can have a negative stigma surrounding it, despite the efforts of charities and individuals trying to promote awareness and acceptance of mental health issues within society.*
>
> *When I first met the class I realised that there was nothing to be nervous about. Living with a mental illness or not, everyone is human and should be treated as such, treated with acceptance and this is something that working with Converge teaches you immediately.*
>
> *It changed my perception of people with mental illnesses, enforced the saying 'treat others how you would like to be treated' (which has become the motto for my work), and inspired me to want to change other people's perceptions also.*
>
> *I feel as though the only way to overcome the stigma surrounding mental health is to break down the divide that can sometimes seem to exist; and this is where I feel Converge has massively come into play.*

Converge also gives participants opportunities to develop as performers, artists and practitioners, by staging performances or taking part in recordings or exchanges. For example, in 2017 Converge was involved in a project in London that brought together groups that use creative practice to support people with mental distress. Bekhi Ostrowska, a Converge student and mentor who took part, wrote a poem to capture the sense of personal and artistic discovery that this brought about.

This Is London

Off we go, our hopes are high!
Anxiety strikes, feel as though I might die!
Tremendous, Tension, Trauma, Tubes, Trains, Testing… my very existence
This is London.

We are arrive in Euston Road—second shittest on the board
Alongside the road we wearily walk,
The writing's on the wall,
THIS MANOR IS SHIT!
This is London.

We navigate these busy roads, passing bridges, red buses and crowds,
North-West.
We're nearly there—we thought we were—none of us really sure.
Hastening hearts—heavy,
This is London.

Heat ever rising, backs are breaking—road after road,
God forsaken—please be close,
Please be near—frightening,
Fearful, ferocious, fear,
This is London.

At last a room to straighten my head.
Wardrobe, desk, a single bed.
Excitement building for what's ahead… new places, new people,
New feelings inside.
Relieved I've managed to ride this tide-
Actual, Achievement, Admirable, Anxiety—Actioned!
This is London.

Then a meeting of people on the Bankside steps, Lewisham,
Knaresborough, Leeds—Chapel FM.
Greetings, smiles, a shaking of hands—coming together in these alien lands.
A conga of people—floating down the river.
Bridges, banners, glorious trees glimmer.
Hopeful, happy, hungry, haste.
This is London.

Off the beaten track waltzes our pack, to a fine feast,
Overlooking the Thames.
Arts Network arrive—faces alive—adding to the vibe,
Take a seat—we eat—now enjoying the heat…
Coming together, complete.
People, Pasta, Pizza, Plentiful, Pleasures.
This is London.

Day two begins after a bountiful breakfast,
Back to the steps for ten.
Now familiar faces—gather around,
None of us knowing where we are bound,
Heat rising from the ground—new confidence in the faces found.
Curiosity, calling, creeping, crawling,
Confidence, coming,
This is London.

Following the leader we set off on the train—destination—
Arts Network base.
Footfall fast—along goes our cast—
Passing a tree depicting a face, pace quickening—winning the race.
We arrive to such an inspirational space!
Magnificent, magical, mosaics, mirroring, mindfulness.
This is London.

More introductions—the rest of the crew
Instructions given on what we're to do
Tie-dye being the task in hand—
We set to work our merry band—safe in the arms of this wondrous land.
The results are amazing—we're proud as punch
Opportune moment to stop for lunch.
Inspirational, ideas, increasingly, industrious, idealistic.
This is London

Back we head for a workshop at the Tate—
Excitement is heady—can we stand the wait?!
En masse we sit—with a glorious view of London—
Talk about the art of conversation—
Take postcards to seek out things in this inspirational location.
Astonishing, amazing, astounding, Awesome, Art.
This is London.

Free time is given to enjoy the pleasures—
Of the incredible Tate Modern and all of its treasures.
Monet, Rothko, Kalinsky are seen,
And Picasso—my favourite—the greatest artist ever been.
My emotions overwhelming, up close to this art—
Only sound I'm hearing is the beating of my heart.
Perfect, pleasures, paintings, Picasso, portraying, Peace.
This is London.

The language of education and discovery and the new identities it encourages are made possible by Converge's university setting, and the next section considers how using the space of YSJ contributes to the initiative's success.

Inviting in, Not Dispatching Out

In an inversion of the usual practice of universities sending their students out to placements or work experience in hospitals, clinics or community centres, a practice that risks maintaining unequal power relations and the 'othering' of people with mental distress (Chupp & Joseph, 2010), Converge instigates a flow of movement in the opposite direction. A foundational part of the initiative is to open up York St John University as a space to be shared by people with experience of mental distress. Spaces and places are not neutral, but are the product of the actions of their users, and as such carry meanings, associations and messages about who we are and how to behave (Massey, 2005; Rowe, 2015). A university is a socially valued, future-oriented place, associated with learning, aspiration and opportunity; and it has the resources that enable Converge to work with people as students—in dance studios, music rooms, black-box theatre spaces and seminar rooms (Rowe, 2015). The social spaces of the university—cafes, bars and reception areas—are also frequently used by Converge students, many of whom also choose to access a library card and associate membership of the student union. Adam Bell, a Converge student, actor in Out of Character, member of Communitas choir and mentor, reflects on his response to the university setting:

> *We are a community of learners here at York St John University. Our identity as students is so much stronger now as we are equally regarded and included on campus. Our social interactions in the wider community help us to break stigma together as one strong voice by having a non-judgmental place to go where there are staff and tutors with experience of mental health issues. It is such a big plus to develop a greater understanding and awareness about this very important subject. The academic setting is crucial to enhance the partnership and creativity. York St John University students come together with Converge students and Discovery Hub learners to help people to reach their goals and aspirations through education in the arts.*

Converge students have the opportunity to perform their work both at the university and beyond, through productions or recitals at York Theatre Royal, the National Centre for Early Music and York Minster. Engaging with the city's wider cultural infrastructure in this way continues our approach of 'opening up' spaces that may otherwise be experienced as off limits to people with experience of mental distress, due to financial constraints or social exclusion. In 2017 Converge sought to build on this by creating six 'Discover Courses' aimed at connecting Converge students to the social and cultural life and institutions of York. The courses, on art; museums; film; theatre; physical activity; and writing and books, were led by experts in their field and held in relevant, socially valorised buildings in the city. For example, there were sessions on understanding the practicalities of a rehearsal room at York Theatre Royal, working with ceramic artists in York Art Gallery, and creative writing at York Explore (libraries and archives).

Initiatives like this, we propose, contribute to a shift in how activities for people with mental distress are positioned, regarded and delivered: away from the '1980s undertones of draughty, poorly equipped spaces, cups of tea on Formica surfaces, murals and the almost bygone whiff of cigarette smoke' (Sagan, 2015, p. 49) associated with the outdated therapeutic activities traditionally on offer, such as basket weaving (Crawford, 2015). The initial hope is that upon completion of the course individuals feel equipped to access the facilities and communities of each establishment autonomously and engage with each building's own programme of activity.

Collaboration and Discovery

It is not just the literal space of a university or cultural organisation that can help facilitate action and change, but the metaphorical 'space' created by a collaborative, dynamic and enquiring approach to learning. Prilleltensky (2003) states that action is only possible under conditions of freedom and plurality, and Converge aims to create the space for these conditions, basing itself around values of inclusivity and reciprocity, and reflecting that any useful interventions must be done 'with' people, not 'to' them (Kagan et al., 2011). Over the years, Converge's developments, such as providing more courses and opportunities for progression, have been informed by students' feedback, suggestions and expertise. Some of the results of this ongoing process of collaborative reflection and enquiry include the mentor scheme, which was set up in response to the informal support seen among Converge students within, and outside of, courses. In 2013, a small group of students who had participated in courses for a year or more came together to create the role of mentor at Converge. Ideas from the group included individual pastoral support and acting as ambassadors. The role of mentor continues to evolve as it is dictated by the skills and experiences of the current team, who meet regularly and problem-solve as a group. It is voluntary and flexible, allowing mentors to give as much time as they wish, as well as enabling them to come back after a period of absence. It can also provide a stepping-stone to further progressions, such as work, through enabling people to take on more responsibilities when they feel ready. This collaborative process arguably constitutes what Freire (1970) calls generative dialogue, one of the basic conditions he proposed as necessary to instigate transformational change. This stresses equality, trust and respect between participants and a commitment to reflexive practices, questioning what is thought or taken for granted. Paul Gowland, Converge student and tutor, likens this participatory learning environment to a pond:

> *A pebble may be small, but once it is thrown into a pond it sinks and lays deep. However the water's surface is disturbed, there is the split moment of impact where the water is thrown up into the air and gravity pulls it back down. It lands back down scattered and chaotic and not in the place where it originally started from. The surrounding surface vibrates and moves a little more swiftly than before; the ripples circling and pushing outwards, expanding wider and wider until they reach their final destination. The water then becomes calm and still, until another pebble is thrown and the effect begins again.*
>
> *Collaboration works in the same way. An idea or concept is formed by an individual. This could be from the facilitator of a group or from a participant. The idea*

may have already been formed, just like the pebble waiting to be thrown into the pond. The idea is thrown into the group waiting as it lands to see where the splash will fall and how far the ripples will reach. Sometimes the first pebble thrown can be enough to spark further ideas, further ripples and even more pebbles thrown. And then at other times a larger pebble may be required to be thrown into the pond. But once the effects take hold multiple pebbles are usually thrown in causing higher intensity, higher enthusiasm and even more ripples. They overlap, crash and collide until finally the very last one is thrown which is the largest pebble. The impact is strong making a solid splash with solid ripples but this time with a lasting effect.

The smallest of ideas can have the biggest of impacts. These impacts vary from changing lives, to fuelling even more creative pebbles to be thrown into the pond. Collaboration can also aid to widen the possibilities and opportunities, hence increasing the size of the pond and adding even more pebbles.

If there is no pond then there is no splash to be made and no ripples to form. Therefore it is vital that there are opportunities made that allow for collaborative work to be formed and created. The success of this collaboration can have an ongoing lasting effect for those who are involved as well as the observer on the side. Ripples expanding out across to every area of the pond, lapping at the edges potentially connecting to the observing pebble to be cast into the mix.

Possibly one of the most valuable elements of Converge's remodelling of the university-mental health services relationship, then, has been this willingness to throw pebbles and see what happens—to wander with curiosity rather than set a direct course and follow it. This has parallels with Kay's (2011) concept of obliquity, which refers to doing or saying something in an indirect way, and which he suggests as an explanation of why the most successful businesses or initiatives are often not the ones who make financial gain their target, but those that concentrate on the actual product or service they provide. Foregrounding enthusiasm and aiming for excellence, Kay argues, is an effective way of working in a world that is complex, uncertain and liable to change. Similarly, Converge was not set up with the specific aim of improving people's mental health, but of creating opportunities for learning and artistic expression. Yet in taking up these opportunities, many participants have reported, both formally and informally, increased confidence, less distress and more engagement with the wider community. For example, in recent research by the Converge Evaluation & Research Team (CERT), which used photo-elicitation interviews to explore the experiences and interpretations of Converge students of two years or less, one participant said, 'I realised I was capable of doing something positive. It helped my mood and how I felt about myself'. Another reported that 'the Discovery Hub linked me to volunteering;

volunteering makes me feel like I'm contributing to the community' (Lambley et al., 2019).

Quantifying and providing 'evidence' for these outcomes, however, is not straightforward. As Sagan (2015) notes, the complexity of participatory arts means they are not suited to assessment by the positivist, quantitative methods favoured by funders; yet the dominance of 'evidence-based practice' in policy and healthcare prioritises randomised controlled trials and systemic reviews over personal accounts, and by doing so tends to promote 'evidence' over experience (Trinder, 2000). Geddes (2000) has argued that evidence-based practice approaches may even lead to poorer services and outcomes as only those treatments or programmes that can produce 'evidence' are considered. This has been an ongoing challenge for Converge but one way we have found to push against it is to measure educational rather than health outcomes, using monitoring and evaluation processes similar to those used by York St John University. This means the data we capture is aligned to the desired outcomes of the activity, unlike the Warwick-Edinburgh Measure of Wellbeing Scale (WEMWBS), favoured by many funders but often resented by mental health service users (Reason & Rowe, 2017). WEMWBS measures such as 'I've been feeling loved' seem to have no relevance to the experience of taking a Converge Creative Writing course, for example; and 'I've had energy to spare' may be counterintuitive to reflect on a Converge Dance class, when the student may be exhausted, but has learned new techniques. More useful is data that tells us about take-up of, and progression from, courses, as this suggests students are engaging in a meaningful and ongoing way with Converge. For example, in the academic year 2016–2017 we found that 81 per cent of people who started Converge courses finished them, with most re-enrolling on follow-up or new courses. Additionally, the aforementioned recent participatory action research by CERT found that a sense of purpose and opportunity was a key theme in Converge students' experiences, with eight out of ten participants reporting that they intend to try different courses (or already had), and/or volunteer as a result of their engagement. One participant called Converge 'a new beginning' for her, explaining her choice of a picture of a compass by saying, '[Converge] helps me find direction, from where I started.... There is always room for that compass to alter and go somewhere else, which gives me hope, even if I just stick to the one course for now' (Lambley et al., 2019).

Challenging Dominant Narratives

A growing body of critical work on mental health links people's experience of distress to structural issues that contribute to or cause them, such as rising inequality and the responsibilising, individualising project of neoliberalism (e.g. Fisher, 2017; Rimke, 2016; Wilkinson & Pickett, 2009). Converge's collaborative, action-oriented approach and the educational and artistic context provided by the university setting arguably put it in a strong position to shine a light on these issues by employing Freire's (1970) concept of conscientisation, the development of a critical awareness of the dynamics of distal power achieved through collective action and reflection. However, there is also a danger that adult education, which is often predicated around personal growth and self-fulfilment, may lack such critical conscientisation (Lloyd, 1972). We have found two concepts useful here: Prilleltensky's (2003, 2008) application of 'psychopolitical validity' in evaluating community psychology initiatives, and Butin's (2010) 'anti-foundational learning' as applied to service learning in students.

Prilleltensky (2003, 2008) advises assessing the extent to which interventions acknowledge people's experiences of oppression, the power dynamics that allow oppression to flourish and the consequences of this oppression at a personal and societal level (epistemic psychopolitical validity). Additionally, he stresses the importance of promoting familiarity with psychopolitical ideas and empowering participants to take action to challenge the status quo—what he calls transformative psychopolitical validity. An opportunity to address psychopolitical validity came in the 'Understanding Happiness' course taught by community psychologist (and co-author of this chapter) Emma Anderson. This course ran for four terms, and while it changed in each iteration, depending on the interests of the cohort, it attempted to critique and open up for debate the dominant narratives around happiness—that it is largely dependent on a positive mind-set, and that it is an individual's *interpretation* of their circumstances rather than the circumstances themselves that leads to unhappiness (Binkley, 2011, 2014; Cromby, 2011). As various authors (e.g. Binkley, 2014; Davies, 2015; Greco & Stenner, 2013) argue, this view, which underpins many positive psychological interventions, serves to reinforce individualising narratives, both obscuring structural reasons for unhappiness, such as poverty or a lack of social justice, and de-legitimising appropriate emotional responses to such situations.

In the Understanding Happiness course we explored ideas about happiness ranging from Aristotle's eudaimonia to Seligman's (2011) 'Flourishing', noting how 'knowledge' is created by the privileged—middle or upper class, usually white and often male—as well as engaging with and debating critical ideas, such as Ehrenreich's (2010) critique of the cult of positive thinking. This approach led to students sharing their own ideas about happiness and suggesting topics for later sessions, such as exploring 'negative' emotions like anger and shame. Kev Paylor, a Converge student, takes up similar themes in his piece about safeguarding in mental health, where he writes about resisting the individualising language of mental health, calling instead for an approach that is grounded in community support, artistic risk and informed anger.

> *Community Care = Safeguarding*
> *Section 136*
> *Community Care = Progressive Care*
> *Liberty*
> *Safeguarding is dependent on policing. Laws, rules and regulation are dependent on an authority. The authority creates a power structure which can be positive or negative, i.e. lead to recovery or install institutionalism. The whole thing depends on legitimizing; again, without the necessary checks and balances, this can be draconian and destructive.*
> *To empower is to give liberty to interact, educate, experience, inform and form wholesome relationships. Allowing a person to take responsibility, gain respect and reconcile themselves to their given environment.*
> *Progressive Care is a mode of operation and democratic in principle, leading to an individual altruism to Connect with the Collective. Co-operation lies at the heart of recovery.*
> *The concept of Liberty is the recognition that instead of language and systems that pigeon hole; each of us is free to express and in turn become a champion racer. To soar above and be happy.*
> *Liberty depends on empowerment given, an impetus or movement, to break the mental chains and respond with anger to legitimating myths.*
> *Anger is an energy, leading to some satisfaction and completion; to always question but never to assume. Neither executioner nor executed.*
> *The ethos of Converge, to challenge, communicate and empower with growth and Liberty is instrumental to Recovery. A focus to interact, to be educated, to experience and form wholesome dynamics with others.*
> *Creativity is the "Formula one" of thinking; to express, question, focus, grow and learn. Mainly through art; individual expression leading to a more complete sense of self. To function amongst peers and enjoy respect in the community leading to friendship.*

Another ongoing challenge for Converge, highlighted by Asghar and Rowe (2017), is how to encourage YSJ students to question the social injustices in mental health and develop awareness of the cultural, historical and political dynamics at work in framing debates around mental health. Butin (2010) refers to this as the 'anti-foundational' strand of service learning. This involves going beyond raising awareness of diversity and exposing students to people who are different, by facilitating critical thinking and reflexivity in students. This, Butin argues, is achieved by allowing meaningful relationships to develop and by fostering a state of doubt in students in which they can question issues of inclusivity and power and the role played by the institution, its practices and beliefs. As Weiner (2015, p. 323) puts it, service learning that fosters genuine collaborative opportunities, such as co-creating a play or piece of music, can encourage students to 'examine axes of power and privilege across social boundaries'. However, while YSJ students are strongly encouraged to develop relationships, collaborate and challenge their own assumptions, this is not something that can be guaranteed and it is possible that some students see their participation in Converge as merely a means to an end goal of employment rather than a genuine opportunity for reflexive and critical thought. A lack of meaningful and transformative engagement will be more likely in larger classes such as the Communitas choir, where the greater numbers of both Converge and YSJ students can lead to a 'silo-ing' off into groups who already know each other. One of the ways of tackling this is to undertake smaller group work within these classes to facilitate people getting to know each other better—something that serves as a useful reminder that Converge's commitment to growing and nurturing a community of learners is not merely about numbers, but relationships between people.

Conclusion

While Converge started as a response to the deepening mental health crisis in the UK, we contend that its strides towards transformational change have affected not just York's population of people with mental distress, but York St John University itself—its spaces and its practices. The ever-developing community of learners that comprises Converge has led to strengthened social bonds, a renewal of hope and meaning in life, more empowering identities and a reimagining of what a university can be, and for whom.

Outcomes such as Converge students becoming mentors, creating their own courses and working as tutors, and the beginnings of a critical awareness of the structural and political forces at work in framing knowledge and debates about mental health in both Converge and university students, could be said to have ensued from praxis, rather than having been pursued by design—side-effects of a particular way of approaching things. By focusing on education rather than therapy, 'opening up' the university as a welcoming space for people with experience of mental distress and the collaborations and discussions that this facilitates, Converge offers a model for how universities can act as a site of resistance to the dominant individualistic understanding of our social world.

However, Converge must also be considered in the context of the ongoing marketisation of higher education, which has created a culture wherein students are recast as 'consumers', universities must compete with each other to attract students and therefore funding, and in which an institution's 'worth' is judged in terms of contribution to economic prosperity (Collini, 2017; Molesworth, Nixon, & Scullion, 2009). While Converge is based on values and aspirations that go beyond the idea of economic and reputational return, there are clear benefits for the university in terms of Converge offering vocational training and increased employability for students, the ability to demonstrate 'impact' both for REF purposes and for the university's Social Innovation goals and economic return in the form of funding from the NHS and other trusts and foundations to maintain and extend the operation of Converge. For other universities wishing to implement a Converge-like initiative, then, these demonstrable and measurable outcomes can be a useful way of making the case for something that can satisfy the demands of university managers to offer added 'value for money' to students and demonstrate impact, while also carving out space for creative and participatory enquiry through community education and mutual discovery.

To finish, we will return to where we began: attempting to bridge the distance between York St John University and Bootham Psychiatric Hospital. A recent play by Out of Character Theatre Company explored historical ideas and approaches to mental health, linking them to current practice in a thought-provoking and sometimes hard-hitting way. *Objects of Terror* lifts the curtain on the inmates of Victorian lunatic asylums and the 'mad doctors' who ran them, asking the audience to watch and consider how these 'human marvels' wrestled with adversity, persecution and the judgement of others. Written by Paul Birch based on stories, themes and characters researched and devised by the cast, it was first performed at York Theatre Royal in November 2016. In the last monologue, the character Carroll has died after an operation to rid him of the 'infection' that caused his madness and is lamented by the character Dr Rideaux:

The Episodes of Dr Rideaux: 6

RIDEAUX is cradling the bloody-sheeted corpse of CARROLL. His keys lie before him. The cast stop. During the final speech they drop the keys, one by one, on the floor and return to their first positions.

RIDEAUX: I have deliriums. They are too many mad in the world. They knock at my door begging to be let in. They need our help. The sadness of this work. The pressure. Highs and lows.

Sometimes I am filled with such tremendous joy that we can welcome the afflicted and shelter poor souls. We wanted to put an end to madness. (Looks at his keys) So many voices! So many solutions! (Picks up a key) Fresh air? (Picks up a key) Exercise? (Picks up a key) Locked in the asylum? (Picks up a key) In the care of the community? (Picks up a key) Shocked back to sanity? (Picks up a key) Opiates for submission? A pill for every occasion…? What do they want us to do! Nolo Contendere. It is so very hard sometimes to remember we are trying to care for people as well as cure a disease because we have so little money and so little time. We must put the past behind us.

He is alone and forlorn. Picking up keys uncertain as to which might open a door.

Ladies and gentlemen… help me.
Please…

Blackout.

References

Asghar, M., & Rowe, N. (2017). Reciprocity and critical reflection as the key to social justice in service learning: A case study. *Innovations in Education and Teaching International, 54*(2), 117–125.

Binkley, S. (2011). Happiness, positive psychology and the program of neoliberal governmentality. *Subjectivity, 4*, 271–394.

Binkley, S. (2014). *Happiness as enterprise: An essay on neoliberal life*. State University of New York Press.

Birch, P. (2016). *Objects of Terror*.

Butin, D. W. (2010). *Service-learning in theory and practice: The future of community engagement in higher education*. Palgrave Macmillan.

Campbell, C., & Jovchelovitch, S. (2000). Health, community and development: Towards a social psychology of participation. *Journal of Community & Applied Social Psychology, 10*(4), 255–270.

Chupp, M., & Joseph, M. (2010). Getting the most out of service learning: Maximizing student, university and community impact. *Journal of Community Practice, 18*, 190–212.

Collini, S. (2017). *Speaking of universities*. Verso Books.

Crawford, P. (2015). *Health humanities*. Palgrave Macmillan.

Cromby, J. (2011). The greatest gift? Happiness, governance and psychology. *Social and Personality Psychology Compass, 5*, 840–852.

Cromby, J., Harper, D., & Reavey, P. (2013). *Psychology, mental health and distress*. Palgrave Macmillan.

Davies, W. (2015). *The happiness industry: How the government and big business sold us well-being*. Verso Books.

Ehrenreich, B. (2010). *Smile or die: How positive thinking fooled America and the world*. Granta.

Fisher, M. (2017). 'It's not your fault': Consciousness-raising as a reversal of magical voluntarism. *Clinical Psychology Forum, 297*, 4–7.

Freire, P. (1970). *Pedagogy of the oppressed*. Penguin.

Geddes, J. (2000). Evidence-based practice in mental health. In L. Trinder (Ed.), *Evidence-based practice: A critical appraisal* (pp. 66–88). Blackwell.

Greco, M., & Stenner, P. (2013). Happiness and the art of life: Diagnosing the psychopolitics of wellbeing. *Health, Culture and Society, 5*, 1–18.

Harper, D., & Speed, E. (2014). Uncovering recovery: The resistible rise of recovery and resilience. In De-medicalizing misery II (pp. 40–57). Palgrave Macmillan

Kagan, C., Burton, M., Duckett, P., Lawthom, R., & Siddiquee, A. (2011). *Critical community psychology*. Wiley.

Kay, J. (2011). *Obliquity: Why our goals are best achieved indirectly*. Profile Books.

Keating, D. P., & Hertzman, C. (Eds.). (1999). *Developmental health and the wealth of nations: Social, biological, and educational dynamics*. Guilford Press.

Lambley, R., Kaley, E., Morris, R., Robinson, A., Rowe, N., Sellar-Edmunds, J., ... & Anderson, E. (2019). 'Wow, it's at the University'! Experiences of people with mental illness of an educational arts programme. *Journal of Applied Arts & Health, 10*(3), 315–332.

Lloyd, A. S. (1972). Freire, conscientization, and adult education. *Adult Education, 23*(1), 3–20.

Massey, D. (2005). *For space*. Sage.

McCubbin, M. (2009). Oppression and empowerment: The genesis of a critical analysis of mental health. In D. Fox, I. Prilleltensky, & S. Austin (Eds.), *Critical psychology: An introduction* (pp. 300–316). Sage.

Molesworth, M., Nixon, E., & Scullion, R. (2009). Having, being and higher education: The marketisation of the university and the transformation of the student into consumer. *Teaching in Higher Education, 14*(3), 277–287.

Prilleltensky, I. (2003). Understanding, resisting, and overcoming oppression: Toward psychopolitical validity. *American Journal of Community Psychology, 31*, 195–201.

Prilleltensky, I. (2008). The role of power in wellness, oppression, and liberation: The promise of psychopolitical validity. *Journal of Community Psychology, 36*(2), 116–136.

Prilleltensky, I. (2012). Wellness as fairness. *American Journal of Community Psychology, 49*(1–2), 1–21.

Reason, M., & Rowe, N. (2017). *Applied practice: Evidence and impact in theatre, music and art*. Bloomsbury.

Rimke, H. (2016). Mental and emotional distress as a social justice issue: Beyond psychocentrism. *Studies in Social Justice, 10*(1), 4–17.

Rowe, N. (2015). Creating a healing campus: A partnership between a university and a provider of mental health services. *University Partnerships for Community and School System Development, 5*, 119–134.

Rowe, N., Forshaw, N., & Alldred, G. (2013). A return to ordinariness: How does working alongside people who use mental health service effect theatre students' attitudes to mental illness? *Journal of Applied Arts & Health, 4*(2), 151–162.

Sagan, O. (2015). *Narratives of art practice and mental wellbeing: Reparation and connection*. Routledge.

Scott, A., & Wilson, L. (2011). Valued identities and deficit identities: Wellness recovery action planning and self-management in mental health. *Nursing Inquiry, 18*(1), 40–49.

Seligman, M. (2011). *Flourish: A New understanding of happiness and well-being – And how to achieve them*. Nicholas Brealey Publishing.

Townley, G., & Sylvestre, J. (2014). Toward transformative change in community mental health: Introduction to the special issue. *Global Journal of Community Psychology Practice, 5*(1).

Trinder, L. (2000). *Evidence-based practice: A critical appraisal*. Blackwell.

Weiner, D. (2015). Across boundaries of privilege: Service-learning for social justice. In V. Jagla, A. Furco, & J. Strait (Eds.), *Service-learning pedagogy. How does it measure up?* (pp. 323–340). Information Age Publishing.

Wilkinson, R. G., & Pickett, K. (2009). *The spirit level: Why equality is better for everyone*. Penguin.

15

The Jannah Tree: An Islamic Faith–Inspired Metaphor and Spiritual Framework for Healing, Co-created by British-Pakistani Women Through Cyberspace Technology

Rukhsana Arshad

Introduction

This chapter will seek to outline a unique online community intervention between British-Pakistani women of the Muslim faith who had been reluctant to access mainstream UK therapy services, or who had negative experiences of it. What formed in response involved a cyber-therapeutic forum using messenger services and email to share thoughts, reflections and journal entries on processing their strengths and difficulties. This evolved into a formation of a shared metaphor and an evolving framework from which to understand their suffering, healing, growth and transformations. Using an Islamic-faith inspired spiritual 'scaffold', the women who participated in this intervention sought to map how Western approaches and understandings could offer support to their Islamic-spiritual formulations. Thus, enabling them to form more connections between aspects of their spiritual worlds previously disconnected or experienced as dismissed from the mainstream therapeutic discourses. This was especially poignant for those who felt unsatisfied with their previous encounters with mainstream therapy services.

UK policy spanning the last decade or so has highlighted the need to improve mental health services for minority ethnic service users (also referred

[Other volunteers wish to remain anonymous.]

R. Arshad (✉)
Birmingham and Solihull Mental Health Foundation, Birmingham, UK
e-mail: rukhsana.arshad@nhs.net

C. Walker et al. (eds.), *The Palgrave Handbook of Innovative Community and Clinical Psychologies*, https://doi.org/10.1007/978-3-030-71190-0_15

to as Black Minority Ethnic (BME) or Black Asian Minority Ethnic (BAME)). This has largely been driven by the poor health outcomes, overrepresentation in severe end services and underrepresentation in psychological or early intervention focussed services. For example, there have been national initiatives and reports calling for cultural competency in the National Health Service (NHS) in being able to work flexibly with service user cultural norms, such as the Inside Outside report by the National Institute for Mental Health England (NIMHE, 2003), the delivering race equality agenda (Department of Health, 2005–2010) and the relevance of the formation of the Equality Act in 2010. The more recent five-year forward view for mental health (NHS England, 2016) policy also raises the importance of continuing to work in meeting the needs of marginalised groups, including minority ethnic communities. The year 2020 has seen the rise of Black Lives Matter pledges across organisations and NHS services, the pandemic having a devastating disproportionate impact on BAME communities and the digital divide impacting those in need including children and new mothers from these marginalised communities. The need to 'build back better' a report and narrative unknowing how far it is taken on by the political powers, if at all. It is important to note that there are many forms of racism that contribute to distress, including institutional and structural racism. The recognition of these processes is an important part of promoting any meaningful or lasting change in equality of service delivery.

The common theme for ethnic minorities across all these initiatives by the Department of Health, NIMHE and others is that there is a need for service users from ethnic minority backgrounds to be better engaged in mental health services. Often Western mainstream services fail to engage or provide adequate access of services that are responsive to ethnic minority community needs (see writings by Fernando, 2010; Fernando & Moodley, 2018). The main issues that are of importance include that ethnic minority communities often draw on communal values and spiritual explanatory models of health and wellbeing. This is in particular for minority communities with connections to eastern/religious societies (see Koenig & Shohaib, 2014; Moodley, Rai, & Alladin et al., 2010). These issues are not to be misunderstood, but meaningfully engaged with in a way that makes services responsive to needs. Since the end of the delivering race equality agenda, there seems to have been less emphasis and less urgency to address BME inequalities in accessing or creating responsive mental health services. This experience may vary from service to service and region to region. In general, however, the message is still the same—the mental health outcomes for BME populations in the UK continue to be poor and require continuing attention (p. 13; NHS England, 2016). The integration of culture, spirituality and religion has been discussed as useful and helpful in coping for BME service users and/or those who identify as religiously committed by several authors. It is also at least implied, if not explicitly stated, by the drivers of the race and culture initiatives mentioned above in the context of improving outcomes for BME service users in the NHS. This issue in itself is not the scope of this chapter, and I have written about this elsewhere in relation to working with service users with a diagnosis of psychosis (see Arshad, 2007).

In regard to British-Pakistani service users' experiences of mental health, the ideas introduced into mainstream literature by Malik (2000) in her chapter on culture and emotions are significant. Her research highlighted that there is no true Urdu translation of the word 'depression' and that instead participants seemed to refer to a metaphor of the 'sinking heart' when describing their feelings. These observations of feelings centred in the heart fit with the model of the QALB (heart) which has been discussed in more detail by others (Skinner, 1989 [2018]; Keshavarzi & Haque, 2013; Kaplick & Skinner, 2017; Rothman & Coyle, 2018; Rothman, 2018). Specific interventions for Muslim communities of Britain have been developed by Mir and her research team (2015). This has been an adaptation of behavioural activation rather than a deep exploration of an indigenous model such as the QALB model. In the meantime, more is being discussed about global and indigenous psychologies (Fernando & Moodley, 2018; Marsella, 2013) which promote the idea that every psychology should explicitly own up to its indigenous foundations. This would mean to acknowledge consequently that Western psychologies are rooted and tailored to the population from which they were developed in the first place. One of the implications of this is that they may not actually be fully applicable cross-culturally as currently positioned and proposed.

In the current intervention, with the spirit of collaboration and cultural/spiritual integration, participants' personal and collective meanings of distress and wellbeing were explored. 'The Jannah Tree' became the prominent metaphor used in the thickening discourse around what healing represented for the participants. This chapter will attempt to summarise the reflections, concepts and processes the women grappled with in arriving at their shared and preferred therapeutic map for healing and change. The chapter will include anonymised diary excerpts, diagrams/sketches and quotes. The author held a facilitator role and specifically helped to contribute towards translation where possible between both worlds of Islamic faith and Western psychotherapy. The author also helped to collate and amalgamate the evolving narratives into one shared 'script' or 'product'. In this process, the facilitator encouraged active participation from all in contributions and in the shaping of the metaphor.

The intervention, therefore, aimed to empower women to form their own formulation map and expand on their personal marginalised explanatory frameworks, although already held by them, were treated as invisible or irrelevant and unimportant in their experience. The metaphor acted as a spiritual framework to help creatively guide them back to using and integrating their 'indigenous' understandings of the self without becoming 'flooded' with only dominant Eurocentric models, which felt incongruent in the first place. Finally, the metaphor allowed the women to judge when and where Eurocentric therapy models could serve them best within their own explanatory framework. The women felt safe to explore these themes online as they could choose selectively who to share with, and therefore, it was a more trusting space in an 'Islamophobic' world (also see Inayat, 2007, for more discussion on how 'Islamophobia' impacts upon therapeutic spaces for Muslim clients).

The women empowered each other to begin thinking outside of Eurocentric biases and drew upon insights within their own minds, whilst also acknowledging a keenness to understand the predominantly eleventh-/twelfth-century Ghazali-based discourses on the psychology of the self (such as described in Keshavarzi & Haque, 2013; or accessed in translations such as al-Ghazali on the marvels of the heart, Skellie, 2010). This perspective holds the spiritual self as a fundamental foundation for change and optimum overall health. It locates fundamental change processes in the heart (QALB).

Method

This online community intervention involved six women of differing educational attainment levels (ranging from holding a certificate to a PhD) and of British-Pakistani nationality. They shared varying degrees of spiritual belief identity—primarily a strong belief in the Islamic faith aligning with Hanafi and/or 'Sufi' interpretations. They reported to practise their faith moderately or strongly. These women were between their late 20s up to 60 years in age, with an average age of 37. The women formed a small group anonymously using cyber technology. This occurred in stages explained below. They were seeking support for their distress (construed as depression, anxiety or trauma) and clarifications about how Western approaches could support them to heal and move forward, whilst not dismissing their cultural and Islamic-spiritual beliefs.

The Formation of the Online Group

The women had contacted the facilitator for advice or support through online forums aimed at Muslim women where the author was already an active online community volunteer member. Initially all participated in individual online communication to clarify the need for support and appropriateness of online contact. This process included discussions on consent for participation and to follow ground rules set by the group. Three of the women had previous experience of therapy (third-wave cognitive-based therapies) and two had minor to moderate experience and knowledge of research skills within the social sciences. The evolution of a shared metaphor and framework involved several stages of online discussion and reflection; this was not as a continuous unanimous group. The process involved individualised online interactions and between sub-groups, and an eventual forming of a larger shared group at later stages. The modes of communication used were congruent with those used in the online forum they were already using (instant messenger service and email).

Analysis

Dialogues were analysed with permission for themes and new issues were interwoven back into discussions until ideas reached a level of adequate density. Participants gave informed consent at each stage where appropriate in the use of their preferred online platform for communication and for results to be shared in written form to benefit other communities in future. These online interactions were largely conducted over a 12-month period. The women consented to share and to take responsibility for what they shared. They all agreed that this work may be published with permission. They were assured that any identifiable details would be changed.

Results

This section is divided into three parts to represent the main themes and processes identified. Part (1) is called 'stimulating growth narratives' and relates to the stirring up of subjugated and hidden concepts related to healing. Part (2) will describe the process of 'scaffolding holistic elements with metaphorical tools'. Here the metaphors are developed and used from core assumptions of growth and beauty of the invisible transformation processes that are not seen to the naked eye. This was felt to be represented by the universal symbol of the tree. The tree represented a symbol of Jannah (paradise) to the women in this intervention. The Lote tree is a particular tree mentioned in the Quran (Islam's Holy book). This is a tree at the end of the seventh heaven and marks the boundary between creation and creator (chapter 53: verse 14). The Jannah Tree metaphor is discussed and used as felt to embody growth and beauty and to symbolise the goal of one working towards the eternal home called Jannah in the Quran. Jannah is notably mentioned to be beautified with gardens and thus befits the symbol of the human growing from a seed originally belonging in Jannah, but planted and growing through Earth; finally the tree finding its place back in Jannah once more at the end of life. Part (3) focusses on how the metaphor is used by 'tracing maps of personal experience onto the Jannah Tree metaphorical framework'.

Part (1) Stimulating Growth Narratives: Rousing—Stirring Up and Stimulating Intimations

A prominent theme amongst all participants was that they were struggling with the deficit (problem-focussed) model of mental health. They felt frustrated by this and found themselves in a process of trying to give words to alternative views. One member shared an exquisite image with a quote. This created a ripple effect of 'inspiration' each time it was shared. It reads, 'And don't think the garden loses its ecstasy in winter. It is quiet, but the roots are down there riotous'—'riotous roots' image and quote attributed to Rumi; retrieved at various site pages via Google and Instagram searches). This quote had been circulating on social media and was attributed to Rumi (famous thirteenth-century scholar). This image and quote wonderfully aroused discussions and reflections from the participant women:

> I am inspired, and I am stirred. I saw the tree and it just hit me right in my heart. Yes! This is me! I look lifeless, but I am growing. I am mad-angry, but I am growing in my pain. I know there is a meaning to all this, and it will reveal itself.
>
> It wasn't just the picture—although it is so beautiful. The quote underneath it just described what I had been meaning to say but could not express. Yes, the image and the quote together were powerful to me. This is my turning point!

Some women started to journal about the image and wrote poems inspired by it. Others wrote messages they would one day like to share with others after feeling stirred by it.

Some women reflected on how the image and quote made potential therapeutic shifts, they reflected on this, and how this had not happened whilst with their own therapist in ways that they had wanted:

> There is no disease except God has also sent a cure—I believe in this, and this gives me hope. There is an internal struggle with the self, and this is the crux. This image is about 'Do not judge what you see'. It is a dead lifeless tree at the top but under the ground it is bursting with growth. It feels like it is saying don't you dare judge me, look at what I am going to become. It is like a spiritual crisis in a way. It gets me depressed, or anxious but it is really all the internal struggles. And when the therapy did not fit me, I just thought—come on there has got to be something better than this. Something in the mix is not right. But I didn't feel brave enough to say that to her straight. I knew my therapist would call me resistant or something in her notes. But I knew she could not fully get me because she does not view the unconscious as I do. And she just seemed unable to hold new ideas and hear them. I just retreated then till I found a new way of knowing how to use what she could offer—but in a way that I was leading and, in a way, that I needed it.

The Role of Dreams and the Subconscious

Participants reflected on their journal entries and about what they thought the meaning of their distress was. They raised the issue of dreams as a tool to the subconscious. This felt like a risky topic to discuss; however, they felt able to do so in this intervention.

> Every morning I try to re-memorise my dream before it fades and then I rush to write it out in my journal. I draw pictures and whatever I want. It really helps. I feel like I am tapping more into my subconscious. Sometimes I may have a dream that I think has a meaning deeper than just the ramblings of my mind or my fears. I think that it is possible to receive guidance and inspiration through dreams, but it is a skill to understand which dream has such a message. And of course, I know that dream interpretation is controversial in many circles.

> I do journal too, and I know I can't afford therapy—it may be free on the NHS, but I can't afford the time and childcare and the travel. So, I just think it causes more stress than good. So, I journal. It helps me to reflect deeply about things.

> I also write my dreams down too. Sometimes I do Quran journaling and try to find the answers to what my feelings may actually mean.

Understanding Wisdom and Inner Inspiration

Participants highlighted the need to develop wisdom to recognise inner inspiration. Both seemed missing in their experience of therapy.

> Some of my dreams actually have given me clues to wisdom and inspiration. I have noticed how my dreams have gradually started to change too.

Participants explicitly used the Quran as a tool for developing wisdom.

> I self-analyse what could be going on and try and work out what wisdom is there. Or what fear is there. I use the Quran to help me. I do Quran journaling. So, I use inspiring passages in the Quran to help heal me.

They used the Quran to help develop positivity and hope about desperate and despairing situations. They linked this to the idea of growth embodied in the riotous roots image.

The Role of Companionship and the Social Environment

Participants started to reflect wider than themselves. They identified that it was not just the internal world of feelings, thoughts, drives, inspiration and dreams—but that the role of companionship and social environment was also fundamental.

> You have to understand it is not just me. It is not just me. It is really what I went through. What happened to me and who did it. You got to understand it is the stress of the bills. The tight kitchen which stinks, and I can't cook in because it is so tiny. I would not be in half as much this mess had I not have to move each year or put up with people who do not respect … the fact that had the community support been in place a lot of things could have been prevented.
>
> I longed for a friend to open my heart too. Instead now I sit in the garden and find a friend in nature. Like God is just watching me. I miss the friends who encouraged me with hope. The voices you hear have a big impact on your heart.

Drives (and Triggers) Impact Balance

The participants moved on to identify that the interaction between the internal world and the external environment influenced the level of balance that they seemed to practice in their life.

Sharing those ideas and thoughts yesterday, really helped me to understand more about my drives. When I am full of an angry energy or full of fear—how things trigger me up. I can see how I lose balance. I snap and can't appreciate my family. … Now I am monitoring when I lose balance and how to get it back. My inner drive for justice and protection can be unhelpful when in extremes.

Spiritual Productivity as Fuel

Participants concluded that they were deeply concerned in a search for the key to balance, equilibrium and internal contentment. They traced events back to 'Gods will' and added that things happened with a deeper meaning to drive for spiritual change and deeper connections to God.

> But here is the solution, for me anyway. I know that spiritual work is my fuel. It is where I get my fill when no one is giving to me. It somehow can drive me when I don't have any support. I don't think that is even recognised by therapists. I mean it is a thing you can put down as a hobby or a value and goal. But it is not seen as integral. But it is integral to my healing for me. Religious spirituality has been given a bad name, but it is essential to me. I mean how do I explain the power of dua (personal prayer) in a CBT session?… help me have less mental overload in trying to patch the two worlds up to make sense in my healing.

Balance, Mistakes, Opportunities and Rebalancing the Whole Self

The women agreed that they were looking for a spiritual therapy that emphasised growth over problems, a model that was filled with hope and effortless connection to their core beliefs that were embedded in their religious and spiritual faith.

> What does it mean to put faith as integral to healing? I think it would add spiritual dimensions at the core. These should not be treated as irrelevant or second-

> ary. Things like eman (faith), intuition, inspiration, messages in dreams, self (nafs) balancing, the love of the prophet and the power of dua (prayer).

> For me I think interventions are at several levels. Not just a thought and feeling level. That is just far too reductionist. Interventions can cover the spiritual level—the inner talk level, good deed activation level, community giving level, emotion or behavioural habit skill level, modelling from good company level, body strength and nutrition level and yes to access 'therapy', or maybe to access a skilled Muslim clinician and imam who can assess the whole thing.

Inspired by these discussions and shared excerpts, the participants decided that they would think (individually) deeper about what they meant. The group agreed to feedback on quotes, books and videos that further inspired them. This unanimously resulted in members mentioning that they had felt inspired by Rumi and Ghazali. The next part discusses the approach that they went on to develop inspired by the traditional Ghazali model of the self (QALB model). This was developed by exchanging ideas and reflecting on its parts over a period of several months. The participants agreed that they wanted to develop the metaphor of the tree, as opposed to inferring directly about the workings of the human body and soul. They felt that speaking metaphorically enabled them to keep a respectful distance from the traditional Ghazali model enough, but also allowed them to use abstract expressions related to it in a creative medium. (One interpretation of the Ghazali model of the self is described in Keshavarzi and Haque, 2012.)

Part (2) 'Scaffolding Holistic Elements with Metaphorical Tools': The Framework and Its Component Parts

This section describes how the women used metaphors to represent a holistic framework for wellbeing. Several smaller metaphors were scaffolded into the overall metaphor of the Jannah Tree which represented growth, beauty, transformation and a hopeful end to their healing journey. The key components of the framework mapped on to the traditional parts of the QALB (heart) model of the self (attributed to al-Ghazali traditional works). This includes aspects of qalb (heart), aql (intellectual abilities), nafs (drives) and ruh (life spirit). These terms were loosely translated by how the participants understood the concepts themselves. These components are consistent with the literature on the QALB model referred to in the introduction to this chapter. The metaphors chosen collaboratively by the women capture the idea of the spiritual energy of the heart as always moving, with the aim of rebalancing itself close to its fitrah (natural) state. It also captures the traditional idea of the heart as a mirror which can become crystal clear or crusted over. Spiritual energy was understood as connecting to the subconscious memory of God, experiencing urges to connect with God, a feeling of high faith and love for God, and an abstract intuition towards 'good deeds'.

'The Jannah Tree Enveloping a Diamond Seat: The Crystal Heart'

What is the Jannah Tree: 'The Jannah Tree—symbolises invisible inner and outer growth. It is strength, resilience, beauty and eternal—connected to

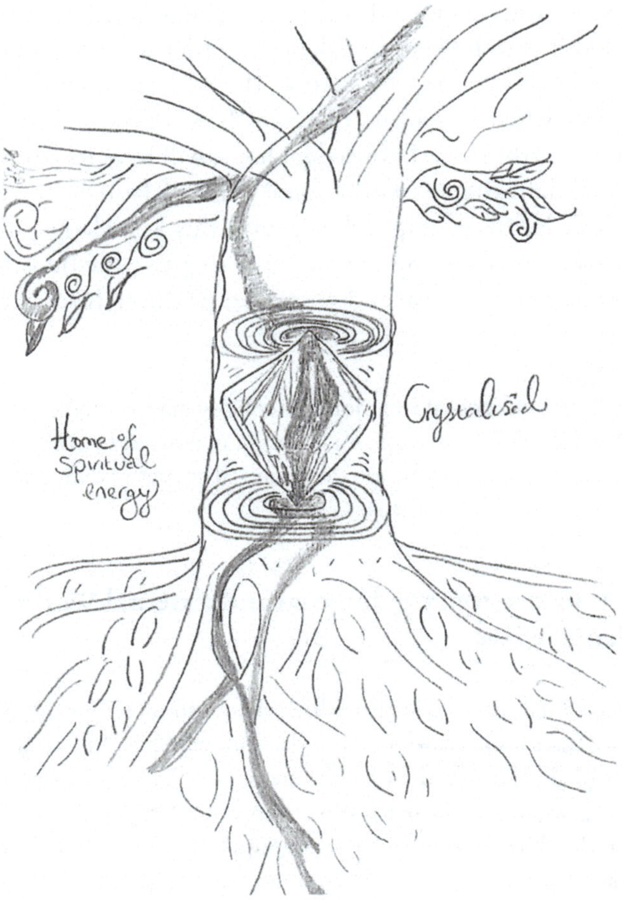

Fig. 15.1 Sketch of The Jannah Tree

prophetic heritage and others who sought to embody it from the past. It blooms in the love of the creator and the prophets. It suffers through its own seasons. It does not cease growth or movement though we cannot always see—its destination is to be connected through its roots and leaves to form the heavenly garden of paradise. Then the true colours and fruits of any suffering is seen, as well as reconnections made with other lost loved heavenly trees. We are those beautiful trees. We make up the garden itself and become the jewels there' (Fig. 15.1).

What happens inside the Jannah Tree?: 'The sap flows through the roots and the branches as if it carries the spiritual energy. This transports healing throughout its being. The sap is churned upwards or downwards by its crystallised form at the base of the trunk, this forms a crystallised diamond. If the diamond becomes too solid, the sap cannot flow. If the sap is too fluid the diamond loses its shape and form. The diamond is the seat of the spiritual energy, and it is to be kept in balance in order for it to keep the whole being in balance in distributing its energy. The tree can bloom and suffer through seasons, but when it appears lifeless it is working and growing inside, and beneath the earth. It has knowledge that it will have its completed form magnified in Jannah where it will become a tree of Jannah. So the tree is hopeful and can recover from despondency with this knowledge. The tree cultivates patience while it is waiting for the seeds to grow, the buds to bloom and the roots and branches to heal and grow over or through rocks that may attempt to bury it.'

> So, when the sap crystal (diamond) is solid—the spiritual energy needs increasing. When it is fluid, the spiritual energy may need to come from other directions, as one source may be too dominant. The crystal diamond is likened to the qalb in all of us—the spiritual heart.

Connection Between the Internal and External World of the Jannah Tree

> In the spiritual seat—(the crystallised diamond representing the heart/QALB), there are three main qalb elements. The ruh which is the essence of life. It is like the spirit part of us which holds the memory of Jannah—from which its original seed came from. It is the place where wisdom is felt and sweet belief enters. Next is the nafs which is a bit like the ego (appetite drives) which may not want to distribute the sap beyond itself. And next is the aql—this is the thinking part of the tree which perceives and analyses. All these elements are connected to the crystal diamond which symbolises the qalb. Harmony and balance within the

diamond is formed when the inner spirit is connected to the memory of Jannah and God. The inner spirit is to lead the inner thinker and inner drives towards serving in a way that it can reach the goal of becoming an ultimate Jannah tree. So it must allow its leaves to fall and nourish the soil, its fruits to feed nearby inhabitants, its branches to make shade and its roots to grow deep and firm to allow it to be a stable habitat for the surrounding creatures to benefit from. In the same way we need to give love and offer stability and compassion, feed the needy and contribute positively to society to keep our qalb in balance.

The crystal is also connected to the outer parts of the tree—the trunk, roots and branches. The tree is a whole system of connections. Connections flowing inwards, or outwards can disrupt balance of the crystal seat. If it causes contamination or erosion or could bring positive strength by nourishment—these processes could either help or hinder balance of the sap flow.

The diamond is at the seat of the tree, and it acts as the heart and house of spiritual energy, and pushes out physical and transformatory growth.

Imbalances in the Crystal Heart of the Jannah Tree

When the nafs is dominant, the crystal may become too hard, and when the aql is dominant the sap may liquidify and run through the veins too fast without nourishing itself sufficiently. It is like the aql is spinning thoughts out too fast, they are racing like the running fluid. It is never silent enough to hear the voice of the ruh.

It is like how the sap in the maple tree drips out as maple syrup. It is not useful to remain trapped, on the other hand if it flows too rapidly it is like it has moved out too quickly before it had the chance to absorb nutrients and be nourished.

Through Transformation: The Jannah Tree in Phases

The women discussed the strength, resilience and 'growth' determination of the Jannah Tree.

Can the tree still grow despite impurities in the soil? The roots don't give up—maybe they wait for leaves to be swept over and nourish the ground and emerge at a different time. Other parts of the tree still grow despite the weaker parts.

> The tree may experience the crystal as Stuck/stagnant. The tree has to find ways of Pushing through—releasing and reshaping—eventually blooming its outer parts and blossoming above and within.
>
> The tree produces flowers which are a sign of the fruits to come. The sweetness of faith flows in the sap. And the sign that the goals are near completion.
>
> I envision that the crystal rotates in rhythm, harmony and balance, and if out of balance a homeostatic response is initiated from one of its other parts to rebalance it. The energy can flow from any branch, root, flower or environmental influence, or from a place within the crystal linked to the memory of its connection to Jannah. So, spiritual energy can pass back into the crystal to restore and re-form balance. The state of the crystal is in regular flux—just as the sun shines on the sap and it flows by noon, then begins to solidify by night if neglected, or if alternative sources of sunlight are not tapped into regularly. Therefore, a holistic approach to managing the balance of the crystal is what enables it to function optimally.
>
> The body affects the heart too. What the roots feel and what the branches see affects the heart. The heart can open wider with signs of God, or it can begin to close if exposed to things which unbalance it.

Part (3) The Embodied Metaphor (Examples of How Participants Embodied and Related the Metaphor to Their Own Healing): Tracing Maps of Personal Experience onto the Jannah Tree Metaphorical Framework

The framework was formed in parts by participants. They used the relevant parts of it to map their own experiences. They predominantly used the notion of hopefulness and the idea of balance to reflect on what directions they could take from the ideas in the metaphor. This process was mainly shared as journal entries between participants (Fig. 15.2).

> The night it all seemed to go wrong was like a sudden storm had hit me hard, and me and my babies were left. I was like a wavering tree in the storm, desperately holding onto my roots. Then we fell and struggled as if part of me snapped in two. I was numb and scared. I had to carry on though. And somehow, we did. And though we looked dead and dirty to others, something was churning inside. I knew it was just a matter of time and these branches would grow back. That image of the tree was exactly how I felt. Dead at the top, but oh so powerful experiences going off inside. I was churning, and I felt through each traumatic

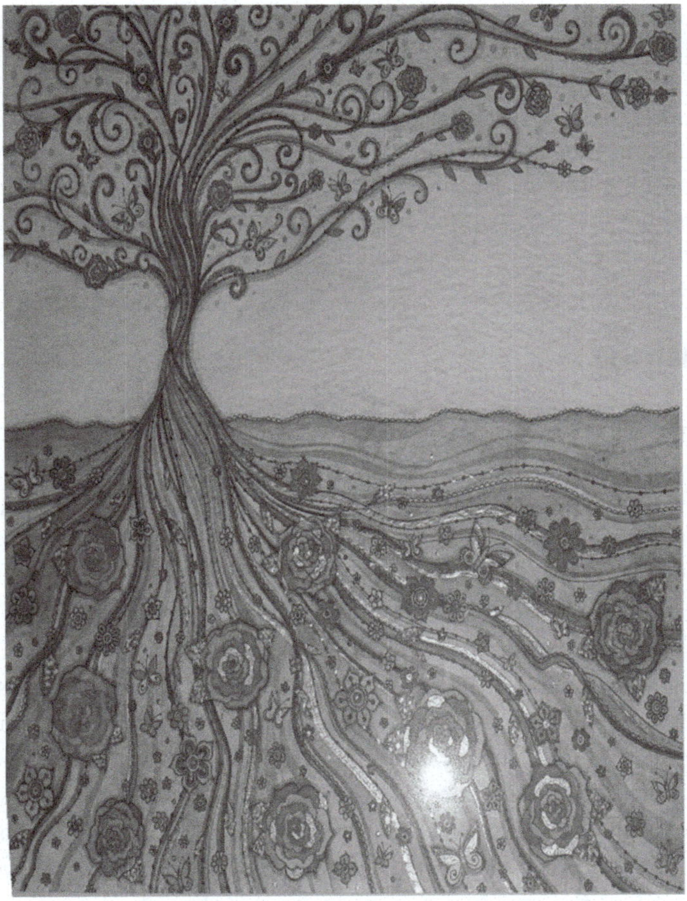

Fig. 15.2 Photo of original comissioned Art -Author's impression of The Jannah Tree blossoming

dream, the mirror of life was reflecting in. I got up and mapped my dreams and studied what they meant....I turned to my prayers to ask, so why and what now. I searched inside me, and I could feel that sap flow, I could feel it flow through my roots and I started to believe that it would grow upwards and not just down below. I saw that I could be strong as my roots broke through stones. I look ugly now. I look dirty now. But my buds will flower, and I will grow. I knew I had to power up my spiritual energy and I found peace in the night. I could not pray, but I sat still in the dark. And then one day I could whisper, and the next day I could cry—and it was like I could feel the movement inside me—like the crystal had pushed free to turn and let the spiritual energy flow in me again. Such relief to find God, such relief. I was so grateful. I knew I needed to work hard to attract butterflies. I needed to work hard to cultivate the soil. I needed to change

> things and people in my environment and home. I knew I needed to work on certain habits and I had to face my fear. … I had to let my aql calm my nafs, and I had to let my spiritual centre reassure my aql—that it did not always need to be in control, because that is what faith in God is about. … And I am awaiting those buds opening and blooming and trying to be very patient with myself as I am growing. I love the Jannah Tree, it makes me cry with its beauty and with the hope that one day that will be me, ultimately my glorious full form will be revealed.

Conclusions

Summary

Here, as author of this chapter, I summarise the metaphor and how it worked as a spiritual framework for balance and healing: 'There is a common saying that "every flower must grow through dirt". The Jannah Tree is the image of this beautiful creation which is growing through the natural dirt of Earth. It is growing by pushing forth the fibres, vines, roots, stems and branches with the turning and flowing of its sap—spiritual energy. The seat of this sap is at the base of the trunk wherein it forms a diamond crystal—which is neither too solid nor too fluid. The rotating motions of this crystal forms the balance in the flow of the spiritual energy (connections to God). The over solidification of the crystal ceases growth temporarily in one or more directions, alternatively, the excessive fluidity of the sap would create a flow too fast which would not allow the spiritual energy to be distributed adequately enough. Thus, it is the balance in the form of the crystal, and in its fluctuations between hard and soft states, which are of primary importance for optimal growth and transformation to occur. Understanding ways to manipulate sap formation (spiritual energy) and flow from all directions is important. However, this alone is incomplete as the nutrition on the ground, nearby trees, inhabitants of life cycle processes, weather, breakages, cracks, drought, blossoms and branch or root regrowth processes are important. As are the natural seasons the tree experiences in which leaves shed and spring brings new growth. Thus, it is a recursive interaction between the outside and the inside of the tree that is important to consider in how it would impact overall health of the Jannah Tree. The participant women used the framework to judge actions required to keep the crystal (qalb) in balance, as this represented optimal health and the best conditions for healing.'

Bridging Eurocentric Models

For the benefit of readers who wish to couch the metaphor into Modern secular psychological literature, in my view the analogies and cross-overs could possibly occur at a schema-narrative level. However, although overlaps are present, the women came to conclude that 'patch-working' theories and models were for the primary benefit of clinicians to feel at ease within their own language systems but could actually remove participants from the closeness of meanings they already have in place. Whereas Western psychology could map as tools in different parts of the framework—they altogether were not sufficient to address the whole spiritually led system of the self described by the women. Therefore, the metaphor became a useful frame to hold where and how Western tools could be used in supporting goals. However, the philosophy for change itself residing in the metaphor chosen was ultimately based on the Ghazali understanding of the self. This holds the spiritual heart as explicitly a central feature—which is not the same as an adaptation of a Eurocentric therapeutic model which may insert the concept if and when required. A critical community psychology approach, however, was felt to appreciate and value resources within communities and support the revival of indigenous methods to resourcefulness and wellbeing. The fact that this kind of intervention can be discussed in a community psychology handbook speaks volumes.

Members of the intervention were keen to voice that the use of narrative, symbolism and metaphor in faith-based scriptures was present before the advent of such formal models and theories in psychotherapy. Finally, participants requested that the Jannah Tree framework that developed is viewed as a creative attempt to simplify and relate easily to the eleventh-century Ghazali-based psychology of the self-model (and for themselves personally). This is explicitly holistic, spiritual, religious and Islamic. The women felt clearer, than they did at the start, about how the use of cognitive, behavioural, systemic or body therapies could help support the balance of the qalb within their new understandings of their original explanatory models. The women reported that the amalgamation of indigenous explanatory models previously held had become much more connected and accessible to them as a result of this intervention.

Cyber-Psychology and Increasing Access

The effects of working creatively online helped to connect isolated women to an intervention which helped them to make sense of their distress, and choose how to move forward with NHS services, or to reassess whether indeed lifestyle changes could work equally well in some cases. They were able to better judge what indigenous resources they already possessed and where Western tools may contribute within their own healing frameworks. The impact of online access also allowed for risky discussions in challenging the norms of Eurocentric psychotherapy and contentious religious topics such as dream interpretation. They openly felt able to question and learn how to situate mainstream psychology resources and tools for their good use when appropriate and timely. The women felt the intervention had not only shifted them 'off the fence' but made clear decisions of how a combination of different tools served them, and how ultimately the spiritual heart was at the core of this—the missing jigsaw piece was found.

In this instance all group members unanimously agreed that the use of cyber technology and social media platforms had enabled them to form connections, seek help and move forward. For some isolated women, cyber community psychology approaches could be an important step towards helping them to take steps to reconnect and access support. In some cases, it was described as a life-line. It is important to recognise online communities as legitimate communities that can be pivotal for people who are very isolated. Online working may also be a useful stepping stone for those who experience extreme shame and guilt as a barrier to accessing help face to face. Please note this work was conducted prior to the pandemic of 2020 and so online working was not a norm in therapy services at the time of writing.

Appendices

Key Learning Points and Benefits of the Developing Framework

The women felt that the intervention had many personal benefits to them including:

- The use of their own ideas in using metaphorical tools to discuss their knowledge and form what symbolised to them a hopeful approach, and a framework for change. The key features being that it was biased towards assumptions on the need for balance/rebalancing and growth rather than towards discovering innate 'deficit and damage'.

- The approach connected them to both worlds and was therefore congruent with their core beliefs, rather than disconnected. As Malik (2000) found, ideas of the heart (QALB) were relevant to British-Pakistani participants, including second-generation British Pakistanis.
- The approach made connections to transformations not seen on the outside and focussed on internal spirituality and its effects. This helped them to verbalise the importance of Islamic spirituality to them in their internal explanatory models.
- It encouraged self-belief and connected them seamlessly to their belief in God. This was what they were seeking from previous experiences of feeling disconnected from God.
- They felt driven to learn about inner balance and felt they received validation about their observations of incongruence in other approaches.
- The women felt that the framework was pivotal to their lives, and at the same time demonstrated the need for a formal Ghazali-based indigenous psychology model to be able to access easily. They felt satisfied that they had been able to interpret what they already knew as an image they could draw on easily in day-to-day life to help them access the principles of such an approach informally.

The core message for community psychologists from this work is that to work within participants' own core assumptions, explanatory models and beliefs is central to engagement and change. Understanding the importance to not dismiss the spiritual realm of core beliefs and experience is central as it is important for their beliefs to be judged as 'equally valid' as any other set of beliefs a client may hold about life and meaning. This should be explored respectfully. Finally, for psychologists to remain curious and to be accountable for their curiosity, especially about indigenous approaches that are resources from within communities. It is crucial to access appropriate training, supervision, guidance and reflective practice to work competently with minority communities.

Next Steps

The women who participated in this online intervention had started to use social media to promote the idea of art and journaling for wellbeing. They hope to use the artistic image of the blossoming Jannah Tree as a logo in future works, which they hope to develop into a project called the 'The Jannah

Tree' of course! If anyone reading would like to support these efforts, please get in touch with the author (drrukhsanaarshad@protonmail.com).

Practical Issues to Consider in Setting up a Collaborative Online Intervention

(a) For this kind of intervention to form, it is usually a good idea to already be an active participant within online forums of interest. This allows for your own natural interest, niche specialist skills and knowledge to be naturally present and available to others through sharing and informal support you may be offering. Therefore, to be knowledgeable on how to use social media platforms safely and competently should ideally not be a big concern and will be less cumbersome to understand once you are ready to form an intervention group.

(b) It is a good idea to access formal training in how to use online mediums for therapy purposes. This will form a good introduction in thinking about general good practice around privacy, safety, boundaries and ways to record online communication. This may be useful information even though you are not intending to offer formal therapy online. It is useful to understand online communication behaviours, for example, how some people can be more disinhibited or discourteous online; or what to do if risk information is unexpectedly shared by a user with a masked online profile.

(c) Similarly, it is important to understand the new General Data Protection Regulation [GDPR] regulations on consent and storing information to ensure that you are compliant if this is relevant to your intervention set-up. The current work was conducted before GDPR came into force in the UK.

(d) Clarify your role. Are you supporting others as a psychologist or are you contributing as a non-professional community volunteer? This will have implications on how you work, participate and are accountable.

(e) You may decide to put a call out for a specific support forum/initiative you have in mind, or you may decide to wait and see if online users naturally contact you. If there seems to be a pattern in the kind of input requested, it may be an indicator of the direction in which to facilitate an intervention.

(f) Clarify participation rules and group boundaries at first contact. Including ongoing consent and confidentiality/respectfulness on issues shared. Inclusion/exclusion criteria. What is your role? Facilitator, participant and facilitator? How many people can you realistically facilitate and attend to? Do you need a co-facilitator, or a way to work with fewer people using a time delay method rather than instant online communication mediums? How will you ensure the process is inclusive and collaborative?

(g) Clarify the timeframe of support and group goal. Define a closure process. Ensure you have appropriate capacity and support for this work.

(h) Decide what mediums you will use—messenger, email, webcam video-calls and so on.

(i) Clarify your intentions, goals and desired outcome. Clarify what will happen to the online group information at the end of the process.

Section 3: Transformative Change Work

> Can we therefore be participative students and agents of change and work together in order to assist in this intellectual and political movement for people's self-reliance and empowerment, for the defense of life and the pursuit of relevant, useful science? Can we commit ourselves as scholars and citizens to this epoch-making task? (Orlando Fals Borda, Participatory (action) research in social theory: Origins and challenges)

Setting the path for structural changes requires time, consistency and dedication to attempt new projects and approaches. In this section we present works that, in diverse contexts, try to design and implement something alternative to the known and codified way of 'doing things' in psychology to foster social justice and enact transformative change. From this perspective, in Chap. 16 Hammond and Palmer outline an alternative person-centred review process within the community to support children with Special Educational Needs and Disabilities (SEND), and transform their educational and professional path. With a similar emphasis on connecting existing community networks, in Chap. 17 Zoli et al. critically analyse a pioneering project where the typically excluded (migrants, prisoners, unemployed and people with physical and learning disabilities) engage in a number of community-supported agricultural projects that benefit directly into the community.

Reflecting on the role of students as agents of change, in Chap. 18 Akhurst and Mitchell discuss the importance of transforming clinical psychologists training programmes using the example of Community-Based Service Learning (CBSL) placements to better equip future psychologists to work with the complex and multifaceted realities of the communities they will serve. On another topic, but strictly connected to enacting local change at the community level, in Chap. 19 Miranda et al. present a collaborative work conducted with multiple stakeholders and Roma in mapping their own needs, in order to transform local Roma health governance. On the line of enabling the oppressed to own their own narrative, in Chap. 20 Richards presents three projects with people with learning disabilities (LD), where the participants became agents of change transforming the discourses and perceptions around their stigmatised group.

With the aim of transforming discourses and policies on youth and poverty, in Chap. 21 V. Johnson et al. explain how they engaged marginalised youth and policymakers to co-create a cross-cultural and collective understanding of uncertainty, community and justice in three sites of post-conflict Nepal. Youth is also the focus of the research and intervention presented in Chap. 22 by S. Johnson, who argues for a radical change from punitive-oriented practices—a strong legacy of the Apartheid era—towards democratic care provision for abused and neglected male youth in Cape Town, South Africa. The work is presented as a mutually transformative journey for the youth as well as for the carers in generating safety, love and acceptance at personal, interpersonal and community level. Transforming the dominant narratives of oppression is one of the aims of the 'Challenging Heights' project to tackle trafficking of children in Ghana presented by Danvers in Chap. 23. The initiative uses the Freirian concept of conscientisation to enable the oppressed communities to understand their own oppression and devising collective practices to resist it. Additionally, Danvers critically reflects on the need for a radical shift of Western care provision from trauma-centred to rights-oriented.

Finally, in Chap. 24 Taliep et al. discuss how Community-Based Participatory Research (CBPR) can be used as a transformative approach to violence prevention interventions, and safety, peace and health promotion in South Africa. Moreover, the authors highlight the importance of being transformative in writing 'about what, and for whom' it really matters. It is with such aim of voicing narratives from the people and for the people, that the chapters in this section present academically informed researches, and transformative initiatives that try to live up to the onerous task set by Fals Borda of pursuing a relevant, useful science to foster transformative change.

References

Arshad, R. (2007). *How do clinical psychologists work with religious themes in psychosis?* Dissertation thesis. DclinPsy. University of Leicester. UK. https://lra.le.ac.uk/bitstream/2381/31235/1/U240464.pdf

DoH. (2005). *Delivering race equality in mental health care, an Action Plan for reform inside and outside services; and the Government's response to the independent inquiry into the death of David Bennett.* Retrieved at http://webarchive.nationalarchives.gov.uk/20130123204153/http://www.dh.gov.uk/en/Publicationsandstatistics/Publications/PublicationsPolicyAndGuidance/DH_4100773

Equality Act. (2010). Retrieved from http://www.legislation.gov.uk/ukpga/2010/15/contents

Fernando, S. (2010). *Mental health, race and culture* (3rd ed.). Palgrave Macmillan.

Fernando, S., & Moodley, R. (Eds.) 2018). *Global psychologies. Mental health and the global South*. Palgrave Macmillan, UK.

Inayat, Q. (2007). Islamophobia and the therapeutic dialogue: Some reflections. *Counselling Psychology Quarterly, 20*(3), 287–293. https://doi.org/10.1080/09515070701567804

Kaplick, P., & Skinner, R. (2017). The evolving Islam and psychology movement. *European Psychologist, 22*(3), 198–204.

Keshavarzi, H., & Haque, A. (2013). Outlining a psychotherapy model for enhancing Muslim mental health within an Islamic context. *International Journal for the Psychology of Religion, 23*(3), 230–249.

Koenig, H., & Shohaib, S. A. (2014). *Health and well-being in Islamic societies: Background, research and applications*. Springer.

Malik, R. (2000). Culture and emotions: Depression among Pakistanis. In C. Squire (Ed.), *Culture in psychology*. Routledge.

Marsella, A. J. (2013). All psychologies are indigenous psychologies: Reflections on psychology in a global era. *Psychology International*. Retrieved August 1, 2018, from www.apa.org/international/pi/2013/12/reflections.aspx

Mir, G., Meer, S., Cottrell, D., McMillan, D., & House, A. (2015). Adapted behavioural activation for the treatment of depression in Muslims. *Journal of Affective Disorders, 180*, 190–199. https://core.ac.uk/download/pdf/82300923.pdf

Moodley, R., Rai, A., & Alladin, W. (Eds.). (2010). *Bridging east-west psychology and counselling: Exploring the work of Pittu Laungani*. Sage.

National Institute for Mental Health England NIMHE (2003). *Inside outside: Improving mental health services for black minority ethnic communities in England.* http://webarchive.nationalarchives.gov.uk/20130105200229/http://www.dh.gov.uk/prod_consum_dh/groups/dh_digitalassets/@dh/@en/documents/digitalasset/dh_4019452.pdf

NHS England. (2016). *The five year forward view for mental health.* https://www.england.nhs.uk/wp-content/uploads/2016/02/Mental-Health-Taskforce-FYFV-final.pdf

Rothman, A. (2018). An Islamic theoretical orientation to psychotherapy. In C. York Al-Karam (Ed.), *Islamically integrated psychotherapy: Uniting faith and professional practice*. Templeton Press.

Rothman, A., & Coyle, A. (2018). Towards a framework for Islamic psychology and psychotherapy. *Journal of Religion and Health, 57*(5), 1731–1744.

Skellie, J. (2010). *Al-Ghazali: The marvels of the heart. Book 21 of the ihya ulum al-din—The revival of the religious sciences*. Fons Vitae: USA.

Skinner, R. (1989 [2018]). Traditions, paradigms and basic concepts in Islamic psychology. Journal of Religion and Health. https://doi.org/10.1007/s10943-018-0595-1

Part III

Transformative Change Work

> Can we therefore be participative students and agents of change and work together in order to assist in this intellectual and political movement for people's self-reliance and empowerment, for the defense of life and the pursuit of relevant, useful science? Can we commit ourselves as scholars and citizens to this epoch-making task? (Orlando Fals Borda, Participatory (action) research in social theory: Origins and challenges)

Setting the path for structural changes requires time, consistency, and dedication to attempt new projects and approaches. In this section we present works that, in diverse contexts, try to design and implement something alternative to the known and codified way of 'doing things' in psychology to foster social justice and enact transformative change. From this perspective, in Chap. 16 Hammond and Palmer outline an alternative person-centred review process within the community to support children with Special Educational Needs and Disabilities (SEND) and transform their educational and professional path. With a similar emphasis on connecting existing community networks, in Chap. 17 Zoli et al. critically analyse a pioneering project where the typically excluded (migrants, prisoners, unemployed, and people with physical and learning disabilities) engage in a number of community-supported agricultural projects that benefit directly into the community.

Reflecting on the role of students as agents of change, in Chap. 18, Akhurst and Mitchell discuss the importance of transforming clinical psychologists training programmes using the example of Community-Based Service Learning (CBSL) placements to better equip future psychologists to work with the complex and multifaceted realities of the communities they will serve. On another topic, but strictly connected to enacting local change at the community level, in Chap. 19 Miranda et al. present a collaborative work conducted with multiple stakeholders and Roma in mapping their own needs, in order to transform local Roma health governance. On the line of enabling the oppressed to own their own narrative, in Chap. 20 Richards presents three projects with people with learning disabilities (LD), where the participants became agents of change transforming the discourses and perceptions around their stigmatised group.

With the aim of transforming discourses and policies on youth and poverty, in Chap. 21 V. Johnson et al. explain how they engaged marginalised youth and policymakers to co-create a cross-cultural and collective understanding of uncertainty, community, and justice in three sites of post-conflict Nepal. Youth is also the focus of the research and intervention presented in Chap. 22 by S. Johnson, who argues for a radical change from punitive-oriented practices—a strong legacy of the Apartheid era—towards democratic care provision for abused and neglected male youth in Cape Town, South Africa. The work is presented as a mutually transformative journey for the youth as well as for the carers in generating safety, love, and acceptance at personal, interpersonal, and community level. Transforming the dominant narratives of oppression is one of the aims of the 'Challenging Heights' project to tackle trafficking of children in Ghana presented by Danvers in Chap. 23. The initiative uses the Freirian concept of conscientisation to enable the oppressed communities to understand their own oppression and devising collective practices to resist it. Additionally, Danvers critically reflects on the need for a radical shift of Western care provision from trauma-centred to rights-oriented.

Finally, in Chap. 24 Taliep et al. discuss how Community-Based Participatory Research (CBPR) can be used as a transformative approach to violence prevention interventions, and safety, peace, and health promotion in South Africa. Moreover, the authors highlight the importance of being transformative in writing 'about what, and for whom' it really matters. It is with such aim of voicing narratives from the people and for the people that the chapters in this section present academically informed researches and transformative initiatives that try to live up to the onerous task set by Fals Borda of pursuing a relevant, useful science to foster transformative change.

16

Towards Social Inclusion: Creating Change Through a Community-Developed Model of Person-Centred Reviews (PCRs) to Support Children with Special Educational Needs and Disabilities (SEND)

Nick Hammond and Nicola Palmer

After our initial training focused largely on experimental psychology and unchallenged mainstream psychologies, we were left despondent by the seemingly over simplification of complex human behaviour and the intrinsic removal of individual behaviour, emotion and thinking from the interplay with systems, structures and power that often create and maintain them. Now, as qualified applied psychologists, it does not sit comfortably with us to apply psychology to others, but rather we strive to apply psychology with others. Initiatives such as person-centred ways of working, allow us to move closer towards this aspiration and empower people whilst reaching some understanding of the systemic, structural, political, historical and social influences on them and their circumstances. Through this we want to redress power imbalances and support individuals and their communities to create sustainable change. We continue to work with and learn from our clients and colleagues as we develop our thinking and practices in this respect.

N. Hammond (✉) • N. Palmer
Department of Psychology & Therapeutic Service, Suffolk County Council, Suffolk, UK
e-mail: nikki.palmer@suffolk.gov.uk

C. Walker et al. (eds.), *The Palgrave Handbook of Innovative Community and Clinical Psychologies*, https://doi.org/10.1007/978-3-030-71190-0_16

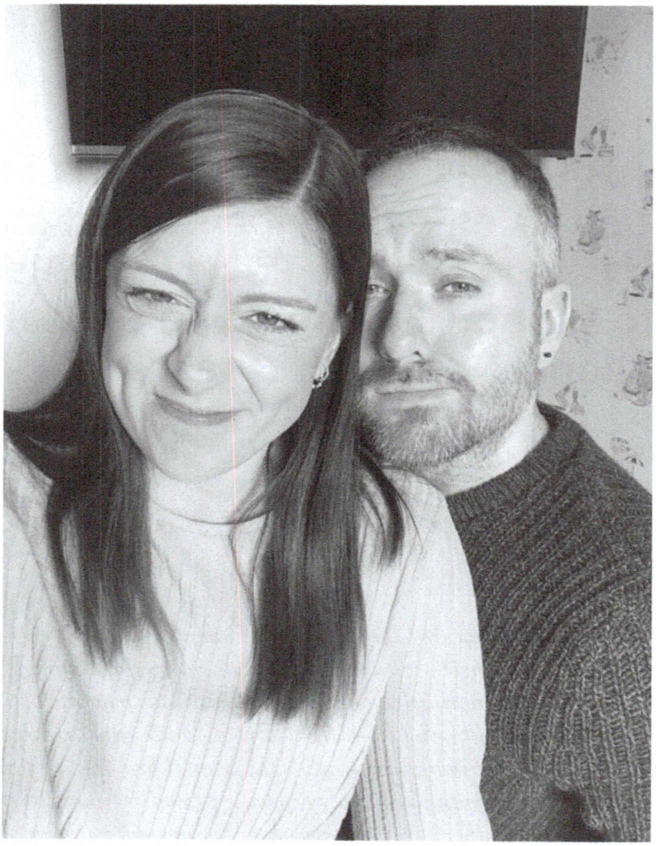

The Children and Families Act 2014 and associated Code of Practice (DfE/DoH, 2015) highlights that person-centred planning should be at the heart of meeting the needs, raising aspirations and improving outcomes for children and young people identified as having a special educational need and disability (SEND). Yet many systems remain entrenched within structuralist ideas of education creating oppressive conditions for these children. In 2015 the authors began a two-year study to develop a person-centred review (PCR) process that puts children, young people and their families at the centre of planning their own futures. This chapter will report on the research process that framed the study. Working with over 60 research partners from children to parents and teachers to health care professionals, we first identified challenges inherent to existing SEND process and then set about developing a process that would, in the eyes of the community, redress these obstacles. The process accumulated in an arts-based installation where community members were invited to review resources developed by local artists, a child-friendly video introducing PCRs created by the authors and experience a mock-up

PCR meeting. The chapter explores the opportunities and challenges of attempting such change.

> *Disabled people are still being treated as second-class citizens. Progress to date is not sufficient, and the road to disability equality is littered with missed opportunities and failures.* (Equality and Human Rights Commission, 2017: 5)

According to the most recent statistics, 6% of people with a learning disability are in paid employment—a steady trend, with a peak of 7%, since 2009 (Public Health England, 2016). A recent government briefing paper shows that 49% of people with any form of disability were in employment, compared to 81% of those without a disability (Brown & Powell, 2018). These extraordinary figures show a grave social injustice in the labour market. We are drawn to the question of why this might be the case. We believe that a diverse workforce relies, firstly, on an education system which is designed to promote confidence in employers, create opportunities for all through participation and building on individual strengths and challenge societal perceptions of (dis)ability (Hammond & Palmer, 2018). This leads us to consider how we might proactively encourage participation and inclusion in education, with the view of long-term social mobility.

Education as a Foundation to Social Inclusion

> *Social inclusion is ... the process of improving the terms of participation in society for people who are disadvantaged on the basis of age, sex, disability, race, ethnicity, and economic and migration status. ... Promoting social inclusion requires both removing barriers to people's participation, including certain laws, policies and institutions as well as discriminatory attitudes and behaviours, and taking active steps to make such participation easier.* (United Nations, 2016: 1)

Social inclusion starts with education. The education system in England is results-orientated and hierarchically structured in a way which creates and maintains division and diminishes the value of specific subjects and people (see Hammond & Palmer, 2018; Hammond, 2015; Robinson, 2006). It is important that all children and young people receive a broad and balanced education which meets individual need and promotes life chances. Yet, by virtue, many children with a special educational need or disability (SEND) may experience highly differentiated curriculum content and design. Where such differentiation takes place in an educational vacuum as a means to an end (i.e. within a classroom setting to fulfil societal expectations as opposed to person-centred, holistic approach with a long-term view of social inclusion), or limits access to subjects held in high regard by societal norms and economic value, it is likely to contribute towards the social exclusion of adults with particular needs (Iannelli, 2013). This is unacceptable and as psychologists working largely in educational contexts, it is an issue we continuously challenge—everyone has the right to have access to opportunities which are socially inclusive. Yet, we recognise that big world changes, such as shifting societal values and norms, are not directly changeable in the immediate future (Equality and Human Rights Commission, 2017; Hammond & Palmer, 2018). Rather, working closely with individuals and those who support them in a person-centred way can identify strengths and opportunities available within the community (Wolfensberger, 1995; Osburn, 1998; O'Brien & O'Brien, 2000). An example would be working with people to help them develop action plans for their educational and social inclusion. As practising psychologists, these kinds of *ameliorative* approaches aim to empower the child or family to make a difference at a, largely, individual level. This is in contrast to *transformative* interventions which are designed to change the very systems and policies which place the individual in the oppressive position in the first place (Fox et al., 2009).

Nevertheless, whilst the changes described here may not prompt immediate cultural or broader systemic change, we hope it will be a step towards changing the person's life, affording them opportunities to achieve and engaging the immediate systems to begin to think differently. Thus, small world changes can be the start of cultural or systemic change—or, in other words, big world change. For example, it has been seen that small changes and initial ideas made at an individual or local community level can, over time, accumulate into radical change (Plowman et al., 2007). We therefore anticipate that the proposed PCR approach would create multiple small world changes, at the individual, family and community level, which over time could influence those big world changes (Hammond & Palmer, 2018).

But what would such a person-centred approach look like, and moreover, how could we engage families and communities in developing the very approach designed to create *their* change? This chapter provides a theoretical rationale before describing the person-centred approach taken and, most importantly, how communities were involved in developing this way of working.

An Education in Social Value

Social Role Valorisation (SRV) is a theory which emphasises the valued role everyone has to play in a progressive and inclusive society and that each person should be given the opportunity to fulfil that role (Osburn, 1998; Wolfensberger, 1995). A basic endeavour of education must be to consider the child's inclusion and participation in their local communities. This begins by systematically planning, collaborating and challenging societal values at the individual, family and local community level (Osburn, 1998).

Many schools, colleges and specialist provision create opportunities for their pupils to engage in meaningful work experience and develop vocational skills. This is particularly helpful for pupils with SEND and provides employers with the skills in how adjustments can be made to support those with SEND in the workplace (Beyer et al., 2014). Indeed, we have seen first-hand through local initiatives, how work-based learning opportunities provide the life skills and sense of achievement not afforded to many children with SEND. These initiatives provide examples of SRV might work in real-world contexts.

However, local employers need to have the capacity, time and willingness to work in collaboration with schools to offer these opportunities. Thus, these opportunities can be limited and, in some cases, unavailable (Beyer et al., 2014). Nevertheless, giving these opportunities to young people experiencing SEND provides a basis upon which they can build their skills and knowledge within a work-based context. In turn, learning becomes embedded, interconnected and focused on the person's strengths and interests. Therefore, chances of successfully entering the labour market and accessing associated rewards—such as a greater financial, social and independent status—are improved and a valued social role achieved.

Moving Towards a Person-Centred Education System

A child-centred education places value on the person at the heart of learning and development, as opposed to a system which is driven by societal and economic values. Shuayb and O'Donnell (2008) found that there is a rather contradictory system in UK primary education, which, whilst in some respects is set up to be inclusive by supporting individual need, also drives children towards achieving economic and social goals, where economically valued qualifications are prioritised—thus establishing the beginnings of exclusion for those children unable to access these modes of learning or content.

A *good education* is that which is considered, by society, to prepare children for the future by emphasising subjects which are most likely going to be valuable to the economy as a whole, such as maths, English and science, as well as modes of learning and assessment thought to be superior, such as exams (Doddington & Hilton, 2007: 56). In contrast, person-centred education provides well-rounded and immersive education focused on each child's needs and experience (Doddington & Hilton, 2007). Whilst it is important to ensure society has the means to provide economic stability and secure skills required to provide a wide range of progressive health, education and social care services, we argue here that other roles are of equal importance and that all children, regardless of individual circumstance, should receive a varied and balanced curriculum which allows them to fulfil their aspirations and play roles in society which are equally as valued. We believe that person-centred education provides opportunities to promote inclusion in schools as well as develop transferable skills for the child's eventual transition to their wider community—which, ultimately, must be the aim of any education system.

Person-centred education focuses on the whole person, developing skills which will allow them to not only acquire academic knowledge and labour-driven skills, but also be equipped with important inter- and intra-personal skills. These skills are believed to be central to the development and maintenance of collaborative, socially just and progressive communities (Kohn, 2015). However, many teachers feel the need to become more confident in person-centred education (Perren et al., 2017). Indeed, children accustomed to more traditional classroom practice may also find person-centred education a challenging shift (Kohn, 2015). This is perhaps reflective of the societal norms and values we not only abide by but are socialised into. This provides an example of the complexities involved in making big world change.

Another key feature of person-centred education is the idea that the child is embedded and embodied in their environment and is provided with experiential learning opportunities (Doddington & Hilton, 2007). For SEND children who often benefit from this type of learning, and more visual learning tasks, this could invoke better engagement and a deeper more personal learning experience. This should be encouraged in both the core subjects and providing skills for independence and inclusion. This could be developing skills through work experience or vocational courses, directly linked to the needs and wishes of the person. Indeed, there are schemes that exist which promote this way of learning, such as *Towards Inclusive Learning Environments* (Smith & Bell, 2015).

Education systems are designed to meet specific social needs set within particular social values and norms (e.g. Boronski & Hassan, 2015). In turn, a system which should fundamentally be hopeful and provide the basis for social inclusion, can, by some, be experienced as disempowering and exclusive (e.g. Hammond & Palmer, 2018; Allen, 2017; Hammond, 2015). As such, we are motivated to understand how education can be personalised in an attempt to move towards a more inclusive, equitable society.

Personalised Education

In the UK as a result of the Children and Families Act 2014 (DfE/DoH, 2015), major SEND reforms ensued. This had a direct impact on how children with SEND were assessed and involved in their own planning. Specifically, it re-focused professionals on person-centred planning, multi-agency working and ensuring availability of information for those working with children with SEND (DfE/DoH, 2015). The SEND Code of Practice (DfE/DoH, 2015) highlighted the importance of capturing the child and parent's voice. Such processes of collaboration can help reduce power imbalances and improve services which better met the needs of the child and their family (Cahn, 2004). Through person-centred practices, it is hoped that one can be better able to focus on the child's strengths and, working as a team, identify meaningful opportunities for the child's immediate and long-term inclusion.

Whilst person-centred practices are important, these approaches do have limitations. For example, such approaches are embedded in Rogerian theory, which has been criticised for being overly simplistic when dealing with complex human situations and taking the basic premise that professionals must accept what a client is saying 'as is', and thus lacks appropriate challenge (Feltham, 2010). Yet we know that, from time to time, it is necessary to challenge clients with whom we work in a sensitive way. Moreover, through our own endeavours, we recognise that person-centred approaches with children must be implemented with care at the risk of becoming child-led and creating additional challenges (Hammond & Palmer, 2018).

Person-centred reviews (PCRs) have been widely used to support adults with additional needs, as well as to support young people transitioning into adulthood (Sanderson & Lewis, 2012). PCRs are based on person-centred, interactionist and social constructionist psychological principles and are part of a family of person-centred tools, which are in turn based on the core belief that every person has a valid role in society and has the right to be respected and placed at the centre of support and care plans that affect them.

A PCR places the focus person in the centre of the process, allowing them to take part in their own planning and prioritises a close working relationship with wider systems to promote multi-agency working and co-construction. The PCR invites everyone working with the child or young person, with the aim of having representatives who are able to meaningfully comment and create links to the wider systems and community. A co-constructed action plan is developed placing an emphasis on the strengths and skills already in the room, and particularly those held by the child or young person.

Previously there has been a focus on using the PCR in cases where a person is undergoing a major life transition, such as from pre- to post-16 education, and adult social care. Whilst PCRs have been used in schools with children and families experiencing SEND (White & Rae, 2016), there is limited empirical research into this specialised area of educational and care planning. This meant that any PCR model we chose to use ran the risk of being out of sync with the needs of the person, family and community it was intending to serve. As such, we embarked on a major two-year study with the ultimate aim to develop a PCR process with and for the community it intended to serve (see Hammond & Palmer, 2018).

We were particularly keen to explore the nuanced issues of the PCR process when used in schools with children and families experiencing SEND, as a form of early intervention and planning. We were also concerned with how the PCR model could be developed with communities. We will now report on this development process.

The Ethical Dilemma of Pseudonyms

The issue of whether to use pseudonyms in research of this nature is a contentious ethical dilemma. Decisions must balance participant voice, ownership and empowerment, with associated risks of removing anonymity. Some of these decisions relate to the ethical and methodological position researchers take to a piece of work, as well as a risk assessment of the possible implications of using or not using pseudonyms.

We were working in a changeable and highly sensitive context. Many of our partners were children, young people and parents, discussing sensitive issues, including challenges within contexts they continued to live. We were keen to capture honest commentary on these issues, and offering anonymity was one way of achieving this outcome (e.g. Crow & Wiles, 2008). These ethical issues and risks were substantial enough to conclude that anonymity and thus the use of pseudonyms was the best way forward. We took a blanket approach to this decision as, given the interconnectedness of our population, revealing one identity may have revealed others.

Whilst we recognise the challenges pseudonyms present to our attempts to empower, full regard was given to our ethical codes of practice, local policies and collective supervision discussions. Despite these changes, the role of the person and their words have not been changed. This for us was significant, as it is by capturing these real voices that we were able to advocate their positions to create systemic change.

Creating a Space for Personalisation

Ensuring the child and those supporting them are engaged in the PCR process is paramount to its success, after all, a one-off meeting is not in itself going to lead to the necessary changes or utilise the available opportunities. This engagement presents in two parts: firstly, in each individual meeting, and secondly, as part of the development of this new way of working. We will first explore the former point, before explaining how the community were engaged in developing this approach within one local authority region.

Whilst it is not a new proposal that children should be allowed to participate by way of being given genuine opportunity for joint decision-making (Hart, 1992), how this is achieved can be problematic. Children and young people with SEND may struggle to participate in the PCR in its most basic form, dependant on presenting needs. For example, we found that young people with needs relating to social interaction and communication struggled to access some of the PCR formalities, but that younger children with similar need did not (Hammond & Palmer, 2018). One explanation for this could be that despite similar engagement opportunities being made available through individual settings, there was a difference in how these settings worked with the child or young person. We noted that those who proactively sought the views of the child or young person by using appropriate elicitation activities (see Hammond & Palmer, 2018; Sanderson & Lewis, 2012) saw far more engagement from the child or young person, compared to those settings which did not use the materials in that way. The importance of including the focus person within the process should not be overlooked as it can be a very empowering experience for both of them, their parents and the process, as the parent of one child, Amelia, explains:

Parent: I thought it was a really good experience ... with some of the comments that Amelia was putting down but then I got to know what things were worrying her, I got to understand more what

> the other professionals, helping her thought about Amelia and the ways that we could come to an agreement on where we would go in the future, which I found really informative. That is the only way I can put it because I didn't know before then what their thoughts on Amelia were; I got reports on this and [that], but nothing mingled together if you know what I mean. Whereas [with] this, everything all comes together [as a] whole—so it made it more convenient for me, and Amelia understands more now as well.

This parent reflects how nice it was to have Amelia included within the meeting, and how this helped her understanding of what she was good at as well as areas requiring support. PCRs work towards rebalancing power distribution that can often occur in an assessment situation. Smale et al. (1993, 2000) proposed three models of assessment: the questioning model, the procedural model and the exchange model. Within the first two models, the expertise lies with the professional, or within the system. There is a sense of doing to and serving the needs of the system, professional or other adult agenda, largely, if not exclusively, separate from the person. This is akin to the way education systems are generally set up, as explained earlier, to fulfil societal needs within unchallenged social norms and values. However, within an exchange model it is recognised that everyone is an expert in their own right (Smale et al., 2000) and that there is a sense of information sharing and co-construction of ideas. The exchange of these ideas and expertise can help create new opportunities and, through making small world changes and focusing on the person, we can challenge accepted social norms and values. This exchange model is, nevertheless, carefully balanced to ensure that the interests of the child are advocated and protected (Sanderson & Lewis, 2012). This is particularly important where peripheral issues, such as safeguarding concerns, are evident.

The PCR process therefore allows for a continuous vision of inclusion within the child's setting, the participation of the child or young person in planning, as well as empowering parents and relevant professionals to move towards strength based and future thinking. Care is taken to consider appropriate ecological systems (Bronfenbrenner, 1989), for example, the community the child lives in and the impact this has on the child's development; it also ensures that connections can be made between education and the wider community.

A Co-produced Community-Practitioner PCR Model

The project was based on a collaborative research process with over 60 research partners including children, young people and their families, teachers and health care professionals. After identifying the challenges inherent to revised SEND systems and processes from parent and professional perspectives, we completed several PCRs based on the model outlined by Sanderson and Lewis (2012) with the view of developing this model to meet the needs of the communities we work with and for children and families experiencing SEND. We will now discuss each element and demonstrate how we involved the community in these developments, which concluded with an arts-based installation presentation.

Using an action research methodology, we were able to take a critical, reflective and collaborative approach to re-imagining the PCR process with the communities we were working with (Nelson, 2013). We wanted to look at the PCR model and ensure that it fits the needs of the children, young people, families and professionals in those communities we work in. The study was made up of three distinctive parts: the first involved focus groups with parent and professionals which aimed to understand how new SEND reforms were being implemented and experienced within the local community. We were particularly keen to understand the context that we were working within and did not simply wish to parachute in ways of working that may have worked elsewhere, but under different circumstances. We wanted to understand how best to involve children, young people and their families in improving outcomes as part of the SEND reforms. The second was to pilot a simple PCR model (Sanderson & Lewis, 2012) to familiarise the community with what a PCR is and how it might work in their local community. Finally, we held interviews, focus groups and a PCR installation event to develop the model and a wide range of practical tools (see Hammond & Palmer, 2018).

These initial focus groups formed the basis of us deciding to pilot the PCR model proposed by Sanderson and Lewis (2012), with some minor adaptations for very young children, such as elicitation activities. The original PCR model involved seven questions written on sheets of paper and placed around the room with a facilitator. Participants are asked to move around the room and answer the questions posed; they write their responses in different coloured pens. These are then discussed and summarised, and a collaborative action plan is agreed to move forward (Sanderson & Lewis, 2012).

The roll out of this PCR model to several local communities formed the basis of the second stage of this action research process. Feedback, using a semi-structured questionnaire, was sought from all attendees at these PCRs including professionals, teachers and parents, as well as a selection of semi-structured interviews with research partners to look further into their experiences of their specific PCR. The feedback and interviews were analysed, using a deductive semantic thematic analysis (Braun & Clarke, 2006) and used to propose a revised PCR model (see Hammond & Palmer, 2018), which was more suited for use within an educational setting, and with children.

Information gathered from cycles one and two were used to critically reflect on the experiences of those exposed to formal and informal SEND reforms and link this to developing practice (Nelson, 2013; McNiff, 2017). The authors were then able to piece together findings and propose a revised PCR model; this was then presented at a special PCR installation event where community members were able to further comment on our thinking and suggested improved model.

Feedback on the Initial PCRs

After each PCR, research partners were asked to provide feedback on their experience. The approach was felt to be largely positive (a mean feedback score of 8.8 out of 10), whilst areas for further development were proposed by those taking part, such as:

Teacher:	For certain children the whole process is daunting, parents found aspects of it hard too. I felt it put a huge amount of pressure on them.
Headteacher:	[My concern is] how to engage children and their point of view, how to make sure this is captured.
Inclusion manager:	Managing expectations of parents in advance.

The original model used is an evidence-based person-centred approach (Sanderson & Lewis, 2012), typically for adults and young people transitioning into adulthood. However, feedback from our study demonstrates how important it is to work with your own community, children and young people, when introducing new initiatives, as no matter how well-founded, parachuting in ways of working is not necessarily fruitful—or at least, as much as it might be when working in collaboration with the communities we are aiming to serve. Our research partner's main criticisms related to how participants were prepared and accessibility of the process to children and their parents:

SENDCo: [I'd like to know] how to help the child not feel overwhelmed and how to help the parent not feel overwhelmed.

During the initial cycle of PCRs, preparation activities were provided to settings to complete with children and young people. However, feedback from those using the materials suggested these were difficult to follow and not helpful for very young children:

Class teacher: The child's elicitation of views was very difficult to fully complete with such a young child—I did alter the way I asked lots of it.

SENDCo: Ways of how a very young child's views can be expressed needs some more thought. I wonder how they be more involved in the meeting.

Indeed, whilst many parents believed the PCR was a positive experience for their child, this was not always the case, as one young person, Emily, commented:

Emily: [There was] way too much information being thrown around at once, I had trouble keeping track of the conversation.

Emily has a social interaction and communication need and whilst several attempts were made to include her, the initially proposed process was not accessible:

Parent: I did read the information sheet beforehand. … I have to say, as a parent of a young person on the Autistic Spectrum it was not an easy process for my daughter and which obviously effects how I would look at things. To put her in a room she has never been in, with a group of people where she only knows me, you are not going to get the best out of her and I think that came over if you look at the sheets that came out of the review. She had put question marks on a lot of them because she was actually put in an uncomfortable situation and although I had read the sheets beforehand and I had spoken to her about what we would be doing as best as I could. You

> say within your process that you expect, and I can understand that you expect, a young person of Emily's age would participate in the meeting, but I think you have to know the young person you are dealing with and I think when the young person on the Autistic Spectrum, quite often there are a complex set of mental health issues there … it doesn't mean to say that your that they are able to deal with that situation.

This parent reflected how nuanced the process needed to be in order to meet the needs of a wide range of children and young people. Indeed, during the pilot of the PCRs we worked with a range of children, many who had social interaction and communication needs and who were able to participate within the parameters of the process—though partly because of how settings had prepared these children and young people. In this case, we accept that the parent may have become detached from the process, as might have Emily, and to that extent our endeavour was not quite as person-centred as we might have hoped. As such, we had to take some time to critically think about how we could address issues of preparation and accessibility and consider how our perceptions of inclusion aligned to the authenticity of being person-centred, which might, for example, mean not involving the focus person in the entire meeting. Equally, we may have also stumbled across an inherent limitation of being 'person-centred' (Feltham, 2010). Indeed, this was one of the first changes we made—offering the focus person and adults who know them best to choose whether they attend none, part or all of the PCR. To achieve this, we needed to ensure that regardless of the choice made, the focus person's views were adequately sought and included. This prompted a major revision of the pre-elicitation activities and documentation that was supplied to settings and parents before each PCR.

Engaging the person and their support network is crucial if we anticipate creating plans which will have an impact on long-term inclusion. How to achieve this when the children and young people we worked with ranged from 4 to 20 years old, in settings ranging from nurseries to Further Education colleges and with a range of complex SEND, was challenging. As such, we re-worked our original elicitation activities and provided a range of options upon which the child, young person and parents could decide to participate. For example, we created leaflets, visual storyboards and introductory film to enhance engagement and accessibility (see Hammond & Palmer, 2018). Letters sent out with invites to meetings contained all of these materials and a telephone number to the PCR coordinator, so that parents could make a judgement on how best to prepare themselves and their child, having ready access to support should they need to talk anything through. Settings were sent versions of preparation packs too, which include reminder sheets, lists of questions that will be asked and how to prepare the room which the PCR would take place.

The aim was to enable the child to share what they felt was important to their education and future goals (Doddington, 2015; Doddington & Hilton, 2007). We also created multiple activities per question, allowing flexibility pending on age and need, and encouraged each setting to nominate a member of staff to be a *PCR Champion* who would be responsible for preparing the child and parents, as well as coordinating the attendance of multi-agency professionals (Hammond & Palmer, 2018). As Emily's case highlighted, we wanted to be sure that if a child or young person choose to attend, that they would have at least one other familiar person in the room who was not their parent or carer. In addition to the child's attendance, it was hoped that the activities would provide a basis upon which the child's views could be incorporated into the PCR meeting allowing for the action plan to be tailored to the experiences and aspirations of the child. There is, however, an onus on the setting and parents to complete the activities prior to a PCR and to this extent, the inherent challenges and unfamiliarity of being person-centred are not removed.

Indeed, we found during the initial piloting of this project that where views are not gathered prior to the PCR can reduce the person-centred aspects of the meeting. In turn, we risk returning to the established equilibrium of adult-dominated agendas set within the parameters of what ought to be. Of course, the facilitator has a key role in managing this process effectively (Hammond & Palmer, 2018), but that role becomes easier when the child's voice is documented in advance. Indeed, where this was the case during the piloting stage, it made a noticeable difference to the feel of the process:

SENDCo: The voice of the child is important; I thought this was a great way to capture this.

Educational Psychologist: I felt there was a real focus on eliciting all the views of the people involved (including the child) in an environment which didn't feel pressured (it felt informal).

We were excited to share our revisions and remained mindful that our interpretation of what our communities were telling us may have differed from their intentions. Continuing to use the action research model, we introduced a third and final cycle, which invited all of our research partners, parents, professionals, local authority workers, to an open-house arts installation. This installation was designed to share our revisions and evidence from the data analysis in an interactive and accessible way, where our research partners could further comment on the PCR model.

Showcasing the Revised PCR Model

The arts installation took part in a multi-room venue, where our research partners were first seated to hear a short presentation of the PCR research followed by a viewing of the child-friendly PCR film. At the end of the film, partners were invited to ask questions before the room was open up into an arts installation. This consisted of displays featuring initial analysed quotes, preparation activities and a mock-up of a PCR meeting as it would look in a real-world scenario. Partners were walked through by members of the research team who were on hand to answer questions and elicit feedback in relation to the displays and interpretation of data.

Action research allows the lead researchers to *bring the story to life* (Nelson, 2013: 193) through means which are accessible to research partners, in this case we utilised the idea of an arts installation to our partners, who were made up of professionals and parents. We hoped that this form of presentation would allow our partners to explore the process that they had helped to create in an engaging way. We anticipated that this informal, yet immersive experience would open a space within which we could continue to co-construct the interpretation of data which led to a revised version of materials and process. Indeed, Broussine (2008) suggests that creative methods of presentation can allow a deeper emotional connection to the work, unveiling preferences and rationales of research partners which may have otherwise being unconsciously informing future revisions. This allowed us to work sensitively with our partners and led to the most appropriate changes being made as well as highlighting areas which may require the mindfulness of facilitators, such as the necessity to signpost and use non-jargon language.

The installation also allowed our research partners to become involved in the critical analysis of some of the data. This allowed us to revise previously interpreted data based on partner comments, as Alvesson and Deetz (2000: 33) suggest, '*people are not considered to be objects … but are active sense makers like the researcher … the key conceptions and understandings must be worked out with the subjects under study*'.

In addition to these discussions, post-it notes were made available at the end and throughout the installation where partners were encouraged to write down their feedback and understanding of the quotes. Research partners commented on the difference a PCR made to their setting and the child; however, they also identified key things which would be helpful in moving forward such as schools having copies of leaflets explaining what a PCR is before it is agreed, that some of the transcripts originally chosen where difficult to understand and one reflected that PCRs were well suited to early intervention.

Again, these were fed into the final analysis and write-up. This collaborative approach allowed the communities that we worked with to be included in the process that would ultimately lead to how the PCR process came to be understood and, indeed, practised within the communities we work.

Research partners also passed comment on the revised preparation activities, enabling us to understand how these materials would be read and understood, and also gave us important insights into how to future develop them to be fit for purpose. The range of backgrounds and professional agencies represented during this presentation allowed us to triangulate issues that were of most concern, and where amendment or further clarification was important. This process led to an equalisation of power, sharing of expertise to develop the most efficient and accessible process (Broussine, 2008; Smale et al., 2000).

The arts installation was chosen to reflect the fact that our research partners were equal stakeholders in the project. The aim was to create something that lived on well beyond the project and that would, ultimately, provide a mechanism within settings that would be used to develop education plans that linked to wider communities and provided the basis for social inclusion. Although, not a typical research community (RC), the essence of an RC was the intention of our endeavours (Wallace et al., 2009).

The installation process afforded us the opportunity to gather a final round of feedback from research partners that led to the final PCR model presented in *Personalizing Education: A Person-Centred Approach for Children with Special Educational Needs* (Hammond & Palmer, 2018) and now features within the local communities that the lead researchers work.

Summary and Conclusion

This chapter started with considering the disparity between the long-term social inclusion prospects of those with SEND by contrasting the employment figures of populations considered disabled and non-disabled. This led us to consider the starting point for social inclusion and long-term social mobility—education. Situation education systems within societal norms and values, we considered the inherent advantages and disadvantages of traditional and person-centred approaches to learning and how such approaches may lead to differences in how communities are involved in the education of different populations, and how skills and knowledge of those people are valued by society as a whole. We concluded that whilst big world changes, such as societal values, were not directly changeable, a series of small world changes, such as personalising education, would be more likely to lead to greater opportunities for all populations of children and, ultimately, lead to greater social inclusion.

We proposed PCRs as one way of achieving a person-centred approach to education and in interconnecting education with the wider community in the hope of long-term inclusion and social mobility. We outlined a PCR model and how we developed this with local communities with this vision in mind and the anticipation that community ownership would create a momentum that might perpetuate this way of working long after the project's conclusion.

We found that PCRs can be a powerful process to be part of, for all involved, as this parent summarises:

Parent: Like Sophia (SENDCo) said it was hard to do it and now I have come out the other end of it, it was well worth it. Because it has made so much difference to me and Kyle's life now, it is so much better for him, for me, well when it's better for his life, it is better for me. So, it has made a huge difference already so what it is going to be like in another year, touch wood, it is just going to get easier and easier for him—so yes, brilliant.

Our endeavour to establish a community-developed PCR model did not quite come to fruition. Whilst we aimed to address some of the social injustice we have discussed in this chapter through multiple small world changes, which we believe was achieved to a point (see Hammond & Palmer, 2018), for some the process led to detachment as we endeavoured to find a way to include everyone. Equally, there were limitations as to how far we were able to fully engage the entirety of the communities we aimed to work with (i.e. all children and young people with SEND and their families). On reflection, taking small samples or focusing on a more well-defined community population, such as one setting, might have been a more fruitful way of allowing the process to be more community developed. However, this too would have created challenges as the wider population within which we work is so incredibly diverse and, as discussed earlier, this may have led us to simply 'parachute' an idea into other adjoining communities—which would not have been satisfactory at all.

Whilst we are confident that we created many small world changes, it will, of course, be many years before we are able to see whether a continued PCR process does lead to big world changes for individual and communities of children. For example, this study was not longitudinal and therefore we are limited by how far we can assess the long-term, big world, changes that occurred from it. However, we are aware that some schools and the Virtual School for Looked After Children within the local region adopted PCRs as part of their approach to improve practice and include children in their communities. We believe that, by changing day-to-day practice, and the lives of individual children and families, we can stimulate changes in culture and wider systems. Over time, we would anticipate recruiting policymakers, service managers and employers, in addition to community groups and individuals, to develop and utilise PCRs further. By promoting participation and engagement, we would want to see an increase in inclusive opportunities for the child and young person, both within education and in the wider community. This might include, for example, a greater confidence amongst teachers in how to include children with a range of needs and disabilities in their classroom, more diversity in school and workplace environments where children with a wide range of needs and none learn, work and play together, and ultimately, an increase in meaningful learning and employment opportunities where the culture plays to a person's strengths and not exclude on difference.

What we do know is that personalised planning for many children and young people across the world is already having a profound impact. A good example of personalised planning from childhood through to adulthood can be found in Franklin and Sanderson (2013), what we have endeavoured to achieve here is a personalised approach which starts in the early years and that sees the child and young person through to meaningful social inclusion. Whilst generally current education systems place value in societal norms and economic value, there is a shift in what is offered to those children with SEND. Social inclusion starts with education, and so it is necessary to promote an inclusive climate early in order to recognise the value of individual contributions to the wider community. PCRs provide a platform to achieve this through planning with the child or young person at its centre and proactively involving community-based stakeholders to be part of that person's support network. We hope that these small world changes will go on to address big world changes and injustices currently experienced by those with SEND.

References

Allen, A. (2017). Psychology and education: Unquestionable goods. In T. Williams, T. Billington, D. Goodley, & T. Corcoran (Eds.), *Critical educational psychology*. BPS Wiley/Blackwell.

Alvesson, M., & Deetz, S. A. (2000). *Doing critical management research*. Sage Publications.

Beyer, S. R., Meek, A. J., & Davies, A. (2014). Supported work experience and its impact on young people with intellectual disabilities and their families. *Journal of Applied Research in Intellectual Disabilities, 27*(4), 372–372.

Boronski, T., & Hassan, N. (2015). *Sociology of education*. Sage Publications.

Braun, V., & Clarke, V. (2006). Using thematic analysis in psychology. *Qualitative Research in Psychology, 3*(2), 77–101.

Bronfenbrenner, U. (1989). Ecological systems theory. *Annals of Child Development, 6*, 187–124.

Broussine, M. (2008). The seductive qualities of creative methods: Critical awareness. In M. Broussine (Ed.), *Creative methods in organizational research*. Sage Publications.

Brown, J., & Powell, A. (2018). *People with disabilities in employment*. Briefing Paper 7540. London, UK: House of Commons Library. Retrieved January 25, 2018, from http://researchbriefings.parliament.uk/ResearchBriefing/Summary/CBP-7540#fullreport

Cahn, E. (2004). *No more throw-away people: The co-production imperative*. Essential Books.

Crow, G., & Wiles, R. (2008). *Managing anonymity and confidentiality in social research: The case of visual data in community research*. NCRM Working Paper. ESRC National Centre for Research Methods (Unpublished).

Department for Education and Department of Health (DfE/DoH). (2014). *Children and Families Act*. Crown.

Department for Education and Department of Health (DfE/DoH). (2015). *Special educational needs and disability code of practice: 0 to 25 years*. Crown.

Doddington, C. (2015). Embodied arts experience: The educational value of somaesthetics. In Fleming, M., Bresler, L., and O'Toole, J. (eds.) *The Routledge International Handbook of the Arts and Education*, pp. 60–67. Routledge: Abingdon, UK.

Doddington, C., & Hilton, M. (2007). *Child-centred education: Reviving the creative tradition*. Sage.

Equality and Human Rights Commission. (2017). *Being disabled in Britain: A journey less equal*. Equality and Human Rights Commission.

Feltham, C. (2010). *Critical thinking in counselling and psychotherapy*. Sage.

Fox, D., Prilleltensky, I., & Austin, S. (2009). *Critical psychology: An introduction*. Sage.

Franklin, S., & Sanderson, H. (2013). *Personalisation in practice: Supporting young people with disabilities through the transition to adulthood.* Jessica Kingsley Publishers.

Hammond, N. (2015). *Forum theatre for children: Enhancing social, emotional and creative development.* IOE Press/Trentham Books.

Hammond, N., & Palmer, N. (2018). *Personalizing education: A person-centred approach for children with special educational needs.* Trentham Books/UCL Institute of Education Press.

Hart, R. A. (1992). *Children's participation: From tokenism to citizenship.* UNICEF, International Child Development Centre.

Iannelli, C. (2013). The role of the school curriculum in social mobility. *British Journal of Sociology of Education, 34*(5–6), 907–928.

Kohn, A. (2015). *Progressive education: Why it's hard to beat, but also hard to find.* Bank Street College of Education. Retrieved March 14, 2018, from http://educate.bankstreet.edu/progressive/2

McNiff, J. (2017). *Action research.* Sage Publications.

Nelson, D. (2013). Action research: An appropriate research paradigm for practitioners. *Language in India, 13*(10), 183.

O'Brien, J., & O'Brien, C. L. (Eds.). (2000). *A little book about person centered planning* (2nd ed.). Inclusion Press.

Osburn, J. (1998). An overview of social role valorization theory. *The International Social Role Valorization Journal/La revue internationale de la Valorisation des roles sociaux, 3*(1), 7–12.

Perren, S., Herrmann, S., Iljuschin, I., Frei, D., Körner, C., & Sticca, F. (2017). Child-centred educational practice in different early education settings: Associations with professionals' attitudes, self-efficacy, and professional background. *Early Childhood Research Quarterly, 38*, 137–148.

Plowman, D. A., Baker, L. T., Beck, T. E., Kulkarni, M., Solansky, S. T., & Travis, D. V. (2007). Radical change accidentally: The emergence and amplification of small change. *Academy of Management Journal, 50*(3), 515–543. https://doi.org/10.5465/AMJ.2007.25525647

Public Health England. (2016). *People with learning disabilities in England 2015: Main report.* Crown.

Robinson, K. (2006) Do schools kill creativity? Online Retrieved March 6, 2018, from https://www.ted.com/talks/ken_robinson_says_schools_kill_creativity

Sanderson, H., & Lewis, J. (2012). *A practical guide to delivering personalisation: Person-Centre practice in health and social care.* Jessica Kingsley Publications.

Shuayb, M., & O'Donnell, S. (2008). *Aims and values in primary education: England and other countries (primary review research survey 1/2).* University of Cambridge Faculty of Education.

Smale, G. G., Tuson, G., Biehal, N., & Marsh, P. (1993). *Empowerment, assessment, care management and the skilled worker.* HMSO.

Smale, G., Tuson, G., & Statham, D. (2000). *Social work and social problems: Working towards social inclusion and social change*. Palgrave.

Smith, A., & Bell, S. (2015). Towards inclusive learning environments (TILE): Developing the roadmap for the inclusion of students with special educational needs in vocational education and workplace settings. *Support for Learning, 30*(2), 150–160.

United Nations. (2016). *Leaving no one behind: The imperative of inclusive development*. United Nations. Retrieved March 14, 2018, from http://www.un.org/esa/socdev/rwss/2016/full-report.pdf

Wallace, B., Leyden, S., Montgomery, D., Winstanley, C., Pomerantz, M., & Fitton, S. (2009). *Raising the achievement of all pupils within an inclusive setting: Practical strategies for developing best practice*. Routledge.

White, J., & Rae, T. (2016). Person-centred reviews and transition: An exploration of the views of students and their parents/carers. *Educational Psychology in Practice, 32*(1), 38–53.

Wolfensberger, W. (1995). Social role valorization is too conservative. No, it is too radical. *Disability & Society, 10*(3), 365–368.

17

Overcoming Marginalisation and Mental Distress Through Community Supported Agriculture: The *Streccapogn* Experience in Monteveglio, Italy

A. Zoli, J. Akhurst, S. Di Martino, and D. Bochicchio

The ultimate goal of farming is not the growing of crops,
but the cultivation and perfection of human beings.
—Masanobu Fukuoka, *The One-Straw Revolution* (2009)

A. Zoli (✉)
School of Applied Social Science, University of Brighton, Hove, UK
e-mail: a.zoli@brighton.ac.uk

J. Akhurst
Department of Psychology, Rhodes University, Church Crookham, UK
e-mail: J.Akhurst@ru.ac.za

S. Di Martino
Division of Psychology, University of Bradford, Yeadon, UK
e-mail: s.dimartino@bradford.ac.uk

D. Bochicchio
Research Centre for Animal Production and Aquaculture, CREA Council for Agricultural Research and Economics, San Cesario sul Panaro, Italy
e-mail: davide.bochicchio@crea.gov.it

C. Walker et al. (eds.), *The Palgrave Handbook of Innovative Community and Clinical Psychologies*, https://doi.org/10.1007/978-3-030-71190-0_17

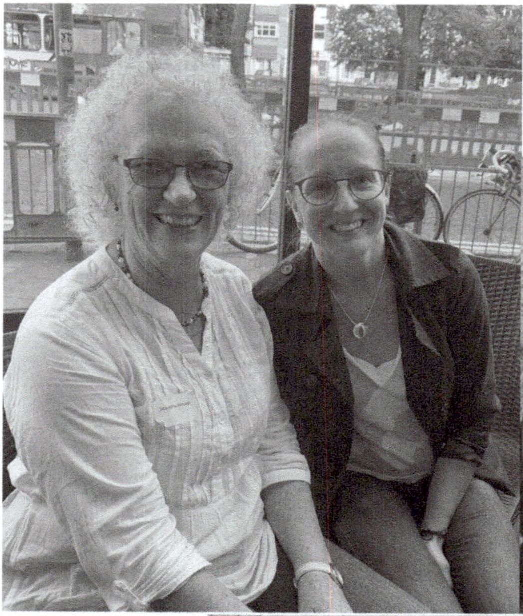

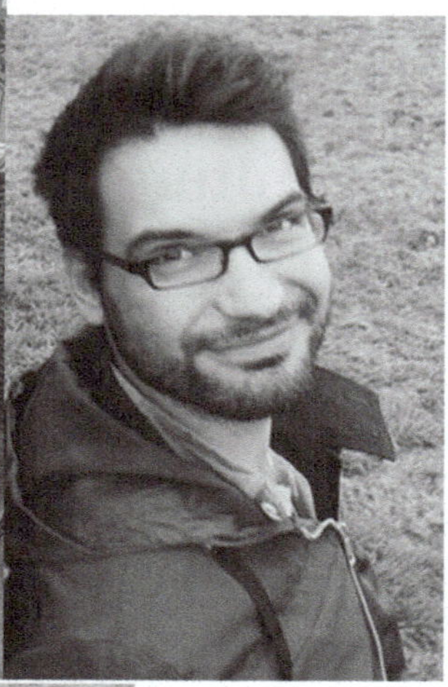

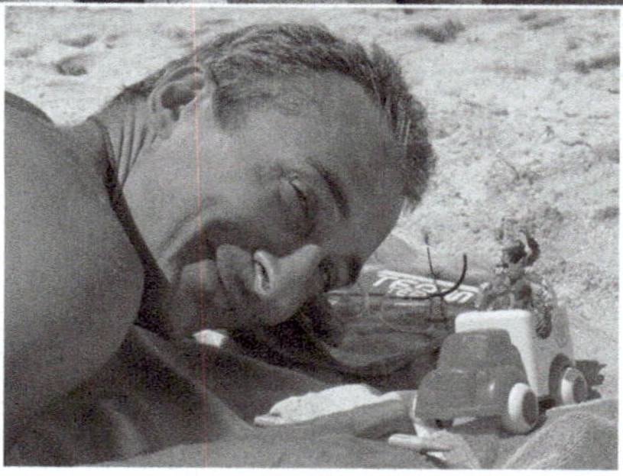

Anna, Jacqui, and Salvatore are colleagues and friends brought together by their love for community psychology and activism, cross-cultural understanding, and the outdoors. You can find Anna and Jacqui running a workshop together to facilitate peer group learning, as well as wild camping in a national park hoping to spot a rhino. Salvatore and Anna have long telephone conversations whenever they can to discuss the status of the CP discipline, their visionary projects about LGBTIQ+ issues, the promotion of happiness and wellbeing worldwide, and also the best prices to fly to Italy. Anna and Davide, who was primarily a gatekeeper in Anna's research in the field, became very good friends from then onwards. They are usually in touch by encyclopaedic emails, and they love discussing anything from food chains to local activism and anthropology, ultimately trying to get their head around the intricacy of being humans.

Anna, Jacqui, Salvatore, and Davide all share the passion for transcending disciplinary boundaries, and they are driven by a strong curiosity and openness to more holistic and comprehensive visions. When they approach new projects or face a new challenge, they search for solutions beyond their individual working environments, they ask for advice from friends, and they love exploring new issues by intertwining their personal previous knowledge with new paradigms, in order to deepen the possibilities to understand 'reality'. All of them put a great deal of personal and intellectual effort into writing an accessible account of the experiences detailed in this chapter, which they hope the reader will find of interest.

Introduction

In this chapter we aim to describe the experience of *Streccapogn*—a community and agricultural project based in Monteveglio (Italy)—through the principles and practice of Critical Community Psychology (CCP), Transition Towns (TT), and Permaculture. In particular, we will show how the initiative unfolded through experiential data gathered in a broader research process (Zoli et al., 2014), which we highlight through vignettes of the marginalised people involved in the project. In this regard our aim is twofold: first, we introduce the TT movement and Permaculture from which the *Streccapogn* vision derives, and highlight the connections to CCP principles. This entails drawing some theoretical connections between CCP, Transition, and Permaculture, before we outline the project itself. Then we describe the experiences of the marginalised people involved in *Streccapogn*, to show how the project developed and to consider what lessons have been learnt in the process. The chapter is based on the first author's (AZ) PhD project, which was co-supervised by the second author (JA). The third author (SDM) is a community psychology scholar and colleague of AZ and JA, who facilitated a critical reflection on the project from an 'external' perspective, while the fourth author (DB) was the main gatekeeper for AZ to access TT and *Streccapogn* in Monteveglio.

The Transition Towns (TT) movement is a cultural movement, a quiet revolution, aiming at shifting society from an economic model based on an illusion of unlimited low-cost fossil fuels and the exploitation of natural resources, to a different economic model aware of both peak oil[1] and climate

[1] Peak oil is the reduced capacity of world oil production to satisfy the demand (Hirsch et al., 2006; Hubbert, 1956).

change[2] (Hopkins, 2008). In line with this ethos, the economy cannot be decoupled from the environment and people's well-being; and the current economic, environmental, and social crises are seen as outcomes of an economic model that exploits resources, destroys the environment, and isolates individuals (Natale et al., 2016). Transition Towns identify communities as the ideal scale and nexus for action to promote the use of local resources and social inclusion (Barnes, 2015). Communities are pivotal in the process of economic re-localisation, and in triggering proactive participation (Connors & McDonald, 2011). The TT movement is rooted in Permaculture sharing its values and principles (Connors & McDonald, 2011; Felicetti, 2013; Hopkins, 2008). Permaculture is an innovative approach to redesigning natural and social environments that are in harmony with nature and sustainable in the long term. As a discipline, Permaculture is centred on the ethical principles of care for people, care for the Earth, and fair-shares (Holmgren, 2002), which strongly relate to CCP values as we show in the following paragraph.

Critical Community Psychology (CCP) embraces a transdisciplinary, value-driven, and systemic approach to tackle individual, community, and social issues (Fox et al., 2009; Kagan et al., 2011). Although CCP values and principles are described differently by diverse scholars, many agree on at least three core values, which are stewardship, community, and social justice (Kagan et al., 2011). Stewardship refers to the careful use of all types of resources, be they human, natural, or economic. Thus, CCP shares the Permaculture principle of 'care for the Earth', including human beings amongst the many creatures and elements inhabiting the planet. Community, as a value rather than a social object, means working with people's strengths and capabilities, disclosing individuals' and collective potential in the reach of respect and inclusion. This seems closely related to the Permaculture principle 'care for the people', in that everyone is considered a valuable member of society, able to contribute to the collective without being left at the margins. In Permaculture, margins are deemed fundamental to productivity, and diversity guarantees eco-systemic richness and long-term sustainability. Similarly, TT has 'inclusion' as its second foundational principle, calling for interpersonal and intergroup dialogical communication (Hopkins, 2008). Furthermore, TT explicitly advocates community-based interventions to overcome individual powerlessness and foster proactive people and communities (Hopkins, 2008). In line with TT and Permaculture, CCP considers social inclusion pivotal to healthier and happier communities (Kagan et al., 2011; Nelson & Prilleltensky, 2010). Moreover, CCP holds that in pursuing community as a value,

[2] Climate change in this context links human activities unequivocally to consequent global warming (Intergovernmental Panel on Climate Change, 2007).

facilitation and mediation skills are key to the maintenance of ongoing relationships with respect for individual needs, hopes, and desires. Finally, social justice recalls "people's right to self-determination; to a fair allocation of resources; to live in peace, with freedom from constraints, and to be treated fairly and equitably" (Kagan et al., 2011, p. 37). This embeds the distributive ethos of the Permaculture "fair share" principle, echoes the TT vision of a "fairer world" (Hopkins, 2011, p. 28), and extends it to all the aspects of social justice, including procedural and retributive justice.

Other pivotal principles that are common to CCP, TT, and Permaculture are social change, systemic thinking, and action. TT and Permaculture promote a systemic approach to radical social change by emphasising the role of communities, and foster collective action at community level in order to transform current Western societies. Similarly, CCP puts a strong emphasis on community interventions that enact transformative social change by tackling social inequalities at the structural level. This is why CCP praxis frames individual experiences of mental distress and marginalisation into the wider socio-economic-cultural and political context and designs interventions that address different ecological levels (Bronfenbrenner, 1979). The psychological focus highlights a special attention for people's feelings, thoughts, and experiences and how these can come together in community actions to resist oppression and create a better world (Burton, Boyle, Harris, & Kagan, in Reich et al., 2007; Harré, 2018). Overall, the clear shift of Critical Community Psychology from the cure of individual suffering located in the mind, to the care for shared experiences of distress and oppression in a community setting created the premises for engaging with the Italian Transition Town of Monteveglio for the first author's PhD research.

By drawing some theoretical connections between Transition Towns, Permaculture, and Critical Community Psychology, we argued how the principles and vision of TT and Permaculture are appealing to a community-minded psychologist. In the next sections we will show how *Streccapogn* attempts to embody Permaculture and TT principles by describing its development and enactment, and discussing the challenges and future prospects of this project from a CCP perspective.

Methodology

Monteveglio is a town of 5282 inhabitants (Italian National Institute of Statistics, 2011), set in the municipality of Valsamoggia in the province of Bologna, Italy. It was selected as the site of the first author's PhD research project (Zoli et al., 2014), which comprised a two-year-long ethnographic case study (Yin, 2009). Monteveglio was chosen for two reasons: first, it became the first official Transition Town in Italy and in continental Europe in 2009[3] and, second, it is the only TT in Italy recognised by an institutional document: resolution n. 92/2009 of the Council of Monteveglio. Data were collected from different sources using multiple qualitative techniques (i.e. semi-structured interviews, observations, and document analysis) and analysed through *hybrid thematic analysis* (Braun & Clarke, 2006; Fereday & Muir-Cochrane, 2008). The research aim was to study intergroup and intragroup dynamics of the Transition Town steering committee. Research questions were: how do people work together in order to take bottom-up action and foster social change in the community? Is there such a thing as a *community* and *sense of community* in Monteveglio? What are the contextual features that enabled the Transition Town initiative to start in Monteveglio? How do people work together to sustain it, and what are the strengths and weaknesses of such process?

The present chapter revisited the data corpus described, in order to outline the experience of marginalised people that were central to the TT experience in Monteveglio, embodied by the *Streccapogn*. As mentioned, we did not directly interview the people described in the vignettes, because they were identified as vulnerable subjects and would have required further ethical steps. However, the material in the vignettes has been gathered from the analysis of the witnesses' voices, and mainly from the thorough field notes of the ethnography and observations. While we acknowledge as a limitation not having a first-hand account of people's voices, we highlight that the triangulation of data from different sources and the familiarity of the first author with the data corpus allowed for voicing people's experience through vignettes that accurately reflect what the author has witnessed and recorded in her two years of ethnography, therefore ensuring rigour and trustworthiness (Guba, 1981; Shenton, 2004).

Down to Town

Transition was started in Monteveglio by a single person recognising the challenge of finding a solution to the multiple global crises affecting the economy, food, and the environment. This person was soon followed by a few people

[3] Monteveglio is registered as 102° official Transition Town in the world, and the first in continental Europe. Before, other Transition Towns were born in the United Kingdom, Ireland, Australia, Aotearoa/New Zealand, Man's Island, the United States, Chile, and Japan (Transition Network, 2013).

sharing the goal of producing local change by experimenting with novel approaches, drawing from the TT ethos. Monteveglio was chosen as a place to start, due to its agricultural territory, small size, and strong network of relationships between local people, a wildlife park, a shared cultural background, and sensitivity to the environment. Moreover, the upcoming election of a new local council created the opportunity for local activists to involve the political candidates who were willing to learn about Transition, and incorporate its vision into their electoral platform. Drawing from TT experience (Biddau et al., 2016), a small group of three created *Streccapogn*, an association focused on agriculture as a tool to support the community and rebuild social ties among people of the area. As we describe in more detail in the chapter, *Streccapogn*'s aim to include a range of marginalised and disadvantaged people created the space for involving several professional figures, such as educational psychologists, social workers, and international scholars.

From Vision to Action

Streccapogn is the name given to a variety of wild radicchio (*Crepis vesicaria*), which is typical of the Monteveglio area. It is usually eaten as a salad or used as an ingredient in local recipes. The name was chosen because it is a resilient plant that is strongly rooted in the ground. Similarly, the *Streccapogn* project aims to be a steadfast example of how to build a resilient community, rooted in its agricultural resources and local people.

Streccapogn started as an association for social promotion (Streccapogn, 2010) with three main thrusts: economic, environmental, and social. The economic aspect refers to re-localising food production and creating local job opportunities, with a focus on the disadvantaged. The environmental aspect encompasses a vision of nature and agriculture as the deepest link between people and the living soil. The social aspect refers to generating and building trustworthy relationships between community members and newcomers. Thus, it addresses people's fundamental needs for sustenance, health, social connection, and well-being. In 2012 a namesake, *Streccapogn* agricultural cooperative, was created to recruit trainees and employ workers in the production, transformation, and sale of products. The association and the cooperative are animated by the same ethos, but their different legal constitutions allow for access to different funding streams and other projects. The Streccapogn (2010) approach incorporates the vision of both TT and Permaculture. Production is local and based on organic farming, people are involved regardless of their status and backgrounds, and incomes are equitably redistributed. Moreover, the parallel with CCP is evident in expressions of the core values of community, stewardship, and social justice (Kagan et al., 2011).

The economic, environmental, and social functions of *Streccapogn* overlap and create a virtuous cycle. Food (ancient varieties of grains, vegetables, fruit, wine, and pork) is produced on local farms and processed by a local miller, butchers, bakers, and the *Streccapogn* members (making jams or pesto). The final products are then sold to the local markets, local businesses (restaurants, hostelries, butcheries, bakeries), directly to families or through ethical purchasing groups (in Italian: *Gruppi di Acquisto Solidale*, G.A.S.). These supply chains revitalise the local economy by hiring local individuals, being a source of income for families, as well as building and benefitting small and medium enterprises (SMEs), whilst reducing the ecological footprint as food is produced and consumed in the same area (known as Kilometre Zero 'KM 0' food), reducing detrimental environmental effects. Moreover, food is produced through the Permaculture principles of biodynamic farming and organic agriculture, aiming to regenerate both the Earth's and people's health. Finally, fair shares in pricing and income are achieved through a constant dialogue with producers and awareness raising with consumers.

Streccapogn draws from the Permaculture principle of valuing the marginal, in line with CCP ethos of working with marginalised people. This is particularly evident where people with various disabilities, prisoners, migrants, and the unemployed take part in agricultural and social activities, countering their conditions of social exclusion through foregrounding their active role in the community. Sharing spaces that are linked to the activities of food production and socialisation is a chance for people to liberate themselves from stigma and to construct positive identities. Furthermore, in line with CCP values, the *Streccapogn* approach focuses on people's strengths rather than deficits, their abilities rather than their limits. This has been shown to have important consequences in overcoming mental distress, increasing the sense of personal control, hope, and self-esteem (Rapp & Goscha, 2011). Thus, whilst neither agriculture nor community is a site of therapy, they have therapeutic effects.

This implies two other important conceptual shifts (Zoli et al., 2014). Firstly, 'from cure to care': marginalised people are not the receivers of cures in the medical sense, as in a one-way direction from experts to patients, but are welcomed in a multidirectional and mutual care-orientated community network. All the participants thus benefit from the building of trustworthy and direct relationships. Secondly, 'from cage to choice': community is not an entity with defined territorial and relational boundaries, not replicating institutionally bounded hospitals, prisons, assistance programmes. Community is a choice, in that people decide freely to enter or withdraw at any time. In the following section we outline how *Streccapogn* is organised as an inclusive community care model implemented in the non-traditional spatial setting of agriculture by providing detailed vignettes of the marginalised people involved in the initiative.

Lived Experiences

The effects of marginalisation are detrimental to the well-being of a number of people who experience discrimination, such as those diagnosed with physical or mental disabilities (Rowe, 2015), prisoners (Bereswill, 2004), the unemployed (Paul & Moser, 2009), and migrants (Bhugra, 2004). To address these, *Streccapogn* aims to expand people's individual capabilities as well as adult community learning (Lewis, 2012). The former calls for resources to address psychological, social, and economic problems as well as opportunities for personal growth and social inclusion (Rose & Thompson, 2012), whereas the latter entails striving for citizen involvement in community life as well as a mutual interest in exchanging knowledge, practices, experiences, and skills (Johnston & Coare, 2003; Packham, 2008). The *Streccapogn* approach aims to develop the individual capabilities and the community of adult learners. *Streccapogn* members hold periodic meetings and self-organised workshops in order to educate themselves to utilise dialogical communication and reflective praxis, and they set the example for the wider community they live and work with. "Essentially, each member becomes an AgroEcological-Educator, teaching others about growing food and the positive impacts that community-based food systems have on personal health, the local economy, and the wider ecology" (Wight, 2014, p. 208). In line with TT pedagogy, the *Streccapogn* project is also an ongoing learning process, where people acquire practical skills together with emotional and relational ones (McGregor & Crowther, 2016).

Streccapogn enacts social change by transforming the food production in the community, and ultimately overcoming marginalisation and mental distress. They try to achieve this dual purpose through a combination of agricultural-based work and socialisation (similar to Fieldhouse, 2012) reflected in the use of spaces related to such activities. Indeed, *Streccapogn* members work both outdoors in fields, wildlife park, and local markets and indoors in schools, homes, and the headquarters (two small rooms and a large one assigned by courtesy of the council of Monteveglio). Everybody, despite their backgrounds, contributes to agricultural activities, which take place in fields that are offered free of charge to *Streccapogn* by farmers or friends who are unable to cultivate them, or in fields that belong to farmers associated with the *Streccapogn* society. The following paragraphs describe how people with different conditions are integrated into the initiative.

People with Disabilities

Between 2010 and 2013, two individuals labelled with a mental impairment (learning disabilities, and diagnosis of mental disorder) joined *Streccapogn*. Giovanni[4] and Marco started as volunteers during their last year of agricultural high school through the 'school-work alternation' programme, a training programme for all school-leavers. It is important to highlight the interaction with the educational system through local schools at the meso-level (Bronfenbrenner, 1979). In this case the agricultural high school fits well with *Streccapogn* activities; thus the programme links with education related to agricultural practice within the community. At the end of the training programme, and after getting the high school diploma, young people with mental disabilities have very few opportunities to enter the labour market and they often end up living at home with their parents without prospects for future employment, especially in times of economic austerity.

In this scenario due to good interconnections, *Streccapogn* identified the cooperative *Accaparlante* as a support partner to include people with learning difficulties in agricultural work. *Accaparlante* is a social cooperative, entitled by the social services and founded in 2004 in Bologna, working with people with disabilities by providing opportunities for social and work activities in the province. *Accaparlante* entrusted the management of continuing activities of Giovanni and Marco to *Streccapogn*, while maintaining professional supervision of the two, and conveyed the funds provided by the social services to *Streccapogn*. Giovanni and Marco are supported daily by non-professional educators that have a mentoring role and enable the match between working and educational outcomes. Giovanni and Marco work together with the other *Streccapogn* group members as peers in the fields and workshops, as well as participating in community events in Monteveglio and the surroundings where *Streccapogn* have a stand, run free workshops, and sell their products.

Other people involved in the *Streccapogn* activities are affected by physical disabilities. Giulio and Camillo also joined the association through the social services of the province of Bologna and *Accaparlante*. Giulio works as an

[4] All the names used in this article are fictitious in order to guarantee anonymity.

accountant and administrative officer for the *Streccapogn* association and the agricultural society. He works at the computer and registers bills, costs, membership fees, and income after every market day and when customers are supplied with the products. He cannot perform his work independently due to his physical impairments; therefore, he works with a supervising mentor. Camillo has a severe physical disability and he cannot move or speak. Thus, he needs constant and intensive support; he relies on computer-based communication whereby he dictates letters to his mentor who puts them together on a screen to compose sentences. However, the communication barrier does not prevent him from being among people and sharing the spirit of the community. Given his condition and the nature of *Streccapogn* activities, concerns have been expressed by members about his inclusion in the project. *Streccapogn* have received feedback that they do not have enough resources to cope with Camillo's condition and need to consider whether they are able to continue. Such situation highlights the contextual limitations that a radical community-led initiative can face. External forces (such as scarcity of resources) can set unavoidable constraints, and *Streccapogn* decided to deal with them case by case. During the periodic meetings, *Streccapogn* members would discuss alternative ideas and possibilities to maintain, expand, or terminate existing projects.

Prisoners

The inclusion of prisoners was possible through the collaboration of the *Streccapogn* association with *Poggeschi per il Carcere* association, which was founded in 2006 with the declared aim of connecting young people with prisoners of the Dozza penitentiary in Bologna. In 2014, the two associations launched the project 'Growing citizenship' with the aim of offering prisoners the possibility to take part in alternative measures to detention, by spending time in agricultural activities outside the prison walls. The prisoners who are eligible to take part in the initiative voluntarily choose to participate.[5] Likewise, the prisoners' activity on the field is on a voluntary basis, meaning that they are not entitled any salary for their work. However, *Streccapogn* and *Poggeschi per il Carcere* cover travel and subsistence costs throughout the project. Moreover, *Streccapogn* offers prisoners a monthly allowance in order to challenge the potential structural exploitation of a free labour force and

[5] According to the art. 21, c. 4 third of the penitentiary Order, prisoners and sectioned can volunteer for projects of public utility at the service of the community.

dignify their work. The allowance comes from the surplus sale of the products, which is fairly distributed among all the *Streccapogn* volunteers.

According to the agreement signed among the parties, prisoners work most days from 8 a.m. to 2 p.m. The prisoners spend the morning working together with whoever is contributing on that day. The president of the *Streccapogn* association is responsible for their constant supervision, mandatory by law. As with those with disabilities, there are professional educators that supervise the progression of the prisoners. However, the dire need for more educational support coupled with the overcrowded Italian penitentiary system—with just 6 educators for 747 prisoners at Dozza penitentiary (approximately 200 inmates over prison capacity, Ministero della Giustizia, 2016)—hinders offering of appropriate support to prisoners, and connections with more associations like *Streccapogn*.

Participating in *Streccapogn* agricultural activities as an alternative measure to detention has two main aims: the first enables the prisoners to enter a relational context in the world outside the prison, where the label of prisoners is not the main feature of their identities (although in this chapter this comes across as the main feature of their identity). Second, they gradually re-acquire autonomy, by travelling autonomously on public transport to and from the workplace, and in case of prolonged activities, staying over for a few days before returning to the prison. Ideally, the goal of the project would be to hire the prisoners at the end of their detention. However, this aim has been proved unrealistic so far, due to the economical sustainability of the cooperative, and the impossibility to generate an income that would pay for a salary. Initially, two prisoners joined *Streccapogn*, one towards the end of his sentence, and the other mid-conviction. The former stayed a few months, then finished his detention and the work with the community. The latter became actively involved in the activities and continued.

After the first year, the project was valued as a positive experience for prisoners (according to the feedback that external social workers received both from the prisoners themselves and from *Streccapogn*), and consistent with the educational outcomes of the law; thus it obtained support for the following years. Another prisoner has recently joined *Streccapogn*, and the project continues. Moreover, given the increasing trustworthy collaboration between the parties, another project, called 'Seeds of freedom', is about to start inside the walls. The project includes professional training in organic agriculture for inmates and will reach all those prisoners who cannot apply for external work, due to their specific convictions. Inmates will grow traditional plants and aromatic herbs with organic certification that will be sold outside. 'Seeds of freedom' and 'Growing citizenship' both work for transformative change in the penitentiary system, as they radically promote a conceptual and practical shift from detention as a punishment towards detention as a space and time for training, work, education, and re-socialisation.

Migrants

Another group of people that collaborate with *Streccapogn* are migrants. Between 2010 and 2015, the number of migrants in the province of Bologna increased at a steady pace, with over 100,000 migrants registered as residents, and the number continues to grow (Fondazione di Ricerca Istituto Carlo Cattaneo, 2015). Therefore, they are increasingly becoming part of the local communities and economies.

Karim is a Tunisian baker who arrived in Monteveglio in 2011 during the 'Arab Spring'. Being jobless, he made contact with *Streccapogn* by word of mouth. Karim joined the group as a volunteer and worked in agricultural activities with other *Streccapogn* members. Since Karim was a baker, this became central to his activities. He was invited to run a series of workshops in the kindergarten and elementary school on how to make bread, tagliatelle, and pizza. This example shows how his existing skills were valued and he was enabled to put them to service in the community. Many other activities worked at the meso-level (a person's immediate surrounding environments, such as peers, school, and work) and at the exo-level (a person's indirect environment, such as the neighbourhood, and the extended family. See Bronfenbrenner, 1979) to connect him with other people and the local context, illustrating the CCP values of community and social justice. Other migrants joined *Streccapogn* for shorter period of times, but we chose to focus on Karim since he spent more time with the association and interacted extensively with the community.

Another example of *Streccapogn* networking to involve migrants is the collaboration with 'Seedbed', a project by a public authority to promote the integration of migrant women in the territory. *Streccapogn* and Seedbed started the project 'The other food of Valsamoggia', an opportunity to gather local and migrant women through the experience of cooking recipes from their countries of origin, using local and organic ingredients. This experience addresses particularly the values of stewardship and community: women get the chance to know each other, discover, and value diversity while encountering new tastes and new people, build relationships through solidarity, enhancing social integration.

The Unemployed

Due to the economic crisis in 2008 and the subsequent recession, many people lost their permanent jobs in Italy (estimates in 2013 of about 150,000 people), with employment conditions becoming increasingly oppressive under the label of 'flexibility' (Eichhorst et al., 2010). They are known as *esodati* (those undergoing an exodus) as they suddenly found themselves jobless and deprived of benefits and pensions (Garibaldi & Taddei, 2013). Whereas the disabled and the prisoners are integrated into *Streccapogn* activities through formal agreements that assign funds to the association, migrants and the unemployed are not recruited through institutional channels.

Streccapogn with their community structure and agriculture-based work quickly became a point of reference for unemployed people in search of a potential occupation or the support of others. Among these were two *esodati* men in their 50s, three enthusiastic young people (two men and a woman) who left their employment to start a new life through employment in agriculture, and two young women doing part-time or freelance work while gradually joining *Streccapogn* activities. Most of them saw in *Streccapogn* a living and working example of Transition and Permaculture, others wished to find a caring community where they could overcome personal difficulties surrounded by the warmth of welcoming people, and for others it was an opportunity to change their lives towards a more sustainable and rewarding lifestyle.

The experience of enthusiasm led people in different directions. One *esodato* left, and the other continued to attend the *Streccapogn* projects irregularly. A young man launched his own agricultural business out of *Streccapogn*, and the other four people (three women and a man: Giulia, Sara, Luisa, and Federico) occupied key roles in the association and the agricultural cooperative taking on multiple tasks. Giulia focussed more on agriculture and attended several courses around Italy on Permaculture and Organic Agriculture. She was responsible for building a greenhouse, selecting the seeds to plant and grow as well as managing the *Streccapogn* farms, and preparing the items for the local markets. Giulia gradually left her freelance job and became permanently employed by the *Streccapogn* agricultural society. Sara was more involved in the organisation and soon was elected by the group as vice-president of *Streccapogn*. Luisa and Federico became increasingly more interested in the educational aspects of *Streccapogn*, working with people with disabilities and the prisoners. They spent all the activity time with them outdoors in the fields and indoors in workshops.

Challenges, Limitations, and Future Prospects

Streccapogn's long-term goal is to (re)connect the community with its agricultural roots while using agriculture as a means to (re)build community ties. This requires continuous care for ongoing relationships and constant attention to all levels of the ecological system (Bronfenbrenner, 1979). Transition Towns' strong focus on pragmatism, as apparent in the slogan "the power of just doing stuff" (Hopkins, 2013) is not exempt from criticisms (Bay, 2013; Connors & McDonald, 2011; McGregor & Crowther, 2016). A major challenge is that *Streccapogn* does not act in a social vacuum and that systemic changes have to be addressed at the exo- and macro-levels. Conflicts with people who do not know the principles of Transition or do not share its values can hinder the project's effectiveness. For example, it has proved difficult to persuade local business owners to employ a migrant or an ex-prisoner. The social effects of stigma create barriers to the inclusion of marginalised people, especially in the employment sector, which is currently undermined by the global economic recession. This is a potential clash with the declared long-term aim of *Streccapogn* to create new jobs for marginalised people and stable occupations. Furthermore, there are also challenges at the meso- and micro-levels.

Sustaining the exo-level requires constant interactions between different stakeholders such as associations, institutions, and businesses. Whenever this is not well handled, it can lead to a series of intergroup conflicts, which were observed in the *Streccapogn* experience. In this scenario, Zoli (2018) identified those elements that thwarted *Streccapogn*'s attempts to interact with a political, economic, and social structure which is not in Transition. What emerged were continuous resistances to change and tensions between the radical *Streccapogn* initiatives and the rigid, slow, and formal institutional structures. A reason for intergroup challenges could be the contrast between the strong pragmatism of TT and the institutional political structure for a number of reasons that go beyond mere bureaucracy. For example, *Streccapogn* (and TT initiatives) do not have the burden of representation; in fact they are not elected bodies representing a collective or tied to governmental instances. If this is a positive aspect in speeding up the realisation of some projects, it has an evident drawback in reaching the wider community. Indeed, *Streccapogn* represents the vision and willingness of a small proportion of the population. As Felicetti (2013, p. 569) points out, "in the relationship between community groups and local institutions, there are also clear power imbalances, largely connected to the obvious differences in terms of legitimacy and available resources".

At the meso-level, interpersonal conflicts and power negotiations also undermined the strength of *Streccapogn*, leading some members to eventually abandon the group. In this context, Zoli (2018) also analysed *Streccapogn*'s difficulty in managing the different needs and expectations of its individual members. For example, in spite of periodic meetings aimed at voicing members' needs and planning future steps, several participants found it difficult to tell "The Truth" (McMillan, 1996),[6] especially when they had uncomfortable feelings towards leading figures. This reinforced a spiral of unexpressed antagonism towards certain individuals, which ultimately escalated into unmanageable conflicts, and reduced participation due to people's withdrawal from the project. Similarly, the centralisation of power in the hands of a competent and keen individual leader may lead to disapproval and discontent from others as well as to a sense of exhaustion for the leader (Zoli et al., 2014). This highlights the challenge of moving towards a participatory model; when people are not well-equipped to take on certain roles, and perhaps due to familiarity with more hierarchical models, they may be passive recipients of the project rather than its masters.

These considerations suggest the paramount importance for similar groups to consider the involvement of professional figures that are well-equipped to work with group dynamics in the project planning phases. It is worth noting that the TT foundational texts do suggest the engagement of external trained professionals, so in Hopkins (2011, p. 191) we read: "Conflict nearly always feels edgy, so don't underestimate yourselves—but do bring in an outside facilitator or other support if needed. Having a neutral person facilitating is a big help to reaching solutions." However, this was not pursued by *Streccapogn*, possibly due to a lack of appropriate needs assessment, or awareness of the initiative's strengths and weaknesses. Seeking external professional intervention, like working with community psychologists, could lead to forging better alliances, strengthening relationships, and facilitating genuine dialogue. This is essential for enduring grassroots initiatives in the long term, and the pursuit of transformative social change.

Although the richness of the data enables a detailed description of *Streccapogn* praxis, the lack of empirical results on participants' well-being is an obvious limitation (as found in Leck et al., 2015). Psychology-related measures would be needed in order to demonstrate an improvement in *Streccapogn* participants' mental health during and after the projects. Further studies could focus on a longitudinal approach to assess the effects of re-socialisation

[6] "What we mean by 'The Truth' is a person's statement about his or her own internal experience" (McMillan, 1996, p. 316).

in alternative spaces through community-supported agriculture and its impact in overcoming mental distress among marginalised people. Moreover, a single case study allows for analytical generalisation, but not statistical generalisation, meaning that similarities and connections can be drawn from different Transition experiences, but no universal claims can be made (Yin, 2009).

Accaparlante and Streccapogn (2016) presented their project plans for the following years. They will consolidate the ongoing projects with social services targeting those with disabilities and prisoners and will maintain the principle of inclusion and social integration by welcoming migrants, the unemployed, and volunteers. However, the relatively small size of the *Streccapogn* structure is a limiting factor for those who are able to take responsibility. Although *Streccapogn* aims at expanding their project, the ideal is that people will learn from their example and start similar projects in other contexts.

Streccapogn continues to collaborate with the local kindergarten and elementary school, to introduce new generations to the values of care, community, and social justice. For the next school year, they will run workshops on 'Learning from Mother Earth'. They will also offer extracurricular activities through workshops called 'Streccakids'. There are also new projects at the planning stage, such as 'social farming' and 'Free entry'. The former consists of creating a small farm of animals that participants will take care of (they are already caring for a female donkey) with therapeutic effects (Hassink, 2003). The latter will map the physical, cultural, and relational accessibility of the territory for the physically disabled. This is about considering what other people see as walls or spatial barriers to participation. *Streccapogn* is thus an innovative initiative, which has the potential to have a long-term impact on human relations and the quality of life of the marginalised. However, we acknowledge the limitations described above, which validate other controversial findings from TT initiatives (Haxeltine & Seyfang, 2009). Finally, at a theoretical level, the psychological work on 'sense of community' also offers insight on community dynamics in particular, with reference to the dimension of *trust* (McMillan, 1996), but it is beyond the scope of this chapter to enter this discussion (see Zoli et al., 2014).

Conclusions

This contribution aimed at describing how *Streccapogn*, an Italian association from Monteveglio, is working to overcome marginalisation and mental distress through community-supported agriculture and alternative spaces. Their ethos is rooted in the TT movement and we have highlighted its connections with Permaculture principles and CCP as a discipline. Our intention was to align the analysis of the *Streccapogn* experience to the recent attempts of the academic literature to adopt multiple perspectives—by enabling dialogue and cross-fertilisation between disciplines—in order to better deal with complex issues (Choi & Pak, 2006). From an action perspective, *Streccapogn* illustrates a radical praxis in the pursuit of environmental, economic, and social change. Although it has intrinsic limitations, the *Streccapogn* initiative is a valuable bottom-up attempt at overcoming marginalisation and mental distress. However, in times where austerity, structural debt, and restrictions on public welfare provisions have a recognised impact on people's mental distress (Walker et al., 2012), it is important to reflect further upon the ability of such initiatives to enact transformative change. In particular, neoliberal policies may find in initiatives like *Streccapogn* powerful allies, as they may use them as a cheap replacement for increasingly underfunded social services. Paradoxically, from this perspective such initiatives could be at the mercy of the very capitalist power they aim to replace, with the ominous result of fostering the same structural social inequalities they tackle. Whilst hoping that other projects with similar values are implemented in different contexts, we point out the systemic challenges at various levels, from the political context to the group dynamics. When considering interpersonal and group-related limitations that constrain action, we highlight the importance of including professionals with group and mediation skills to support the community in assessing needs, planning future directions, and implementing changes at all levels.

References

Accaparlante and Streccapogn. (2016). *PROGETTO PER IL LABORATORIO SOCIOCCUPAZIONALE AGRICOLO 2016*. http://www.streccapogn.org/16/wp-content/uploads/2014/06/PROGETTO-LABORATORIO-SOCIOCCUPAZIONALE-AGRICOLO-2016final.pdf.

Barnes, P. (2015). The political economy of localization in the Transition movement. *Community Development Journal, 50*(2), 213–326.

Bay, U. (2013). Transition town initiatives promoting transformational community change in tackling peak oil and climate change challenges. *Australian Social Work, 66*(2), 171–186.

Bereswill, M. (2004). Inside–out: Resocialisation from prison as a biographical process. A longitudinal approach to the psychodynamics of imprisonment. *Journal of Social Work Practice, 18*(3), 315–336.

Bhugra, D. (2004). Migration and mental health. *Acta Psychiatrica Scandinavica, 109*(4), 243–258.

Biddau, F., Armenti, A., & Cottone, P. (2016). Socio-psychological aspects of grassroots participation in the transition movement: An Italian case study. *Journal of Social and Political Psychology, 4*(1), 142–165.

Braun, V., & Clarke, V. (2006). Using thematic analysis in psychology. *Qualitative Research in Psychology, 3*(2), 77–101.

Bronfenbrenner, U. (1979). *Ecology of human development: Experiments by nature and design*. Harvard University Press.

Burton, M., Boyle, S., Harris, C., & Kagan, C. (2007). Community Psychology in Britain. In S. M. Reich, M. Riemer, I. Prilleltensky, & M. Montero (Eds.), *International Community Psychology: History and Theories* (Chap. 10, pp. 219–237). NY: Springer. https://doi.org/10.1007/978-0-387-49500-2_11

Choi, B. C., & Pak, A. W. (2006). Multidisciplinarity, interdisciplinarity and transdisciplinarity in health research, services, education and policy: 1. Definitions, objectives, and evidence of effectiveness. *Clinical and Investigative Medicine, 29*(6), 351–364.

Connors, P., & McDonald, P. (2011). Transitioning communities: Community, participation and the Transition Town movement. *Community Development Journal, 46*(4), 558–572.

Eichhorst, W., Escudero, V., Marx, P., & Tobin, S. (2010). *The impact of the crisis on employment and the role of labour market institutions.* Discussion paper series: Forschungsinstitut zur Zukunft der Arbeit, No. 5320. https://www.econstor.eu/bitstream/10419/52004/1/668782129.pdf

Felicetti, A. (2013). Localism and the transition movement. *Policy Studies, 34*(5–6), 559–574.

Fereday, J., & Muir-Cochrane, E. (2008). Demonstrating rigor using thematic analysis: A hybrid approach of inductive and deductive coding and theme development. *International Journal of Qualitative Methods, 5*(1), 80–92.

Fieldhouse, J. (2012). Mental health, social inclusion, and community development: Lessons from Bristol. *Community Development Journal, 47*(4), 571–587.

Fondazione di ricerca Istituto Carlo Cattaneo. (2015). *Cittadini Stranieri nell'area Metropolitana di Bologna: Caratteristiche e Tendenze 2015. Il profilo socio-demografico dei cittadini stranieri nell'area metropolitana di Bologna (Prima sezione).* http://www.cittametropolitana.bo.it/sanitasociale/Engine/RAServeFile.php/f/Documenti/Rapporto_completo_Anagrafico_2015.pdf

Fox, D., Prilleltensky, I., & Austin, S. (2009). *Critical psychology: An introduction* (2nd ed.). Sage Publications Ltd..

Fukuoka, M. (2009). *The one-straw revolution: An introduction to natural farming* (C. Pearce, T. Kurosawa, & L. Korn, Trans.). Other India Press.

Garibaldi, P., & Taddei, F. (2013). *Italy: A dual labour market in transition* (Employment Working Paper No. 144). International Labor Organization.

Guba, E. G. (1981). Criteria for assessing the trustworthiness of naturalistic inquiries. *Educational Technology Research and Development, 29*(2), 75–91.
Harré, N. (2018). *Psychology for a better world: Working with people to save the planet.* University Press.
Hassink, J. (2003). *Combining agricultural production and care for persons with disabilities: A new role of agriculture and farm animals.* Paper presented at the Farming and rural systems research and extension. Local identities and globalisation. Florence: Wageningen University/Fifth IFSA European Symposium (pp. 332–341).
Haxeltine, A., & Seyfang, G. (2009). *Transitions for the people: Theory and practice of 'Transition' and 'Resilience' in the UK's transition movement.* Tyndall Centre for Climate Change Research, Working Paper 134.
Hirsch, R. L., Bezdek, R., & Wendling, R. (2006). Peaking of world oil production and its mitigation. *American Institute of Chemical Engineers Journal, 52*(1), 2–8.
Holmgren, D. (2002). *Permaculture: Principles & Pathways beyond sustainability.* Holmgren Design Services.
Hopkins, R. (2008). *The transition handbook: From oil dependency to local resilience.* Green Publishing.
Hopkins, R. (2011). *The transition companion. Making your community more resilient in uncertain times.* Green Books.
Hopkins, R. (2013). *The power of just doing stuff.* Green Books, UIT Cambridge Ltd.
Hubbert, M. K. (1956). *Nuclear energy and the fossil fuel.* Paper presented at the Drilling and production practice, American Petroleum Institute.
Intergovernmental Panel on Climate Change (IPCC). (2007). *Climate Change 2007: Synthesis Report. Contribution of Working Groups I, II and III to the Fourth Assessment Report of the Intergovernmental Panel on Climate Change.* Core Writing Team, R. K. Pachauri, & A. Reisinger (Eds.). IPCC, Geneva, Switzerland. http://www.ipcc.ch/pdf/assessment-report/ar4/syr/ar4_syr_full_report.pdf
Italian National Institute of Statistics (ISTAT). (2011). Censimento della popolazione e delle abitazioni 2011. http://dati-censimentopopolazione.istat.it/index.aspx?queryid=1694
Johnston, R., & Coare, P. (2003). *Adult learning, citizenship and community voices: Exploring community-based practice.* NIACE.
Kagan, C., Burton, M., Duckett, P., Lawthom, R., & Siddiquee, A. (2011). *Critical community psychology.* Wiley-Blackwell.
Leck, C., Upton, D., & Evans, N. (2015). Growing well-beings: The positive experience of care farms. *British Journal of Health Psychology, 20*, 745–762.
Lewis, L. (2012). The capabilities approach, adult community learning and mental health. *Community Development Journal, 47*(4), 522–537.
McGregor, C., & Crowther, J. (2016). The Transition movement as politics and pedagogy in communities. *Community Development Journal, 53*, 1–17.
McMillan, D. W. (1996). Sense of community. *Journal of Community Psychology, 24*(4), 315–325.

Ministero della Giustizia. (2016). BOLOGNA—Casa circondariale. https://www.giustizia.it/giustizia/it/mg_data_view.wp?liveUid=2014DAPCARD&Nome=UFF56804

Natale, A., Di Martino, S., Procentese, F., & Arcidiacono, C. (2016). De-growth and critical community psychology: Contributions towards individual and social well-being. *Futures, 78*, 47–56.

Nelson, G. B., & Prilleltensky, I. (Eds.). (2010). *Community psychology: In pursuit of liberation and well-being*. Palgrave Macmillan.

Packham, C. (2008). *Active citizenship and community learning*. Learning Matters.

Paul, K. I., & Moser, K. (2009). Unemployment impairs mental health: Meta-analyses. *Journal of Vocational Behavior, 74*(3), 264–282.

Rapp, C. A., & Goscha, R. J. (2011). *The strengths model: A recovery-oriented approach to mental health services*. Oxford University Press.

Rose, V. K., & Thompson, L. M. (2012). Space, place and people: A community development approach to mental health promotion in a disadvantaged community. *Community Development Journal, 47*(4), 604–611.

Rowe, N. (2015). Creating a healing campus: A partnership between a university and a provider of mental health services. In B. Cozza & P. Blessinger (Eds.), *University partnerships for community and school system development* (pp. 119–134). Emerald Group Publishing Limited.

Shenton, A. K. (2004). Strategies for ensuring trustworthiness in qualitative research projects. *Education for information, 22*(2), 63–75.

Streccapogn. (2010). Statuto dell'associazione di promozione sociale Streccapog. http://www.streccapogn.org/16/wp-content/uploads/2012/10/statuto_streccapogn_final.pdf

Transition Network. (2013). *Official initiatives by number*. https://www.transitionnetwork.org/initiatives/by-number

Walker, C., Johnson, K., & Cunningham, L. (2012). *Community psychology and the socio-economics of mental distress: International perspectives*. Palgrave Macmillan.

Wight, R. A. (2014). The AgroEcological-Educator: Food-based community development. *Community Development Journal, 49*(2), 198–213.

Yin, R. K. (2009). *Case study research: Designs and methods* (4th ed.). Sage.

Zoli, A. (2018). Un approccio psicosociale e di comunità allo studio delle Transition Towns in Italia. In P. Nicolini & S. Porcu (Eds.), *Una mente sociale: Contributi in ricordo di Barbara Pojaghi*. FrancoAngeli.

Zoli, A., Pojaghi, B., & Akhurst, J. (2014). *Community development in the Transition Towns. The case study of Monteveglio*. PhD Thesis in Behaviour and Social Relations Sciences, Dep. of Political Sciences, Communication and International Relations, University of Macerata. Retrieved May 11, 2016, from http://ecum.unicam.it/766/1/TESI.pdf

18

Community-Based Service Learning During Clinical Psychology Training: Working at the Critically Reflective Interface

Jacqueline Akhurst and Carol Mitchell

"If you want to build a ship, don't summon people to buy wood, prepare tools, distribute jobs, and organize the work, rather teach people the yearning for the wide, boundless ocean." Antoine de Saint-Exupery. In our work with students in community psychology, we have aimed to teach them the yearning for the wide, boundless ocean. Students have few opportunities to experience 'psychology in action' within the 'ponds' of their programmes; and given the current strident calls to 'decolonise' the curriculum, our challenge is to move from predominantly westernised approaches to more transformational knowledge creation. Working in communities stimulates broader yearning as the raw and real problems of the world stir up the desire to learn and research, to answer complex and complicated questions that are not easily resolved in traditional academic ways. This way of knowing, doing and being, also challenges us, as we are not the experts of these multiple, unpredictable situations; and so we too learn from our students and our community partners. We all therefore hope to contribute as critical citizens, to the social justice imperatives in our discipline and country. Working in this way allows space for innovation and the generation of new doubt, which leads to more questions, which leads to more yearning…

J. Akhurst (✉)
Department of Psychology, Rhodes University, Makhanda, South Africa
e-mail: J.Akhurst@ru.ac.za

C. Mitchell
Leading Change Psychology, Townsville, QLD, Australia
e-mail: carol@leadingchangepsychology.com.au

C. Walker et al. (eds.), *The Palgrave Handbook of Innovative Community and Clinical Psychologies*, https://doi.org/10.1007/978-3-030-71190-0_18

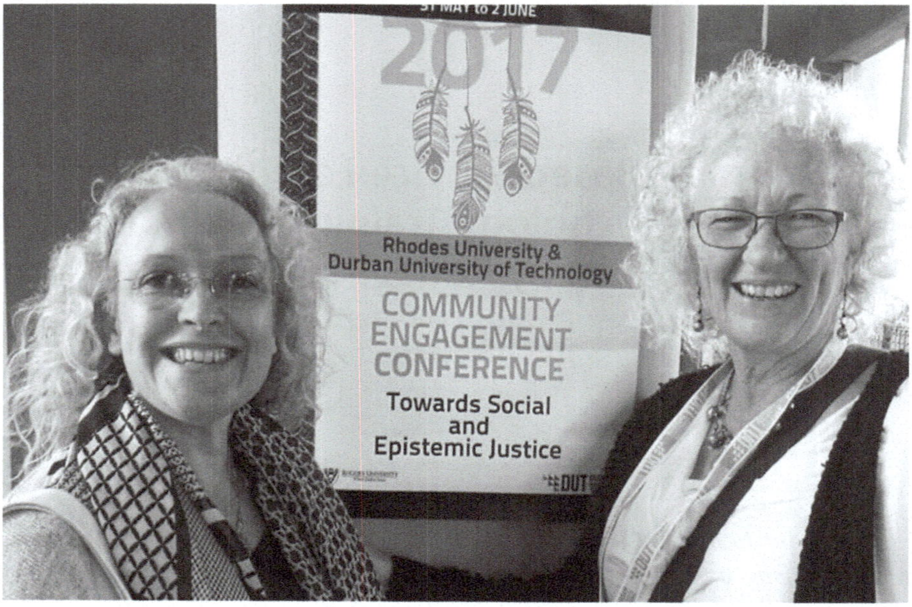

Introduction

As we write this chapter and reflect on the title 'new ideas for new times', we (Jacqui and Carol) are challenged to critically reflect on our own practices in South Africa (SA) and their relative successes and failures. I (Carol) cannot help but think of the Biblical parable of pouring new wine into old wineskins, where the old wineskins burst and cannot hold the new wine, leaving both the wine and the wineskins wasted and ruined. This may seem an odd way to introduce this chapter on working more critically in community psychology with clinical psychology trainees, but we want to honestly share our stories in the hope that these will help to generate innovative new 'wineskins'.

The work of poststructuralist French philosopher Michel Foucault (1983) encourages us to ask how things could be otherwise. His perspectives on power and knowledge remind us "not that everything is bad, but that everything is dangerous, which is not exactly the same as bad. If everything is dangerous, then we always have something to do" (pp. 231–232). Thus, if we withhold judgement, or more realistically, if we suspend our tendency to rush to pronounce ideas and practices as good or bad, we can perhaps ask how we can work in that 'dangerous' space of training our trainees in particular ways of knowing, doing and being.

This chapter frames our stories through relevant critical community psychology (CCP) and community-based service-learning (CBSL) literature. Thereafter we describe our contexts and efforts to promote community psychology with clinical trainees through community-based placements. In these placements, trainees are discouraged from individual work with service users, rather they need to work in group-based and consultative ways, building community partnerships and supported by critical reflective processes. Our relative successes and failures are discussed in the light of trying to innovate, to produce outcomes that move beyond amelioration at an individual level, hoping to promote greater social justice.

Theoretical Frameworks

Critical Community Psychology

Bearing in mind the assertions of Fryer and Laing (2008) that there are various forms of community psychologies, soon after forming the Community Psychology Section (CPS) of the British Psychological Society (BPS) in 2010, the committee at the time (chaired by Jacqui) (accepted deletion by reviewer here) spent time deliberating about the features that distinguished British community psychology from other manifestations of the sub-discipline. It was clear that a central theme drew from critical approaches to the impact of power and the structures of political and socio-economic influences, which promote inequality and a lack of social justice. The following working definition was thus proposed:

> Community Psychology (CP) views individual behaviour, health and well-being within a broader social and political context. It offers an alternative paradigm to the individualism that dominates much of psychology. In particular, it focuses on where power lies and how it is exercised in ways that maintain privilege and discriminate against certain groups. In practice, those committed to CP principles of collaboration and sharing of 'knowledges' work in negotiated partnerships, striving to build on the assets of participants. In this way, collectives of people inform themselves, recognising and gathering information about oppressive social arrangements in order to challenge these. Activities include the amelioration of the effects of societal inequalities and working preventatively, but aiming for the transformation of policies and interactions, to promote empowerment, liberation and social justice. (BPS CPS Committee, 2011)

This definition foregrounds the importance of the contextual and societal influences that impact upon mental health and distress, challenging the pathologising of individuals typical of much mainstream psychology (Cromby et al., 2013) and locating aetiology firmly in social structures that promote discrimination against and systemic oppression of certain people, with resultant inequalities. This highlights the importance of the social justice agenda: a way of working collaboratively with groups of people, valuing their attributes and knowledges, striving to work together to build mutual consciousness and solidarity focused towards systemic action and change.

In CCP then, 'social justice' is of central concern, representing desires to promote greater equity in the way societal resources are distributed, where people are able to live peacefully without externally imposed constraints, and with expectations of fair treatment and the rights to self-determine their progress. Kagan (2015, p. 16) thus recommends that trainees further their 'critical consciousness'; to consider how to create 'new forms of social relations (new social settings)'; the 'development of alliances and counter systems'; taking on roles of 'accompaniment, advocacy and analysis of policy'. In addition, Lazarus et al. (2015) write about the need to consider the profound influence of power dynamics on knowledges, resources and relationships when envisaging participation and partnership-building in the very unequal South African context.

In the definition above, the term 'community' was not interrogated to the same extent, but followed the ideas of Kagan et al. (2011), where 'community' is not seen as an entity circumscribed geographically (though not excluding such), but rather the active promoting of 'community', incorporating elements that draw individuals together into groups, whether formally or informally. Kagan et al. (2011) included 'social justice' as their second component, and also added as a third component the inherent respect of people and the planet, formulated into the concept of 'stewardship'.

One of the key features of the BPS definition is that it does not place amelioration in opposition to transformation (in contrast to Nelson & Prilleltensky, 2010), but rather sees a continuum of psychologists' practice as moving between these aspects, depending on the focus, systemic level and effects of the work. All of the above ideas resonate in the even more unequal and socially divided context of SA, where the imprints of the oppression and racial discrimination of the apartheid era are still very evident, more than twenty years after the dawn of democracy. Here in SA (as in the UK), clinical psychology has predominantly been associated with individual pathology and treatment, strongly associated with psychiatry, even though there have been regular calls for shifts in focus (as in Ahmed & Pillay, 2004; Carolissen, 2006; and Seedat, 2014).

Naidoo et al. (2007), in an important text outlining the history and applications of community psychology in South Africa, describe the challenges of moving from a more 'top-down' 'mental health' approach to community psychology (which seems to emphasise amelioration and the expertise of the psychologist, but with little impact systemically), towards a social action approach and beyond that to applications that are informed by Liberation Psychology (see Kagan et al., 2011). This is represented in Fig. 18.1 (developed by Jacqui), which distinguishes between three models (also see Arumugam, 2001, for further explorations) and shows how these 'operate' differently in terms of focus, levels of impact and engagement with power, to inform practice.

A CCP approach would be located firmly in the social action and social-liberation models. In SA, CCP could provide participatory asset-based approaches to promote (through critical reflection) deeper awareness of social asymmetries, still so evident, including spatial and resource-access inequalities; the effects of discriminatory practices; increased levels of poverty due to the neo-liberal policies of recent years and the impacts of the highest levels of HIV-infection globally. However, the translation of these ideas into practice has mostly been rhetorical (Carolissen, 2006; Seedat, 2014), rather than there being widespread evidence of the influence of CCP on psychologists' practice. An important way that practice could be changed is through clinical psychologists' training, and our particular interest is in projects that strive to translate these principles into action.

	Mental Health	Social Action	Social - Liberation
Focus	Groups, the bio-psycho-social interconnections, working within the system for amelioration and prevention	Self-determination for freedom and justice working within the system through social support / cooperatives	Political and social knowledge generation, work for political change via collective action & building social capital
Impact levels	Changes in social systems incidental and may evolve (but not the main aim); strong interconnections with medical and social care systems	Greater emphasis on structural inequalities and pressure on those in power to be more responsive through self-help groups, advocacy	Change through information sharing and intersectional campaigning for transformations at higher levels
Power	May unintentionally reinforce traditional systems of power because these are not critically analysed / challenged	May encourage systems and structures to be more responsive and invest more in human rights and existing policy delivery	Leads to political shifts, changes in policy and resource allocation towards greater social justice

Fig. 18.1 Comparison of three models of community psychology-based interventions

Community-Based Service Learning

Service learning is mainly understood to have originated in the USA in the 1980s and has gained popularity there over the last three decades. The pedagogy/practice is known by other names in different contexts—community-based learning (see Hart & Akhurst, 2017, for UK-based accounts), academic service learning, community service learning or academic community-based learning. Our preference is for 'community-based service learning' (CBSL) since this highlights the community-based partnerships that are essential to this work.

CBSL is intended to challenge trainees to use both the theory and skills they have learnt in training, to apply these to local knowledge from their work in communities. In addition, the service-learning experience is an attempt to alert trainees to social injustices and to reflect on their role as agents of change in these communities (Mitchell, 2008). Critical reflection is essential to enhance learning from these experiences (Gilbert & Sliep, 2009). Without critical reflection, trainees are unlikely to ask deeper questions about inequality and injustice and may therefore not question the status quo. CBSL is therefore more than just a practicum, internship or chance to apply theory. CBSL presents the unique opportunity for trainees to be both deeply engaged in a community and also to meta-reflect on this engagement in a way that challenges them to be active citizens (Akhurst et al., 2016). CBSL also has a number of other benefits for trainees and communities (Akhurst, 2017). It is designed to be a mutually beneficial exercise. Trainees require guidance to ensure that this happens. They also require assistance with developing the skills of critical reflection, since these require dialogical opportunities (Mitchell & Humphries, 2007).

Mezirow's (2000) model of transformational learning has been appropriated in service learning. He proposed a non-sequential learning process involving:

1. a disorienting dilemma,
2. self-examination with feelings of fear, anger, guilt or shame,
3. a critical assessment of assumptions,
4. recognition that one's discontent and the process of transformation are shared,
5. exploration of options for new roles, relationships and actions,
6. planning a course of action,
7. acquiring knowledge and skills for implementing one's plans,
8. provisionally trying new roles,

9. building competence and self-confidence in new roles and relationships,
10. re-integration into one's life on the basis of conditions dictated by one's new perspective. (p. 22)

The important disorienting dilemma usually results in disequilibrium or dissonance that motivates the people involved to re-evaluate their assumptions and beliefs, resulting in new understandings that change practices. Researchers have found that participation in service learning can sometimes have this transformational impact on trainees (e.g. Deeley, 2015; Eyler & Giles Jr., 1999; Rhoads, 1997). Eyler and Giles Jr. (1999) however warned that this kind of transformation of perspectives was not common in trainees, since many resist the process of critically assessing their worldviews.

The emphasis on social justice that we raise above has been debated in CBSL literature (e.g. Mitchell, 2008). Should service-learning activities be understood as located along a continuum—with charity at one end (seen as somewhat more self-serving, perhaps assuaging guilt) and social justice at the other? Or should these concepts be considered discrete entities, not overlapping? Some practitioners see the virtue of a continuum, allowing for more permutations. Strain (2007) usefully proposes that service learning is more complex than the continuum model is able to capture. He argues that trainees are capable of moving along and across paradigms in an integrative way, with service learning being a multilinear endeavour, which he likens to moving like a starfish. He rejects the duality of self and other and claims that when we are in touch with others, an awareness of our interconnectedness "scours away any sense of noblesse oblige, any patronising or condescending attitude, any trace of moral superiority" (p. 5). Thus, a student may be engaged in an act of 'charity' in one dimension, but may be engaged in multiple other ways of being at the same time.

The core values of CBSL may thus depend on the positioning of the practitioner (as is the case with community psychology). Nguyen (2016, p. 7) interrogates five core values of service learning as originally proposed at Duke University in the USA, to guide their programmes: 'rigor, reflection, relationship, reciprocity, and real life'. It is important to consider that some of these 'values' may actually reflect the needs of academics and trainees, rather than encompassing communities' perspectives. How then do these intersect with the three CCP dimensions of social justice, community and stewardship?

Jacqui has described intersections of CCP and CBSL in the South African context in more detail (Akhurst, 2017), highlighting some of the challenges of service users' expectations of trainee psychologists and the impact of oppressive social relations on being able to build more equal partnerships. The trainees reported knowledge exchange and the immersive learning of CBSL as enabling their conscientisation (Freire, 1970). We explore trainees' accounts of CBSL further in this chapter, after briefly locating their training contextually.

The Local SA Context and Clinical Psychology Training

Post-apartheid resource constraints and the imperatives of the SA context as a developing country demand responses that are wide-reaching and well beyond individually focused traditional psychologists' training. A number of authors (e.g. Naidoo et al., 2007) illustrate community psychology's broad applicability to societal reconstruction post-1994. Most SA master's degree training programmes for psychologists integrate community psychology into the core coursework of professional training (Yen, 2007), because it has applications in all categories of psychology. Trainees on such programmes have various levels of prior learning about community psychology (from minimal exposure through to extensive NGO-based work). After the first year of master's training, clinical psychologists complete an internship year (usually in a psychiatric hospital); but of particular relevance to this topic, this is then followed by a compulsory final 'community service' year, where the trainee is employed as a psychologist by the Department of Health in settings such as correctional services, local hospitals, community mental health services, HIV- and TB-intervention and prevention facilities. It is thus important that they have had training in CCP, to equip them for work in settings with the majority of people who were previously disadvantaged by discriminatory structures and systems, and where many may still experience unequal access to resources, exposure to violence and crime (both linked to widespread unemployment and poverty; Lazarus et al., 2015) and the devastating consequences of the HIV pandemic.

Project Descriptions

UKZN Masters Trainees' Community Interventions Projects in 2017

At one UKZN campus, thirty-two masters-level trainees from four of the professional training categories (clinical, counselling, educational and research psychology) worked across their registration categories in project teams. Thus, trainees in different specialisms were in the same project team. There were seven clinical masters trainees in this cohort. It is their reflective reports that provided data for this chapter.

In their respective projects, trainees worked with:

- An organisation that supports LGBTI communities: the trainees assisted with research directed at ascertaining the value of a programme run by the organisation.
- An organisation that provides support to educators from rural and township schools: one group developed and ran a two-day strengths-based educator development workshop during the July school holidays; the other group worked with two pilot schools to determine the usefulness of a tool designed for early identification of learning difficulties in children.
- A community-based organisation that provides care for people affected by HIV, through community-based workers. They assisted the organisation with a programme of care for the workers.
- A community initiative that promotes science development in schools and communities, where trainees conducted community-based research.
- An association that assists the elderly, with trainees exploring how the preferred model of care was being implemented.

The trainees worked in these project teams for the academic year. Sessions for reporting on progress and reflecting on experiences in the light of theory were scheduled regularly over the course of the year.

Rhodes University (RU) Trainees' Community Intervention Projects in 2017

The annual cohort comprises twelve trainee masters-level clinical and counselling psychologists. They pair up by category, enabling them to work on six projects in the year (from June to the end of October). The six trainee clinical psychologists' accounts of their work in three settings, in pairs, are the focus for this chapter. During 2017, they worked in the following community placements:

- A day centre for people discharged from the local psychiatric hospital, where participants engage in craft-work and psychosocial skills development, where the trainees provided group therapeutic support;

- A school for learners who had been excluded from mainstream schools due to their intellectual and socio-emotional needs, where the trainees provided group psycho-education;
- A peer counselling programme provided at a local youth centre, where the trainees facilitated regular peer support groups for the volunteer counsellors.

The group of six clinical trainees met weekly over the course of their projects for structured peer group supervision (Akhurst & Kelly, 2006), which provided a critical reflection space to review their work. In addition, the pairs sought additional supervision with Jacqui at points of decision-making. The data were collected from an end of year focus group with the six trainees, as well as their inputs into a day-long reflective colloquium held in conjunction with another regional university's trainees.

Methodology

We have drawn from two groups of trainees' experiences in two different university settings on the eastern seaboard of South Africa (one in KwaZulu-Natal, KZN, and the other in the Eastern Cape, EC, over 750 km apart). The language of instruction in both is English, although trainees come from backgrounds representing a number of the eleven official languages of SA, with many studying and working in English as an additional language. Following ethical clearance and informed consent processes, we collected data from three sources: at UKZN, seven written individual critically reflective reports were accessed; the RU data were from the transcriptions of focus group discussions and the presentations of six clinical trainees in a colloquium. All data were analysed using thematic analysis (Braun & Clarke, 2006). We did not draw from the final written project reports, however: since the UKZN submissions were from the cross-specialisation groups, we could not determine which reflections were the clinical trainees' perspectives, and the RU reflective reports were not all available at the time of writing.

Participants

UKZN: 6 females, 1 male; ages 23–52
RU: 4 females, 2 males; ages 22–32

Since many of the trainees do not originate from the local areas around these two campuses, none of them had worked previously in the specific community settings described above, so had not established prior relationships with these community partners.

Reflexive Note

As authors, we need to acknowledge our own variety of positionings in this endeavour: as academics, practitioners, researchers and activists. All of these positions influenced our roles in facilitating the students' experiences and assisting them to reflect on their learning. In our discourse, we promote the ways of being and doing that we wish to see in our students. Our passion is likely to indicate to students how to say the 'right' things. Thus, the trainees' accounts and our choices of excerpts need to be read with this in mind. In addition, in SA it is impossible to engage in this kind of work without considering issues of race and gender. As white women we are positioned in particular ways by the trainees we work with, by the communities they engage with and by ourselves in the academy. Having each worked in CCP for well over a decade, we are very aware of our positions as white female academics in the current South African context of interrogating white privilege (Urson & Kessi, 2018). Our trainees represent a very diverse group across racial, ethnic and language categories, and thus, it is an important opportunity to explore and problematise these factors.

At this point we would also like to acknowledge the lack of communities' voices in this chapter. Most community partners were not engaged in formal feedback about the trainees, but throughout the programme there were occasions where UKZN partners would provide feedback or request clarity regarding the activities of the trainees. Generally, these queries involved miscommunication or confusion regarding the role of the trainees. For example, one organisation wanted the trainees to provide individual de-briefing to approximately eighty-five field workers, which was beyond the brief to trainees. In another instance, an organisation's lack of communication with trainees indicated resistance to the process (despite having requested assistance earlier).

Where feedback was possible, the RU partners constructed their roles as contextual mediators, noting the collaborative decision-making and their resultant sense of agency. They valued regular communication and trainees' flexibility in adjusting plans when needed and their sense of being co-determinant, influencing the evolving processes and resultant interventions. Those interviewed appreciated trainees' preparedness, passion and energy. The gains for their organisations included being able to rely on trainees due to the bonds established, strengthening their work; they appreciated networking and referrals to appropriate agencies as well as learning together, where they assisted trainees with culturally sensitivities and in turn they gained insight into psychological work. The project difficulties that partners reported related to the shifting needs of the context as the processes unfolded, with some sense of dependency on the trainees' input since there were no other resources, and regret that they could only work together for six months. At UKZN, after completion of the projects and following the trainees' feedback, some community partners specifically requested more input from trainees in the future.

Findings

In the analysis below, *anon org* represents the times when trainees used the name of the organisation with whom they partnered. The trainees' identities are also anonymised, and their words are shown in italics, with participant code after the quotations. P1–P7 are used for the UKZN group and P8–P13 for the trainees from RU. The findings are separated into two broader themes; *viz.* the benefits to the trainees and the challenges they encountered.

Benefits to Trainees

The themes to emerge from the data include learning about and applying community psychology; learning from and supporting each other and a greater awareness of their positioning and the system, with its inequalities.

Learning About and Applying Community Psychology

Some trainees reflected upon their lack of knowledge at the beginning of the projects and the ways that their learning progressed through engagement. Examples are:

- *community psychology was a concept that I did not fully grasp. I did not have clear idea of what might be expected of me as a student psychologist, and of what I can contribute … However, the interaction with* *anon org* *and their staff members, the service that we provided and everything that I learned in the process changed my perspective* (P7)
- *Initially … I'm not known and how are they going to receive me as a psychology student … So it was very important I think … for us to create rapport and … collaborate … so it shifted from just being unknown people to becoming part of the community* (P10)

- *starting with community psychology I felt very unsure, as if I didn't know anything...there's this initial sense of anxiety and not knowing and being unsure, going into the unknown* (P8)

A number of trainees echoed the above comments on being unsure or anxious early on, but once they had initially engaged they realised that their 'people skills' could be usefully applied and that taking a non-expert position was helpful:

- *we formed connections with people, real authentic meaningful connections... bringing our own personhood to the work* (P8);
- *the community that we went into was sort of receptive of us, so that helped. I was less anxious going there rather than if they were not accommodating ... so if I think if the community wants people to come from the outside, ... it helped with whatever anxieties ... and the fears I might have had* (P12);
- *trying to understand their community from a point of not being an expert, so ... I wasn't under too much pressure to sort of change things, or to come up with solutions* (P11).

The participants saw the value of doing an initial collaborative needs and assets evaluation, in a way that enhanced participation:

- *we can only work out what people need when one builds the relationship* (P13);
- *we focused more on strengths and what was positive* (P9);
- *the importance of understanding what the community you are working with needs. It is not about going into a community ... and providing them with resources and delegating... Rather, it is about collaboratively working together, using each other's resources and skills, to enhance their community in the way they think will benefit ... the most* (P5).

A number reported needing to be flexible and responsive to what evolves organically in the work. This was contrasted with previously only reading about the work; when actively engaging they mentioned the resources they had used or required. For example:

- *helped me realise the realities of community work as opposed to what is cited on paper. ...Community psychology is an avenue ... which not only needs time but also dedication, passion, understanding, resourcefulness, resilience, communication and general motivation to not give up* (P4);

- *it's different to therapeutic work, it can be administrative … organizational management, like managing people and meeting times and paper work* (P13);
- *we used the CBT model of substance abuse as a basis for psychoeducation, role plays, making resources available, giving psychology away … pictures … cards* (P10);
- *the use of breathing exercises, mindfulness techniques, playing with clay, group members interviewing each other* (P8).

The following comment summarises not only what trainees offered, but also what they gained:

> *to do community psychology is a complex process that requires access to different resources, which sometimes might be a difficult process. It is also … a fulfilling process whereby one is able to provide a service that benefits some number of individuals (a community) while learning about that community in the process.* (P7)

Certain trainees noted the value of the experiential learning that CBSL had provided, expressing opinions about what could and could not be planned beforehand:

- *we actually had to experience the feeling of being uncertain, the anxiety that comes with that… we actually had to sit with this uncertainty … 'cause it doesn't always turn out the way you hope, or that we expect that things would turn out. … I think with every community project that's going to be different … you can't really pre-plan the skills I'm going to need for this community project, because depending on the community, depending on the needs of the community* (P11);
- *so you're going into community and we experience it then first hand, but until we engage with community work and actually do it, … then, only then I think, I feel that we can really learn* (P10);
- *feeling like this uncomfortability actually opens me up to experience a bit more… and to new things, that I wouldn't have, I think experienced* (P8).

This last comment highlights the sense that the work is imbued with uncertainties, but if the trainees can find ways to cope with those (through the various strategies that they note), there is the potential for creativity with their partners (both other trainees and community participants), as noted in the next theme.

Learning from and Supporting Each Other

The UKZN trainees were working on their projects in a group, whereas the RU students worked as pairs. Two UKZN students reported as follows:

- *During this process and involvement with* *anon org* *I have learned how to work well within a group, to respect other people and see value in other group members' contributions. I learned that one needs to be considerate of others' opinions, time, and sensitivity to group members' circumstances. Furthermore, I have learned empathy and understanding* (P7);
- *not all members may have been getting along but the group should have been able to work collaboratively in order to achieve set outcomes* (P1).

These divergent views illustrate the tensions between members experienced by one group, as contrasted with a group where the dynamics appeared to work more effectively. Ways of dealing with difficult group dynamics are addressed further in the discussion.

The pair-work at RU enabled trainees to experience support from each other, for example:

- *to know that there was someone that was there going into the community with me, 'cause I think I might have been more anxious if I worked there alone; and maybe sometimes if I got stuck at something, then there's someone who picked that up and then continued* (P10);
- *at least having your partner to share the frustration with, definitely helped* (P11).

The RU students also met in a more structured mode of peer group supervision (as described in Akhurst & Kelly, 2006), with one member of each pair presenting a challenge each week. The trainees all appeared to appreciate this forum, as noted in:

- *when I had feelings come up … to have others' comments … so they're giving their, in a sense, objective impression and by hearing those views at least helped me to provide more clarity in areas that I'm more concerned about or anxious about* (P12);
- *We've had to experience, support one another … having people who are also sharing similar experiences as you are, sort of validated the difficulties* (P11);
- *Every single one of you thought about what I struggled with … supportive … and not being observed* (P8);

- *Community psychology has disquiet with the role of the expert, so* (peer) *supervision is more like the practice … equal power distribution and group generation of ideas* (P13).

In comparison to their therapy supervision, one noted a freedom from being 'observed' and they concurred that the group process enabled a greater sense of *independence* (P11) and *autonomy* (P8), was *empowering* (P11), provided *different minds, different expertise* and being more *relaxed* (P9).

This theme has highlighted the value gained by most trainees in relation to working with their peers and in groups. The following theme reflects their reports of learning about social systems.

Greater Awareness of Their Positioning and the System with Its Inequalities

The next excerpt summarises trainees' developing consciousness of their roles and power (and its limits), in relation to the societal systems they encounter. This highlights the sensitivities required and the need for enhanced awareness of their own and their partners' needs and positions:

- *while community psychology interventions can offer important opportunities for community members to empower themselves, it is also a delicate balance… is very important for the community psychologist to be mindful of: the context …; identifying the community's needs vs. their own needs; …the potential to abuse their power derived from frequently having greater education, wealth and/or privilege; … the importance of not imposing or intruding on a community without their consenting to the proposed intervention; …the risk of patronizing community members* (P3).

The structural and systemic challenges faced by people became clear to a number:

- *… even though we live in a democratic society … other communities within the country still face prejudice, discrimination, a lack of adequate resources to address the needs* (P7);
- *The environment around the school is not conducive for learners and gives a message to them about being placed on the margins* (P10);
- *I realised the need of psychological services especially in the under-resourced areas and I wish to be involved with clusters such as* *anon org* *to help empower our communities and expand access to psychological services* (P4);

- *The most striking thing I learnt, is the amount of struggle and hatred this community actually goes through, which has not turned them into bitter people, but rather has made them more accepting, open and loving to everyone* (P5).

The trainees thus had first-hand experiences of people's struggles and the final comment shows the value of trainees' exposure to groups of people they may not previously have encountered. The following reflection illustrates trainees' compassion for and appreciation of the people whom they encountered:

- *I was very humbled by the load, the women in the community we worked with, carry. One woman created a vivid image of the demands she deals with, describing herself carrying her daughter's infant on her back, helping another person with homework, preparing supper, and trying to meet targets at work and the emotional needs of the population she works with* (P3).

Some of the trainees mentioned their frustrations with the limitations of their capacities to influence the system, for example:

- *Even us as trainee psychologists, there are very limited things that we could do … especially getting to be advocate and things like that* (P8);
- *whilst we worked from a mental health model, coming from a preventative approach, we would have liked to take a social action model approach that would lead us to mobilizing and activism with the department of education to make a broader impact … but with only two of us, we're not sure what our contributions could assist in making a difference* (P12).

The above threads are drawn together in the following summative comment from one, where she highlights the need to draw from the voices of the service users:

> *What I learnt about community psychology is about hearing the voices of the people on the grass-root level. There is presence of power dynamics in all communities and it is imperative that the voices that are heard are those of the people being serviced. In our community project intervention, what was communicated to us by* *anon org* *management was not necessarily the need of the* *anon org* *facilitators. I further saw the value of immersing oneself with the community and their culture as it aids in implementing a successful intervention. Furthermore … as a community psychologist it is important to respect the community's diversity in culture and knowledge.* (P2)

The above excerpt emphasises the nature of some of the challenges encountered, explored further below.

Challenges Encountered

Even when the first negotiations made clear the trainees' roles, the limits of what they could offer along with people's hopes, needs and perceptions of how psychology 'works', led to other expectations. This work is unpredictable and time-consuming, without clear boundaries or rules; this can lead to trainees experiencing various discomforting feelings and having to cope with unexpected challenges, for example:

- *We had an initial meeting with the* *anon org* *management which … was very intimidating. The meeting was structured in an interview manner which left us feeling belittled as we had hoped it would be a collaborative journey* (P2).

One RU pair described how although local partners were keen for them to begin an intervention in the local centre, the regional organisational gatekeepers placed numerous barriers in the way, meaning that their proposed project could not begin and they then needed to change to a totally new project. This led to them needing to cope with unexpected feelings and re-assessment of their positioning:

- **anon org* was not that receptive … based on our training and the individual work, we get into this somewhat privileged position of being needed, of being this person who's got all of the skills, so we're kinda used to being needed* (P13);
- *hoping to be accepted by the community … we actually had to sit with this uncertainty … it felt like … something that you're doing, … 'cause it doesn't always turn out the way you hope, or that we expect that things would turn out* (P11).

Without prompting about CCP evaluative models, some of the RU trainees commented on how difficult it was to evaluate the impact of their work. One said:

- *it's like working on the grey areas all the time … you think that you're not making a transformative impact, but maybe over time it does* (P9).

There are also risks of community partners' over-dependence and of trainees' over-investment, as noted by one pair:

- *We build this relationship now and then we just left. And I know it is important to ... give things over to them, it is also part of transformation to not take everything on ourselves, but it is difficult. I'm left with a feeling of what did we do? What's going to happen now?* (P8).

In the SA context of enduring structural and race-based inequalities, establishing more equal partnerships was challenging, inhibiting sustainability and community 'ownership' of initiatives.

The trainees raised concerns about the implementation of the mental health model that supports amelioration rather than transformation, for example:

- *sometimes the kind of context of community project is in and our own capabilities meant, means that we had to almost work in a particular kind of mental health model ... and not being able to work in other kinds of models. Because of our own teaching and what we could do, or meant that we have to ... take on an aspect of psycho-educating, of being an expert at times* (P12);
- *not to be so black and white in my thinking ... about what community psychology is and what a mental health model is and ... what transformation is, and to see it more on like a spectrum* (P9).

This indicates their sense of not feeling able to break free of the predominant model.

Programmatically, one group member commented that community psychology became marginalised in comparison to other modules:

> *in the beginning I felt I was very dedicated and eager to work hard on this and ensure that my contributions were valuable and up to standard. However, as my workload increased from other modules, I found that I became more lenient on myself when it came to putting in effort ... on* *anon org* *community project.* (P5)

A further potential risk was that peers tended too much towards being supportive, perhaps not being challenging enough:

- *Operating in a group with peers, if they may not be ... almost attempting to ... engage in a bit of ... group think, ... but might affect trying to look at something ... critically* (P12).

These excerpts describe the many learnings of trainees through their participation in the CBSL community psychology modules, illustrating benefits and challenges. It is noteworthy that issues of social justice and challenging the status quo were not foregrounded in their reflections, with little mention of advocating for systemic and structural change. Thus, while it is interesting to reflect on what students reported, it is possibly more useful to interrogate what was not stated, particularly in the light of our intentions to educate students who are critical community psychologists.

Discussion

The findings about benefits to trainees highlight the value of this form of experiential learning, as noted by Nguyen (2016). These include the fundamental of building 'relationships' and the 'rigour' needed to work in CBSL. The trainees valued the 'reflective' spaces provided to assist in processing the material and they comment on the 'real life' experiences that CBSL provided. However, Nguyen's item 'reciprocity' was more difficult for them to achieve. In relation to the links between these and the features of CCP identified by Kagan et al. (2011), it would appear as if there are resonances with developing 'community' with each other and their community partners through relationships and reflectivity and with certain features of 'stewardship' (through rigour and real life developments); however, it is much more challenging to be able to aspire to creating spaces for promoting greater social justice (in reciprocity and equal partnerships), due to inequities in power and the relatively low status of clinical psychology trainees in the systems.

The processes implicitly appear to follow some aspects of Mezirow's (2000) model of transformation. The trainees reported initial anxieties about their roles, the expectations of them and their concerns about making adequate contributions, which all seem to resonate with the idea of a 'disorienting dilemma'. They then explain some of their coping strategies, including forming relationships and the relief at feeling welcomed by community partners, as well as the need to work collaboratively with their peers and partners, establishing needs and assets to make realistic contributions. They note ways of utilising both their personal attributes and applying their skills and knowledge, drawn from other aspects of their training. Mezirow's (2000) model is thus supported to some extent by the findings, except that their journeys do not seem to proceed in the linear way proposed by the ten items as listed. So, whilst the model appears to have value, the trainees' experiences, awareness and learning might be more multilinear (Strain, 2007), dipping in and out of some of the elements and progressing at different rates, depending on the complexities of the different partnerships and settings.

More than fifteen years ago, Pillay (2003) questioned: whether clinical psychology trainees had the necessary training and skills to engage in communities; whether their training prepared them to practice in communities; and what training and skills would be needed to make them confident in the practice of community psychology. It is clear from the findings above that the trainees believe that their experiential learning equipped them in different ways compared to their individually focused work, but the shift towards more actively promoting social justice and taking a social liberation approach remains challenging in our context. Some possible reasons for this are explored below.

Time, Timing and Partnership-Building

Whilst CCP would appear to enhance CBSL, with there being coherence of focus on participation, positionality and power, taking such an approach led to trainees feeling frustrated that their work had been only at micro- and meso-levels (Bronfenbrenner, 1994), with limits on the potentials to shift from a small group focus to advocacy or broader activism in the system. Nguyen's (2016) reminder to work with rigour in relationships rooted in the real world seems to have been reflected, emphasising the basis of the work on relationships that can be sustained over time. However, the modular designs of South African university programmes only allow for time-limited interventions, undermining the potentials and the trainees' capacities to work towards greater equality with community partners. Thus, finding other ways of 'bridging' the time gaps between trainees' engagements becomes important, and careful ongoing communication with partners is important for 'two-way' sharing, to guard against unmet expectations or potential exploitation.

With regard to partnerships, the trainees also learned the difficulties of group work within their teams. This is an important aspect of the experience, since the real world demands the professional to interact and collaborate with peers. The trainees were provided with a theoretical frame for their experiences (the 'forming, norming storming, performing and adjourning' model of Tuckman & Jensen, 1977) and could call on their supervisor to resolve conflict within the group. At UKZN the groups of trainees were formed across training categories and at least some of the conflict revolved around the higher status of clinical psychology (discussed further below).

Underdeveloped Critical Reflection Skills

Most trainees also find it difficult to employ critical reflection skills. The cultivation of these skills, through dialogic encounters (Gilbert & Sliep, 2009), requires far greater, resource-intensive investment from faculty, earlier in the trainees' tertiary education. However, this is not possible in our current higher education context where we are under pressure to 'massify' (Subotzky, 1999). The result is that in SA we continue to produce psychologists who want to go into private practice, where the realities of our situation and context remain somewhat at a distance.

Hegemony of Traditional Models

The trainee reflections show that mental health models of community psychology are still the default mode for interventions. One possible reason for this is the time-limited nature of the trainee involvements, which makes it very difficult to effect any kind of systemic or sustainable change. Systems take years to develop and years to shift (Kidd et al., 2018; Rodgers et al., 2017). In a context of limited resources (like many SA communities), challenging the status quo might also result in negative consequences for the challenger, like the removal altogether of what little resources were available. In our interventions we therefore strive to work with systems, and not against them; even when we try to diplomatically suggest how things could be better.

From the university systems' perspective, there is no doubt that CBSL activities are more staff- and resource-intensive than traditional training modes; CBSL therefore requires institutional commitment that is more than 'lip-service'. From within the discipline of psychology, the old wineskin is thus the most popular. This is evidenced by the number of applications we have for our clinical psychology programmes, where there are five to ten times the number of applicants compared to other 'streams'. Clinical psychology in its more traditional forms is thus still dominant: with individual and pathology-focussed interventions having the most credibility and psychological assessments and therapy thus being reified over other kinds of interventions.

Community psychology approaches challenge these ways of working, and this does not sit comfortably with many of our colleagues or some trainees. As noted in Fig. 18.1, the mental health approach serves to (unintentionally) reinforce these traditional systems of power. Shifting further towards social action and social-liberation models constructs even more of a challenge, becoming risky. CBSL thus risks being marginalised and not assigned status or resources. In this context, asking questions about power, positioning, benefit and the status quo is troublesome; it is generally not rewarded by the structures whose interests are served by things remaining the same.

Concluding Thoughts

These meta-reflections on our work leave us with many questions: So what do we do? How might things be otherwise?

Given the complementarity of the core values of the CBSL and CCP approaches (as noted in the literature review), it is perhaps useful to use them as mirrors to elucidate the shortcomings in each field. For example, from what we know of both approaches, using categorical thinking (e.g. charity versus social justice) is not helpful and it is better to think of continuums, for example, between amelioration and transformation in CCP, just as there is a continuum between social justice and charity in CBSL. This kind of thinking allows us to recognise that we and our trainees can occupy different positions in the process of community psychology. Sometimes an ameliorative approach is necessary to build relationships so that we and our community partners can move into more transformative work at later stages. It is clear that this work is enhanced by investing in developing genuine relationships with community partners that are long term and sustainable, such that power differentials are minimised. As psychologists, one of core skills is the development of relationships with our 'clients'. We should use such skills to enhance and challenge our current practices in communities.

Related to this is the importance of recognising the bi-directional nature of the community-university relationship. We influence each other. Many western texts emphasise the centrality of moving this relationship from one of communities being dependent on community psychologists towards independence. From an African perspective, we would argue that the aim is for an interdependent relationship (Arumugam, 2001)—where we discover that we need each other. Acknowledging that higher education institutions are dependent on the communities in which they operate (to challenge traditional academic ways of thinking, doing and being; to keep curricula relevant to context; to challenge dominant discourses) could result in a kind of humility and a realisation that we do not hold the monopoly on knowledge construction. Ideally this would assist in challenging hegemonic notions of how clinical psychology should be practised.

CBSL emphasises the centrality of critical reflection to enable students to learn from their experiences. We would benefit from programmes that encourage the development of critical thinking skills in trainees earlier, so that these skills are not absent at the postgraduate (fifth year of study) level. How can we produce trainees who are able to think and question, when our current system is focused on increasing the units of production for government subsidy purposes? How can we argue for courses that challenge trainees to confront their own assumptions, values and biases and how these impact on their work? We therefore make the following recommendations for consideration by programme designers.

Recommendations for Developing CBSL in Practice

In SA, CBSL integrated into clinical psychologists' training has real traction in that the trainees will all do an additional 'community service' year (Ahmed & Pillay, 2004), employed by the Department of Health, following their internships. In addition, should the structural and systemic barriers be removed (which currently inhibit clinical psychologists' work in primary settings), CBSL has great potential to enable more preventative and transformative work closer to the provision of services 'in communities', thus reaching well beyond the current ambit of clinical psychology services. Whilst we cannot comment on the situation in developed countries such as the UK, it would seem from our standpoints that the contraction of formal service provision as a result of austerity measures could lead to a re-conceptualising of the work of clinical psychologists closer to communities.

Where CBSL is integrated into clinical psychology training programmes, we recommend that consistency be built into relationships with community partners through various means that straddle the briefer work that trainees can do in their time-limited placements. Carol and Jacqui have acted in this capacity as links to our partners; however, such work is not necessarily included in their academic workloads.

There needs to be investment from training settings in persons who can sustain these partnerships over periods of time. Such ideas could promote sustainability and shift the sense of agency of community partners: so that the work becomes more participatory, valuing their inputs and providing greater potential for more equal knowledge exchange. These kinds of partnerships could also generate opportunities for applied research. Finally, there needs to be 'buy in' from other staff members on a training programme, in order that messages are not conveyed that CBSL is somehow marginalised and of lesser importance.

Clinical psychology programmes can have an influence on honours-degree-level preparation of candidates for professional psychology. Given our experiences of those trainees who had not been exposed to CCP before their community psychology modules having to make up a great deal of ground philosophically, theoretically and practically, we would strongly recommend that trainees are encouraged to have earlier exposure to community psychology, whether through an honours degree elective or other means. The capacity to critically reflect should also become a key outcome of programmes earlier in the clinical psychology training.

Trainees need to be taught to manage the complexity of CCP in practice. Personal skills and relationships are crucial, capacities to 'sit with uncertainties', flexibility as well as administrative, logistical and organisational capabilities are all important (for any 'competences' debate). These should not be seen as separate from other clinical psychology work. Supervisory arrangements and opportunities for ongoing reflection must be built into the CBSL from the start. Since we prefer a model where trainees work in pairs or groups, the means of dealing with any conflicts/disagreements need to be provided, through supervision arrangements or mentoring.

We hope that these examples of our work and our resultant dilemmas have stimulated readers to consider how things could be otherwise in their own practices. We would welcome comments and ideas of how we can develop the 'new wineskins' we need, to advance our work in our communities, including innovative practice ideas or radical case studies. In classic Foucauldian tradition, we are left with more questions than answers.

References

Ahmed, R., & Pillay, A. L. (2004). Reviewing clinical psychology training in the post-apartheid period: Have we made any progress? *South African Journal of Psychology, 34*, 630–656.

Akhurst, J. (2017). Student experiences of community-based service learning during Masters' level training, as related to critical community psychology practice. *Journal of New Generation Sciences, 15*(1), 1–20.

Akhurst, J., Solomon, V., Mitchell, C., & van der Riet, M. (2016). Embedding community-based learning into psychology degrees at UKZN, South Africa. *Educational Research for Social Change, 5*(2), 136–150.

Akhurst, J. E., & Kelly, K. (2006). Peer group supervision as an adjunct to individual supervision: Optimising learning processes during psychologists' training. *Psychology Teaching Review, 12*(1), 3–15.

Arumugam, S. (2001). *A Discussion of the Ecological Indigenous, Organisational, Mental Health, Social Action and Liberatory Models of Community Psychology.* Unpublished manuscript, University of Zululand, KwaDlangezwa.

Braun, V., & Clarke, V. (2006). Using thematic analysis in psychology. *Qualitative Research in Psychology, 3*(2), 77–101.

British Psychological Society Community Psychology Section Committee. (2011). *Working definition of Community Psychology*. Unpublished minutes.

Bronfenbrenner, U. (1994). Ecological models of human development. *International Encyclopaedia of Education, 3*, 37–43.

Carolissen, R. (2006). Teaching community psychology into obscurity: A reflection on community psychology in South Africa. *Journal of Psychology in Africa, 16*, 177–182.

Cromby, J., Harper, D., & Reavey, P. (Eds.). (2013). *Mental health and distress*. Palgrave Macmillan.

Deeley, S. (2015). *Critical perspectives on service learning in Higher Education*. Palgrave Macmillan.

Eyler, J., & Giles, D. E., Jr. (1999). *Where's the learning in service-learning?* Jossey-Bass.

Foucault, M. (1983). The subject and power. In H. L. Dreyfus & P. Rabinow (eds.), *Beyond structuralism and hermeneutics* (2nd ed.) (Afterword). University of Chicago Press.

Freire, P. (1970). *Pedagogy of the oppressed*. Penguin.

Fryer, D., & Laing, A. (2008). Community psychologies: What are they? What could they be? Why does it matter? A critical community psychology approach. *The Australian Community Psychologist, 20*(2), 7–15.

Gilbert, A., & Sliep, Y. (2009). Reflexivity in the practice of social action: From self- to inter- relational reflexivity. *South African Journal of Psychology, 39*(4), 468–479.

Hart, A., & Akhurst, J. (2017). Community-based learning and critical community psychology practice: Conducive and corrosive aspects. *Journal of Community and Applied Social Psychology, 27*, 3–15.

Kagan, C. (2015). Community psychological perspectives and counselling psychology. *Counselling Psychology Review, 30*(3), 12–21.

Kagan, C., Burton, M., Duckett, P., Lawthom, R., & Siddiquee, A. (2011). *Critical community psychology*. BPS Blackwell.

Kidd, S., Davidson, L., Frederick, T., & Kral, M. J. (2018). Reflecting on participatory, action-oriented research methods in community psychology: Progress, problems, and paths forward. *American Journal of Community Psychology, 61*, 76–87.

Lazarus, S., Bulbulia, S., Taliep, N., & Naidoo, A. (2015). Community–based participatory research as a critical enactment of community psychology. *Journal of Community Psychology, 48*(1), 87–98.

Mezirow, J. (2000). Learning to think like an adult: Core Concepts of Transformation Theory. In J. Mezirow & Associates (Eds.), *Learning as transformation. Critical perspectives on a theory in progress* (pp. 3–33). Jossey-Bass.

Mitchell, C., & Humphries, H. (2007). From notions of charity to social justice in service-learning: The complex experience of communities. *Education as Change, 11*(3), 47–58.

Mitchell, T. (2008). Traditional vs. critical service-learning: Engaging the literature to differentiate two models. *Michigan Journal of Community Service Learning, 14*(2), 50–65.

Naidoo, A., Duncan, N., Roos, V., Pillay, J., & Bowman, B. (2007). Analysis, context and action: An introduction to community psychology. In N. Duncan, B. Bowman, A. Naidoo, J. Pillay, & V. Roos (Eds.), *Community psychology: Analysis, context and action* (pp. 9–23). UCT Press.

Nelson, G., & Prilleltensky, I. (2010). *Community psychology: In pursuit of wellness and liberation* (2nd ed.). Palgrave Macmillan.

Nguyen, C-H. (2016). Partners for success. *Journal for Service-Learning, Leadership, and Social Change, 5*(2), Art 3.

Pillay, J. (2003). Community psychology is all theory and no practice': Training educational psychologists in community practice within the South African context. *South African Journal of Psychology, 33*(4), 261–268.

Rhoads, R. A. (1997). *Community service and higher learning: Explorations of the caring self.* State University of New York Press.

Rodgers, M. A., Grisso, J. A., Crits-Christoph, P., & Rhodes, K. V. (2017). No quick fixes: A mixed methods feasibility study of an urban community health worker outreach program for intimate partner violence. *Violence Against Women, 23*(3), 1–22. https://doi.org/10.1177/1077801216640383

Seedat, M. (2014). Mobilising compassionate critical citizenship and psychologies in the service of humanity. In S. Cooper & K. Ratele (Eds.), *Psychology Serving Humanity: Proceedings of the 30th International Congress of Psychology: Volume 1: Majority World Psychology* (pp. 1–17). Psychology Press.

Strain, C. R. (2007). Moving Like a Starfish: Beyond a Unilinear Model of Student Transformation in Service Learning Classes. *Journal of College and Character, 8*(1), 1–12. https://doi.org/10.2202/1940-1639.1150

Subotzky, G. (1999). Alternatives to the entrepreneurial university: New modes of knowledge production in community service programs. *Higher Education, 38*(4), 401–440.

Tuckman, B. W., & Jensen, M. C. (1977). Stages of small-group development revisited. *Group & Organization Studies, 2*(4), 419–427.

Urson, R., & Kessi, S. (2018). Whiteness and non-racialism: White students' discourses of transformation at UCT. *Psychology in Society, 56*, 46–69.

Yen, J. (2007). A history of 'community' and community psychology in South Africa. In N. Duncan, B. Bowman, A. Naidoo, J. Pillay, & V. Roos (Eds.), *Community psychology: Analysis, context and action* (pp. 51–66). UCT Press.

19

Health Inequities of Silent Roma Ranks from a Social Justice Perspective

Daniela E. Miranda, Marta Escobar-Ballesta, Emilio Vizarraga Trigueros, María Jesús Albar Marín, and Manuel García-Ramírez

Overcoming Health Inequities of Roma Silent Ranks from a Social Justice Perspective

> Against us, the worst and cruelest form of discrimination occurs, and I would categorize this as indifference. Roma are warmly applauded when artists emerge and are capable of filling a stage with their art and interpretive capacity. But there is indifference to the starvation that occurs in the suburbs of our cities, there is indifference to the 400,000 Roma who do not have vital elements to survive. (Heredia-Ramírez, 1978)

This quote, from a speech made by Juan de Dios Ramirez-Heredia—the first Spanish Roma congressman—shed light on the social injustices faced by this population. These words continue to deeply resonate within Roma

The study presented in this chapter was funded by the International Organization for Migrations' EQUI-HEALTH project. It is part of the first author's PhD dissertation. We would like to thank our colleagues at FAKALI, and a special thank you to our community partners and Roma neighbors in Polígono Sur.

D. E. Miranda (✉) • M. Escobar-Ballesta • M. J. Albar Marín • M. García-Ramírez
Social Psychology, CESPYD, Coalition for the Study of Health, Power and Diversity, Universidad de Sevilla, Sevilla, Spain
e-mail: danimiranda@us.es; mja@us.es; magarcia@us.es

E. Vizarraga Trigueros
Studio 41013, Sevilla, Spain

C. Walker et al. (eds.), *The Palgrave Handbook of Innovative Community and Clinical Psychologies*, https://doi.org/10.1007/978-3-030-71190-0_19

communities and to be emblematic of their realities. Roma are still subjected to stigma and negative public perception attached to their heritage and ethnic group.

Immersed in a permanent struggle against abandonment and persecution, Roma people have managed to survive and persevere by hiding the signs of their identity ingrained in symbols and traditions, rites and social norms, showing a unique talent for embedding their Roma identity into the dominant social norms and the communities where they have settled for centuries (Sasao & Sue, 1993). While this struggle has allowed them to survive over centuries, it has excluded them from benefiting from political, economic, and social resources. Consequently, the health gap between them and the rest of the population is one of the worst outcomes of this struggle. Today, this gap is one of the most shameful pieces of evidence of the long journey that Europe must travel to become a fair, respectful, and dignified society (Boscoboinik & Giordano, 2008; Cahn & Guild, 2010; FRA, 2012; MATRIX, 2014).

The World Health Organization's policy framework Health 2020 commits European member states to address Roma' health inequalities and ensure participatory governance, especially for the most disadvantaged ranks (World Health Organization, 2013). More recently, the United Nations' 2030 Agenda revisits these commitments in order to ensure that shared political efforts address inclusiveness in economic, social, and political spheres for Roma (United Nations, 2015). As a result of the European Union expansion between 2004 and 2007, which included countries with high Roma populations (e.g., Bulgaria, Romania), governments and civil societies became interested in Roma rights, their multiples inequities, and the ways to integrate them into an enlarged and open Europe (Hajioff & McKee, 2000; Vincze, 2014). Despite Roma populations being included in policy agendas and non-binding, "soft policy" instruments aimed at addressing institutional discrimination, they have not had a significant impact in improving their engagement in economic, social, and political areas (Mirga-Kruszelnicka, 2017).

The Open Society Foundations, the World Bank Group, and the European Union Agency for Fundamental Rights (FRA) have marshaled the implementation of these efforts and have alerted their limited impact in responding to systematic concealment of Roma across Europe (FRA, 2017; Gatti, Karacsony, Anan, Ferre, & De Paz Nieves, 2016; Mirga-Kruszelnicka, 2017). These think-tanks have attributed failures to policy development for Roma without Roma and anti-gypsyism has direct effects on health outcomes. Experts argue that these are neoliberal policies intended to Europeanize and turn Roma into a labor force by depoliticizing the actual causes of marginalization, focusing on cultural differences and racializing poverty (Vincze, 2014). Hence, there is a need for a social justice approach that encourages the engagement of the most silent and hidden Roma communities in a process that incorporates participation and agency in addressing health inequities. This chapter adopts a social justice approach based on the principles and values of Liberation Psychology. This perspective gives a voice and power back to the most invisible ranks by (a) developing critical consciousness to understand and identify conditions of oppression, (b) developing empowering settings ensuring the capacity to act, and (c) identifying potential mechanisms that can be levers of change and collective action (García-Ramírez, de la Mata, Paloma, & Hernández-Plaza, 2011; Martín-Baró, 1994; Montero & Sonn, 2009; Watts & Serrano-García, 2003). In this chapter we present a pilot study which aims to unveil local health inequities and ensure Roma health governance through community capacity building for empowerment and accountability. First, we will describe how and why Roma in Spain have developed as a hidden community. Second, we will propose Roma Liberation Psychology as a useful framework to analyze and overcome unfair health conditions. Third, we will present an experience developed in a Roma community in Southern Spain. Finally, lessons learnt will be presented.

Hidden Roma in Spain

Roma have been the largest, poorest, and most persecuted ethnic minority group in Spain since their arrival in the country in the fifteenth century. In a Catholic state, they were persecuted for their traditions and were forced to assimilate (Ringold, Orenstein, & Wilkens, 2005). Following this era, they lived through a short period of political tolerance under King Charles III but returned to face persecution under the dictatorship of Francisco Franco between 1939 and 1975. The restoration of democracy finally brought the recognition of Roma as full citizens but not as a national minority—despite accounting for nearly a million of the 12 million Roma living in Europe (Real Academia Española, 2015; Ringold et al., 2005).

Nevertheless, in the last few years, the upsurge of anti-Roma discourses within political and mass media spheres keep perpetuating and justifying the cycle of segregation and persecution against them among Spanish and European societies (Council of Europe, 2012; Fundación Secretariado Gitano, 2013; Ignăţoiu-Sora, 2011; Kroon, Kluknavská, Vliegenthart, & Boomgaarden, 2016). As a result, Roma face several difficulties to access formal employment opportunities, forcing them into poverty and being dependent on welfare services (FRA, 2014; Fundación Secretariado Gitano, 2012;

Guy, Liebich, & Marushiakova, 2010). Discrimination continues at educational levels where many Roma face segregation and many more are condemned to abandonment (Brüggemann, 2012; Gay & Blasco, 2016). Similarly, they are forced to move into settlements on the outskirts of gentrified urban areas with no social services and inhumane living conditions (Bancroft, 2001; FRA, 2009). The healthcare system also discriminates against Roma through accessibility barriers, low responsiveness of services, racist attitudes of providers, or the lack of compliance with their rights to health (Aiello, Flecha, & Serradell, 2018; Escobar-Ballesta, García-Ramírez, & De Freitas, 2018; Janevic, Sripad, Bradley, & Dimitrievska, 2011; La Parra, Gil-González, & Jiménez, 2013).

From generation to generation, Roma have learned to invest in their cultural and social capital (i.e., music, dance, trade) in order to survive. The impossible effort of overcoming prejudices made them develop a positive and distinct identity, strong networks, and tight social support (Boscoboinik & Giordano, 2008; Kolarcik, Geckova, Reijneveld, & Van Dijk, 2015; Reysen, Slobodnikova, & Katzarska-Miller, 2016). In this sense, family—both immediate and extended—is not only a central protective factor against discrimination but also a facilitator of positive and healthy adjustment of their members. Family is therefore the strongest structure through which Roma find a "mobile community," the core of a symbolic nation with its own rules and laws that all Roma are impelled to follow in order to be recognized as part of their collectivity (Dimitrova, Chasiotis, Bender, & Van de Vijver, 2014).

The historical separation between Roma and non-Roma has bred mistrust and misconception between both groups. Nonetheless, the systemic and oppressive mechanisms used at institutional and societal levels against Roma have contributed to normalizing asymmetrical power relations as well as perpetuating marginalization. The coping strategies used by Roma have been misunderstood and used to characterize them often as a subhuman collective (Dalsklev & Kunst, 2015).

Liberation Psychology

Liberation psychology offers a praxis which helps frame and direct action toward the multiple mechanisms of oppression collaboratively with hidden Roma communities (Kyuchukov, 2011). Studies and reports highlight that racism and violence against Roma are systematic and structural; the services responsible for its prevention, detection, and punishment fail in these tasks by victim blaming, thus creating fear, low self-esteem, and defenselessness among at-risk Roma (Briones-Vozmediano, Parra, & Vives-Cases, 2018). A simple but significant example is that, in Spanish, the word *gitano* is often used synonymously as thief (Real Academia Española, 2015). Discriminatory mechanisms have legitimized and sustained a social ecology in which Roma without entitlement and access to community resources and public services. Hence, they experience much worse health than that of the rest of the population in the lowest socio-economic positions, and it continues to be so even if they upgrade their social status (La Parra, Gil-González, & de la Torre, 2016). This has led to fatalistic attitudes toward Roma communities by both non-Roma populations and themselves. Liberation psychology frames normalized conceptions of society in terms of oppressive social, economic, and political patterns that are responsible for unjust indicators while giving silenced Roma communities the tools to resist.

Liberation psychology allows to understand how Roma, like any other group, have the potential and capacities to resist through transforming day-to-day manifestations of oppression and resistance into opportunities to claim their rights. The process of reflection, sharing narratives, and examining the power dynamics embedded can be reversed by developing critical consciousness and building critical knowledge (Freire, 1970). This conscientization is the process of developing awareness of one's relation to the unjust conditions as a result of oppression. Liberation psychology offers the methodological tool of problematization—or new knowledge and way of understanding unjust social structures—that allows for oppressed communities to challenge accepted dominant narratives and norms. Individual and collective narratives and social structures need to be reconstructed and can be understood as an empowerment process that strengthens oppressed communities to challenge and change oppressive contexts and their position in the social order (Montero & Sonn, 2009).

Therefore, liberation psychology is not only a way to think, it is also a way to act. There is a pressing need to overcome this unfair situation by emphasizing advocacy actions led by a multi-level partnership (e.g., researchers, Roma organizations, and policymakers) to identify oppressive mechanisms and to make Roma's needs visible and valued and to ultimately bring about change (Escobar-Ballesta et al., 2018; Fésüs, Östlin, McKee, & Ádány, 2012). Roma leadership in this process needs to be ensured through community capacity building and development for the redistribution of power and resources (Carlisle, 2000; Wolff et al., 2016). To this end, community psychologists have the responsibility to accompany groups as co-researchers and adopt three fundamental roles: (1) to act as instigators who develop critical thinking in passive attitudes from both institutions and Roma communities; (2)

mediators who build bridges between civic society, organizations, and institutions; and (3) advocators who take action and represent hidden communities in the face of injustice (Balcazar, Garate-Serafini, & Keys, 2004). These roles ensure continuous checks and balances between researchers, Roma organizations, and policymakers to ensure real participation and liberation of Roma in developing policies and programs.

With these targets, liberation psychology focuses on critical reflection and community mobilization by building on community strengths and resilience (García Ramírez, Escobar-Ballesta, Lizana, & Albar, 2016). This praxis works at the personal, interpersonal, and political levels in order to bring about collective action. At the personal level, developing resources and skills while at the same time bringing individuals to work together and commit to collective action. Community-based participatory research (CBPAR) methods are a useful method for this goal because they focus and prioritize the local needs of underrepresented populations and develop participatory processes in order to influence and develop policies and programs that ensure equity (Balcazar et al., 2012). By supporting communities through CBPAR, we can facilitate multiple levels of empowerment to optimize existing resources and develop the ability to create new ones. Through a liberation psychology lens, CBPAR for advocacy is a way to develop personal and interpersonal capacities to transform discriminatory structures. This study focuses involving Roma neighbors and other key stakeholders in an impoverished local context to identify the mechanisms through which local Roma are hidden, as well as promoting their health and leadership in safe spaces.

Unveiling the Roma in Polígono Sur

This section presents CBPAR processes based on liberation psychology values that allow at-risk Spanish Roma locals to defend their health rights through active participation. To that end, a university-community alliance was built to implement an iterative process that included the following phases: (1) building alliances; (2) mapping Roma assets; (3) building advocacy capacity among Roma neighbors; and (4) empowering Roma settings. In this section we will describe the context of the study and the four phases from this pilot study and provide lessons learned (Fig. 19.1).

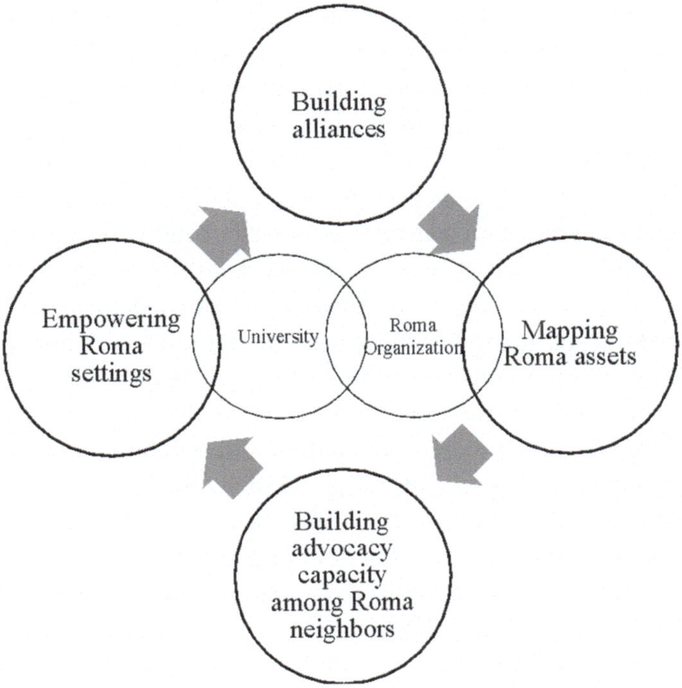

Fig. 19.1 Community mobilization process for local Roma health governance

The Context

Polígono Sur (PS) is representative of a marginalized community resulting from gentrification and forced displacement of disadvantaged populations in the 1960s in Seville, Spain (ABC, 1977). Nowadays, approximately 20,000 people live in PS of which an estimated 25% are of Roma descent. Geographically, PS is a district located on the outskirts of the city center, tucked away and enclosed by two highways and train tracks. Although PS is composed of six neighborhoods, the majority of Roma live in the most disenfranchised (Martínez Montañés). Despite being less than a kilometer in distance, reports show that in 2005, La Oliva—the neighborhood closest to the city center—had almost half the unemployment rate of Martínez Montañés and a significant difference in economic activity. Both neighborhoods present different tendencies in the use of social services and other community resources which have been attributed to the contrast in the populations living in each (Ayuntamiento de Sevilla, 2016).

These physical boundaries are further amplified by the political boundaries recognized by the City Council, defining PS as an area in need of social transformative change due to the alarming differences in health status, unemployment, and school absenteeism in comparison to the rest of Sevilla. In order to respond to these unjust social conditions, the district has its own local policy coordinating entity whose objective is to integrate efforts in improving conditions in PS under a local plan (Maeztu, 2006). The presence of this institution has allowed PS to be the subject of many social interventions, which has made for a strong social welfare network that serves the area. However, this network is blind to Roma health challenges. The PS Roma community attributes this to the absence of real participatory spaces in local policy-making and interventions, which are dominated by non-Roma professionals working in public institutions and local organizations.

PS has often been at the center of negative media attention, contributing to stigmatizing the area and those living there through images and stereotypes of poverty, violence, drugs, and gangs (Barba, 2018; Lerida, 2018). News reported that public transport in Martínez Montañés was being limited because of potentially threatening situations for bus drivers (Lerida, 2017). Media further divides a stigmatized population from the rest of the city, thus perpetuating the gap and differences that separate them and victim blaming the Roma for their inequities. As stated by a Roma neighbor, "the problem is that the non-Roma community has built this image of us that is based on negative stereotypes, they do not want to recognize that because it is much easier to assume that the crime problem is a problem of the Roma community." In this fragmented context Roma are obligated to remain underground.

Phase 1: Building Alliances

A pilot study was done in a partnership between university researchers and Roma-based organizations settled and/or working in the neighborhood (henceforth the partnership). The objective was to build a multi-level alliance with the community and their key stakeholders to uncover the realities of Roma living in PS. Identifying and building these relationships were essential to have a space where we could reframe local Roma health problems and define actions to work together toward a common goal. The health director of the local policy coordinating committee facilitated the partnership contact information with local health stakeholders. A group of ten key health providers were identified, including representatives of community-based organizations, public institutions and services (i.e., housing and primary healthcare centers), and local policymakers. To overcome coordination challenges and show commitment, our role as community psychologists was to slowly build this networking group through visiting providers in their organizations, weekly phone calls and emails, adapting our agenda to theirs, and offering support. Proactivity was key since these providers previously had negative experiences with university-based professionals regarding inconsistency and lack of follow-up.

Meetings between key health providers and the partnership were held over a period of seven months with two fundamental transverse objectives: to raise awareness on Roma health status and to dismantle dominant narratives through an interactive and reflective problem-based learning method. Problem-based learning develops high-order thinking through sharing experiences and dialogue (Hmelo & Ferrari, 1997). Shared experiences regarding local Roma were discussed. The partnership led dialogue in order to identify sources of discrimination and build commitment for Roma health. In each meeting partnership shared information regarding anti-gypsyism, health policies, and local best practices to initiate conversations. Key health providers expressed their concerns with their understanding of the Roma community, the lack of evidence and consolidation of best practices to adapt their protocols and services to specific needs, and the lack of support received from the system and local policymakers to improve services based on their location and users. These meetings were imperative in order to ensure a group of key health providers who were committed to working toward local Roma health equity. Table 19.1 provides quotes from these initial meetings.

Table 19.1 Key health providers' narratives regarding PS Roma health

Quotes
"We try to work with Roma because it is a priority in Polígono Sur, and we understand that they have particular needs. We are conscious that we lack mediation to better understand them, it is challenging."
"The 'I am a social victim' is a persistent problem of the population here. 'By being a Roma I have a right to everything', and this is not the reality. Because there are non-Roma people who have much greater needs and we have to be provider in a wide spectrum."
"There is no continuity in providers. Associations come and go and the population is abandoned, so what relationships can they give to Roma? They cannot. There is no time."
"It's not only a cultural problem but a marginalization problem. We are treating Roma like outsiders. It is not a problem of not knowing what to do, it is a problem of not knowing how to do it."
"The problem is culture, discipline and prevention are not health practices of the Roma. They have to change their attitudes."

Phase 2: Mapping Roma Assets

Through an assets-based approach, university researchers partnered with Roma neighbors to identify and assess strengths within community resources to respond to Roma needs (Morgan & Ziglio, 2007). In order to gather all available evidences and incorporate the voices of local Roma, the mapping process was developed in three stages:

Evaluating the Roma Sensitivity of Local Assets

Researchers conducted a search of all health plans, policies, and programs that were being implemented in PS through initial stakeholder interviews and a systematic online search. We searched for keywords that are proposed within European and national frameworks for Roma integration to provide a set of specific actions that hold national, regional, and local governments accountable for implementing appropriate interventions (García-Ramírez, Escobar-Ballesta, & Lizana, 2015). In order to assess the sensitivity toward Roma, we developed an instrument based on the Roma Health Integration Policy Index (Escobar-Ballesta et al., 2018). The Evaluation Index for local Roma health assets in Polígono Sur (Table 19.2) comprised the following categories: (a) entitlement as the right to health resources; (b) accessibility as the facilitators and barriers to accessing health resources; (c) responsiveness of resources and their adaptability to respond to health needs; and (d) developing and sustaining future actions through participatory platforms and multi-stakeholder involvement.

Results show that local policies, plans, and programs in PS homogenized the target population under the principle of equality, ignoring that an equality perspective is not an equity option for diverse populations. This is supported by the fact that these local assets are not evidence-based within the context, making it difficult to obtain exact data on Roma health. In fact, this creates a barrier to adapting policies and services to respond to Roma needs, making them invisible and further perpetuating the institutional discrimination against them.

Table 19.2 Evaluation Index for local Roma health assets in Polígono Sur

Category	Indicator
Entitlement	Components of health service
	Entitlement requirements
Accessibility	Utilization of at-risk Roma groups (type, context, provider, objectives, time)
	Accessibility barriers
	Identify Roma non-users of services
	Roma health mediator
Responsiveness	Health inequities identified by the National Roma Integration Strategies health component
	Health service satisfaction of at-risk Roma
	Mechanisms to confront barriers and more sensitivity to Roma at-risk groups
	Mechanisms for professionals to adapt services for at-risk Roma
	Mechanisms to adjust health services to respond to particular needs of Roma users
Developing and sustaining future actions	Participation of at-risk Roma in the implementation of programs
	Collaboration between stakeholders

Note: Adapted from Aday and Andersen (1974), Escobar-Ballesta et al. (2018), Spanish Ministry of Health, Social Services, and Equality (2012)

Evaluating the Roma Sensitivity of Providers and Their Organizations

The objective was to assess if health providers in PS (e.g., healthcare professionals, community organization professionals) were responding and adapting services to Roma as well as if their organizations were creating flexible and socially fair climate for their staff and Roma users. For that, we conducted 40 surveys on a five-point Likert scale of providers regarding their personal value of work (e.g., "my work is important in my organization's functioning"), adaptations of services (e.g., "I am able to adapt my work to Roma needs"), and Roma sensitivity of their organizations (e.g., "My organization actively identifies accessibility barriers for the Roma"). Overall survey results show that providers—especially those in educational settings and community-based organizations—scored highest on Roma sensitivity. However, many of these providers evaluated their organizations as not sensitive to Roma needs. Please see Table 19.3 for results.

Table 19.3 Sample of health providers and organizational Roma sensitivity by asset type

Asset	Professional score	Organizational score
Healthcare center 1	4.3	3.6
Healthcare center 2	3.3	3.7
Center for drug rehabilitation	4.3	1.6
Primary school 1	4.3	4.2
Primary school 2	4.1	4.1
Employment office	3.7	2.3
Community organization	4.1	3.6
Roma community organization	4.6	4.6

Note: The scores shown are an average of the surveys collected for each asset displayed on a 5-point Likert scale

Identifying Areas of High Roma Density and Incorporating Their Evaluation of Organizations

Through the initial key health providers group, we identified Roma neighbors to collaborate with the research team as community agents, thus facilitating access to the hard-to-reach population. We conducted a survey—mostly in the PS' outdoor market run by the Roma community—to explore and to evaluate what services they use the most and what neighborhood of PS did they live. A total of 200 surveys were conducted by self-identified Roma neighbors.

All information collected during the three stages (i.e., identified local assets and providers' and neighbors' survey results) were coded to a geographic information system (GIS) using the software QGIS. The goal was to have a visual tool we could share with community to understand the strengths and gaps of local Roma health assets in order to define actions directed to improve those gaps. As is evident in Fig. 19.2, 80% of Roma respondents were living in the most hidden area of PS, the Martínez Montañés neighborhood. Another interesting evidence was that they did not travel outside of PS often. Regarding services, educational settings scored the highest as sensitive to Roma needs, and respondents were overall satisfied with primary healthcare centers. Local Evangelical churches were identified as the most frequented asset as opposed to other more proximate organizations and interventions.

In summary, this phase incorporates a mixed-methods approach to gathering all local available evidences while incorporating Roma perspectives regarding their relationship to local assets. Results reflect that policies, plans and programs developed by public institutions and community resources intend to respond to the population of PS as a whole; however, their impact within

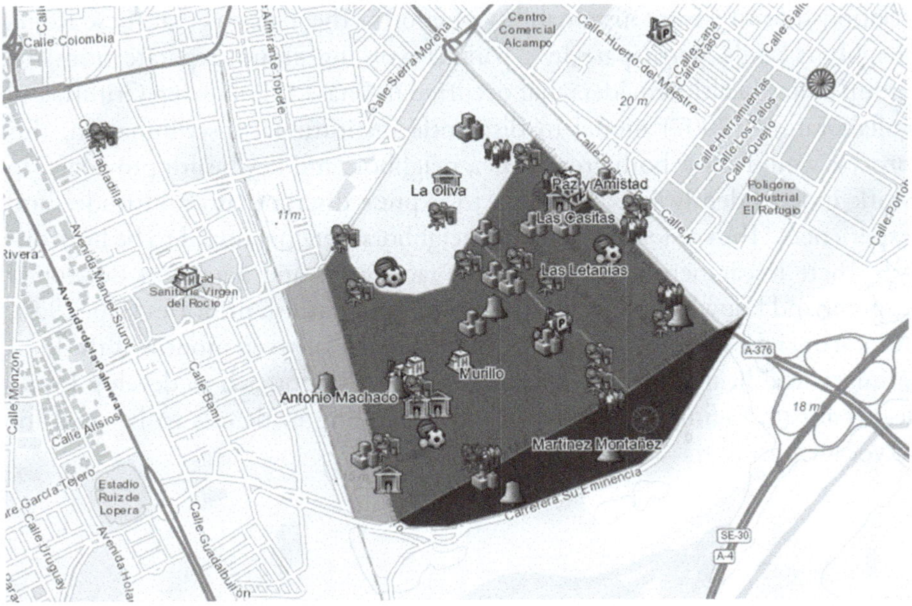

Fig. 19.2 Map of identified Roma assets in Polígono Sur. This example presents density of Roma population in the area and community resources. The darker gradient reflects high density of Roma and icons represent different resources available in the district

the Roma neighbors is limited since did not identify them as an asset. These gaps maintain Roma's status as a hidden community who are highly dependent on religious services to respond to their needs instead of the public institutions that are responsible for ensuring health and wellbeing.

Phase 3: Building Advocacy Capacity Among Roma Neighbors

The objective of this phase was to develop advocacy capacity among Roma neighbors in order for them to identify needs and influence change within their community through collective action. With the assistance of key health providers and Roma organizations who acted as community gatekeepers, researchers identified and selected Roma according to the following criteria: (a) have a relationship with key health providers, (b) identify themselves as Roma, (c) reside in the most impoverished areas of PS, and (d) demonstrate leadership skills and capacity to influence among their neighbors. It was important to select neighbors through key health providers who had a history working with the community as a deliberate strategy to build on existing relationships to ensure sustainability of efforts. The idea was that these Roma neighbors could participate in a parallel working group, separate from the group of key health providers that occurred in Phase 1. Following Griffith and collaborators' (2007) model to dismantle institutional discrimination, this process would allow both groups (i.e., neighbors and key health providers) to work independently in safe spaces to express discriminatory attitudes and experiences. The sessions with Roma neighbors were organized to be horizontal, where researchers acted as dialogue facilitators and neighbors developed content and knowledge around their community health priorities (Fig. 19.3). A total of eight sessions took place over the course of seven months at the local primary healthcare center. We utilized a CBPAR approach to develop Roma leadership in defining local needs and generating evidences to be used for advocacy purposes.

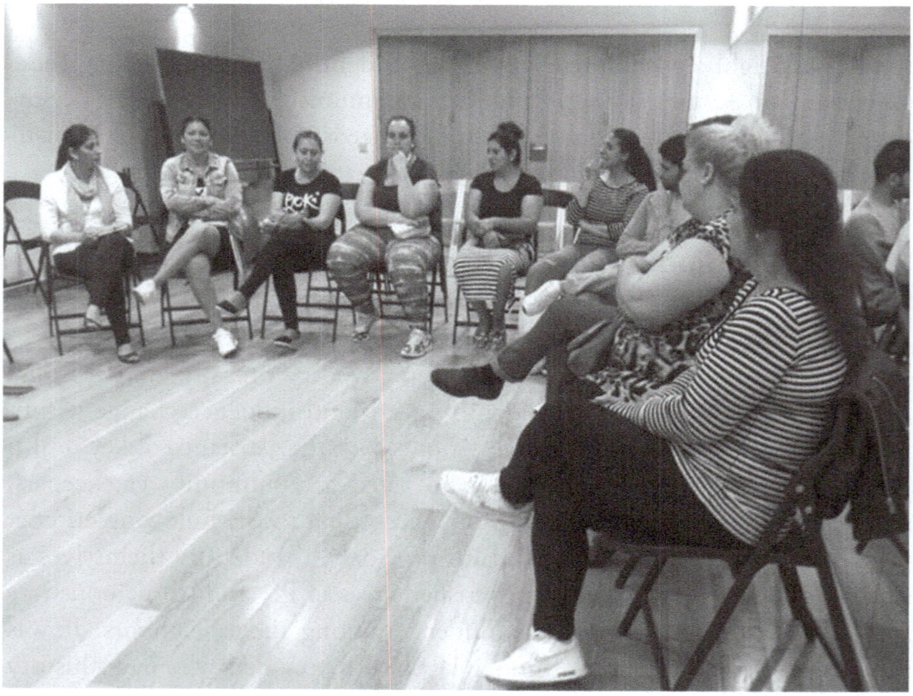

Fig. 19.3 Weekly meetings to build advocacy capacity among Roma neighbors

Liberation PhotoVoice

Roma neighbors expressed their desire to photograph local health concerns of their neighborhood in order to be shared with the group of key health providers. For that, researchers adapted and facilitated a CBPAR method, the PhotoVoice, which uses photographs to develop critical thinking and helps to build community narratives through group analysis and reflection. It has proved to be an effective tool to advocate for marginalized groups' health by generating an empowerment process that helps communities solve detected problems and share with the wider community (Foster-Fishman, Law, Lichty, & Aoun, 2010; Jurkowski & Paul-Ward, 2007; Wang & Burris, 1997). An innovate feature of our PhotoVoice method is that photographs were taken on personal phones and shared through the smartphone application WhatsApp. This idea emerged and was consented to in an initial meeting between researchers and neighbors since both groups already communicated through this application to schedule their meetings. The optimization of this existing resource also allowed for social learning to be a process that went beyond sessions and shifted daily experiences through a health equity lens. Regarding ethical concern, neighbors were trained to not take identifiable photographs of other neighbors and were guaranteed anonymity outside of meeting spaces.

Roma neighbors defined categories that were considered important and detrimental to their overall health and wellbeing: (1) plazas; (2) leisure; (3) commercial space; (4) public services; (5) absence of services; and (6) risk factors. Over the course of two sessions the photographs elicited dialogue between them, reflecting on the different sources of discrimination in everyday life. See Figs. 19.4, 19.5, 19.6, and 19.7 for photographs and excerpt examples.

Neighbors grouped the photographs into three main challenges: (1) unhealthy public spaces, (2) neglect from public services, and (3) urban problems. To develop this activity we used a thematic methodology which allowed us to create a local theory of health inequities suffered by Roma in PS (Foster-Fishman et al., 2010). This information would be consolidated by the group to be presented in the meeting with the group key health providers. Roma neighbors expressed that this experience was useful to develop a group identity, share experiences, and learn to generate evidences and build knowledge regarding their rights and discrimination.

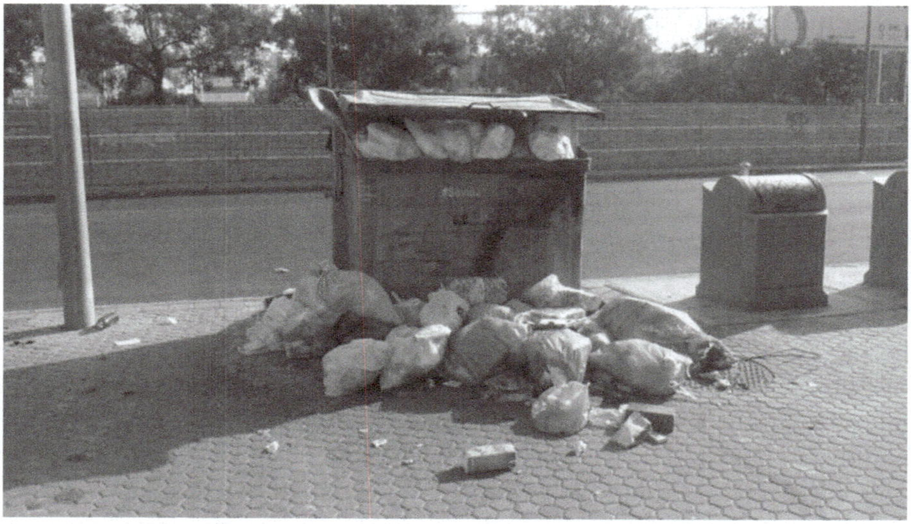

Fig. 19.4 Photograph of trash bins and discussion excerpt from group reflection: "We live amongst trash and its saturating. Why? Because it's not only the trash but what surrounds it. It is not the same waking up in the morning and see a park all clean than it is waking up surrounded by trash and that influences your mental state. Why? It is really depressing, you can't even go downstairs in the summertime...the insects, the cockroaches"

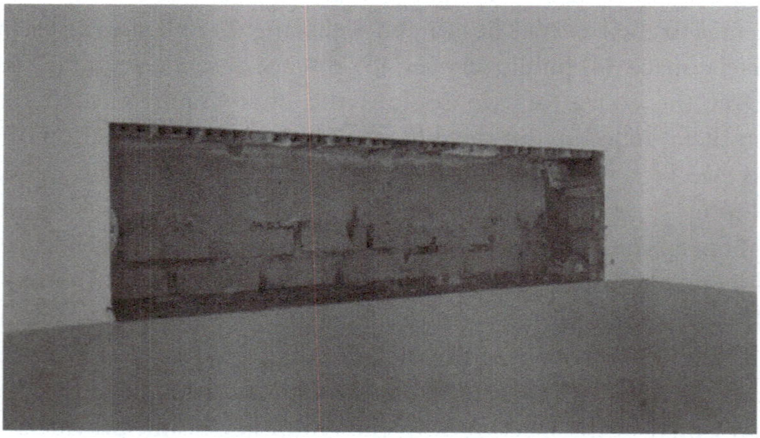

Fig. 19.5 Photograph of mailboxes and excerpt from group reflection: "These are the mailboxes of my building...it has been like this for years..., we have to go to the post office to pick up mail since they do not come here"

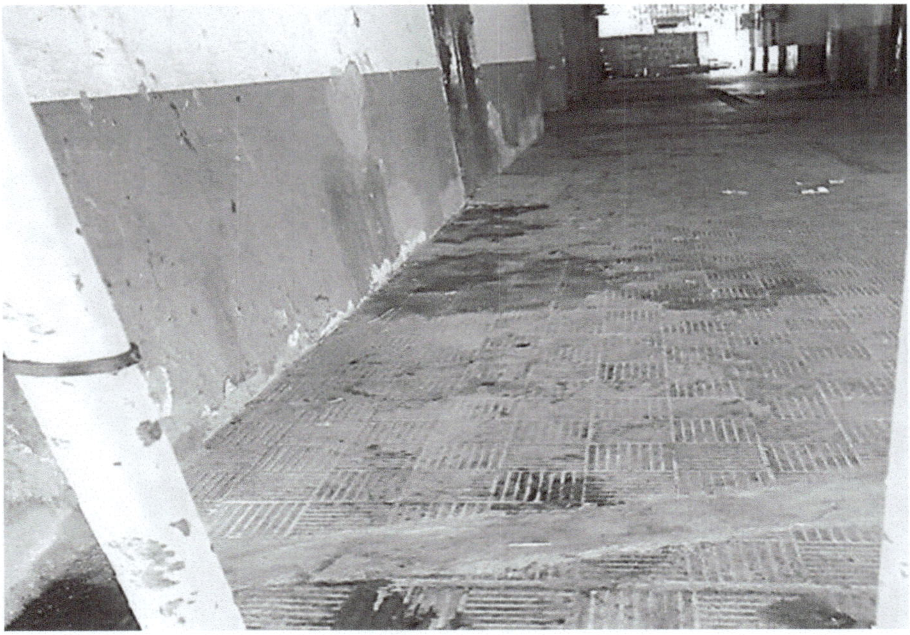

Fig. 19.6 Photograph of commercial spaces and excerpt of group reflection: "There are no shopping spaces in the area. So what do people do? They build informal shops outside apartment building or in their homes...spaces for real shops have no activity, so the physical state is undesirable...the roofs break when it rain, they are full of insects, cockroaches, rats...we are talking about spaces where people sell food and where people go to have a cup of coffee"

Phase 4: Empowering Roma Community Settings

The target of this phase was to create a safe space for key health providers and Roma neighbors to develop a common agenda, renegotiate available resources, and plan future actions to advocate for Roma health. This space allowed constructing new narratives and rebuilding trust between hidden communities and local providers.

A meeting was organized at the same primary healthcare center where neighbors had gathered during the project so they could feel comfortable. A total of 21 participants attended this meeting: 8 key health providers, 5 Roma neighbors, and 8 members of the partnership. The role of the researchers was to facilitate and guide discussion between participants and support Roma neighbors in securing their leadership throughout the meeting. This encounter developed as it follows.

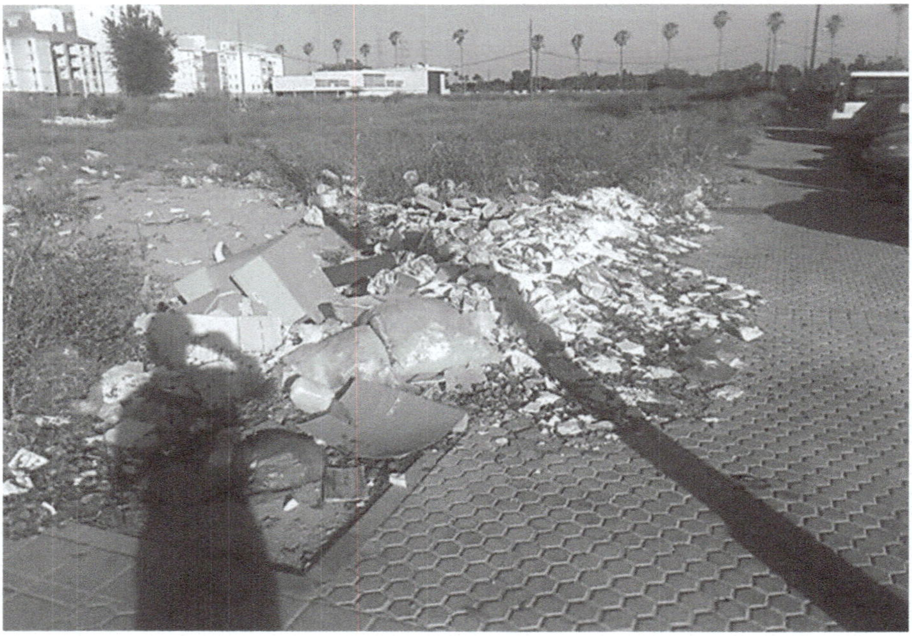

Fig. 19.7 Photograph of an empty space near neighbors' apartment building and group excerpt: "This used to be a football field... I used to look out the window to watch people play and go with my son. Later they removed it to build a park but they never did and this is how it was left...a space filled with trash, rats, insects and broken bottles"

Dissemination of the Evaluation of Plans, Programs, and Policies

Researchers led the conversation regarding the evaluation of local plans, programs, and policies relevant to Roma health. Key health providers and Roma neighbors had complementary reactions. As a provider expressed, "[local plan] tries to give certain orientations that are a reductionist vision of the complex dynamics in the PS." A neighbor also stated that "administrations continue to develop plans and projects from a distance, forcing professionals to work almost as they did before, without offering the possibility to adapt their work to the reality that they face on a daily basis, and without the vision of neighbors' realities."

Presentation of PhotoVoice Results

Roma neighbors had the opportunity to share their PhotoVoice activity to voice their frustrations, "I think this is where we can all agree, that all of the people are tired of unfulfilled promises, initiatives that begin and never finish." Concerns regarding their need to participate were also reflected, "It is necessary to create strategies with neighbors, if technicians already have a thousand working groups, the problem is that citizens should participate in these working groups, which helps transformation."

Group Reflection

Key health providers expressed the challenges of their work and lack of structural support. In fact, they stated they were making informal adaptations of official programs and protocols, but these adaptations were neither supported nor evaluated by the institutions. This lack of evaluation converted these practices into evidence-free areas and—again—made Roma users invisible. As a provider stated:

> PS has many health assets for Roma, there are many programs that are being implemented that, if evaluated, would at least develop formal protocols. This implies that a rigorous evaluation model is needed, that this will allow the Roma community to be visible and the professionals working with them to benefit more than they are now, and receive recognition and compensation.

Roma neighbors described their need to participate in the available spaces since they do not see results, "if there is a working group where these people are responsible and it has not been solving these issues, something is not working" (Fig. 19.8).

Building a Common Roma Health Advocacy Agenda

Both Roma neighbors and key health providers verbally committed to moving forward together. One neighbor said:

> As neighbors we are going to commit to participating with you, to complete projects and also to work in our own contexts. It is fundamental that we find a space where both neighbors and administrations can sit down to talk about problems and how we solve them, but on equal terms. That is to say we can develop proposals in which the two groups can feel satisfied and more or less cover the needs that we all consider important.

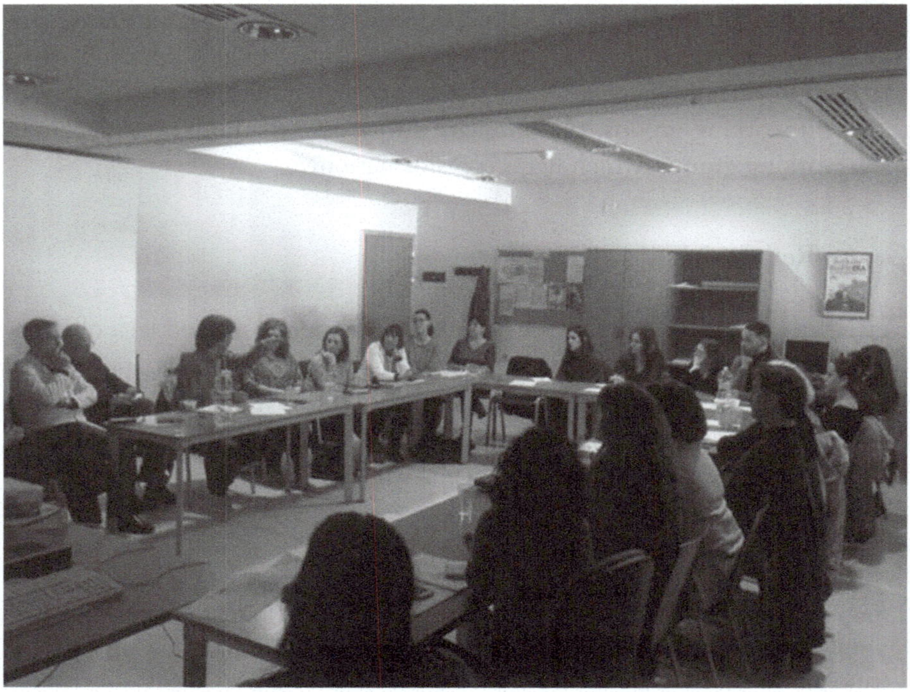

Fig. 19.8 Group reflection between Roma neighbors, university-community partnership, and key health providers

In the same vein, a provider expressed, "what we can do is to continue working so that what is done in the future will continue to have the sensitivity we have acquired here today."

This phase consolidated key health providers and Roma into one Roma health advocacy group that shared concerns, reshaped group objectives, and collectively defined actions for the future. Some of these were the exchange of contact information between neighbors and providers, providers offering navigational support of different resources within the community, and a follow-up meeting and invitation to existing health working groups. Please see Table 19.4 for a list of summarized recommendations and Fig. 19.9 for an example of a recent initiative led by a PS Roma-based organization which developed spaces for PS Roma to create art through Flamenco as a call to action.

Table 19.4 Empowering Roma community settings-specific commitments, strategies, and recommendations

Stakeholder	Commitment, strategy and/or recommendation
Healthcare center director	Open channels for communication with healthcare staff and neighbors
Local policymaker	Neighbors to be included in existing participatory platforms
Housing representative	Develop strategies with neighbors to work on identified priorities
University	Systemize good practices and commit to seeking funding opportunities
Neighbors	Recruit other neighbors and participate in existing spaces

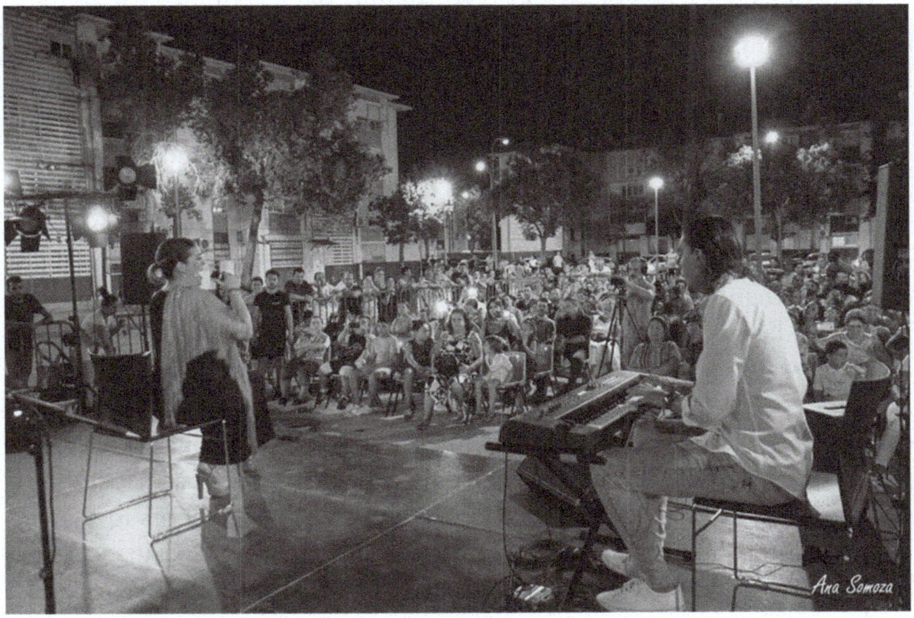

Fig. 19.9 The recent PS Sur initiative "*3000* DeSCencias" led by the Roma community-based organization, Studio 41013. Flamenco music and dance were used by PS Roma neighbors to tell their stories and defend their rights as citizens. This is an example of using community strengths as a source for liberation

Lessons Learned

This chapter describes a liberation psychology praxis that foster CBPAR processes to dismantle mechanisms that sustain Roma health inequities at at-risk local contexts. Roma across Europe have been forced into hiding through oppressive mechanisms that are sustained by policies, institutions, and societal discourses that exclude them (Matache, 2014). This is also visible at the local level. PS Roma neighbors express the scarce predisposition of policymakers and providers to recognize the Roma community, their services are the same and available to everyone without specific strategies. As community psychologists we have the responsibility of instigating processes with hidden Roma communities to gain capacity to become active citizens in order to ensure the fair distribution of resources and holding institutions accountable (García Ramírez et al., 2016). Without Roma in defining those policies and interventions, resources will continue to have a limited impact and contribute to the failures of these initiatives on the Roma population itself (Escobar-Ballesta et al., 2018).

Through the partnership we identified local allies and built collaborative capacity at multiple levels. Evidences show that this kind of partnership is beneficial to understanding and working with hidden, hard-to-reach communities (Benoit, Jansson, Millar, & Phillips, 2005). Learning and engaging with the community can ensure knowledge transfer and the incorporation of Roma voices for new evidences (Goodkind, 2005). Having access to these new evidences helps to hold communities accountable and ensure responsiveness of multiple stakeholders. This process supports identifying potential liberating mechanisms through an asset-based approach as potential levers for liberation. Future initiatives need to transcend traditional methods of research and interventions in order for transformative change to occur. Following Nelson's (2013) transformative policy change framework, community psychologists can lead processes that (1) shape problem definition; (2) reallocate power and resources; and (3) ensure democratic channels of participation. In our study, we incorporated the voices of hidden Roma neighbors in shaping PS health problems and negotiating resources in spaces for participation with key health providers. By incorporating the interests and voices of many actors we have a constant renegotiation and regeneration of objectives and goals, allocation of resources, transparency, and accountability. Community psychologists have the responsibility to guide local mobilization processes through regenerating relationships within the community and working with oppressed members to tell their story by engaging them in the problem-solving process as equal partners. Shifting the welfare paradigm from a "paternalistic" treatment toward Roma in current initiatives to a liberating paradigm as equal partners should be adopted in future actions.

We understand liberation occurs through sociopolitical development in which hidden communities develop critical awareness of unjust mechanisms that sustain oppression and then, they actively advocate by themselves and promote social transformation according to their values and lifestyles (Moane, 2010). Our study proposes that advocacy processes can be understood as liberating processes that give a voice and meaningful participation to hidden communities to defend their rights. In this sense, CBPAR methods can be a useful tool to develop narratives, organize action, and provide evidences to advocate for change. Also, it allows for hidden groups to become active members through developing critical thinking regarding daily injustices and defining actions to take collective action (Lykes & Mallona, 2008). This supports working for Roma with Roma.

It is essential to dismantle existing Roma negative social constructs through meaningful participation of Roma and engaging actors at multiple levels who have the responsibility to transform the public discourse, practices, and policies. The challenge of ensuring the sustainability of these efforts depends on commitment of local policymakers, providers, and Roma neighbors. Although the space created for local Roma to participate was solid in creating a new group identity and sharing experiences, continuity depends on funding. We believe that our work has to target existing participatory platforms and community organizations to include Roma neighbor groups at their tables and in their agendas. Identifying allies within organizations and health services can facilitate pressuring this action. Setting agendas without Roma might perpetuate the misrepresentation and misconstruction of their identity and needs at the policy level. It is a very common and perverse consequence when policymakers and providers focus on the program rather than the people, turning policies into devastating weapons against the people instead of a tool for their wellbeing. By creating empowering Roma settings, led by the Roma for their own change, their dignity and rights can be restored.

References

ABC. (1977). *Gregorio Cabeza ha pedido la desaparición de la secretaría de viviendas y refugios*. Retrieved from http://hemeroteca.abc.es/nav/Navigate.exe/hemeroteca/sevilla/abc.sevilla/1977/06/23/057.html

Aday, L. A., & Andersen, R. (1974). A framework for the study of access to medical care. *Health Services Research, 9*(3), 208.

Aiello, E., Flecha, A., & Serradell, O. (2018). Exploring the barriers: A qualitative study about the experiences of Mid-SES Roma navigating the Spanish healthcare system. *International Journal of Environmental Research and Public Health, 15*, 377. https://doi.org/10.3390/ijerph15020377

Ayuntamiento de Sevilla. (2016). *Diagnóstico de zonas con necesidad de transformación social.* Retrieved from https://www.sevilla.org/servicios/servicios-sociales/publicaciones/diagnostico-de-las-zonas-definitivo-para-publicar-3.pdf

Balcazar, F. E., Garate-Serafini, T. J., & Keys, C. B. (2004). The need for action when conducting intervention research: The multiple roles of community psychologists. *American Journal of Community Psychology, 33*(3–4), 243–252.

Balcazar, F. E., Suarez-Balcazar, Y., Adames, S. B., Keys, C. B., García-Ramírez, M., & Paloma, V. (2012). A case study of liberation among Latino immigrant families who have children with disabilities. *American Journal of Community Psychology, 49*(1–2), 283–293.

Bancroft, A. (2001). Closed spaces, restricted places: Marginalisation of Roma in Europe. *Space and Policy, 5*(2), 145–157.

Barba, E. (2018). *Nuevos clanes de narcos se disputan el control de las Tres Mil Viviendas.* Retrieved from http://sevilla.abc.es/sevilla/sevi-nuevos-clanes-narcos-disputan-control-tres-viviendas-201804010053_noticia.html

Benoit, C., Jansson, M., Millar, A., & Phillips, R. (2005). Community-academic research on hard-to-reach populations: Benefits and challenges. *Qualitative Health Research, 15*(2), 263–282.

Boscoboinik, A., & Giordano, C. (2008). Roles, statuses, positions. Social categories and multiple identities of Roma in Romania. In C. Giordano, A. Boscoboinik, M. Curelaru, S. Gog, A. Neculau, T. Niţu, F. Ruegg, D. Tarnovschi, D. Zaharia (Eds.) Roma's Identities in Southeast Europe: Romania, EthnoBarometer, 7-2, 3, .

Briones-Vozmediano, E., La Parra, D., & Vives-Cases, C. (2018). Healthcare providers' narratives on intimate partner violence against Roma women in Spain. *American Journal of Community Psychology, 61*, 411–420. https://doi.org/10.1002/ajcp.12235

Brüggemann, C. (2012). *Roma education in comparative perspective. Analysis of the UNDP/World Bank/EC Regional Roma Survey 2011. Roma inclusion working papers.* United Nations Development Programme.

Cahn, C., & Guild, E. (2010). *Recent migration of Roma in Europe.* Council of Europe. Retrieved from https://www.osce.org/hcnm/78034?download=true

Carlisle, S. (2000). Health promotion, advocacy and health inequalities: A conceptual framework. *Health Promotion International, 15*(4), 369–376.

Council of Europe. (2012). *Human rights of Roma and travellers in Europe.* CoE Commissioner of Human Rights.

Dalsklev, M., & Kunst, J. R. (2015). The effect of disgust-eliciting media portrayals on outgroup dehumanization and support of deportation in a Norwegian sample. *International Journal of Intercultural Relations, 47*, 28–40.

Dimitrova, R., Chasiotis, A., Bender, M., & Van de Vijver, F. J. (2014). Collective identity and well-being of Bulgarian Roma adolescents and their mothers. *Journal of Youth and Adolescence, 43*(3), 375–386.

Escobar-Ballesta, M., García-Ramírez, M., & De Freitas, C. (2018). Taking stock of Roma health policies in Spain: Lessons for health governance. *Health Policy, 122*, 444–451. https://doi.org/10.1016/j.healthpol.2018.02.009

European Union Agency for Fundamental Rights. (2009). *Housing conditions of Roma and travelers in the European Union. Comparative report.* Office for Official Publications of the European Communities.

European Union Agency for Fundamental Rights. (2012). *The situation of Roma in 11 EU Member States. Survey results at a glance.* FRA. Retrieved from http://www.undp.org/content/dam/undp/library/Poverty%20Reduction/UNDP_Roma_Poverty_Reduction_Roma_Survey.pdf

European Union Agency for Fundamental Rights. (2014). *Poverty and unemployment: The case of Roma in 11 EU member states.* FRA.

European Union Agency for Fundamental Rights. (2017). *Chapter 4: Roma Integration.* FRA.

Fésüs, G., Östlin, P., McKee, M., & Ádány, R. (2012). Policies to improve the health and well-being of Roma people: The European experience. *Health Policy, 105*, 25–32.

Foster-Fishman, P. G., Law, K. M., Lichty, L. F., & Aoun, C. (2010). Youth ReACT for social change: A method for youth participatory action research. *American Journal of Community Psychology, 46*, 67–83.

Freire, P. (1970). *Pedagogy of the oppressed.* Seabury Press.

Fundación Secretariado Gitano. (2006). *El reconocimiento institucional de la población gitana en España.* Madrid: FSG. Retrieved from http://www.gitanos.org/publicaciones/reconocimientoinstitucional/documentobase.pdf

Fundación Secretariado Gitano. (2012). *Población gitana, empleo e inclusión social. Un estudio comparado: población gitana española y del este de Europa.* FSG.

Fundación Secretariado Gitano. (2013). *Discrimination of Roma communities. Spain National Report.* FSG.

García Ramírez, M., Escobar-Ballesta, M., Lizana, T., & Albar, M. J. (2016). El reto de la equidad en las políticas sanitarias dirigidas al pueblo gitano en España. *Global Journal of Community Psychology Practice, 7*. Retrieved from http://www.gjcpp.org/en/article.php?issue=21&article=118

García-Ramírez, M., de la Mata, M. L., Paloma, V., & Hernández-Plaza, S. (2011). A Liberation Psychology approach to acculturative integration of migrant populations. *American Journal of Community Psychology, 47*(1–2), 86–97.

García-Ramírez, M., Escobar-Ballesta, M., & Lizana, T. (2015). *Implementation of the National Roma Integration Strategy and other national commitment in the field of health, Spain: A multi-stakeholder perspective report on 2005–2014 developments.* International Organization for Migrations. Retrieved from http://equi-health.eea.iom.int/images/NRIS_Spain_final.pdf

Gatti, R., Karacsony, S., Anan, K., Ferre, C., & De Paz Nieves, C. (2016). *Being fair, faring better: Promoting equality of opportunity for marginalized Roma. Directions in development; Human development.* Washington, DC: World

Bank Group. Retrieved from http://documents.worldbank.org/curated/en/292771468196732276/Being-fair-faring-better-promoting-equality-of-opportunity-for-marginalized-Roma

Gay, P., & Blasco, P. (2016). 'It's the best place for them': Normalising Roma segregation in Madrid. *Social Anthropology, 24*(4), 446–461.

Goodkind, J. R. (2005). Effectiveness of a community-based advocacy and learning program for Hmong refugees. *American Journal of Community Psychology, 36*(3–4), 387–408.

Griffith, D. M., Mason, M., Yonas, M., Eng, E., Jeffries, V., Plihcik, S., & Parks, B. (2007). Dismantling institutional racism: Theory and action. *American Journal of Community Psychology, 39*(3–4), 381–392.

Guy, W., Liebich, A., & Marushiakova, E. (2010). *Improving the tools for the social inclusion and non-discrimination of Roma in the EU*. EC DG for Employment, Social Affairs and Equal Opportunities.

Hajioff, S., & McKee, M. (2000). The health of the Roma people: A review of the published literature. *Journal of Epidemiology and Community Health, 54*, 864–869.

Heredia-Ramírez, J. (1978). *Discurso en las Cortes 1978*. Unión Romaní. Retrieved from https://unionromani.org/audios/

Hmelo, C. E., & Ferrari, M. (1997). The problem-based learning tutorial: Cultivating higher order thinking skills. *Journal for the Education of the Gifted, 20*(4), 401–422.

Ignăţoiu-Sora, E. (2011). The discrimination discourse in relation to the Roma: Its limits and benefits. *Ethnic and Racial Studies, 34*(10), 1697–1714.

Janevic, T., Sripad, P., Bradley, E., & Dimitrievska, V. (2011). "There's no kind of respect here": A qualitative study of racism and access to maternal healthcare among Romani women in the Balkans. *International Journal for Equity in Health, 10*(1), 53.

Jurkowski, J. M., & Paul-Ward, A. (2007). Photovoice with vulnerable populations: Addressing disparities in health promotion among people with intellectual disabilities. *Health Promotion Practice, 8*(4), 358–365.

Kolarcik, P., Geckova, A. M., Reijneveld, S. A., & Van Dijk, J. P. (2015). The mediating effect of discrimination, social support and hopelessness on self-rated health of Roma adolescents in Slovakia. *International Journal for Equity in Health, 14*(1), 137.

Kroon, A. C., Kluknavská, A., Vliegenthart, R., & Boomgaarden, H. G. (2016). Victims or perpetrators? Explaining media framing of Roma across Europe. *European Journal of Communication, 31*(4), 375–392.

Kyuchukov, H. (2011). Roma girls: Between traditional values and educational aspirations. *Intercultural Education, 22*(1), 97–104.

La Parra, D., Gil-González, D., & de la Torre, M. (2016). The social class gradient in health in Spain and the health status of the Spanish Roma. *Ethnicity & Health, 21*(5), 468–479.

La Parra, D., Gil-González, D., & Jiménez, A. (2013). Los procesos de exclusión social y la salud del pueblo gitano en España. *Gaceta Sanitaria, 27*(5), 385–386.

Lerida, A. (2017, October 29). *La Inspección de Trabajo prohíbe la circulación de tres líneas de Tussam por apedreamientos en las Tres Mil.* Retrieved from http://sevilla.abc.es/sevilla/sevi-inspeccion-trabajo-prohibe-circulacion-tres-lineas-tussam-apedreamientos-tres-201711291624_noticia.html

Lerida, A. (2018, March 29). *El barrio más pobre de España se pudre en Sevilla.* Retrieved from http://sevilla.abc.es/sevilla/sevi-barrio-mas-pobre-espana-pudre-sevilla-201803282343_noticia.html

Lykes, M. B., & Mallona, A. (2008). Towards transformational liberation: Participatory and action research and praxis. *The Sage Handbook of Action Research: Participative Inquiry and Practice, 2*, 106–121.

Maeztu, J. (2006). *Plan Integral del Polígono Sur.* Sevilla: Ayuntamiento de Sevilla. Retrieved from http://www.poligonosursevilla.es/opencms/opencms/

Martín-Baró, I. (1994). *Writings for a Liberation Psychology*. Harvard University Press.

Matache, M. (2014). The deficit of EU democracies: A new cycle of violence against Roma population. *Human Rights Quarterly, 36*(2), 325–348.

MATRIX. (2014). *Roma Health Report: Health status of the Roma population data collection in the member states of the European Union.* European Commission.

Mirga-Kruszelnicka, A. (2017). *Revisting the EU Roma framework: Assessing the European dimension for the post-2020 future.* Retrieved from https://www.opensocietyfoundations.org/sites/default/files/revisiting-eu-roma-framework-20170607.pdf

Moane, G. (2010). Sociopolitical development and political activism: Synergies between feminist and Liberation Psychology. *Psychology of Women Quarterly, 34*(4), 521–529.

Montero, M., & Sonn, C. (2009). About liberation and psychology: An introduction. Psychology of liberation. *Theory and Applications*, 1–11.

Morgan, A., & Ziglio, E. (2007). Revitalising the evidence base for public health: An assets model. *Promotion & Education, 14*(2), 17–22.

Nelson, G. (2013). Community psychology and transformative policy change in the neo-liberal era. *American Journal of Community Psychology, 52*, 211–223.

Real Academia Española. (2015). Diccionario de la lengua española (23a ed.).

Reysen, S., Slobodnikova, A., & Katzarska-Miller, I. (2016). Interaction of socio-structural characteristics to predict Roma's identification and desire to challenge low status position. *Journal of Applied Social Psychology, 46*(7), 428–434.

Ringold, D., Orenstein, M. A., & Wilkens, E. (2005). *Roma in an expanding Europe: Breaking the poverty cycle.* World Bank Publications.

Sasao, T., & Sue, S. (1993). Toward a culturally anchored ecological framework of research in ethnic-cultural communities. *American Journal of Community Psychology, 21*(6), 705–727.

Spanish Ministry of Health, Social Services and Equality. (2012). *Process to integrate equity into health strategies, programs and activities.* Retrieved from http://www.msssi.gob.es/profesionales/saludPublica/prevPromocion/promocion/desigualdadSalud/jornadaPresent_Guia2012/docs/Guia_metodologica_Equidad_EPAs.pdf

United Nations. (2015). *Transforming our world: The 2030 Agenda for Sustainable Development.* Retrieved from http://www.un.org/ga/search/view_doc.asp?symbol=A/RES/70/1&Lang=E

Vincze, E. (2014). The racialization of Roma in the 'new' Europe and the political potential of Romani women. *European Journal of Women's Studies, 21*(4), 435–442.

Wang, C., & Burris, M. A. (1997). Photovoice: Concept, methodology, and use for participatory needs assessment. *Health Education & Behavior, 24*(3), 369–387.

Watts, R. J., & Serrano-García, I. (2003). The quest for a liberating community psychology: An overview. *American Journal of Community Psychology, 31*(1–2), 73–78.

Wolff, T., Minkler, M., Wolfe, S., Berkowitz, B., Bowen, L., Dunn Butterfoss, F., et al. (2016). Collaborating for equity and justice: Moving beyond collective impact. *Nonprofit Quarterly, 9*, 42–53.

World Health Organization. (2013). *Health 2020: A European policy framework and strategy for the 21st century.* Retrieved from http://www.thehealthwell.info/node/583943

Daniela E. Miranda is a PhD Candidate of the University of Sevilla. Marta Escobar-Ballesta is a PhD from the University of Sevilla. Emilio Vizarraga-Trigueros is a leader of the Roma community-based organization Studio 41013 in Polígono Sur. Maria-Jesús Albar, PhD, is a Nursing Professor at the University of Sevilla. Manuel Garcia-Ramirez, PhD, is a Community Psychology Professor at the University of Sevilla. All of them are members of CESPYD, the Center for Community Research Action at the University of Sevilla.

20

'I Am Not Disabled, I Just Need Some Help': Are Critical Community Psychology Approaches a Promising Way to Engage with People with Learning Disabilities?

Michael Richards

Psychology has a troubled past for marginalised individuals and groups in our communities. I have heard many people in community settings say how much they hate working with psychologists because of their ignorance and arrogance. The traditional methods Psychologists employ when working with people are arguably outdated and do not allow the voices of the most marginalised influence change, particularly for people with learning disabilities. However, whilst I empathise with people who feel that way, and indeed, I have felt frustrated about the individualising and pathologising nature of Psychology myself for many years, I do believe that if we work with rather than on the most marginalised people in society and be prepared to be innovative and creative in our methods, Psychology can be a greater force for good.

M. Richards (✉)
Department of Applied Health and Social Care, Edge Hill University, Ormskirk, UK
e-mail: Richarmi@edgehill.ac.uk

C. Walker et al. (eds.), *The Palgrave Handbook of Innovative Community and Clinical Psychologies*, https://doi.org/10.1007/978-3-030-71190-0_20

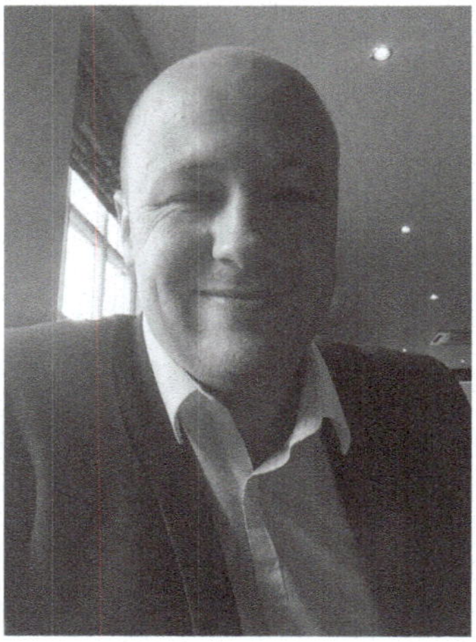

Introduction: The Problem with Psychology!

For over ten years, I have worked in many different community contexts and with different types of organisations, including social services, care homes for teenagers and housing associations. One of my first major pieces of work in the community involved being funded to work as part of The Teenage Pregnancy Strategy Programme in Manchester, with the overall aim to halve the under-18 conception rate by 2010 and to improve the health and social care outcomes for teenage parents and children. I was funded to work with boys and young men aged 13–25 years in the poorest areas of Manchester. I delivered workshops exploring themes relating to teenage pregnancy, including sexuality, relationships, domestic abuse, identity and masculinity (Kagan, Duggan, Richards, & Siddiquee, 2011; Lawthom, Kagan, Richards, Sixsmith, & Woolrych, 2012). My brief was to provide sex education with the aim to reduce teenage pregnancies as well as help young people to become more aware of the consequences of unprotected sex. However, rather than provide sex education that focused on handing out condoms or watching young people squirm as they looked at images of sexually transmitted infections (STIs), the aim was to provide a space, ideally somewhere they felt comfortable, where they could leave their macho image behind and say what they really felt about aspects of their lives and contexts.

Whilst my work with the young men was positive in many ways—that is, engaging in conversations and learning more about their lives—it is important to be clear that the workshops, whether one off or a series, were ameliorative because trying to build relationships and sustain projects over a long period of time was very difficult, if not impossible because of the lack of funds, resources and personnel. The aim to reduce teenage pregnancies was difficult to achieve and is a contested aim because the issue of 'teenage pregnancy' is a complex phenomenon that needs a more complex solution than informal education with young men. Just handing out condoms and talking about STIs is simply not enough. Instead, the workshops, even if only delivered for a short period of time, aimed to foster a greater critical awareness and build dialogical relationships (Freire, 1972) to help understand the deeper contexts and complexities of being a young man (Fig. 20.1).[1]

Aside from exploring issues related to unprotected sex and teenage pregnancies, one of the deepest and most complex issues many of these young men faced that emerged in this project work was that the young people were angry about the labels attached to them. These labels would often be negative, stereotypical and judgemental, often attached to them by professionals, and not necessarily related to their behaviour or how they viewed themselves. The most problematic label that was regularly attached to young people, particularly young men, was any label associated with 'Autism'. For example, so many of the young men I worked with had been diagnosed with Autism Spectrum Disorders, and at the time, often Asperger Syndrome. In some cases, from the descriptions provided by community workers, the label of Autism was attached because a young person was constantly shouting loudly or was always quiet,

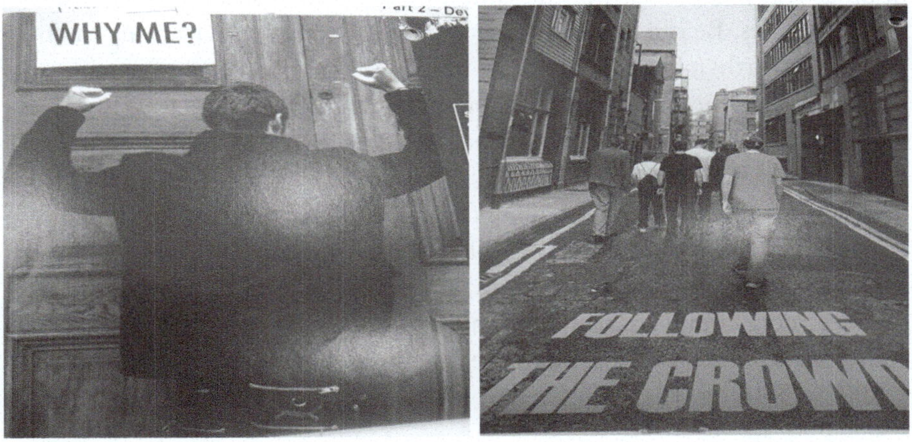

Fig. 20.1 Some of the young men I worked with expressing their frustrations in life through photography (see Lawthom et al., 2012)

[1] All individuals in the photographs presented in this chapter have provided consent at the time the projects took place and were happy for the photographs to be published.

and even when some of the young people put themselves into a dedicated, regular routine of aiming to get into education, or have an organised home, there were judgements made relating to the fact they wanted to stick to a structured routine. Furthermore, other professionals I worked with on occasions gave some of these young men a 'diagnosis' even if they had not met the young man/men I was working with. This sometimes occurred in team meetings and particularly with social workers and student social workers. Once, I witnessed a qualified social worker make a 'diagnosis', based on a page from Wikipedia on Autism to a young man who had started taking drugs. This kind of example made me frustrated about the label of 'learning disabilities' because fundamentally what was being ignored was the skills, talents and aspirations the young men had, and it seemed to me that the problem was contextual, not the young men themselves (Richards, 2014). For example, studies have found that it is social determinants that surround young men that ensure their chances in life are less positive, relating to education, living conditions, work, worklessness, money and resources (Featherstone, Robbt, Ruxton, & Ward, 2017; Hardgrove, McDowell, & Rootham, 2015; Sadler, Akister, & Burch, 2014).

With these concerns emerging, I started to think more about the label of 'learning disabilities' and what it might mean for people, particularly men, as that was on whom my work was based. Having worked with so many young men throughout Manchester at the time, I wanted to explore if what I was finding with young men was the same with adult men and the label of learning disabilities. Before discussing my work with adults with learning disabilities, it is worth reflecting on what influenced my decision to pursue this project. It stemmed from my Psychology undergraduate days learning about 'Critical Community Psychology' at Manchester Metropolitan University (Kagan, Burton, Duckett, Lawthom, & Siddiquee, 2011), in particular from my frustration with Psychology at the time. I was troubled by the way a Forensic Psychologist might psychopathologically analyse a 'criminal' or how a Cognitive Psychologist structures 'thinking' instead of considering the broader, more complex nature of thinking with people coming from different contexts and backgrounds, and hence my thinking was similar to what Parker (2007, p. 3) states below:

> The discipline of Psychology pretends that it is a science, but it draws its images of the human being from culture and from everyday life to construct its object. And part of the de-construction of Psychology is the study of the way ideology in society is the 'condition of possibility' for psychology to exist. Psychological theories do not come out of nowhere. They do not fall from the sky. (Parker, 2007, p. 3)

In other words, for me, Psychology was too simplistic, and it normalised and de-contextualised the many things that make us who we are. For example, in relation to disability, some have suggested that the normalising nature of Psychology has enhanced the power and knowledge of institutions that provide psychological services, providing negative and disempowering experiences for people with disabilities (see Foucault, 1972, 1977). In addition, Goodley and Lawthom (2008, p. 191) suggested that Psychology continues to adopt a form of Positivism that 'privileges a view of disability as impairment', thus implying that Psychology focuses on the problematic individual rather than the problematic environments people live in. However, Watermeyer (2012, p. 162) suggested that despite Psychology being 'limited and awkward', particularly in relation to understanding disability, there have been inroads of representing the 'psychological'. Watermeyer (2012) proposed that instead of simply seeing the history of disability and Psychology in terms of the 'pathological', scholars/disability activists should instead be looking inside Psychology and attempting to understand psychological concepts, to get a better idea of the issues that come with this. Accordingly, ignoring psychological approaches is potentially a mistake, but it cannot be ignored that Psychology and its processes, directly and indirectly, have generated fear, torture and death, not just historically. For example, Connor Sparrowhawk, a man with learning disabilities, drowned in a bath, a death that was preventable in 2014, under the care of Southern Health NHS Foundation Trust and a Psychiatrist (the organisation accepted they were responsible for his death in 2017). Therefore, these psychological approaches instead need to form part of the critical analysis to understand oppression and disability better. Whilst many people with disabilities consider Psychology to be about 'pathologising' and being 'impairment-obsessed' (see Chappell, Goodley, & Lawthom, 2000), a more positive perspective about the future of Psychology and disability is needed. On that basis, the ideas and practices behind Critical Community Psychology gave me a new lease of life in how I felt about Psychology and how Psychology could work for the better for marginalised groups.

Critical Community Psychology approaches helped me to view people in context, and unlike other forms of Psychology, one of the distinct features is that it is value-driven. For example, Kagan (2004 in Lawthom, 2011) conceptualised Critical Community Psychology as being focused around a set of values such as justice, stewardship and community (Kagan, Burton, et al., 2011). In setting these values, Critical Community Psychology attempts to depart from traditional approaches in Psychology in that it places problems and issues individuals, groups and communities face, in their contexts (Nelson & Prilleltensky, 2005). Additionally, another departure from the laboratory-based type Psychologist that focuses on the individual level of analysis is the varied and complex role of a Critical Community Psychologist. For example, during the projects to be presented, my role was constantly negotiated and renegotiated to suit the flexibility of the participants and the type of project. My roles were a web of being a researcher, volunteer, facilitator, Psychologist, confidante, resource person and cameraman, ensuring that I was not set in a permanent role, and instead, my role was on a continuum that was continuous and changeable (Bartunek, 2008; Ritchie, Zwi, Blignault, Bunde-Birouste, & Silove, 2009). The fluidity of these positions stemmed from the social and cultural processes within the projects, ensuring that being a Critical Community Psychologist is not stagnant, but always in flux to meet the demands of the participants within the community projects, helping to embrace the values of justice, stewardship and community.

With the changing nature of roles and values set out by Critical Community Psychologists in mind, this chapter will consider three projects that were influenced by Critical Community Psychology approaches that I jointly facilitated and created with local organisations/partners and their members with learning disabilities. The chapter aims to explore the relationship between Critical Community Psychology and people with learning disabilities. I argue that Critical Community Psychology has the potential to build a strong relationship with people with learning disabilities, and through this it may help to build bridges and provide spaces where the voices of people with learning disabilities can be heard and have influence.

The Realities for People with Learning Disabilities Living in the UK

Before I focus on the three projects, it is worth putting into context some of the hard realities for people with learning disabilities living in the UK. When I first started to work with people with learning disabilities in the community, particularly with adults, it was not long after the 2008 financial crisis. The consequences of this led to many community projects and services for people with learning disabilities closing down due to austerity (Power, Bartlett, & Hall, 2016). Alongside this, people with learning disabilities faced an angry media who portrayed people with disabilities/learning disabilities as 'scroungers' and 'benefit fraudsters' (Briant, Watson, & Philo, 2013; Garthwaite, 2011; Richards, Lawthom, & Runswick-Cole, 2018; Runswick-Cole & Goodley, 2015). Indeed, this was at a time when there were expected increases in the number of people with learning disabilities (Emerson & Hatton, 2008), with many facing complex health issues and barriers to participation in health-related activities.

All of this is a major concern, and it seems that people with learning disabilities are facing more problems than ever before, problems that are preventable and non-medical. From this, we can surely say that support and care will need to become broader and will need to emerge in ordinary spaces within the community, beyond the traditional 'day centres' (see Power & Bartlett, 2015). Previous research has highlighted that community work and projects are usually top-down and formulated around meeting targets and objectives (Laverack & Labonte, 2000; Perez, Lefevre, Romero, Sanchez, & Van der Stuyft, 2009). However, when bottom-up and focussed on participation, collective action is likely to have a greater impact on well-being (Campbell & Murray, 2004). It is on this basis that the following projects aimed to help people with learning disabilities to participate and to take collective action in exploring their identities, challenging some of the misconceptions about their understanding for health and the stereotypes associated with learning disabilities.

Critical Community Psychology Approaches in Action

Project 1: Creating a Community Exhibition with Men with Learning Disabilities in a Museum

Previously, I stated that I worked throughout Manchester, building relationships with various organisations and services to work collaboratively with the people who used their projects for support. I also approached a local learning disabilities charity in Manchester to discuss the possibility of exploring the label of 'learning disabilities' from the perspective of people with learning disabilities and to develop a health promotion project in the community. After many positive conversations with support workers and members of the organisation with learning disabilities, a decision was made that a health promotion project should be developed, and a local museum was contacted to see if they would collaborate with us and provide a space for this project to develop. From the beginning of this process, men with learning disabilities were involved in decisions and presented their ideas and insights into how this project was to be structured. The meeting with the museum was a success because they were keen to work with me and the charity to develop a project based at the museum. Subsequently, the stakeholders planned an initial five-month project, with a possible extension, which would cover the whole year. The museum also suggested that the work of the men could be displayed in a community exhibition at the museum. The charity and I felt that this was a good way to help sustain the project for as long as possible. This fitted in with the museum's agenda of making their organisation accessible to local groups within Manchester, forming part of their mission statement and having funds to work with local groups to create a community exhibition (see Fig. 20.2, which presents one side of the community exhibition created by the participants).

Ultimately, the aim of the research involved working with a group of approximately 30 adult men aged 21–68 years with intellectual disabilities to explore their experiences of working on a health promotion project they helped to create. The initial plan was that the group were to attend every other week to take part in filming and other activities within the museum. The alternate week would involve being out in the community doing activities or being based at other locations. However, soon after the project started the men wanted to keep attending the museum rather than be in different

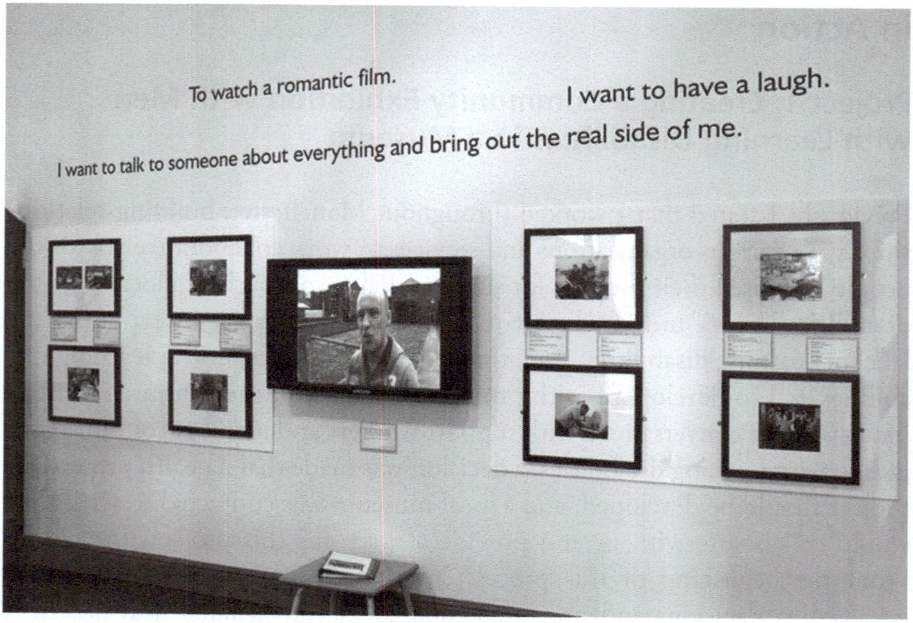

Fig. 20.2 A photograph presenting one side of the community exhibition where poetry and photography were displayed, created by the men who participated in Project 1 (also see Richards et al., 2018)

locations all the time and the museum had suggested that because the work the men created would form part of an exhibition, the project should remain there for the whole year, therefore, attending each week. Consequently, the structured timetable did not work and instead the 45 workshops were planned week by week rather than weeks in advance, which made it easier for activities to be based on what the men wanted to do. This fitted in with the values of participatory approaches in enhancing collaboration and communication between myself (the researcher) and participants (Nelson, Poland, Murray, & Maticka-Tyndale, 2004). The project ended with a six-month community exhibition at the museum, which showcased the work of the men including the presentation of films, art, poetry, sculpture and a giant comic strip depicting their understanding, knowledge and experiences of health (Richards, 2014; Richards et al., 2018) (Fig. 20.3).

Witnessing the men engage with visual methods to explore concepts of health was a powerful experience. For example, one of the main aims of the project was to consider themes on the subject of 'health' including diet, healthy eating and 'being clean'. I found that the men felt comfortable in this context to share their knowledge, but importantly this was not just knowledge they had learnt in the project, but knowledge they had brought to the group. This contrasts with the issues related to the reluctance of people with learning disabilities to seek health care, due to the negative experiences associated with stigmatisation (World Report on Disability, 2011, p. 77). Here, the men were happy to share their knowledge with one another (see Fig. 20.2). The evidence in this research would indicate that if there were fewer problems associated with choice and more focus on listening and sharing experience with people labelled with learning disabilities, more learning could take place about health promotion and awareness (Richards, 2014). In this research, the men wanted to make choices about health for themselves, considering knowledge about health, but without the intervention of 'health promotion' activities. In Fig. 20.4, one participant demonstrates through art that he understands the importance of brushing his teeth. However, he clearly already knew that, indicating that it is important to respect the knowledge of people with learning disabilities rather than assuming they do not know or do not understand. Overall, for the men to make choices, share expertise and participate in health-related activities, suggested that being empowered to do things they wanted to do was important, and not something they experienced much in their day-to-day lives (Richards, 2016).

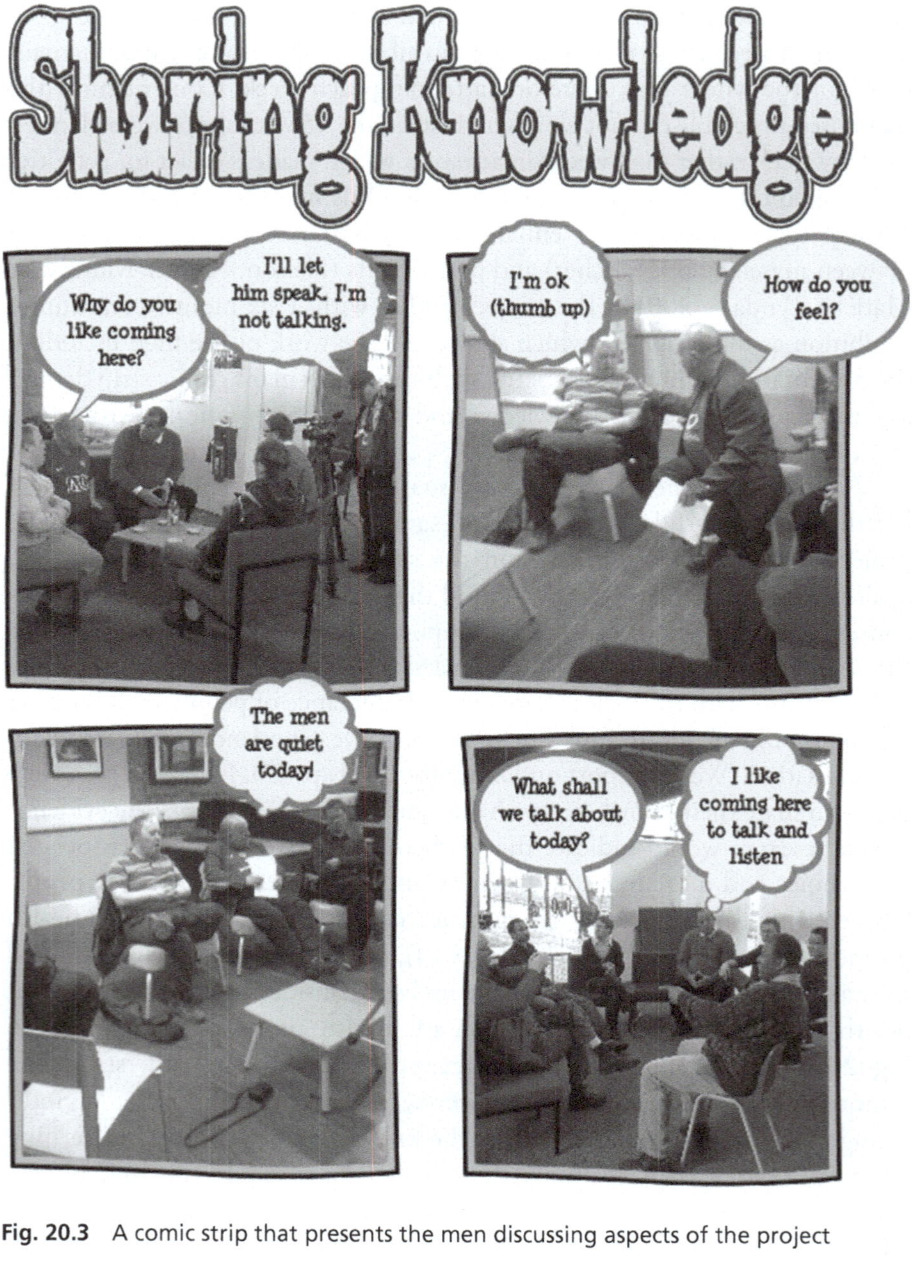

Fig. 20.3 A comic strip that presents the men discussing aspects of the project

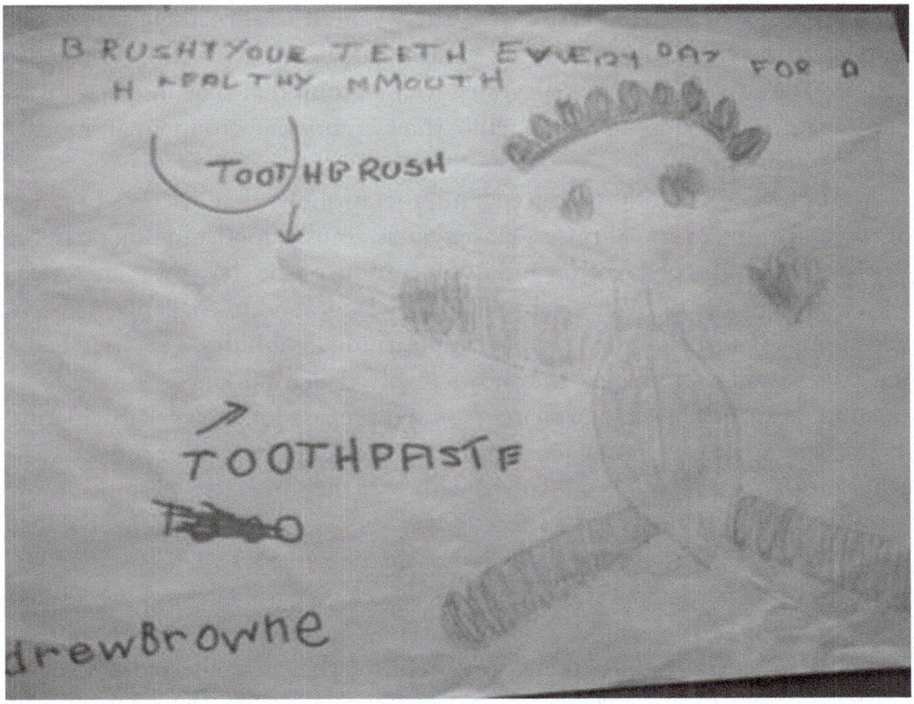

Fig. 20.4 Andrew's art work depicting himself brushing his teeth

Project 2: Developing and Producing Radio Shows at a Local Community Radio Station

When Project 1 ended, and the community exhibition was displayed, some of the men, in collaboration with women members of the learning disability charity, wanted to form a group that continued in a similar way as Project 1. The group started to think about the ways they could challenge the negative perceptions towards people with learning disabilities because their own experiences over the course of their lives had been mostly negative and prevented them from being how they wanted to be. For example, the label of learning disabilities prevented them from getting jobs, having romantic or sexual relationships and making friends. To help counter some of this, the group discussed the best ways of how to have fun and engage more with the community. From these discussions, one of the advocacy workers from the charity had links with a local radio station, in the heart of the local community in Manchester. Here the radio station provided training for marginalised groups, including for people who were unemployed or with learning disabilities, which interested the members of this new group. The group decided to call itself 'Our Advocacy', indicating that they wanted to own their spaces and work with people in their contexts rather than being 'worked on' by other people. The advocacy worker suggested to the group that they might want to participate in developing some radio shows, and the group unanimously agreed to participate.

Accordingly, the group produced a number of shows that discussed a range of topics relating to sexuality, sex, employment, music, food and other day-to-day life topics. The preparation and live recording of the shows was energised, with a strong sense of eagerness to share knowledge, and to challenge negative perceptions that surrounded people with learning disabilities. Everyone had a fun time because producing the shows involved sharing jokes, visiting local restaurants and socialising, to share ideas and prepare for shows. Participating in this activity meant fewer tensions and constrictions often experienced in other projects they had been involved with over their lives. For example, most members felt that their experiences of day services were restrictive because they were regularly told what to do rather than be asked.

A show was prepared a week in advance because parts of the show needed to be edited in. For example, parts of the show involved collecting the opinions of the general public; therefore, an editor (based at the radio station) needed to prepare the best bits of the opinions collected. The group would fuse the opinions into different parts of the show, alongside the discussions and presentation of music. The shows would last for one hour and take place in a small studio, where the group would crowd into the room, sitting down or standing up. This was not as uncomfortable as it seems, and instead made the production of the show more intimate. When the group first started presenting the shows, people were nervous about speaking into the microphone, but once they had done it, there was no stopping their enthusiasm to express their opinions.

Producing and broadcasting the radio shows in the local community helped the members to develop their confidence because they could decide what they wanted to discuss. The members of Our Advocacy could express their perspective on day-to-day issues and topics, and arguably with thousands of people through the radio. Participants in this activity had control over the content and delivered the shows, based on their interests, in a space where they could say what they liked, how they liked, in the heart of the local community. Working with the radio station and producing shows dispels, to an extent, the myth that people with learning disabilities cannot communicate or cannot do 'what other people do' (Fig. 20.5).

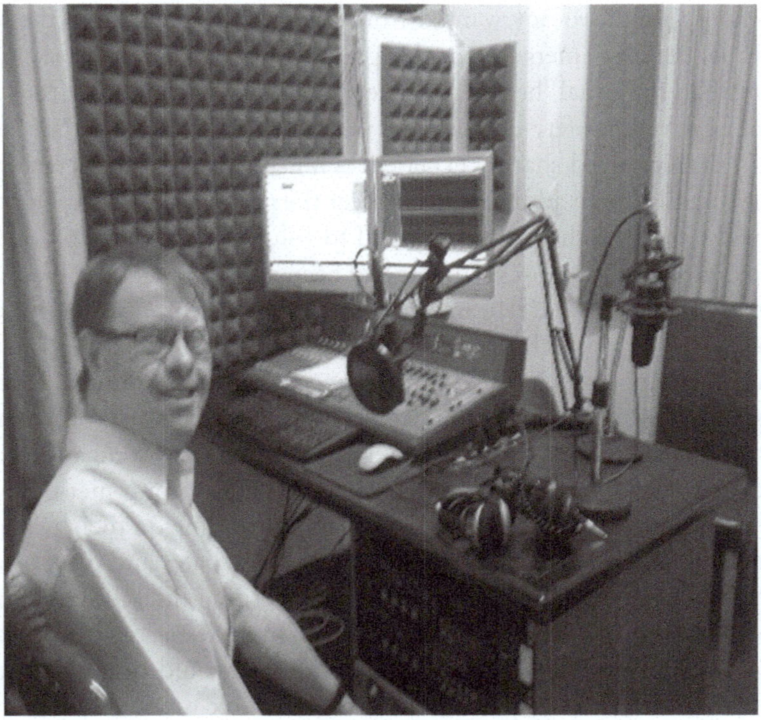

Fig. 20.5 One of the producers of the radio shows in the studio preparing to go live on air

Project 3: Self-Advocacy Work and Training Volunteers

Another part of the Our Advocacy group concerned working alongside a long-running citizen advocacy project, with the learning disability charity. The aim of the citizen advocacy project was to set up partnerships between volunteers and adults with learning disabilities, who were men and women over the age of 18 years, living in the local area. By building up a relationship between the volunteers and members of the project, the members could access the community more, take part in activities, meet new people and have support when needed.

Members of Our Advocacy had expressed that they wanted to meet more people, and they wanted to take part in more activities, rather than just waiting, sometimes every fortnight, for a meeting with their partner (the volunteer from the citizen advocacy project). An idea emerged from one of the members of the group that it might be more productive if volunteers learned more about the lives of people with learning disabilities, and what the members of Our Advocacy wanted from their partnerships with the volunteers. Thus, the idea emerged that this group could deliver a type of training, different than the usual 'health and safety' training (not ignoring the significance of health and safety because this was provided at another time for volunteers), that involved sharing experiences and knowledge about living with learning disabilities. In addition to the ideas the group discussed about changing how the training should be delivered to volunteers, the group decided to develop drama scenes (most members had been members of some local drama projects). The scenes were rehearsed at different, local community spaces and included issues to do with the control of money, sexuality, sex and relationships and bullying, which lasted for no longer than two minutes. Resources such as film-making equipment or cameras were provided by group members and/or by the facilitators. This equipment was used to film some of the activities including drama scenes and poetry readings. The group met on average once a week, sometimes more, sometimes less, depending on their availability. The aim of the scenes was to engage volunteers in debates and discussions, to help them become aware of how people with learning disabilities are treated and how they wanted to be treated, that is with more respect. Once the drama scenes were completed, the group and volunteers would discuss what took place, with the aim to help the volunteers to think more about the issues people with learning disabilities face daily. The drama scenes were preceded by informal interviews for new volunteers, facilitated by the members of the project and followed up by some poetry readings from one member, who wrote poems that discussed his views and feelings on his day-to-day life (Richards, 2017).

Most volunteers who took part said it helped them to think more about what it was like to have learning disabilities, and this would help them to view people with learning disabilities differently in the future. Other volunteers were confused about what the drama scenes concerned and how they related to them, but were willing to learn more to facilitate understanding, which they felt was important in their role as a volunteer. Overall, the members of Our Advocacy felt frustrated by the lack of understanding shown by their volunteer partners (unintentional in most parts) because members of Our Advocacy wanted to participate more in the community and feel more independent. Our Advocacy decided to take action and developed the idea to deliver training that was informal and creative, allowing the members of the group to express their views on how they wanted to be treated and how they think other people with learning disabilities should be treated. The training was split into three parts. First, several drama scenes were performed depicting some of the member's negative stories/experiences that they had experienced in life such as people taking money from them and violent attacks. Second, one man recited a series of poems he had written about his life and sexuality and then explained what these feelings and experiences had meant to him in the context of his life (see Richards, 2017). Third, the members and volunteers would sit together to discuss the performances and how the sharing of these experiences can help to enhance the understanding of how to work with people with learning disabilities.

The training was presented in a relaxed atmosphere, but one in which people could be challenged on their views of learning disability. It helped the people involved to build relationships from the start. The members of the group enjoyed dramatising their scenes because they felt that people were listening to their views and experiences, and the training experience felt like it involved people taking their perspectives seriously.

Are Critical Community Psychology Approaches a Useful Way to Build Bridges with People with Learning Disabilities?

Challenging Stereotypes, Reflecting on Diverse Identities and Creativity

The three projects highlighted in this chapter demonstrate that people with learning disabilities are eager to share their knowledge and expertise about a range of subjects, through a variety of methods, including radio, drama, art and photography. By using these methods, they were able to challenge some of the stereotypes relating to people with learning disabilities, usually related to labels that underestimate their knowledge and understanding of the world. Thus, using Critical Community Psychology approaches helped them to do this, as they could address social and individual change, in concurrence with people in the community (Kagan, Burton, et al., 2011). This is significant because ordinarily, in relation to disability, most people remain confused about defining disability, not least psychologists. This may affect the way in which disability is conceptualised, determining the type of interventions used by psychologists (Finkelstein & French, 1993), including by those who aim to apply Critical Community Psychology approaches. This can lead to the development of stereotypes and unwanted labels for people with learning disabilities. In this respect, Psychology needs to arguably align itself collaboratively with the progress and development of the disability movement concerned with political change (Campbell & Oliver, 1996), and Critical Community Psychology approaches are pathways that can lead to this happening. For example, in Project 3, the members of the group enabled themselves to take action to tell their stories of what it is like to be labelled with learning disabilities through dramatic scenes. These scenes helped the group to convey their reflections and to inform volunteers that the lives of people with learning disabilities are often dominated by control, abuse and fewer opportunities than others to make choices, share experiences and participate fully in everyday life occurrences. This is important because people with learning disabilities often talk about how their experiences of hospitals and services can fill them with anxiety and feelings of disempowerment (MacArthur et al., 2015). Thus, the value-driven epistemology of Critical Community Psychology complements ideals such as standing up for people's rights, making changes, resisting oppression and challenging power, which are important values for people with learning disabilities and other marginalised groups (Aspis, 1997; Ignagni, Fudge Schormans, Liddiard, & Runswick-Cole, 2016). In this respect, Critical Community Psychology approaches may contribute to a strong partnership with people with learning disabilities. In doing so, it challenges the stereotypes and conditions of being labelled with learning disabilities and may enable more research to be done with people with disabilities as co-researchers (Goodley & Lawthom, 2005). Project 2 was another great example of men and women with learning disabilities challenging stereotypes relating to the way they communicate. The shows they produced and created were done in collaboration with non-disabled people and epitomised their skills in imagination, creativity and organisation.

Furthermore, in Project 1, the group of men used creative and visual methods as ways to communicate their thoughts on health promotion and their place in the society. It was clear that they had much knowledge and experience to share—knowledge and experience that is too often ignored because they are judged by the label of learning disabilities rather than the people that they are. It may also be related to the negative history between people with disabilities and aspects of Psychology discipline, because of Psychology's obsession with individualising and pathologising people with disabilities (Oliver, 1990). However, the major shift and break from mainstream Psychology that Critical Community Psychology approaches offer is that people are considered within the contexts they live (Kagan, Burton, et al., 2011; Prilleltensky, Nelson, & Peirson, 2001). The men themselves pinpointed the problems they faced in their lives, relating to the label of learning disabilities in their personal contexts and the experiences they have faced in society. Here, the men used a variety of visual methods to represent their identity, emotions and feelings. Consequently, a strong link between people with learning disabilities and

Critical Community Psychology approaches can provide an interdisciplinary and practical understanding of the causes of oppression, which can be a guide to take action (Goodley & Lawthom, 2005; Richards, 2014).

Whilst I have highlighted some of the positives within the three projects, including features relating to how adults with learning disabilities have empowered themselves to engage with the community, share expertise and participate in activities that helped to develop the spaces where they could have a voice, the projects did not always run smoothly. In Project 1, there were issues relating to the extent to which participants were fully participating, particularly when it came to making major decisions about how the workshops should be facilitated. Similarly, this was the case in Project 2 when deciding the content of the radio shows, and in Project 3 deciding on the type of training that they wanted to facilitate. It was difficult to facilitate projects and to be full inclusive with everyone at all times, with different stakeholders having different agendas that did not suit everyone. For Critical Community Psychology approaches to be as effective as possible, participants need to be able to talk openly and to feel they can be reflective in safe spaces, which will help to ensure there is higher chance of full participation and that people feel empowered to be able to raise their voices to share their valuable expertise and knowledge. This can be done by ensuring that participants, such as people with learning disabilities, can make decisions by being in roles that have power and being in a position to decide how a project should work and function from the ideas stage of the process to the end of the project.

Critical Community Psychology Approaches Can Be Problematic, but They Bring Hope and Innovation for People with Learning Disabilities

Whilst I advocate that Critical Community Psychology approaches can be beneficial for people with learning disabilities, Critical Community Psychology is not without its critics. For example, Parker (2007, p. 145) summed up Community Psychology from a Critical Psychology perspective:

> Community psychology, then, often glues together the two terms 'community' and 'psychology' in such a way as to psychologise what a community is—to treat the community as something that can be conceptualised and studied by psychologists on their own terms—and then to use that psychologised image of the community to understand the individuals that comprise it.

In the same text, Parker (2007) described how Critical Community Psychologists often work within the limitations of a funding agenda, with funders prescribing and controlling how projects work, that is pressure on professionals/professions in the 'Arts for Health' field to apply quantitative evaluation (Staricoff, 2006). In addition, Critical Community Psychology essentially uses qualitative methods, but these types of methods within Psychology are still being dismissed as unempirical (Maracek, 2003) and are taught in few institutions (Camic, Yardley, & Rhodes, 2003), which prevents a discipline like Critical Community Psychology from developing and being influential. Parker (2007, p. 146) further states:

> The concern with turning the dumb non-psychologists into good citizens who would be grateful to those in the discipline who have given away their knowledge is a conservative response to political problems in psychology. It not only betrays the hopes of those outside the discipline who thought that psychology would something interesting and useful to say about alienation, it also betrays the activities of those who have really tried to put politics on the agenda.

The problem I have with Parker's (2007) critique is that it is not very hopeful for the future, and, it may not reflect on how some people in the community or non-psychologists feel, certainly not in my experience. I feel that Parker (2007) rejects any kind of hope in making changes to enhance Psychology and hopes to strengthen the relationship between Psychology and disability. In fact, I feel that Critical Community Psychology is not only values driven but also a reaction against the individualism of Psychology (Goodley & Lawthom, 2008). For example, in the three projects presented, there was an eagerness to reflect on participants' multiple identities. There was a desire to present their skills, talents and opinions through creative means, and whilst doing so, challenge some of the myths and stereotypes about people with learning disabilities through art, photography, drama, debate and radio.

Overall, my advice is that by working harder to listen and engage with people with learning disabilities, and Critical Community Psychology approaches can help to do this, people with learning disabilities can emerge and more focus can be placed on the knowledge and experiences they have to share. This in turn can help to ensure that they are able to make more choices and participate at every level to increase the chances of them having more control over their own lives whilst making an important contribution to wider society (Richards, 2016). My advice would be that if this is to be achieved it is important to develop relationships that are equal at all levels, and this can be helped by accepting the fluid and flexible nature of working collaboratively in community projects, where a common empathy, friendliness and transparency can help to achieve what participants and Psychologists set out to do. By doing so, Critical Community Psychology approaches have the potential to develop a strong relationship with people with learning disabilities, and through this it may help to build bridges and provide spaces where the voices of people with learning disabilities can be heard and have influence.

References

Aspis, S. (1997). Self-advocacy for people with learning difficulties: Does it have a future? *Disability and Society, 12*(4), 647–654.

Bartunek, J. M. (2008). Insider/Outsider team research: The development of the approach and its meanings. In A. B. Shani, N. Adler, S. A. Mohrman, W. A. Pasmore, & B. Stymne (Eds.), *Handbook of collaborative management research* (pp. 73–91). Sage.

Briant, E., Watson, N., & Philo, G. (2013). Reporting disability in the age of austerity: The changing face of media representation of disability and disabled people in the United Kingdom and the creation of new 'folk devils'. *Disability and Society, 28*(6), 874–889.

Camic, P., Yardley, I., & Rhodes, J. E. (2003). *Qualitative research in psychology: Expanding perspectives in methodology and design*. APA Publications.

Campbell, C., & Murray, M. (2004). Community health psychology: Promoting analysis and action for social change. *Journal of Health Psychology, 9*(2), 187–195.

Campbell, J., & Oliver, M. (1996). *Disability politics: Understanding our past, changing our future*. Routledge.

Chappell, A., Goodley, D., & Lawthom, R. (2000). Connecting with the social model: The relevance of the social model of disability for people with learning difficulties. *British Journal of Learning Disabilities, 28*, 1–7.

Emerson, E., & Hatton, C. (2008). *People with learning disabilities in England*. Centre for Disability Research.

Featherstone, B., Robbt, M., Ruxton, S., & Ward, M. (2017). 'They are just good people…generally good people': Perspectives of young men on relationships with social care workers in the UK. *Children and Society, 31*, 331–341.

Finkelstein, V., & French, S. (1993). Towards a psychology of disability. In J. Swain (Ed.), *Disabling barriers – Enabling environments* (pp. 26–34). Sage Publications.

Foucault, M. (1972). *The archaeology of knowledge*. Pantheon Books.

Foucault, M. (1977). *Discipline and punish: The birth of the prison*. Pantheon Books.

Freire, P. (1972). *Pedagogy of the oppressed*. Penguin.

Garthwaite, K. (2011). The language of shirkers and scroungers? Talking about illness, disability and coalition welfare reform. *Disability & Society, 26*, 369–372.

Goodley, D., & Lawthom, R. (2005). Epistemological journeys in participatory action research: Alliances between community psychology and disability studies. *Disability and Society, 20*(2), 135–151.

Goodley, D., & Lawthom, R. (2008). In defence of disability studies: A responses to Forshaw (2007) In defence of psychology: A reply to Goodley and Lawthom (2005). *Disability and Society, 23*(2), 191–192.

Hardgrove, A., McDowell, L., & Rootham, E. (2015). Precarious lives, precarious labour: family support and young men's transitions to work in the UK. *Journal of Youth Studies, 18*(8), 1057–1076.

Ignagni, E., Fudge Schormans, A., Liddiard, K., & Runswick-Cole, K. (2016). 'Some people are not allowed to love': Intimate citizenship in the lives of people labelled with intellectual disabilities. *Disability & Society, 31*(1), 131–135.

Kagan, C. (2004). *What are community psychologists?* Community Psychology UK website (Online). Retrieved April 21, 2014, from http://www.compsy.org.uk/compsyleaflet2004.doc

Kagan, C., Burton, M., Duckett, P., Lawthom, R., & Siddiquee, A. (2011). *Critical community psychology*. Blackwell Publishing.

Kagan, C., Duggan, K., Richards, M., & Siddiquee, A. (2011). Community psychology. In P. Martin, F. Cheung, M. Kyrios, L. Littlefield, M. Knowles, B. Overmier, & J. M. Prieto (Eds.), *The IAAP handbook of applied psychology* (pp. 471–500). Blackwell.

Laverack, G., & Labonte, R. (2000). A planning framework for community empowerment goals within health promotion. *Health Policy and Planning, 15*, 255–262.

Lawthom, R. (2011). Developing learning communities: Using communities of practice within community psychology. *International Journal of Inclusive Education, 15*(1), 153–164.

Lawthom, R., Kagan, C., Richards, M., Sixsmith, J., & Woolrych, R. (2012). Being creative round health: Participative methodologies in critical community psychology. In C. Horrocks & S. Johnson (Eds.), *Advances in health psychology: Critical approaches* (pp. 204–220). Routledge.

MacArthur, J., Brown, M., McKechanie, A., Mack, S., Hayes, M., & Fletcher, J. (2015). Making reasonable and achievable adjustments: The contributions of learning disability liaison nurses in 'Getting it right' for people with learning disabilities receiving general hospitals care. *The Journal of Advanced Nursing, 71*(7), 1449–1740.

Maracek, J. (2003). Dancing through minefields: Toward a qualitative stance in psychology. In P. M. Camic, J. E. Rhodes, & L. Yardley (Eds.), *Qualitative research in psychology: Expanding perspectives in methodology and design* (pp. 49–69). American Psychological Association.

Nelson, G., Poland, B., Murray, M., & Maticka-Tyndale, E. (2004). Building capacity in community health action research. *Action Research, 2*(4), 389–408.

Nelson, G., & Prilleltensky, I. (2005). *Community psychology: Towards liberation and well-being*. Palgrave Macmillan.

Oliver, M. (1990). *The Politics of Disablement.* Basingstoke: Macmillan and St Martin's Press.

Parker, I. (2007). *Revolution in psychology: Alienation to emancipation.* Pluto.

Perez, D., Lefevre, P., Romero, M. I., Sanchez, L., & Van der Stuyft, P. (2009). Augmenting frameworks for appraising the practices of community-based health interventions. *Health Policy and Planning, 24*, 335–341.

Power, A., & Bartlett, R. (2015). Self-building safe havens in a post-service landscape: How adults with learning disabilities are reclaiming the welcoming communities agenda. *Social and Cultural Geography*, 1–22.

Power, A., Bartlett, R., & Hall, E. (2016). Peer-advocacy in a personalised landscape: The role of peer support in a context of individualised support and austerity. *Journal of Intellectual Disabilities*, 1–19.

Prilleltensky, I., Nelson, G., & Peirson, L. (2001). The role of power and control in children's lives: An ecological analysis of pathways toward wellness, resilience and problems. *Journal of Community and Applied Social Psychology, 11*(2), 144–158.

Richards, M. (2014). *Confessions of a community psychology: The tale of a group of men challenging the perceptions of health promotion and learning difficulties.* Unpublished PhD thesis, Manchester Metropolitan University, UK.

Richards, M. (2016). People with learning disabilities need a commissioner and a legal charter of rights – No they do not! *Disability and Society*, 1–5.

Richards, M. (2017). 'Angry, when things don't go my own way': What it means to be gay with learning disabilities. *Disability & Society, 32*(8), 1165–1179.

Richards, M., Lawthom, R., & Runswick-Cole, K. (2018). Community-based arts research for people with learning disabilities: Challenging misconceptions about learning disabilities. *Disability and Society, 34*(2), 204–222.

Ritchie, J., Zwi, A. B., Blignault, I., Bunde-Birouste, A., & Silove, D. (2009). Insider-outsider positions in health-development research: Reflections for practice. *Development in Practice, 19*(1), 106–112.

Runswick-Cole, K., & Goodley, D. (2015). DisPovertyPorn: Benefits street and the dis/ability paradox. *Disability & Society, 30*(4), 645–649.

Sadler, K., Akister, J., & Burch, S. (2014). Who are the young people who are not in education, employment or training? An application of the risk factors to a rural area in the UK. *International Social Work, 58*(4), 508–520.

Staricoff, R. (2006). Arts in health: the value of evaluation. *The Journal of the Royal Society for the Promotion of Health, 126*(3), 116–120.

Watermeyer, B. (2012). Is it possible to create a politically engaged, contextual psychology of disability? *Disability and Society, 27*(2), 161–174.

World Health Organisation and World Bank. (2011). *World report on disability* (Online). Retrieved April 25, 2012, from http://www.who.int/disabilities/world_report/2011/en/

21

Marginalised Youth Navigating Uncertainty: Reflections on Co-construction and Methodology in Nepal

Vicky Johnson, Andy West, Sumon Kamal Tuladhar, Shubhendra Man Shrestha, and Sabitra Neupane

The team of YOUR World Research carried out rights-based and youth-centred research starting from the perspectives of marginalised youth. To even understand the terms 'Uncertainty', 'Insecurity' and 'Marginalisation', we engaged with young women and men and young people who are genderfluid, aged 15–25 years, to co-create translations and methods that would make sense in local contexts and allow youth to feel comfortable and valued.

V. Johnson (✉)
Centre for Remote and Sustainable Communities, UHI, Inverness, Scotland
e-mail: Vicky.Johnson.ic@uhi.ac.uk

A. West
Independent Researcher and Writer; Community Research Fellow, University of Brighton, Brighton, UK

S. K. Tuladhar
Independent Education Specialist, Equity Consultant, Kathmandu, Nepal

S. M. Shrestha
PhD Student at Goldsmiths, Researcher in Nepal, Lalitpur, Nepal

S. Neupane
Independent Researcher, Brampton, ON, Canada

C. Walker et al. (eds.), *The Palgrave Handbook of Innovative Community and Clinical Psychologies*, https://doi.org/10.1007/978-3-030-71190-0_21

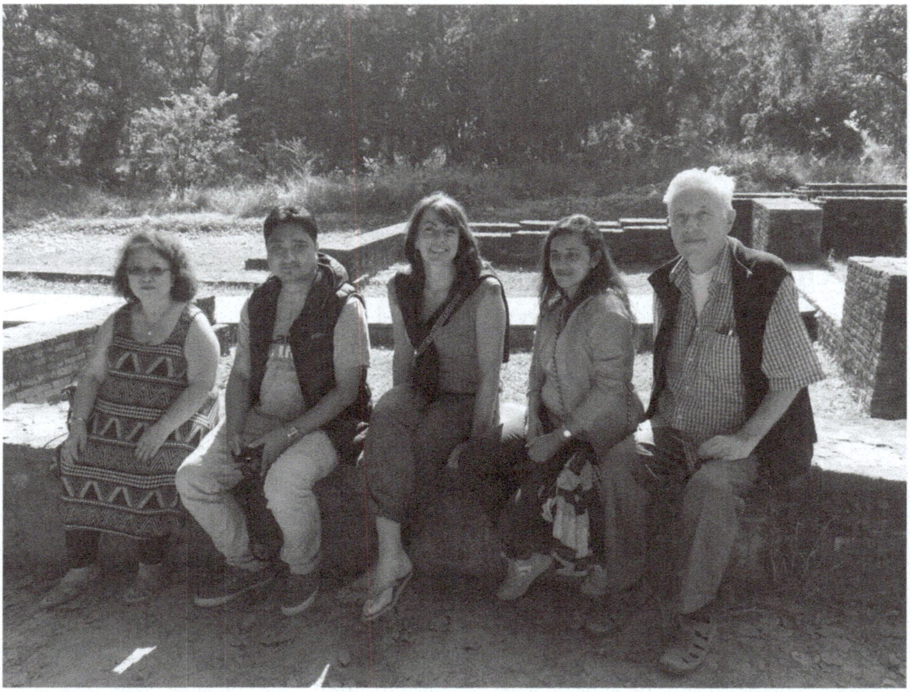

Introduction

Research on youth and uncertainty has been co-constructed with partners and marginalised young people in Ethiopia and Nepal. This Youth Uncertainty Rights (YOUR) World Research, over three years (2016–2019), is part of an Economic and Social Research Council and Foreign and Commonwealth Office (ESRC-FCDO) Poverty Fund programme to find pathways out of poverty—for young people facing poverty and extreme processes of marginalisation and exclusion within fragile and conflict-affected societies. This chapter focuses on the initial project work of co-construction and co-production and approaches aiming to impact policy and practice in Nepal. The chapter discusses the co-constructed methodological approaches and emerging findings produced from the research in post-conflict Nepal. The three research sites: the streets and slums of Kathmandu; the environmentally fragile earthquake-affected area of Sindhupalchowk; and Kapilvastu on the Plains, highly affected by the armed conflict (1996–2006) and later by communal riots (2007), and where fear of retaliatory violence remains high.

This chapter provides an outline of the key Nepal context, including diversity, conflict, change, inequalities and the circumstances of young people, as background to a focus on the research production and intended policy impact processes. The fundamental methodological approach has been co-construction by and through a national research team based in Kathmandu and marginalised children and young people in the research locations. Creative visual, mobile and narrative methods developed and explored in the initial phases of facilitated co-construction were subsequently employed in the research production and impact phases. This approach has been the key to understanding the core concepts and perspectives of marginalised young people about uncertainty in their complex lives. Some examples of emerging findings are provided, indicating the importance of the creative, participatory co-constructive approach in eliciting ideas on uncertainty and resulting actions taken by marginalised young people.

Nepal Context: People, Place and Change

Nepal has a varied geography and a diverse population. The land rises from southern plains bordering India, to the hills and the mountains of the Himalayas in the north bordering Tibet. The 26.5 million recorded people include 125 different caste/ethnic groups who speak 123 different languages (CBS, 2012). Nepal's history continues to influence a hierarchical social structure with differential access to economic, political and socio-cultural resources, the marginalisation of some groups and continuing inequalities (Chapagai, 2016). Exposing and addressing social inequalities, including legislation to address discrimination based on caste and religion and to help ensure equality and universal access (DoE, 2014), have been a feature of the post-conflict period.

The research in Nepal is conducted in four locations across three areas, selected to reflect key aspects of the contemporary context. The locations were chosen on the basis of having been affected by the previous conflict and are environmentally fragile or prone to disasters. Two locations are rural and two urban: one in part of Kathmandu, the urban capital; another in rural Sindhupalchowk, to the north, a principal site of the 2015 earthquake; and both a rural and an urban research site in the southern plains (Terai) in Kapilvastu. These locations are particularly impoverished (NPC, 2015) and show diversity in terms of, for example, religion and ethnic group (CBS, 2014), and so enable exploration of how different processes of marginalisation and vulnerabilities affect uncertainty among young people.

Change: Governance, Conflict and Disaster

Key aspects of the contemporary Nepal context are conflict aftermath, its resolution and the enactment of a new constitution, consequent changes in government and the post-earthquake situation. In addition to the processes of change arising in the period post conflict and earthquake, important factors are levels of poverty in different rural and urban environments, with a consequent high rate of national and international migration, and the hierarchical social structure including ethnic/caste and religious diversity. These add to uncertainties and the complexity of responses made by young people and their families and communities, as well as policy at national level.

The post-conflict peace-building process began following the overthrow of the monarch by a people's movement and the establishment of a Democratic Republic from 2008, with national elections in 2008 and 2013 (Tuladhar, 2014) and again in 2017 following the adoption of a new constitution. The process of disarmament, demobilisation and reintegration included integration of armed forces of rebel groups into the Nepal Army (Subedi, 2013). A new constitution was promulgated through a Constituent Assembly as part of a Comprehensive Peace Agreement. However, several disgruntled and armed groups continued to operate under the cover of political parties in several parts of the country threatening national security (UN, 2010). Elections held under the new constitution at the end of 2017 led to a new government, but the situation lacks stability, among ongoing political and policy change.

The conflict context is particularly significant for youth. Many young people face circumstances of uncertainty because of political conflict and the recent governance vacuum, coupled with lack of employment opportunities, which has led to high migration rate from rural to urban areas and abroad (British Council and AYON, 2011). Young people were at the core of the conflict, both as perpetuator of human rights and as victims of civil war (Gupta et al., 2011); among the 19,000 Maoist combatants, approximately 3000 were identified as minors (below 18 years of age) during the verification process (NIPS, 2013). A culture of impunity developed, with an increased crime rate through former youth combatants who became criminals and got political protection (The Carter Centre, 2011).

The major earthquake of 2015 damaged and destroyed buildings, including houses built with their savings by migrants returned from work abroad (NPC, 2015). Although by late 2016 the local situation was seen as becoming normal, the work of the National Reconstruction Authority had been delayed due to the fragile post-conflict political environment (Awale, 2016). This led to frustration and distrust towards government as a result of delay in responding to reconstruction needs (The National, 2016). Local employment opportunities were created but in practice only provided work for a small number of skilled personnel (Wendelbo et al., 2016). Meanwhile, family livelihood mechanisms were broken due to earthquake, which resulted in more young people likely to migrate out from their home (Randolph & Agarwal, 2017). Although some policies and programmes were developed to address the needs of youth, the lack of effective implementation meant they were not able to retain young people in their own surroundings. Women and girls were found to be more severely affected by earthquake compared to male counterparts (CDPS et al., 2015).

Co-construction Approaches and Methodologies

The methodology for the YOUR World Research aims to co-construct processes of engagement between researchers, national and local agencies, marginalised young people and adult representatives of communities; and for the findings, experiences, ideas and issues subsequently produced to have impact on policy through further engagement of young people with agencies and policymakers in processes for co-production of appropriate and relevant solutions. The method involves a principal investigator (PI), co-investigator (CI) and research officer based in the UK, national research teams in both Ethiopia and Nepal, partnerships with national and local agencies, reference groups involving policymakers from the outset of the project and marginalised young people drawn from poorer communities in urban and rural locations.

A framework for core approaches of co-construction was established, and a set of creative methods, including visual and mobile methods, subsequently co-constructed through piloting in situ; detailed processes for co-production of analysis and subsequent engagement of young people, researchers, agencies and policymakers on findings, ideas and solutions are underway at the time of writing—national seminar processes are planned in each country, as part of the key project aims for impacting policy and practice.

The Framework

YOUR World Research is phased, and this chapter concentrates on the initial phase from which the rest of the large-scale qualitative case study research emerged. This phase involved workshops with marginalised youth held in all of the proposed research sites. These were designed to be open and explore how to talk about uncertainty with young people and what methods they would most enjoy to explore uncertainty in the different aspects of their lives. The national teams from Ethiopia and Nepal tested different ideas using visual and mobile methods, and developed creative ways of understanding and analysing uncertainty with marginalised youth. This initial phase was based on a youth-centred approach to research using Johnson's Change-scape (see Johnson, 2011, 2017); this builds on young people's ideas and takes into account their degrees of inclusion and their multiple and shifting identities. It also connects research with youth to the context in which the research is taking place, so that methods are adapted to political, physical and cultural context and that the research plan incorporates spaces for young people to communicate with researchers to co-construct and with decision-makers to influence analysis, policy and practice. For example, youth workshops in the initial phases helped the research team develop plans for design of detailed case studies, and the national youth seminars to be held at the end of the three years.

The research also utilises concepts of 'Living Rights' from the reconceptualisation of child rights in international development (Hanson & Nieuwenhuys, 2013). This helps to understand rights for young people not just as universal rights in international agreements but rights that need to be translated into how they can be realised in their complex realities in very different global cultural and political contexts. Bauman's (2001) ideas about community and insecurity helped YOUR World researchers understand how youth may seek uncertainty in a positive sense by pursuing new social bonds and breakaway from more traditional bonds, relationships and expectations within communities.

Researchers' Roles and Reflexivity

Having a mix of national researchers who have come predominantly from non-governmental practitioner backgrounds in Nepal and academic institutions in Ethiopia has provided grounds for reflection in the full international team meetings. Skills-training has been facilitated by having full team meetings where those with academic research training emphasise the importance of open interviewing with rigorous note taking, recording and detailed analysis of complex qualitative findings, whilst those with practitioner backgrounds can facilitate sharing on pathways to impact and developing academic–non-academic partnerships. Johnson (PI) and West (CI) as lead researchers have set up a structure whereby there is national leadership in teams, national research assistants and PhD students. Full team meetings provide sharing and skills development between team members and joint reflexive learning across countries.

During the full team initial review meeting, the detailed case study phase of the research was co-constructed across national teams from the participatory research undertaken with marginalised youth. In the full team analysis meeting, a framework for thematic analysis was agreed and key themes discussed and elaborated through intensive comparative debate across the team. Ensuring and producing impact for the project was also discussed and further work with policymakers and practitioners planned. Individual stories from team members provided initial indications on how the researchers themselves had learnt from the process of sharing. For example, two team members had migrated and become street connected, working to develop their education and eventually becoming charity organisation staff and lecturers and successfully applying and joining the YOUR World Research team. To co-produce policy and practice impact, the team have worked consistently with policymakers and service providers from non-governmental partners and government ministries with various responsibilities for youth, and a national youth seminar is planned for the final stages of the project. This will actively engage young people to further develop action towards changes they feel necessary to support their pathways out of poverty.

National Partners

National non-governmental partners have been important in making the research meaningful and impactful at a local and national level. Partners are also critical in helping research teams to identify and access the most marginalised young people, and in ensuring ethical protocols and procedures were robust and included referral to appropriate local services when sensitive issues were raised such as abuse or criminal activity. In some locations the partners also helped with local languages spoken by the most marginalised and other necessary logistical support. National partners in Nepal (ActionAid Nepal and CERID, Research Centre for Educational Innovation and Development at Tribhuvan University) and in Ethiopia (CHADET Organisation for Child Development and Transformation and Addis Ababa University) also help connect the project to local and national decision-makers and service providers. For example, CERID at Tribhuvan University is organising eight dialogue sessions on various themes every month to discuss issues of marginalised youth with academicians, policymakers and practitioners in relevant fields of work.

Youth in Nepal

The National Youth Policy 2010 is the first instance where any policy in Nepal has spelled out a clear definition of youth in terms of age. It categorises young people as those aged 16–40 years, including males and females and the 'third gender'. Conflict and migration appear to have affected this youth population profile. According to the 2011 Census, the total youth population, 16–40 years age group, in Nepal is 10,689,842 (40.3% of the total population), but of these over 54% are female (CBS, 2012). However, the young people in YOUR World Research are those identified aged 15–24 years (following the UN definition on youth) in order to understand changing transitions from childhood (under 18 years as defined in the United Nations Convention on the Rights of the Child (UNCRC), 1989) and early adulthood. The child and youth population in Nepal is growing: in 2011 there were 6.4 million adolescents aged 10–19, nearly a quarter (24%) of the total population, an increase of one million for this age group since the census of 2001 (CBS, 2012).

Major issues affecting young people include: early marriage—37% of girls marry before age 18 and 10% by age 15 (Human Rights Watch, 2016); education—of 1.3 million children enrolled in Grade 1 in 2003, only 30% succeeded to reach Grade 10 in 2012, and of these, only 47% passed school leaving certificate, the majority of unsuccessful cases skewed towards the rural poor, and many Dalit not progressing (DoE, 2015); unemployment, underemployment and migration—nearly 1.5 million youth found to be abroad for employment and education (MoYS, 2014). A 2010 report suggested there is direct relationship between low levels of education, participation and employment and the risk of violent conflict (DFID-CSO, 2010).

Youth movements have also been significant. Resources were captured by political groups in the name of youth wings. The youth population has always been the driving force behind major political shifts including the change to a republican and secular nation. But when political change has been achieved, government has remained passive in institutionalising the potential of youth (Gupta et al., 2011).

Youth Co-construction: Marginalisation and Methods

The overall methodology is interpretivist in epistemology but combines aspects of more participatory and less participatory qualitative research approaches in working with 500 young people and around 150 adults and policymakers in each country. It is a larger scale qualitative case study impact project combining participatory co-construction and action research with marginalised young people leading to youth engagement with decision-makers at national seminars. It builds on Johnson's and West's previous participatory research with marginalised children and young people (e.g. Johnson & West, 2018, Johnson, 2018, Johnson et al., 2014a and b; also see the development of participatory techniques with children, e.g. O'Kane, 2000). ActionAid Nepal is familiar with employing participatory appraisal in their ongoing programme work and in detailed research with children (Johnson et al., 1995). However, unlike participatory appraisal in programme work, the visual and mobile methods used in YOUR World Research were not initially action-orientated or intended to reach consensus on how to move forward. Instead the methods used were open and flexible in order to construct new knowledge about the complex realities of youth, and build an understanding of changes over time, that are important in impacting policy and practice. This knowledge and understanding is derived from rigorous and detailed analysis across case studies in different parts of the country, with young people who express different, multiple and shifting identities. During a process of gaining informed consent, youth profiles were also captured in order to ensure analysis could be linked to different aspects of young people's identity and marginalisation including, for example, age, gender, ethnicity and caste, family and living situation and experiences of working, education and migration.

Marginalised Youth

The Government of Nepal has a particular conception of who is marginalised, as indicated below, which can be understood largely as by caste and ethnicity alongside economic poverty and remote location. Although the project partners and team initially defined marginalisation by following government understanding of this term, the researchers soon felt that there was a need to broaden out in order to work with the poorest, most excluded and vulnerable: to understand marginalisation not only by caste, extreme poverty and location but also by experience, disruption and crisis in personal lives and communities and by young people being excluded by not feeling included as they developed their communities and established relationships with their peers.

The National Youth Policy identifies six categories of youth who are marginalised or vulnerable or priorities, a categorisation that reflects issues of social hierarchy, diversity, inequalities and recent political change. These categories are:

1. Priority Group—women, indigenous nationalities, *Dalit, Madhesi* or youth living in undeveloped regions;
2. Special Priority Group—youths who are victims of conflict, vulnerable, disabled or members of marginalised minority groups;
3. Youth Victims of Conflict—who belong to those victim families who have died, who have been disabled and who have been displaced because of the ten-year armed conflict;
4. Vulnerable Youth—who are infected with HIV/AIDS, who are narcotic drug users, who are involved in the sex trade, youths living in the streets, youth who belong to bonded-labour families and youth who are involved in foreign employment in countries of unsafe destination;
5. Youth with Disabilities—youth with all kinds of physical and mental disabilities;
6. Youth of Marginalised Minority Groups—youth who are deprived of state and non-state services and facilities, who are marginalised and who remain out of the mainstream of national development because of geographical remoteness or because of ethnicity, language, culture, region, class and gender (MoYS, 2010).

In the first phases of YOUR World Research, partners identified poor areas and the Nepal team worked in local schools and organisations and with smaller groups of young people working on rural farms and urban streets. From this initial engagement, young women and men who are not in school were generally regarded as being more marginalised, and those young people who are not attached to any organisation regarded as being more alone and excluded. The research team therefore worked with this initial purposive sample of youth to snowball out to other young people by asking them who were the most marginalised and where would we find them.

Young people themselves helped the research team to define who they felt was or was not marginalised. This co-construction of 'marginalisation' was part of the methodology and research process, and so also an aspect of findings. So this research includes processes of marginalisation that incorporate young people's experiences of abuse and feelings of belonging or exclusion as they develop their identities, and feel they do or do not fit into the social norms and traditional expectations of their communities. Young people express their feelings of exclusion in their shifting and multiple identities. In this project, this included young people's sexual identities as third gender, a refusal to follow beliefs about what they should or shouldn't do during menstruation, a reluctance of girls to accept their expected, often early, marriages or accept gender discrimination to forgo their education in order to work for the household. Young men and women felt they could not always meet their own aspirations or the expectations of adults in their households to follow older conventional practice and stay at home to look after their families while there were better life chances and paths out of poverty for their families if they migrated to the cities and then abroad for work. Even if they risked not being paid or being in situations of modern slavery, some saw little option, in both fragile and conflict-affected areas of Nepal, to get the education they need or obtain work beyond being street connected and earning little money.

Marginalised Youth and the Use of Creative Visual and Mobile Methods

Understanding the lives of marginalised young people, and production of knowledge about their circumstances, expectations, aspirations and ideas, used a range of creative visual and mobile methods. These methods were piloted and co-constructed, aiming to be engaging with young people and suit their time, interests and creativity, whilst also being robust, consistent and rigorous in terms of research in order for the findings and statements produced to have the credibility necessary in current conditions for impacting policy in. This section provides examples of methods and co-construction and some of the experiences of young people emerging.

Roads and Rivers of Life/Timeline: Growing up and Transitions

In order to understand youth transitions as they grow up, how they see their journeys to where they are now and future pathways out of poverty and exclusion, young men, women and young people of the third gender were asked to draw their road or river of life. This method has been used quite extensively in the global south (e.g. in Nairobi with street-connected girls; Johnson et al., 2015) and the global north (e.g. in the UK with the YWCA and youth not in employment, education or training; Johnson & Percy Smith, 2007). This method is effective and fun for young people. They can, for example, represent trouble in their journeys by drawing crocodiles or rapids in the rivers or a bumpy road, and positive aspects with bridges or traffic signs/directions. It provides an opening for discussion rather than an end in itself, but can also help in larger scale work if positive and negative aspects of growing up/transitions are recorded systematically on the visual with the young person so through analysis it can be compared with other youth within the same context and from other places.

This method was piloted in the research location heavily affected by earthquake, Sindhupalchowk, with youth excluded from school because of their household work and paid labour. It was found to help not only talking about young people's experiences growing up but also about their positive and/or negative feelings of uncertainty at moments of their lives when they didn't know what was going to happen. Examples included: experiences of insecurity and uncertainty during the earthquake crisis, when many turned the experience into a positive opportunity by helping out with reconstruction alongside youth movements across the country; or when one young woman was going to marry and felt excited but also some apprehension; or when migrating with often positive feelings of potential creativity and fulfilment to find a different future and to leave their difficult working lives in more remote mountainous areas.

This method is being used across all eight case study areas in Nepal and Ethiopia because young people enjoyed it, and it provided meaningful individual evidence about complex and changing transitions. In other places it was found that, with some marginalised young people, such as street-connected children, this method was complex for them to represent all their thoughts and experiences in symbols on the paper. The process was changed to 'free drawing' so they instead drew whatever they wanted to tell the story of their growing up, and used these as the basis of explanations and discussions with the researchers.

Place and Space: Insecurity and Uncertainty Mapping, Mobility Mapping and Youth-Led Walks

Another method piloted in Sindhupalchowk was participatory mapping, where differences between mapping for programme action and mapping for broader perspectives became apparent. At first researchers used a mapping technique similar to what they had used in the earthquake reconstruction. This technique, used by ActionAid partners, aimed to get fairly accurate mapping of location and particular changes in remote areas from local people's view. Instead, YOUR World Research used much more open community mapping, also widely practised in participatory research: rather than getting an 'accurate' map of an area, it was critical to understand different perspectives on places and spaces which young people inhabit. Groups of young women and young men drew maps and then discussed with researchers their feelings about safety/security/insecurity and their feelings about uncertainty. An example of insecurity in this rural earthquake-affected area was the forests where girls did not walk in case of attack, or areas that were still unstable due to the earthquake. An example of uncertainty was the river which may or may not flood in different seasons and would affect the local livelihoods and mobility. This method changed in the Ethiopia co-construction phase, where young people drew maps and led 'youth-led walks' (see below). They used local materials to construct physical maps rather than use pens/paper to discuss migration for work.

Mobility diagrams were tested with groups of young people in Kathmandu to help understand migration and mobility for work and education. Many youth migrate from rural to urban areas in search of work, and some for education. Instead of a map this method uses connected lines to discuss different locations for mobility and migration, journeys taken and feelings about experiences. Again, these can be drawn on paper or created using physical objects and connecting them with sticks or string so that young people can move them around and discuss their journeys and stories. (Also see Johnson et al., 2014a and 2014b.) (Fig. 21.1).

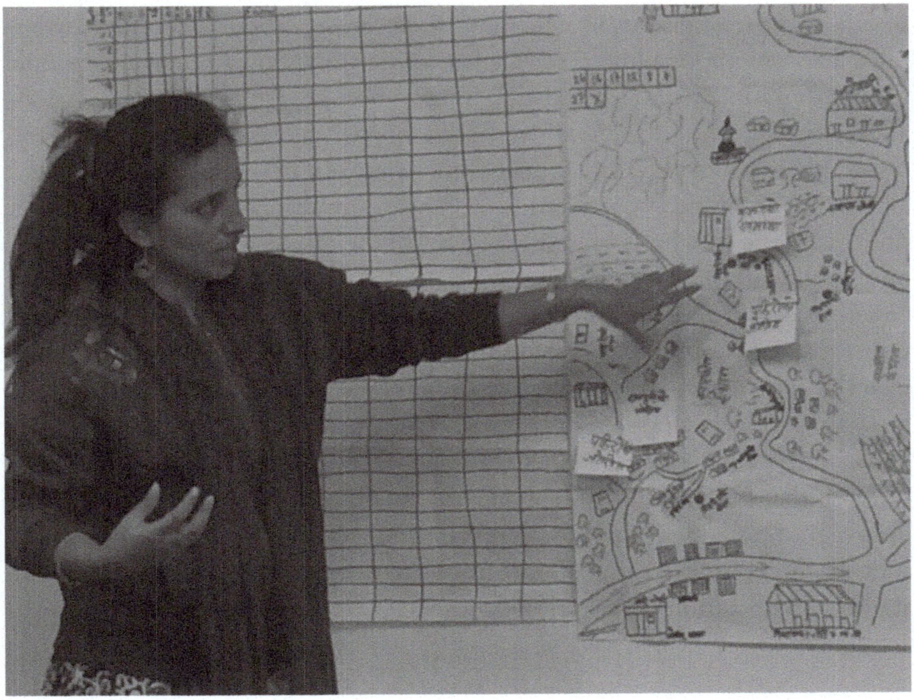

Fig. 21.1 Nepalese researcher presenting research to the National Reference Group

An interactive and popular method has been the youth-led walks, especially in the urban research sites. These were piloted in Kathmandu and then in Addis Ababa. Young people are in control of where they take researchers and it was an effective way for them to discuss issues of uncertainty in the places where they live and in their lives. Young people can also direct which photos are taken of their local environment and narrate stories about their experiences in different locations.

In Kathmandu young women expressed concern about travelling through wooded areas to reach the temple and also discussed abuse they had experienced at the bus terminal. In Addis young men took researchers to the railway bridge where they slept and worked to set up temporary toilets—they discussed how they embraced uncertainty and wanted to migrate to work in 'the gulf' as their only certainty is poverty (Johnson et al., 2021).

Relationships, Autonomy and Support

Different visual and photo methods were developed with young people in Kapilvastu to understand their feelings about their roles and relationships in families and communities. Methods included support network diagrams, photos and presentations to talk about their feelings about rights and autonomy. These methods allowed the team to understand how some young people in the community, who had existing links to non-governmental organisations and who were going to school, were seen by peers as being less marginal and more able to access their rights. Those that were out of school and doing hard labour, for example, were identified as being more marginalised. A greater understanding of who is marginalised, and how to access and work with out of school, working and migrating young people, was developed in this initial co-construction and piloting phase of the research. More detail on youth relationships and support was also an important part of YOUR World Research into the experiences and feelings of young people of the third gender as they grow up and seek support.

This aspect of young people's complex lives requires focused and action research that is creative and imaginative. The next phases of research will dig deeper into processes of youth marginalisation and on initial findings which suggest young people gain support from peers, are tending to question more traditional transitions to adulthood and seek to change social norms.

Co-production: Youth and Migration

The co-construction experience from Nepal was combined with that of Ethiopia to plan the next phases of the project so that larger-scale comparative research could be conducted and produced with the most marginalised youth, as identified by young people. This section presents some emerging findings produced in early phases of research in earthquake-affected Sindhupalchowk. Those presented here mainly concern migration, which was a large feature of youth discussions. Quotes are from interviews from the 'rivers and roads' that young people drew about their lives since the earthquake and their futures (Fig. 21.2).

Preliminary emerging findings from young people include issues around dreams and aspirations, changing perceptions of social norms, values and practices, and problems of alcohol, violence and discrimination, as well as concerns about education and employment. All of these issues are interconnected in various ways, and individual young people highlight aspects from their perspectives. For example, many of the tensions can be illustrated in experiences around migration, such as overt and underlying reasons for

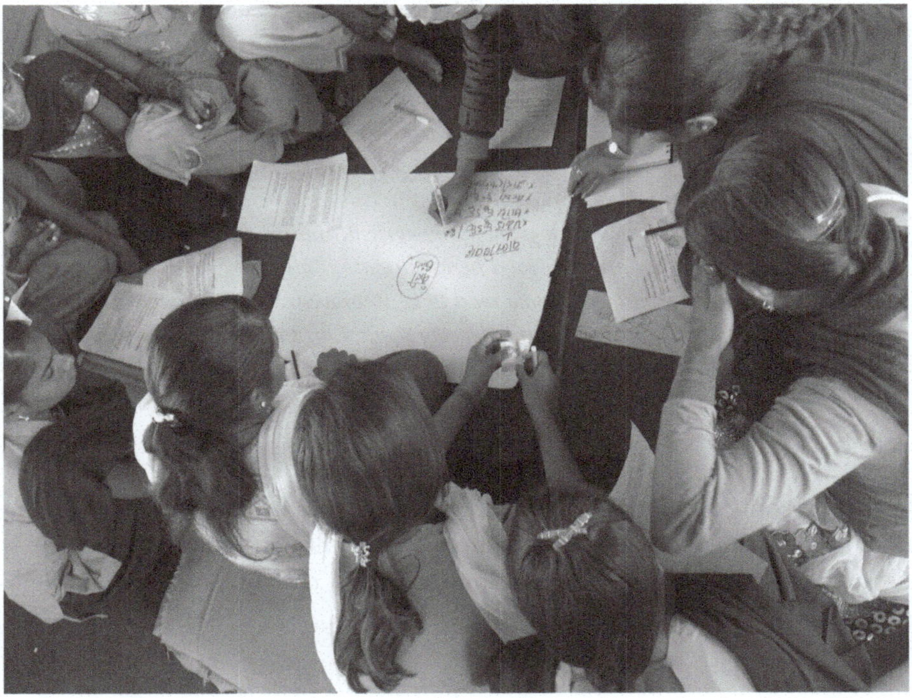

Fig. 21.2 Co-production with young people

departure. One 16-year-old young woman in Sindhupalchowk explained concerns about domestic violence exacerbated by alcohol as contributing to migration: "*When my father comes home being drunk, I feel very scared and I think that is why my elder sister went to Dubai for work.*"

It is particularly noticeable how many young people and their families see migration out of the country as a shorter-term solution to building their future in their own communities. The earthquake in Sindhupalchowk was a crisis that pushed local youth into feeling that working abroad is their only solution although many cannot find the money to travel and feel fairly desperate.

> *Most painful time in my life is now, especially this year. I have a small baby and a wife to feed in my family. I am living in a small wooden hut. I want to build a house but there is no support from the family. I do not have decent job. No organisation wants to help me. They said I cannot get support from the government also because I separated from the family before earthquake. I want to go abroad for work, but I have no money even to go abroad.* (Resham, young man, 20 years)

When young people do migrate, it does not always work out and their journeys and experiences are not always positive as we can see from Man Bahadur's cousin below. Some young people feel that if they had support in making the area more accessible then they would like to stay in their area.

> *My cousin has gone to Saudi thinking of earning more, but he is not doing good. He could not even pay off his loan that he took to go to Saudi. He does not have money to come back. So we have raised some money to send to him. He is going to come back soon and will stay here. If you do hard work, you can earn here, too.*
>
> *Our place is very good. We can grow many agricultural products, like cardamom, orange, and coffee. They are very good here. Climate is also very good, not too cold not too hot to live. We just need some road to be improved. We have to work hard to coordinate the fundraising process and develop roads. Our soil has some problems due to chemical fertilisers and some agricultural products are affected with disease. This is frustrating. If we can take care of those, this is best place.* (Man Bahadur, young man, 24 years)

It is not only males that migrate, but also females for domestic work. This does not only involve youth but their parents, resulting in transnational families and lack of contact between mothers and daughters except through social media.

> *My mum went to Kuwait when I was 8 years old. She came back to Nepal after 9 years when I was about to leave for Kuwait. We met for 16 days and she went to*

> *Lebanon and I went to Kuwait. Then we talk and get to know her better when the employers let me use the internet and we used to skype each other. Now we are meeting face to face after 16 years. She is now with us on her 4-month leave.* (Kuntee, young woman, 22 years)

For those left behind, who do not migrate, life can be hard tending to homes and farms; especially girls and young women do not have access to education or drop out of school and feel powerless to take control of their lives.

> *My father died when I was about 9–10 months old. I have three older sisters. Two of my sisters are already working in foreign countries—eldest one in Kuwait and the second one in India. The third one is preparing to go abroad for work. When I was 13 years old and studying in 8th grade, my mum was sick with gall stone. She was taken to Kathmandu hospital for treatment. Then I was left alone at home with cattle. I have to look after the house, farm and cattle and go to school, which was a great pressure for me.* (Chenga, young woman, 18 years)

> *We were very poor when I was a child. We have no property, and my parents were working for others and staying in other people's land. My elder brother went to Malaysia but returned due to earthquake in Nepal. My younger brother went to India looking for job and he is still there. My mum went to Kuwait for work when I was 8 years old. I was left alone with my father at home and was responsible taking care of all household chores. When I was studying in grade 8th, I had much homework given by school, but no time to do it at home. I had to use my recess time to do my homework. As the school was far, I have to walk more than an hour there and hour back. The school closes at 4 p.m. when I reach home it is more than 5 p.m. In the winter time, it gets dark soon. I have to take care of cattle, as well as other household chores. This has made my life quite difficult. When I am in the class, I think of household chores and when I am at home, I worry about the homework. I could not cope with this so I quitted the school, although my family and relatives were advising me not to quit.* (Kuntee, young woman, 22)

Individual young people of varied age, gender and caste/ethnicity are responding to crisis in different ways, but pressure seems to be increasing for youth to travel out of rural areas for both education beyond primary level and employment. In Nepal many seem to want to come back to invest in their family homes in the hills, although YOUR World is continuing to research the changing relationships and experiences that young people have pre-, during and post-migration. In Ethiopia many young people also migrate to cities from drought and conflict-affected areas of the country and then to gulf states from what they see as a certainty of poverty on the streets (see Johnson et al., 2021).

Conclusion

The creative methodology for YOUR World Research has been co-constructed with national teams of researchers and marginalised youth from Nepal and Ethiopia. As part of the process, particularly to engage concerned sectors, practice and policymakers, further partnership with national non-government organisations (NGOs) and universities was embedded into the design of the programme. The relationship with national NGOs, ActionAid Nepal and CHADET in Ethiopia means that, on the one hand, researchers can access, engage and ensure follow up with some of the most marginalised and vulnerable youth affected, and understand how structural inequalities intersect with their feelings about uncertainty with regard to their transitions growing up, the fragility of their local environments and conflict situations. In addition, partnerships with national universities, Tribhuvan University in Nepal and Addis Ababa in Ethiopia, mean that the team interacts with seminar programmes and national and regional discourses around youth, poverty and the changing political and cultural context. On the other hand, partnerships through national reference groups engage with national policymakers and practitioners, including government, with possibilities for youth influence and impact on policy. The national teams and partners helped to build up national reference groups and interactions with policymakers and service providers so that the research feeds directly into and can influence practical programme interventions and policy debates in both countries. The international team including the PI and Co-I (Johnson and West) initiate innovative and creative cross team processes, support and mentor national implementation of the co-constructed research, working also with partners to ensure systematic, rigorous and comparative research processes and dissemination of findings produced. This co-construction and co-production of processes and findings aims to work with and influence policymaker discussions nationally and have impact internationally.

There are always challenges relating to how participatory research processes can be when scaled up and have policy and practice impact. This large-scale qualitative methodology has been designed in order to contribute to new knowledge about uncertainty in the complex lives of young people and how this interplays with their shifting and multiple identities and rapidly changing and challenging contexts, but it is also important to the researchers that it influences policy and practice to improve the lives of some of the most marginalised and vulnerable youth.

There is often a trade-off between understanding complexity using creative methods and the politics of evidence (Johnson, 2017). People in positions of power may need to see that evidence is coming from sufficient numbers of young people to warrant a change in national policy, and with this in mind the project aims to ensure robust and rigorous qualitative methods but also involve several hundred young people in each country not only to demonstrate complexities, but also common themes and strands of experience, and for youth to engage with agencies and government.

By phasing the research and beginning with a phase of co-construction YOUR World has attempted to start from the perspectives of youth even in designing the larger scale qualitative interviews for the comparative case study research. Later phases also engage with youth with visual, moving and creative methods, to gain details on solution and action-orientated ideas. The planned national youth seminar aims for young people to verify the analysis in the YOUR World Research process and also to directly engage with policymakers. The planned national youth seminar will be held with key partners and government ministries to impact policy and practice, so that pathways out of poverty are based on the realities of young people's strategies to navigate uncertainty and improve their lives.

References

Awale, S. (2016, June 27). Delays continue to plague NRA performance. *The Himalayan Times*. https://thehimalayantimes.com/kathmandu/delays-continue-plague-nra-performance/

Bauman, Z. (2001). *Community: Seeking safety in an insecure world*. Polity Press.

British Council and AYON. (2011). *Youth survey of Nepal*. British Council in Association with Association of Youth Organisations Nepal.

CBS. (2014). *National population and housing census 2011 (village development committee/municipality), SINDHUPALCHOWK*. Government of Nepal, National Planning Commission Secretariat, Central Bureau of Statistics.

CBS (Central Bureau of Statistics). (2012). *National Population and housing census 201*. Government of Nepal, National Planning Commission Secretariat, Central Bureau of Statistics.

CDPS, MoPE, UNFPA, & IOM. (2015). *Highlights from Nepal earthquake 2015: A socio-demographic impact study (with reference to the 14 most affected districts)*. Kathmandu: Central Department of Population Studies (CDPS), Tribhuvan University for the Ministry of Population and Environment (MoPE) with support from the United Nations Population Fund (UNFPA) and the International Organization for Migration (IOM).

Chapagai, R. P. (2016). State *accountability for ESCR in Constitution of Nepal: An overview. Reflections on participatory democracy: With reference to Constitution of Nepal.* Kathmandu: Institute for Governance and Development (IGD) and ActionAid Nepal.

DFID-CSO. (2010). *Youth participation in development: A guide for donor agencies and policy advisors.* DFID-CSO Youth Working Group.

DoE (Department of Education). (2014). *Consolidated equity strategy for the school education sector in Nepal.* Government of Nepal, Ministry of Education, Department of Education.

DoE (Department of Education). (2015). *Flash I report 2072 (2015–2016).* Government of Nepal, Ministry of Education, Department of Education.

Gupta, P., Kumar, R., & Katwal, S. (2011). *National Youth Policy, 2010: Evolution, definition and implementation.* Retrieved February 26, 2018, from http://www.youthpolicy.org/national/Nepal_2011_Youth_Policy_Paper.pdf

Hanson, K., & Nieuwenhuys, O. (Eds.). (2013). *Reconceptualizing children's rights in international development: Living rights, social justice and translations.* Cambridge University Press.

Human Rights Watch. (2016). Our time to sing and play. In *Child marriage in Nepal.* Human Rights Watch.

Johnson, V. (2011). Conditions for change for children and young people's participation in evaluation: 'Change-scape'. *Child Indicators Research, 4*(4), 577–596.

Johnson, V. (2017). Moving beyond voice in children and young people's participation. *Action Research, Special Issue: Development Aid and Social Transformation, 15*(1), 104–124.

Johnson, V. (2018). Hesitating at the door: Youth-led research on realizing sexual rights informing organizational approaches. In C. Morris, A. Cornwall, P. Boyce, L. Harvey, & Y. Huang (Eds.), *Researching sex and sexualities: Methodological reflections.* Routledge.

Johnson, V., & Percy Smith, B. (2007). *Give us a chance! Young people's reflections on work choices and support.* Oxford: YWCA, cited in Waldren, J. and Kaminski, I-M. (2012). *Learning from the children: Childhood, culture and identity in a changing world.* Oxford: Berghahn Books.

Johnson, V., & West, A. (2018). *Children's participation in global contexts: Beyond voice.* Routledge.

Johnson, V., Hill, J., & Ivan-Smith, E. (1995). *Listening to smaller voices: Children in an environment of change.* ActionAid.

Johnson, V., Getu, M., Getachew, M., Ahmed, A. and West, A. (2021), 'Trapped Bodies, Moving Minds: Case Study Research on Uncertainty, Place and Migration with Marginalised Youth in Ethiopia', Children and Society, Wiley-Blackwell

Johnson, V., Hart, R., & Colwell, J. (Eds.). (2014a). *Steps to engaging young children in research: The guide.* The Bernard van Leer Foundation.

Johnson, V., Hart, R., & Colwell, J. (Eds.). (2014b). *Steps to engaging young children in research: The toolkit.* The Bernard van Leer Foundation.

Johnson, V., Johnson, L., Magati, B. O., Kiwanuka, A., & Walker, D. (2015). *UNGEI case study summary: The role of girls' education in Pendekezo Letu's interventions in Nairobi*. UNGEI.
MoYS (Ministry of Youth and Sports). (2010). *National youth policy 2010*. Ministry of Youth and Sports.
MoYS (Ministry of Youth and Sports). (2014). *Nepal youth in figures*. Government of Nepal, Ministry of Youth and Sports, the United Nations Population Fund and Restless Development.
NIPS (Nepal Institute for Policy Studies). (2013, July). Nepal's peace process: A brief overview. *Policy Paper*, Issue 1, Vol. 8. Kathmandu: Nepal Institute for Policy Studies.
NPC (Nepal Planning Commission). (2015*). Nepal earthquake 2015: Post disaster needs assessment, Vol. A: Key findings.* : Government of Nepal National Planning Commission.
O'Kane, C. (2000). The development of participatory techniques: Facilitating children's views about decisions which affect them. In P. Christensen & A. James (Eds.), *Research with children: Perspectives and practices* (pp. 136–159). Routledge/Falmer.
Randolph, G., & Agarwal, P. (2017). *Rebuilding Nepal: Creating good jobs amid reconstruction and migration*. New Delhi/Washington, DC: JustJobs network Inc. April.
Subedi. (2013). War to peace transition in Nepal: Success and challenges ahead. *Small Wars Journal*. Retrieved February 26, 2018, from http://smallwarsjournal.com/jrnl/art/war-to-peace-transition-in-nepalsuccess-and-challenges-ahead
The Carter Centre. (2011). Carter Center: Clashes between political party youth wings have decreased but YCL and UML youth force continue to seek financial gain. February 28, 2011, for immediate release. Retrieved February 26, 2018, from https://www.cartercenter.org/resources/pdfs/news/peace_publications/democracy/nepal-political-party-youth-wings-022811-en.pdf
The National. (2016, April 24). Nepal marks one year since quake as frustration mounts: Some four million survivors are still living in temporary shelters one year on, with frustration against the government mounting. *The National*, Retrieved February 26, 2018, from https://www.thenational.ae/world/nepal-marks-one-year-since-quake-as-frustration-mounts-1.138345
Tuladhar, P. R. (2014). A continuing transition. In *Development Advocate*, year 2 issue 3, December 2014–June 2015. Lalitpur: United Nations Development Programme (UNDP).
UN. (2010). Report of the Secretary-General on children and armed conflict in Nepal (S/2010/183).
UNCRC. (1989). *United Nations convention on the rights of the child*. UN.
Wendelbo, M., China, F. L., Dekeyser, H., Taccetti, L., Mori, S., Aggarwal, V., Alam, O., Savoldi, A., & Zielonka, R. (2016). *The crisis response to the Nepal earthquake: Lessons learned*. Research Paper May 2016. Belgium: European Institute for Asian Studies—EIAS a.s.b.l.

22

Finding Safety in Trauma Recovery at a South African State Care Centre for Abused and Neglected Youth

Sharon Johnson

Introduction

Key principles of love, acceptance and appreciation provide safety (Ziegler, 2018) for recovery from trauma for abused and neglected youth. This study considers the application of these principles in an education-managed male residential state care centre in Cape Town, South Africa (SA). Retrospective meaning-making (Chase, 2005) in categorical transcriptions of care (Schiff, 2017) utilise both text and photographs in various forms of narrative enquiry, from poetry and case studies to photo-elicitation.

Narrative strategies are descriptive tools to systematically examine people's lives to discover meaning. Sensitive, multifaceted and multicoloured portraits of sense develop fine-grained theories of human experiences, which are credible, useful and trustworthy (Schiff, 2017). By taking into account what people say and do in a particular context at a specific time, a transformed psychology of meaning emerges, creating a vision of the person in their social and cultural world (Schiff, 2017).

Love is considered a basic need, but is largely absent in the critical formative years of neglected and abused youth and is under-researched in psychology (Ziegler, 2018). In order to believe in traumatised children, it is necessary to look beyond the dysfunctional protective layers built up and, with love,

S. Johnson (✉)
Cornerstone Institute, Cape Town, South Africa

C. Walker et al. (eds.), *The Palgrave Handbook of Innovative Community and Clinical Psychologies*, https://doi.org/10.1007/978-3-030-71190-0_22

help them to access their higher selves. Love should provide a consistent and unwavering focus on what is best for the child (Ziegler, 2018).

Acceptance counteracts the negative experiences of youth being in state care, such as loneliness, rejection and being alone (Ziegler, 2018). With firmness and consistency, the adolescent starts to experience their needs being met. Acceptance through attachment involves a neurological brain change for children who have been neglected and abused, requiring "consistent hard work" (Ziegler, 2018, Kindle location 679) to help a troubled child head in a positive direction. Nurturing self-acceptance helps them discover who they are, rather than a focus on how they act.

Appreciation involves disaffirming negative thoughts and creating self-belief from disempowering past experiences (Johnson, 2019b). By meeting basic needs of care and safety, youth are able to consider higher aspects of self-development towards self-actualisation (Maslow, 1962). They appreciate their own abilities and the efforts of others to guide them towards their life goals.

This narrative research on finding safety in a community setting for trauma recovery with principles of love, acceptance and appreciation was considered on multiple levels: youth; teachers and carers; management and policymakers. A main question for the youth was: What has impacted your life at the centre? For the teachers and carers the focus was: How has work with maltreated children affected you and what are your notions of care? For management the question was: How have you survived threatened closure? Policymakers were asked: What are future directions for vulnerable children in SA?

Firstly, Reuben (16) introduces youth narratives with a love poem, followed by insights of 17-year-old Tlali's rebirth at the centre (Johnson, 2019d). Acceptance is studied through self-care narratives of teachers and carers in groups in participatory action research (PAR) (Johnson, 2019c). A legal narrative then examines the response of Mr M, the manager, who lost a legal battle for survival, and changing government policy for care and educational practices also shed light on acceptance. Finally, appreciation is then expressed through selected institutional photographs of the boys, with captioned interpretations, give visual care insights from a variety of participants, offering a different type of information in memories and feelings (Collier, 1957; Harper, 2002).

Photographs, selected in this study, provoke different emotions, feelings and insights, impacting older evolutionary parts of the brain than verbal expression. They are part of collective memories, enabling a participant to relate to events in which they may not have been directly involved.

Historic black and white photographs at the youth care and education centre (YCEC) therapeutic hostel were selected by staff from an archive of images to depict notions of appreciation, with handwritten descriptions of the meaning of these images. Black and white photographs are paradoxically more evocative than colour, creating an onrush of memories because more has been left out, challenging the imagination (Berger, cited by Harper, 2002).

Participants provided photofeedback of images depicting a range of scenes of youth engaging in institutional and outdoor activities in a variety of settings. Ethically, only photographs concealing the identity of the boys were deemed suitable, to ensure confidentiality. In the cases of possible identification, faces were blurred to guarantee anonymity. The question asked was: Which photograph best captures the meaning of care and how would you describe the importance of the activity?

All these insights add up to a variety of challenging community perspectives on providing safety for youth-at-risk in state care in violent, impoverished contexts. A trauma protocol for teachers and carers is being developed collaboratively with staff in high-risk schools for the provision of safety on multiple levels as a possible care resource going forward (Johnson, 2019a).

Background and Context

The YCEC is located on the Cape Flats, one of the most notorious areas of SA in terms of gangsterism, drug trafficking and violence. Established in 1948 as an industrial school for indigent, coloured youth (Badroodien, 2001), YCEC reflected the harsh history following on from slavery, apartheid, colonialism and discrimination. As a detention centre for justice boys who had committed crimes, it also accommodated neglected and abused youth from neighbouring impoverished communities, with no distinction being made between these different backgrounds.

Incarceration, corporal punishment and sexual abuse were features of punishing practices of former times (Johnson, 2019c). The centre recently lost a legal battle after years of a protracted court case, with their role for vulnerable youth being reconceptualised. They are emerging from former punitive practices into more enlightened restorative care, with safety for recovery on multiple levels becoming the focus for different types of trauma of staff and boys (such as historic, intergenerational, continuous, post-traumatic stress disorder, complex, secondary and vicarious traumas).

Three years of post-doctoral PAR research and two subsequent years of academic and consulting work involved a wide range of data collection—from conversations, interviews, experiential workshops, evaluation questionnaires, reflective writing and discussions to photographs, institutional records, emails, letters, WhatsApp messages and observation with different groups and individuals. Weekly, 10–30 men and women took part in a PAR open group out of 45 staff, teachers and interns (aged 20–70), responsible for the care of 70–80 boys (aged 11–18) in three hostels.

First Safety Principle: Love

Loving care took many forms at the YCEC, such as the manager's literal open door policy. Passing boys appeared at his outside door at all times of the day, receiving a piece of fruit or sweet, getting a hug and short greeting, encouraged to say what was on their minds. As researcher and consultant, I was mindful of the importance of modelling love through kindness and compassion, whilst acutely aware of differences, being a mature white woman from a privileged background. Some staff had been there for over 30 years. During apartheid, the institution was racially classified as coloured, but for 25 years since democracy it had become a melting pot of diversity, with boys from not only SA but all parts of Africa, representing many races, religions and cultures.

Reuben's Poem

I met Reuben (16) as an academic supervisor, observing two female undergraduate Psychology students in their fieldwork from a non-profit community college. He had nowhere to go in the school holidays, attending a group programme with ten others who also had no home or caregivers. During school these boys attended class, also gaining practical skills in workshops and participating in extra-mural outdoor activities. The students asked the boys to express themselves in poetry and/or rap.

> **"Love"**
> Love is just a word.
> Love is painful.
> It means something.
> It means nothing.
> It comes out of your heart.
> Love is true.
> Don't abuse it.
> Don't lose it.

Reuben stood up and self-consciously delivered this moving poem in a quiet room. Each boy listened intently, seemingly deeply touched by the pain and hope expressed. Some new arrivals were faced with many challenges—not knowing their birth date or age, unable to read or even write their name. Seated among them were adult visitors from a neighbouring Christian-based rehabilitation centre. They had come as mentors to assist the boys to leave the world of drugs, violence and crime.

Together the group began an exercise on goal setting. A visitor described his goals as getting married, being successful and giving up drugs and gangsterism. A participant, Antonio, who looked no older than ten, said his goal was to have a relationship with his mother, a reminder of the bitter, sweet love poem. The boys joked together as each spoke their truth. During conversation time Antonio approached a visitor and asked him how he could extricate himself from the gangs. They had given him six months to join and his time was up. He was likely to be shot if he went home. I watched the two in intense conversation, considering the power of restorative connection, as the visitor attempted to help the boy to transcend a violent and fearful world.

It was hard to identify these seemingly compliant, vulnerable and sensitive boys with those in teachers' reflections in my counselling wellness groups. They described students who refused to be seated in class, pacing the floor or jumping out of windows. I learnt of petty crimes as cell phones were stolen and lack of respect as youth swore at and hurled abuse at their carers. Not all staff agreed with restorative care, believing instead in harsh disciplinary measures involving punishment and violence, practised during apartheid. Youth were isolated then in detention cells and made to endure corporal punishment.

The educational psychologist explained the care metaphor of darkness versus light:

> As practitioners, conceptually that darkness is where we…find ourselves when we are under pressure, or egos are at risk, or power is being displayed. We venture back into those kinds of spaces that contaminate the light that we are trying to have here. The residual effect of that darkness is almost in your DNA and you have to keep a waking eye at the conscious level. Shadows are always lurking somewhere in us, and sometimes they can be overpowering when the ego is not strong.

In attempting to create safety, participants in the wellness groups developed a quiet inner peace and strength, sharing practices like journaling, mindfulness meditation, calming exercises and group sharing. This helped them to deal with their disruptive environment and model care to youth who did not seem capable of love and respect. By showing loving care to teachers, they were able to connect positively to boys in distress, providing a supportive relationship to those deprived of early attachment with a primary caregiver.

Tlali Found Love

Tlali, a 17-year-old Sotho from the rural Eastern Cape, had only been at the YCEC for 8 months when preparing to leave. In a short time, he felt that his life had turned around, ascribing change to meaningful connection. He felt loved by everyone who worked at the centre, and received respect, which he then modelled back to others. He contrasted his time at YCEC with being in a lock-up facility for boys in conflict with the law:

> There you see a leaf outside but you don't touch it—you live in a cement prison and you may connect to one or two people. Here you connect to everyone. You connect to people in the kitchen, in the garden. I can say you are in heaven. You get love everywhere. Even those people not working in the school, there by the gate, as part of security, they love you too!

Tlali had a dramatic life story of abusive and neglectful caregivers, including his mother, father, three step-mothers, aunt and grandmother and multiple homes, from his village to a township, dropping out of schools and suffering from substance addictions like glue, alcohol and drugs. He committed many crimes and by the age of 17 feared for his life. After being in different institutions, such as street shelters and a juvenile secure centre, he was sent to the YCEC, which he said turned his life around. Mr M, the manager, took a leap of faith in accepting Tlali, as the centre no longer shelters boys with criminal records. This is a remarkable story of transformation in a broader context of SA struggling to emerge from decades of exploitation and community disintegration from factors such as poverty, domestic and community violence, crime, substance abuse, discrimination, unemployment and illiteracy.

Tlali described his healing journey as being "pulled back" from criminal behaviour, with the care centre removing the uncontrollable anger within him. He reflected that he was most impacted by the love and respect he received. He admitted that loving experiences sometimes frightened him. He clapped his hands and described his transformation being like a "boom"; it was so dramatic and sudden.

"I came here and I talked to Colin (educational psychologist). He touched my heart and I started to change. What I saw outside, they use people to get something—like back in the days of slaves, they use you to get something. When I was in prison, they locked me up. The boys stay there too long; they are trouble, forming gangs. The teachers and carers protect those in the gangs.

"What I like about them here—even a carer who was an ex-American (gangster) boy—they pull you back…. He doesn't say I am not in his gang. They just give us love. Here many people play a part. What I saw the most, which scared me, was a person who was the father I wanted, the father who could understand me, who was true. This person, Mr X, is a unit manager. He said, "When I see this boy, he reminds me of myself. When I am angry or shout, he said: 'Don't pull your finger, don't be angry. Go to him and ask forgiveness and hold his hand and show him what kind of man you are.'"

"…They really give you love. They really change your life. That is what I like about this school….I want to be a good father. I would like to become a security guard….The centre is helping me….To be honest, what I want in life is to prove…that I have really changed."

He went on to describe his dramatic transformation:

"It was like a boom (clapping his hands). I never saw I had it. Mr M used to look at me and say: 'Tlali, don't worry about what happened in your life'. They coached me to let this meneer (person) see me. They steal a person's heart—they can take out the thing that is in me. They did that. Respect is a most important quality for helping boys. This is what I have experienced here, and what I saw in myself—I respect you because I want you to respect me. I respect you first."

Tlali's response to restorative care practices at YCEC reflected the focus of teachers and staff to develop an ethos of healing, with love and respect. Self-care took many forms, from teacher psychoeducation and training to wellness groups.

Second Safety Principle: Acceptance

YCEC teachers and support staff, like those in public schools, are trained in the Western Cape Education Department's (WCED's) Circle of Courage as a foundational attitude. Originating from research with Indian Americans (Brendtro et al., 2002), this philosophy aims to foster acceptance of youth by developing belonging, mastery, independence and generosity in young people for resilience and self-worth. However, gangsterism is rife in Cape Flats' schools, with a high drop-out rate (Plato, 2012), with youth suffering multiple effects from exposure to life traumas.

The focus of previous mixed-methods M and PhD research (Johnson, 2010, 2013, 2015; Johnson & Naidoo, 2013, 2016, 2017) was on interventions for teachers in high-risk schools, based on evolutionary brain responses to threat.

At the YCEC, a community psychology approach was taken, with a primary goal to assist teachers and staff to accept the youth, seeing them as survivors, with behaviours appropriate to manage their abusive and/or neglectful backgrounds. The centre's care goals focused on alleviating complex trauma symptoms, such as developing capacity for secure organisational attachments, overcoming developmental deficits and acquiring skills for emotional experiencing and self-regulation (Courtois & Ford, 2009).

Teachers and staff took charge of the PAR process, deciding on location, structure and content. Cycles of observation, reflection, planning and action took place over two years. Co-established self-care goals were to reduce self-reported stress and prevent burnout, assisting participants to deal with their greatest work stressor—disruptive learner behaviours. Staff gathered from all over the vast premises, connecting, sharing and relaxing. Multiple techniques were introduced, such as trauma release exercises for somatic destressing (Berceli, 2008) and psychoanalytic psychoeducation to understand the youth better (Canham, 2006). The teachers learnt about temperament and labels (MacGuire, 2008) and the benefit of living values in the classroom (Tillman, 2000).

Group structure and content changed according to participants' needs. Most sessions comprised a counselling support group of 90 minutes, with initial quiet time of 15–20 minutes of journal reflective writing and 15 minutes of mindfulness meditation. An extract from a teacher's reflective journal is: "I feel contented with myself not upsetting myself, and I listen, trying to listen to what others are telling me". Thereafter the group chose a physical activity, like Tai Chi (Cane, 2000), to physically destress, contextualising the movements to their issues.

Sometimes the group just sat in silence. Being a main form of communication, there could be multiple interpretations of silence and in the presence of others; it is always interactive (Haddock, cited in Schlapobersky, 2016). Sharing mostly involved feelings about the learners and responses to boys in the classroom; at other times participants spoke about personal stressors.

Reflections on Acceptance

Teachers struggled to respond to some youths' lack of self-worth: "One learner said: 'Why bother about me? I am rubbish; I come from nothing and I will be nothing.'" The calming, relaxation techniques and group discussions and support gave them tools to manage better. For example, the woodwork teacher explained in his journal:

> "Two weeks ago a learner, who was reluctant to co-operate in the workshop, was very upset because his wood for a project disappeared. He took a piece of wood and damaged other learners' projects. After I stopped him…he broke a bottle in the workshop. It made me very upset, but I calmed myself by taking very deep breaths and counting to 10. I explained to him that damaging other learners' projects won't solve the problem. I promised him I would recover his timber. He seemed to calm down a bit."

Teachers were able to model sharing in the group with the boys, taking practices learnt together into the classroom: "I try to encourage them and speak to them in such a way that they change their attitude for the best"; "The time I spend here I learn a lot, because the children can stress a person out"; "(I) feel good about myself"; "I am always thinking about what we did in sessions"; "I am thinking more of my actions".

A reformed former gangster, who was a hostel carer, described the impact of the self-care group sessions in a focus group reflection: he moved from punishment to care with the boys in his charge.

> "I just needed the sessions…to give me a wider understanding about where the boy comes from, what (do) they need in their lives and what (does) it mean(s) to be a child care worker.…So that programme changed my thinking and it changed my way of handling the boys.…I realised my boys were responding from the survival brain, coming from fear as a result of being oppressed and abused on the outside. (They were) sent here to be better—(they) don't need more oppression and abuse—they need love, compassion and care."

Court Battle

YCEC's future has been uncertain for years. After receiving ongoing closure notices from local government, it turned to the courts for protection. In 2014, the High Court ruled in its favour. This decision was later overturned at the Supreme Court of Appeal on the grounds that these centres fall under the jurisdiction of the provincial departments, who have decision-making powers. In addition, the court cautioned that it was not their place to intervene in such decisions (Minister of Social Development [DSD], 2016).

For Mr M, the principal and manager, strong attachment to boys in their care meant a commitment to acceptance, consistently being present despite the odds. His name means one who extracts, and when musing on the meaning he compared the ability to draw water out of stone with the seemingly impossible task of running a centre legally earmarked for closure.

> "My name being Moses means to take water out of stone. Perhaps I took (it) too seriously. My dad had difficulty in finding an appropriate name. He told my mum: 'With this one I need some guidance, so I trust the process'. My dad was a Sufi—saints and prophets practise through Quawali—in the one song he spoke about Nabi Moosa—and as those lines opened up, I got my name.
>
> "It's been forever that we have tried to be closed, but (it has been) formally since 2012. Prior to that, in the first round in 1995, we were also earmarked for closure and we were one of the schools that remained out of the 18. There were six that remained in early 2000 and now we are the only one—the only youth care centre grounded in an educational model.

When asked if he has come to terms with losing in the Supreme Court of Appeal and what it means for the future, he considers the benefits of the experience.

> "When you fight a very good fight in literally a David and Goliath type of way—the benefits that have accrued from this engagement with lawyers and the amazing support that we got from senior counsel really have been unbelievable. The fact that we have walked such a long path, and while all that has happened at a legal formal level, still to maintain the care paradigm and look at the rhythm and practice of the centre, and how we go about our duties—that to me is the major achievement."

He reflected on the uncertainty of the political times in SA. Having survived colonial domination and apartheid injustice, the struggle in the post-democratic era is one of diminishing resources, increasing demands and economic survival. He acknowledged the toll of the court case, including giving up his academic studies, but appreciated the experience's benefits. He connected his spirituality with fatalism and a belief that right things are happening at the right time. With a temporary order to remain open, the courts continue to send youth to YCEC's residential academic and therapeutic programmes.

> "I have to acknowledge that the court case did impact profoundly as these are not easy processes that you go through—but…it has strengthened our resolve, it has given us a level of tenacity and depth of belief in what we are doing….
>
> "It is a blessing, a privilege to be able to serve. And also to come through this with a kind of protection and because of my belief system—I am not at any place by chance—there is nothing incidental. I am deeply rooted in spirituality, so for me there is so much more going on than at the formal work level. I think one thing that has clearly happened (is) that I have never been a principal, because role definition did not match with what was needed of me."

Mr M has completely accepted his uncertain fate and that of the centre. He is vulnerable, in the hands of provincial stakeholders who have various models for the care of abused and neglected children, including foster care, child and youth care centres without educational facilities, incarceration and temporary shelters. Dalal (2012) describes the morality of care, with considerate attitudes and behaviours, as making our lives meaningful. Courtois (2015) suggests that, ethically, dealing with those who suffer from trauma is to do no *more* harm

> "So the role in this interim period is not an easy one….Predemocracy dealt with a retributive and containment environment, not easily accessible to community participation programmes through developmental perspectives. Access was limited and we now see a potential return to these conditions under the guise of a notion of care."

The Western Cape Education Department's focus on inclusivity and streaming in education gives insights into future directions for abused and neglected children who need institutional care. Centres like YCEC may continue, with educational facilities depending on the child's needs. High support will offer residential facilities, giving children access to a range of appropriate professionals, from occupational therapists to educational psychologists. Medium support will involve working with children in their communities, monitored by suitable professionals collaborating in specialist teams. Low support will offer psychoeducation and continuous training in groups for teachers, parents and support staff.

Third Safety Principle: Appreciation

It will take many years of planning and implementation before national effective care programmes protect vulnerable children in SA. In the meantime, YCEC has implemented after-care programmes offering a wide range of experiences, encouraging appreciation of talents and interests and offering the possibility of achieving newly formed life goals.

In obtaining 53 black and white laminated photographs of youth involved in activities in their time at the centre, captured by staff and kept in a therapeutic hostel, 11 were selected by male (2) and female (3) staff and professionals for captioning. Participants were asked to briefly explain their choice of photograph/s in writing. Photofeedback generally involves photographers commenting on their own work (Harper, 2002), but in this case comments were made on the images of others. The following photographs and captions offer insights into the range of after-care activities at the YCEC; examples of what the educational psychologist described as "caring in the light".

Connection and Transformation: Educational Psychologist/WCED Support Services Official (Female)

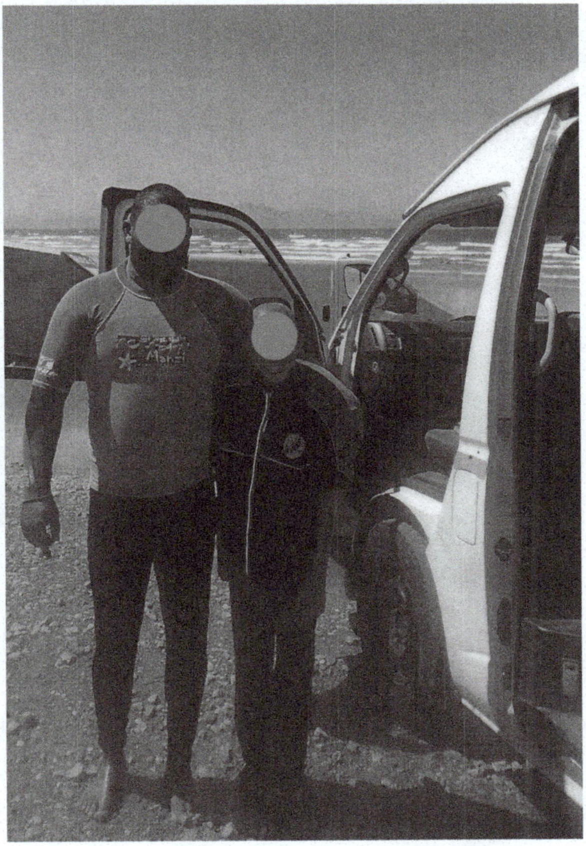

Fig. 22.1 Connecting with nature at the sea and feeling safe and comfortable with my "big brother"

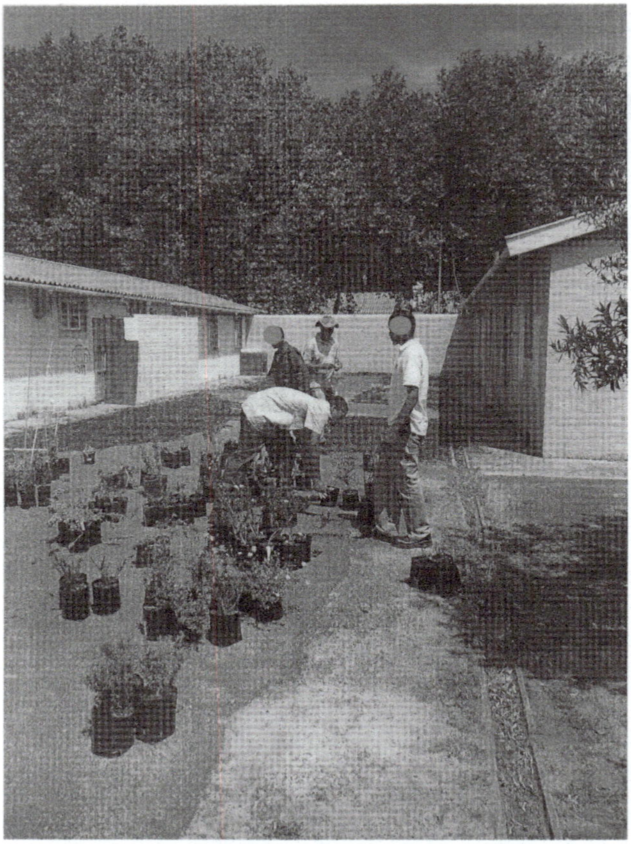

Fig. 22.2 Connecting with nature…tending these plants like we are being tended and growing in this place

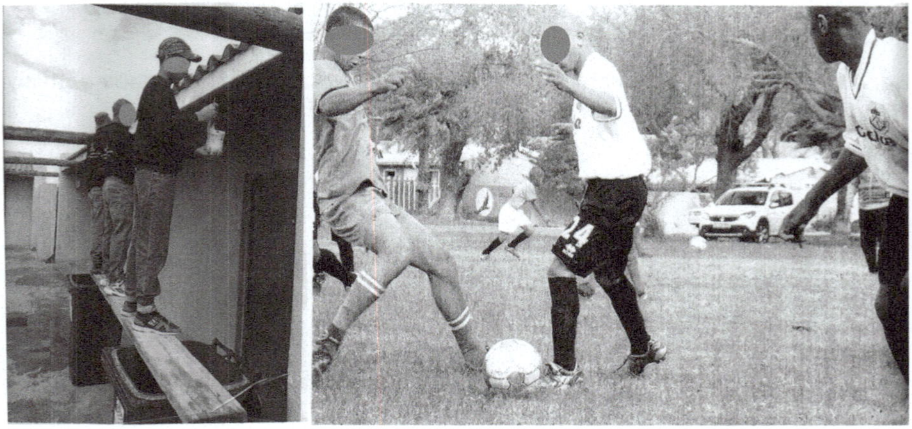

Fig. 22.3 (**a**) and (**b**) Transforming the place that we are living in…as the staff of the centre are transforming us

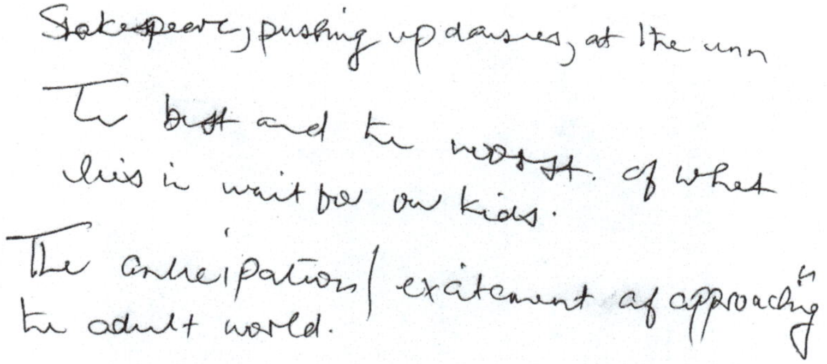
Shakespeare, pushing up daisies, at the inn
The best and the worst. of what lies in wait for our kids.
The anticipation/excitement of approaching the adult world.

Fig. 22.4 Shakespeare pushing up daisies at the inn: YCEC counsellor (male)
This photograph represents for Mr B, the counsellor, "the best and worst of what lies ahead for our kids". It shows "the anticipation and excitement of approaching the adult world" as they enjoy a ball game. (The boy on the left has a talent for the stage and acting—hence being called Shakespeare.) He is still searching for work in his community. The centre boy is dead, fatally stabbed in the heart by a gang member. The third boy works in a liquor store. Mr B reflected that often the least flamboyant boys find their niche and get along best in the outside world.

Circle of Courage skills of mastery, belonging and independence: Education psychologist (male)

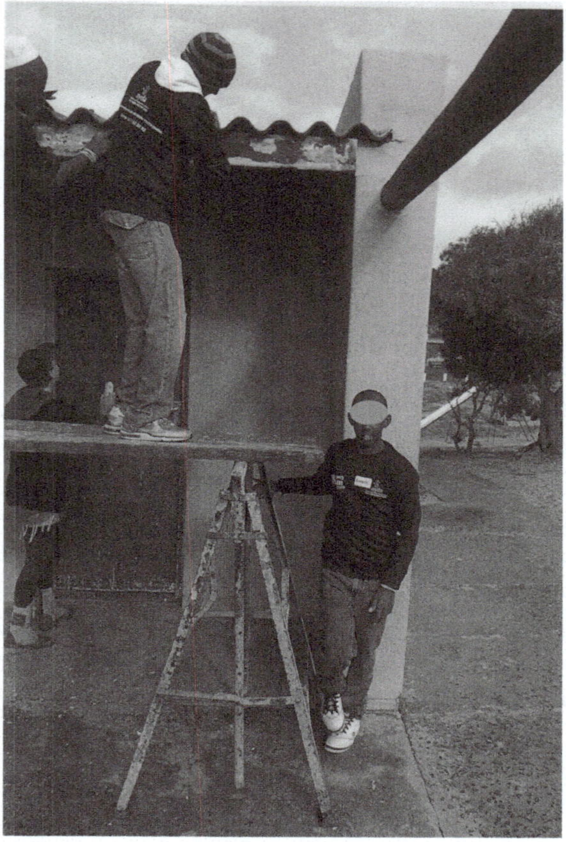

Fig. 22.5 Portability of skills (work skills)

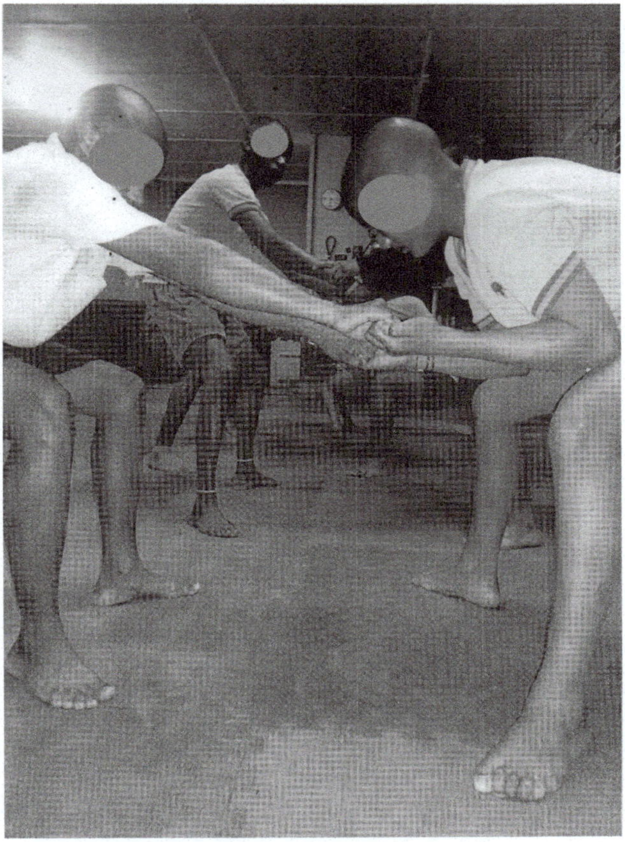

Fig. 22.6 Trusting is a big issue in training (belonging)

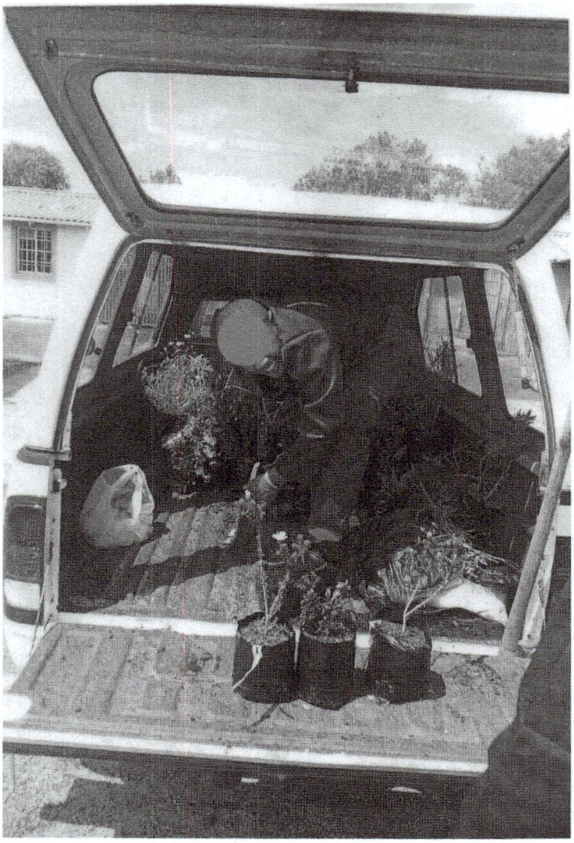

Fig. 22.7 Taking care of nature as a transferable skill to taking care of self (belonging)

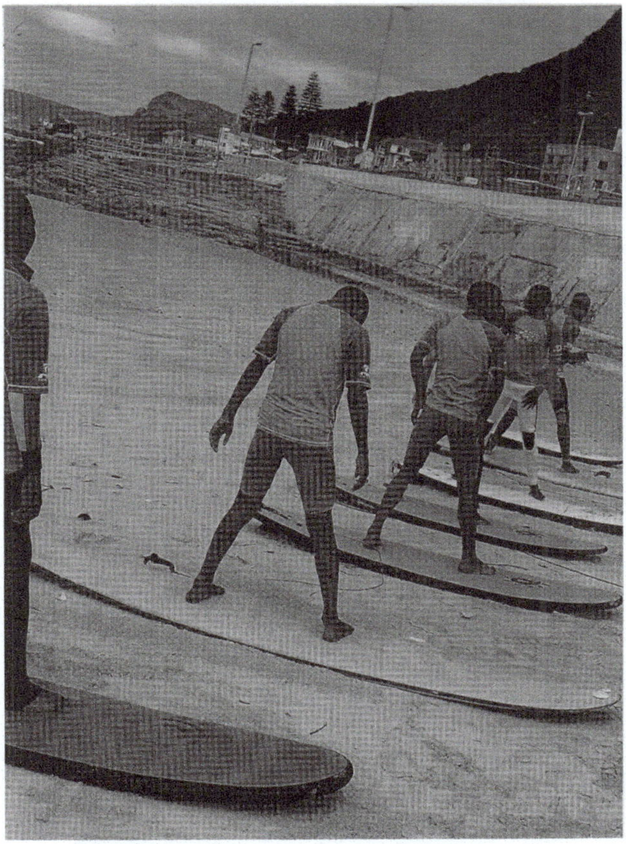

Fig. 22.8 Mastery skills for self-image, with a “can do” attitude

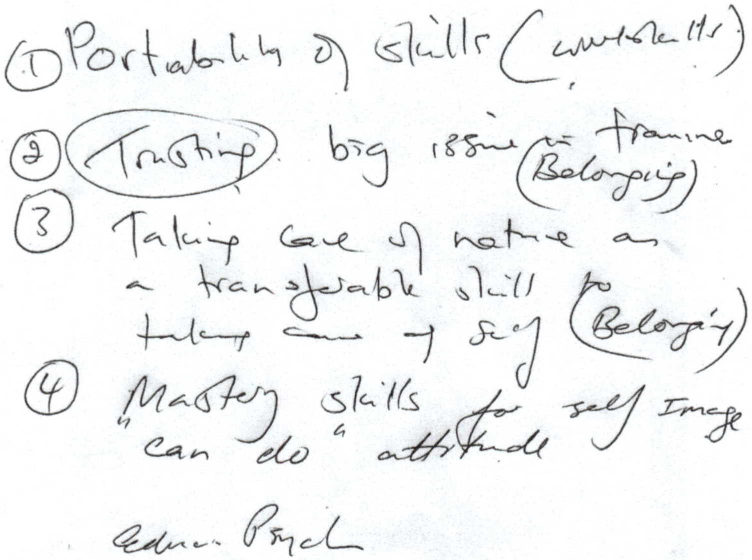
(1) Portability of skills
(2) Trusting big issue in trauma (Belonging)
(3) Taking care of nature as a transferable skill to taking care of self (Belonging)
(4) Mastery skills for self Image "can do" attitude

Fig. 22.9 Fishing…a positive recreational activity—Occupational therapist (female)

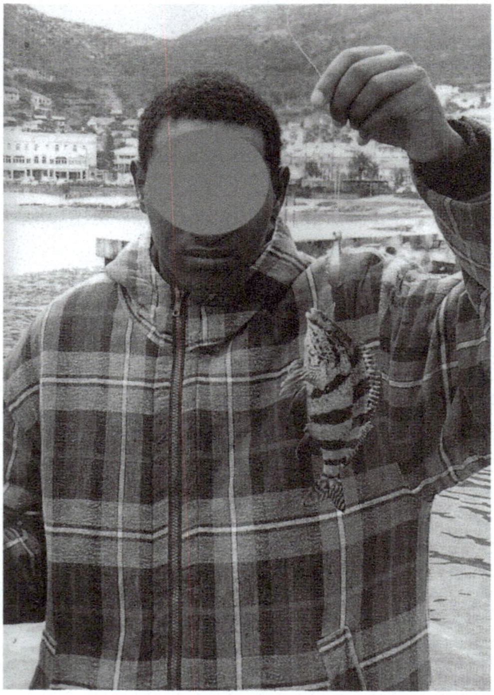

Fig. 22.10 This picture shows (to) me that the boys are now being exposed to other possible recreational activities that (is) are available to them other than substance (abuse) and gangsterism

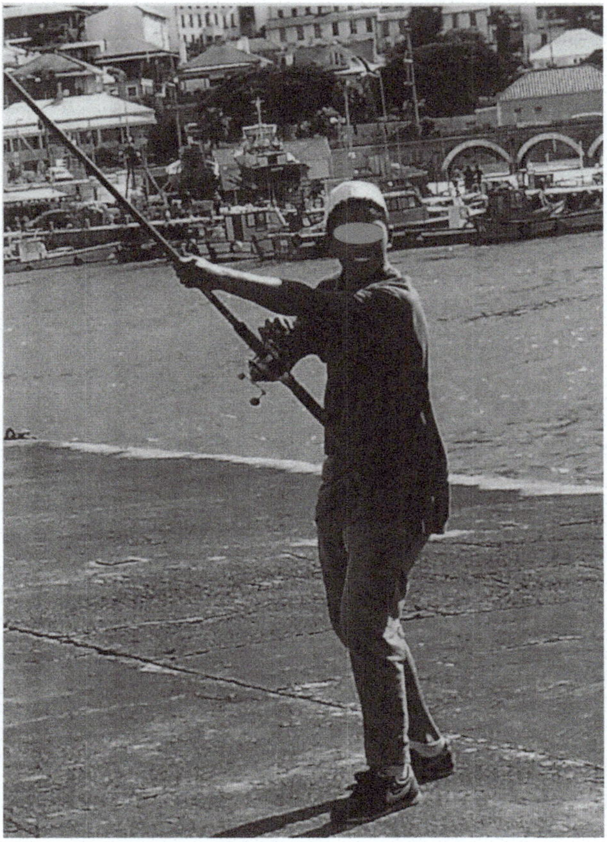

Fig. 22.11 The look on his face as he learns how to use the fish line and preparing to go and catch fish shows that he is a bit (in) shock, as he probably didn't think that he would ever do this, as well as happy learning a new activity skill

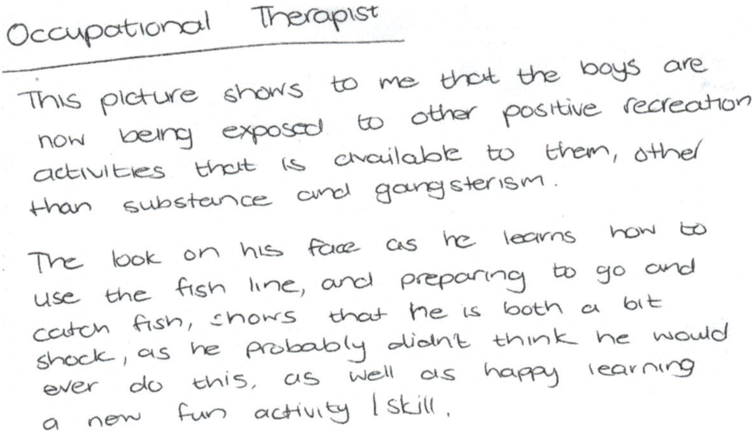

Occupational Therapist

This picture shows to me that the boys are now being exposed to other positive recreation activities that is available to them, other than substance and gangsterism.

The look on his face as he learns how to use the fish line, and preparing to go and catch fish, shows that he is both a bit shock, as he probably didn't think he would ever do this, as well as happy learning a new fun activity / skill.

Fig. 22.12 On the quayside—Admin Clerk (female)

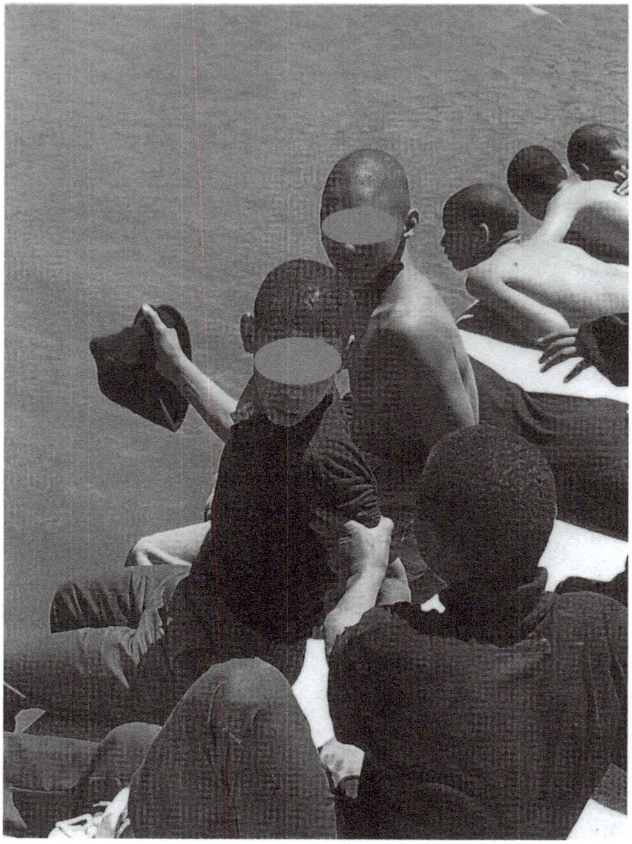

Fig. 22.13 I have chosen this pic because I can see the care shown from one boy to the other. I get the sense that the one boy is telling the other boy to be careful not to fall in the water

I have chosen this picture as I can see the care shown from one boy to the other. I get the sense that the one boy is telling the other boy to be careful not to fall in the water.

Discussion

WCED is considering multilevels of support for vulnerable youth in Cape Town's ganglands. As a high-level centre, YCEC has become a restorative care model of providing safety for traumatised youth, treating them with love, acceptance and appreciation. By surviving, despite ongoing traumatic threats of closure and protracted court battles, it has modelled for the boys the very resilience and strength needed for trauma recovery. The concept of inclusivity means youths are not labelled and isolated, but integrated back into their schools and communities as enabled young men after home visits, sporting activities and family days as well as gaining practical skills. There will be nationally recognised qualifications, giving youth an improved chance of employment.

In caring for high-risk youth, teachers and staff needed to manage their own stress and burnout, especially as role models of love and respect, exposed to the same continuous traumatic contexts of their charges. In PAR, carers were able to take responsibility for their healing, determining what worked for them, enjoying quiet and reflective time together, sharing triumphs and tragedies and gaining psychological insights. Connection and calm were achieved through bodywork and emotional processing in groups, which led to greater attachment to the boys and appreciation of their talents beneath the protective armour of dysfunctional behaviour.

Losing a protracted court battle has done little to deter the determination of staff to accept boys in need of care into the centre and strive to give them optimal opportunities to thrive going forward. In dealing with multiple traumas presented by learners on a daily basis, a teacher trauma tool is being developed collaboratively with Cape Flats schools, based on this research in the centre and a pilot trauma project in primary schools (Johnson, 2019a). It is hoped that educators and carers can prevent further harm to the youth in their care. Based on the goal of providing optimum safety on physical, emotional and cognitive levels, the principles of love, acceptance and appreciation were factors taken into consideration in the protocol design.

Future Directions

While focusing on people in a specific context at a moment in time might seem fleetingly incomplete, narrative strategies provide a creative space to make interpretive acts part of a dynamic interaction (Schiff, 2017). Making connections in varied forms and contexts results in greater understanding.

Multiple narratives and photographic perspectives of love, acceptance and appreciation provided insights into the meaning of safety for trauma recovery of staff and boys at YCEC. Reuben reflected on love and connection, gaining support from peers and mentors. Tlali was able to develop an improved sense of self, integrating attachment to staff and teachers back in his community, establishing improved relations with significant others. Self-care of staff enabled the modelling of restorative care for others. Having survived the legal battle, the centre is considering its inclusion in future educational models. The YCEC may face uncertainty, but the determination of staff to protect the boys in their care and the success of their restorative care programmes suggest a new roadmap of hope for society's most vulnerable at a critical developmental stage of late adolescence.

SA has historically experienced some of the worst atrocities but the country has also led the way in morality with the former president, Nelson Mandela, who reflected: "History will judge us by the differences we make in the everyday lives of children" (Special Report, 2014). Apartheid-era punitive disciplinary practices as a school of industries have been replaced by positive attachment in a restorative care centre, based on principles of safety for vulnerable youths. In large centres with many boys and limited staff, this familial-type care can be logistically hard to practise. In addition, the DNA of "dark age" practices are ever present, threatening the success of more enlightened youth-centred psychological understandings of care, which can make a meaningful contribution to progress in social upliftment projects. As this study showed, it is in the small gestures and daily genuine connections that healing takes place. Hopefully, with the ability to draw water out of stone, the YCEC team will find innovative ways to continue as change agents in times of serious drought.

Afterword

YCEC has been formally closed as a result of the economic hardships of the Covid-19 pandemic effecting government programs. Remaining staff are considering their future role in newly developing care spaces for neglected and abused youth in Cape Town.

References

Badroodien, A. (2001). *A history of the Ottery School of Industries in Cape Town: Issues of race, welfare and social order in the period 1937 to 1968*. Doctoral dissertation, University of the Western Cape.

Berceli, D. (2008). *The revolutionary trauma release process: Transcend your toughest times*. Namaste Publishing, A.A.

Brendtro, L. K., Brokenleg, M., & Van Brokern, S. (2002). *Reclaiming youth at risk: Our hope for the future*. Solution Tree Press.

Cane, P. M. (2000). *Trauma healing and transformation*. Capacitar International.

Canham, H. (2006). Where do babies come from – What makes children want to learn? In B. Youell (Ed.), *The learning experience – Psychoanalytic thinking in education*. Tavistock Clinic.

Chase, S. (2005). Narrative inquiry: Multiple lenses, approaches, voices. In N. K. Denzin & Y. S. Lincoln (Eds.), *The Sage handbook of qualitative research* (3rd ed., pp. 651–679). Sage.

Collier, J. (1957). Photography in anthropology: A report on two experiments. *American Anthropologist, 59*, 843–859.

Courtois, C. A. (2015). *First do no more harm: Ethics of trauma treatment*. Retrieved May 12, 2017, from www.goodtherapy.org

Courtois, C. A., & Ford, J. D. (2009). *Treating complex traumatic stress disorders – An evidence based guide*. Guildford Press.

Dalal, F. (2012). Specialists without spirit, sensualists without heart: Psychotherapy as a moral endeavour. *Group Analysis, 45*(4), 405–429. https://doi.org/10.1177/0533316412461862

Harper, D. (2002). Talking about pictures: A case for photo-elicitation. *Visual Studies, 17*(1), 13–26.

Johnson, S. (2019a). *Circles of care: Developing a teacher trauma tool in high-risk South African schools*. [Manuscript in preparation].

Johnson, S. (2019b). From disempowerment to self-belief: A centre of hope for abused and neglected youth in Cape Town. In M. F. Diaz & B. Shepard (Eds.), *Narrating practice with children and adolescents*. Columbia University Press.

Johnson, S. (2019c). *Lessons of care: Triumph over trauma and tribulation*. [Manuscript in preparation].

Johnson, S. (2019d). Psychobiography as an effective research methodology for the advocacy of abused and neglected youth in South Africa. In C. Mayer & Z. Kovary (Eds.), *New trends in psychobiography*. Springer.

Johnson, S. M. (2010). *Transpersonal practices as prevention intervention for burnout amongst HIV/Aids coordinator teachers*. Unpublished master's thesis, Stellenbosch University.

Johnson, S. M. (2013). *Impact of stress and burnout interventions on educators in high-risk secondary schools*. Doctoral dissertation, Stellenbosch University.

Johnson, S. M. (2015). Reducing teacher stress and burnout in high-risk secondary schools with Transactional Analysis. *International Journal of Transactional Analysis Research, 6*(1), 70–85.

Johnson, S. M., & Naidoo, A. V. (2013). Transpersonal practices as prevention intervention for burnout among HIV/Aids coordinator teachers. *SA Journal of Psychology, 43*(59), 70.

Johnson, S. M., & Naidoo, A. V. (2016). A psychoeducational approach for prevention of burnout among teachers dealing with HIV/AIDS in South Africa. *AIDS Care*. https://doi.org/10.1080/09540121.2016.1201193

Johnson, S. M., & Naidoo, A. V. (2017). Can evolutionary insights into the brain's response to threat suggest different interventions for perceived stress and burnout of teachers in high-risk schools? *SA Journal of Psychology, 47*, 401–415. https://doi.org/10.1177/0081246316675588

MacGuire, P. (2008). *Never assume – Getting to know children before labelling them*. Outskirts Press.

Maslow, A. H. (1962). *Towards a psychology of being*. Harper & Row.

Minister of Social Development Western Cape and Others v Justice Alliance of South Africa and Another (20806/2013) [2016] ZAWCHC 34 (1 April 2016) para 39.

Plato, D. (2012). *Gangsterism in South African schools*. Public dialogue address by Minister for Community Safety in the Western Cape. Cape Town: Centre for Conflict Resolution.

Schiff, B. (2017). *A new narrative for psychology*. Oxford University Press.

Schlapobersky, J. R. (2016). *From the couch to the circle: Group-analytic psychotherapy in practice*. Routledge.

Special Report, "Twenty-five years of children's rights." (2014). Advertorial, 21 November. http://mg.co.za/article/2014-11-21-00-twenty-five-years-of-childrens-rights

Tillman, D. (2000). *Living values activities for young adults*. Sterling Publishers.

Ziegler, D. (2018). *Mental health therapy for children*. Jasper Mountain.

Sharon Johnson is in the Psychology Faculty of non-profit community college, Cornerstone Institute. She holds a PhD in Psychology from Stellenbosch University, South Africa, where she also completed a three-year post-doctoral fellowship in 2016. For the past few years she has been actively involved as a researcher and consultant at a Youth Care and Education Centre, Western Cape Education Department and has conducted workshops on crisis and trauma in high-risk schools. Her community psychology focus is on the stress and burnout of teachers, and institutional restorative care for abused and neglected youth. Johnson has written numerous papers which have been published in peer-reviewed journals on her research in schools. She has chapters published in academic books in the USA and Europe and is writing her own books on the restorative care of vulnerable youth in state care and trauma work with educators in high-risk schools. Johnson runs her own counselling practice and consults to NGOs and Government Departments.

23

Collaborating with Social Justice Activists in Ghana's Fight Against Modern Slavery: A Case Study of Challenging Heights

Kate Danvers

By rescuing others, I feel I am rescuing myself. I feel that I am correcting the injustice that was done when I was young.
—James Kofi Annan (President of Challenging Heights)

Starting out as a Clinical Psychologist, I felt a strong responsibility to share knowledge that enables people to alleviate pain and distress. I also have a desire for adventure, which is why I first left the NHS to go to Jaffna, in Northern Sri Lanka, with VSO. Working in partnership with local colleagues and living in a war affected community forever changed my understanding of mental health. Seeing the impact of the Asian Ocean tsunami and eventually having to leave my home on the resumption of hostilities were life changing experiences, and I learned so much about the benefits and limitations of psychology in extreme situations.

My awareness of the need for systemic changes, rather than medicalising people's problems, grew further working with refugees on my return to the UK. I eventually took time out to complete an MA in Community Psychology in Brighton, cementing my identity as a values-led practitioner. I was fortunate enough to be able to turn my beliefs into action, working with a community-based child rights NGO in Ghana to develop rehabilitation practices for trafficked children. I currently support looked

K. Danvers (✉)
North East London NHS Foundation Trust, London, UK
e-mail: k.danvers@nhs.net

C. Walker et al. (eds.), *The Palgrave Handbook of Innovative Community and Clinical Psychologies*, https://doi.org/10.1007/978-3-030-71190-0_23

after children and child refugees in London, taking a trauma informed, rights-led approach to my clinical work. My activist inspirations are the Only Us campaign, Drop the Disorder, and Psychologists for Social Change, and I continue to try to live my values, despite the limitations of an NHS role.

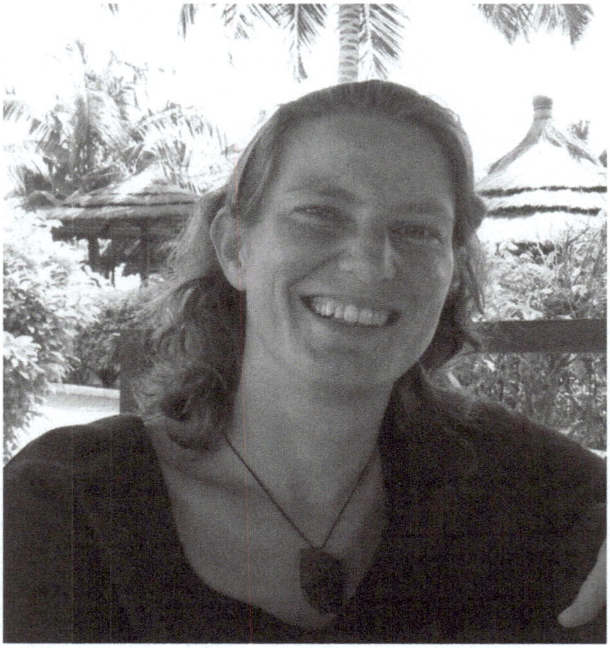

Joining a Grassroots Movement

James Kofi Annan is one of those inspiring, charismatic leaders full of ideas and energy, passionately committed to social justice, and convinced that each of us can and should make a difference in the service of the oppressed. From 2014 to 2016 I was privileged to work in Winneba, Ghana, with James, a social entrepreneur, psychologist, the Founder and President of the non-governmental human rights organisation Challenging Heights, and winner of many awards, including the World Children's Prize and an Honorary Doctorate of Humanitarian Letters.

James is also a survivor of modern slavery, trafficked at the age of six to work in the fishing industry on Lake Volta, where he experienced torturous conditions. James escaped from slavery at age 13, and returned to his home town of Winneba, determined to get an education. Like many from Winneba, James comes from a very large family where education is a luxury that is rarely afforded. Even once reunited with his family, he was not able to rely on parental support to help him flourish. James worked odd jobs to put himself through school: key to his success was his willingness, as a life-scarred teenager, to start again, alongside kindergarten students, asking them for help with basic literacy skills. His persistence paid off, and James successfully completed high school, eventually achieving a University degree in Psychology.

James went on to post-graduate study and a successful career in publishing and banking, but found himself drawn back to the problems in his home community, and the need to rescue trafficked children. In 2005, he began a grassroots community organising project that was to evolve into the now internationally respected child rights charity, Challenging Heights, which he formally founded in 2007.

Unlike James, my upbringing in the UK was privileged: my community was predominantly white, middle-class, safe, and economically stable, with full access to free health care and education. I trained in clinical psychology, qualifying in 2000, when most courses actively discouraged political thought and action, aiming instead for a neutral, non-judgemental, scientist-practitioner, evidence-based approach (Teo, 2009). Soon, I began to feel concerned about a system that often turned away those in greatest need, as their housing/economic/social situation was judged "too unstable" for them to benefit from psychological intervention, but it was not until 2004, when I spent two years working for Voluntary Service Overseas in an impoverished conflict-affected area of northern Sri Lanka, that I fully engaged with alternative approaches to "mental health".

In Sri Lanka, I learned valuable lessons about participatory practice in international development (Chambers, 1997), community responses to collective traumatisation (Somasundaram, 1998) and the rights abuses endured as a result of the organisation of our international political system (Black, 2002). Tamil colleagues who'd experienced displacement during the war taught me to turn Maslow's (1943) hierarchy of needs on its head, arguing "How are we expected to access our basic needs if our minds are full of our trauma?", and I became a fan of "rough-and-dirty" psychological interventions in "unsafe" situations. I continued my interest in rights-focussed Clinical Psychology (Kinderman, 2007) on my return to the UK, choosing to work with refugees, and completing an MA in Community Psychology in 2014.

On joining Challenging Heights, I recognised in the model James had created a community psychology approach, although it was not formally labelled as such (Perkins, 2009). I was inspired to see how this might work in action, and curious to know what I could bring from my more traditional mental health training to aid the charity's rescue, rehabilitation and reintegration work.

The Problem

The unexpectedly large, shallow lake created in the 1950s by the hydroelectric damming of the River Volta produced a thriving small-scale fishing industry in a region of Ghana which had previously been predominantly agricultural. The initially vast fish stocks resulted in large-scale migration from coastal fishing communities, despite the extremely hazardous conditions on Lake Volta.

Winneba is a source community for the trafficking of children to Lake Volta. The coastal fishing communities have strong cultural, familial and economic links with the communities of Lake Volta, and seasonal migration of fishing families is common. In Ghana, males making multiple marriages is common, and traditionally very large family sizes have been prized. Even in wealthier families, it is common for children to live outside of the nuclear family, in order to study, work or support a family member with household chores.

In Ghana, there is also a strong tradition of child labour. There are over 2.4 million "economically active" children aged 5–17 (Ghana Statistical Services, 2010). More than a million children cannot access education because of their need to work, and an estimated 240,000 are engaged in hazardous child labour (Kukwaw, 2013). Ghana is a source, transit and destination country for men, women and children subjected to forced labour and sex trafficking (United States State Department, 2014), and around 193,100 Ghanaians live in conditions of modern slavery (Hope for Children, 2014).

Poverty and poor access to education are the main drivers of child trafficking and slavery identified by Challenging Heights. Many families do not know about the poor conditions on the lake, and may genuinely believe they are sending their children to safely learn a valuable trade. Some families may give their children to traffickers in order to repay a debt, or because they have too many children to feed and care for (Schley et al., 2015).

Estimates suggest that there are 49,000 children working in the fishing industry on Lake Volta, and 21,000 are forced to undertake hazardous labour that may pose a risk to their life (Kukwaw, 2013). The situation for children working on Lake Volta is bleak: they lack access to health care facilities, education, running water, sanitation and electricity (Schley et al., 2015). Fishing work on the world's largest human-made lake can be deadly: storms, accidents and infections all often lead to loss of life (ibid.).

Challenging Heights' own research (Danvers & Osabutey, 2016, unpublished) showed some of the dangers trafficked children working on Lake Volta face: of 183 children rescued in the three years to 2015, 73% of children had at least one experience where they believed they might die, and 55% had actually seen another person die whilst fishing.

Physical abuse is common in Ghana, with caning legal in schools and homes (Danvers & Schley, 2016), and unsurprisingly, 89% of our children described severe physical abuse from their masters and from older children (Danvers & Osabutey, 2016). Often trafficked children are stigmatised in the fishing communities. Eighty-nine per cent experienced verbal abuse, such as name calling, insults and curses (ibid.). We also know that a proportion of our boys and girls are sexually abused by masters, or sometimes older children during their time as slaves, but it is very difficult for them to disclose this abuse, in a society with strong moral teaching against sexual activity, especially same-sex activity. Eighty-one per cent of our children had lake-acquired infections (including bilharzia, malaria, typhoid and hepatitis B) at the time of rescue, and malnutrition and water-related skin damage were very common.

The children rescued by Challenging Heights were between the ages of 5 and 17+, with the majority being male (72%) and aged 13 or younger (69%). On average, our children had spent 4½ years in slavery before being rescued, with a range of 6 months to 17 years (Danvers & Osabutey, 2016).

The human rights abuses endured by children on Lake Volta are an example of structural violence (Farmer, 2005): a process by which suffering is organised by historically and internationally determined laws, processes and economic relations. The poverty and practices of child labour which drive present-day child trafficking in Ghana are directly related to historical British exploitation: British policies encouraged migration from rural areas to mining areas along the "Gold Coast" and used children as a cheap source of labour (Okyere, 2017).

Later, neoliberal policies within international development led to the imposition of structural adjustment programmes by the International Monetary Fund (IMF), forcing the Ghanaian government to reduce spending on citizens' welfare and open up markets to international trade (Okyere, 2017). These policies have been shown to have worsened poverty and held back development in many sub-Saharan African countries (Brecher et al., 2000; Sloan, 2010). This continues today: for example, in 2016, a condition for ongoing US developmental aid was the privatisation of Ghana's electricity supply, leading to an immediate hike in prices for all.

Box 23.1 Voices of Survivors (Osabutey, 2015)

"Sometimes where I go to remove the tangled net is very far, so by the time I come from under the lake there will be blood from my nose." *Boy, aged 12, 6 years in slavery*

"Diving became my core responsibility on the lake and when I am unable to get the net and come up to take air, my master beats me with the fishing rope on the head and back until I remove the net." *Boy, aged 15, 4 years in slavery*

"There were days I was beaten and pushed into the lake to get drowned and when others around interfered, the master only dragged me into the boat like pulling a fish on board." *Boy, aged 14, 4 years in slavery*

"I saw the smallest of the boys beaten badly by my master, and later I heard that he was molested too. My master used to call me a 'foolish child' and insult my parents, calling them 'irresponsible' and disrespectful terms for genital parts." *Boy, aged 14, 4 ½ years in slavery*

"Several times I saw people going to remove stuck nets and they never came back and for that I am sometimes afraid that I might also die." *Boy, aged 16, 1 year in slavery*

"A boy was hit with a paddle and fell into the lake and got drowned and died. I was afraid." *Girl, aged 11, 2½ years in slavery*

"When I was going under the water, I could not breathe well because I was afraid. I thought I was going to die." *Boy, aged 15, 4 years in slavery*

"I was always frightened on the lake when there was a storm and I thought I was going to die. Once I went to the bush to attempt suicide. I tied the rope on the tree but started crying." *Girl, aged 14, 5 years in slavery* (Fig. 23.1)

The Growth of a Movement

James' Early Interventions and the Roots of Challenging Heights

Child Rights Clubs

James' inspiration was always rights-focussed, based on the principles that no child should work on the lake and all should be in school. He began with community-based child rights clubs: getting children together to talk about trafficking and their rights. Gradually, local children became empowered to know their rights and resist trafficking: if they heard of a child due to be sent to the Lake, they'd let James know, and he would visit the family to persuade them to change their minds. Using a participatory approach (e.g. Singh, 2001), he joined with children and key adults, such as religious leaders, teachers and community elders, to come up with activities, such as marches and speeches, to raise local awareness of child trafficking in the communities.

The early roots of Challenging Heights exemplify conscientisation in action. Freire's (1972) concept of conscientisation describes a process where

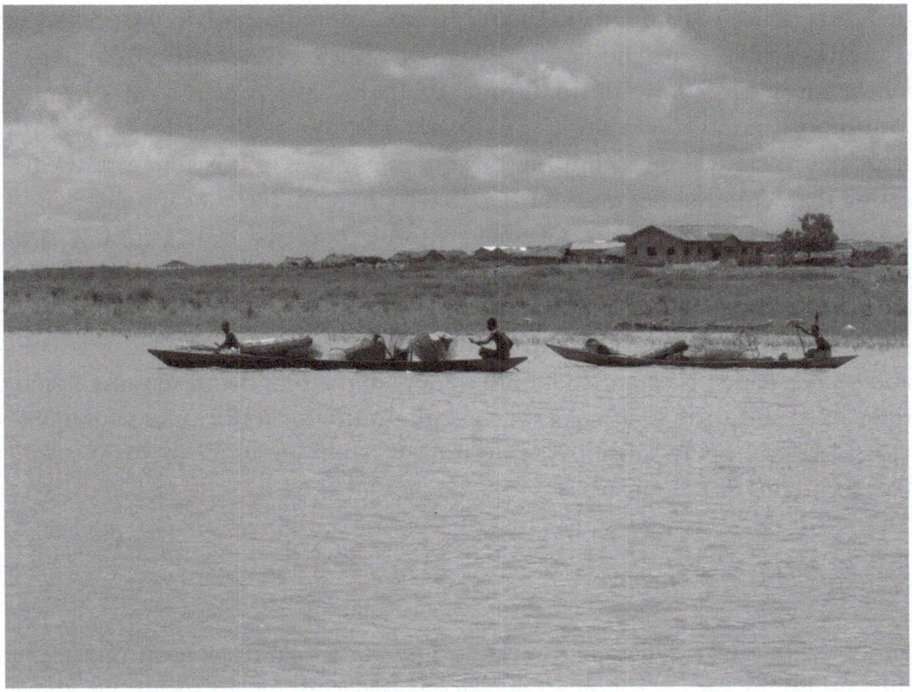

Fig. 23.1 Children working on Lake Volta

groups or communities become aware of their own oppression through a process of discussion and questioning of the status quo, as a first step towards liberation (Martín-Baró, 1994).

Key to the success of James' approach was his status as community member and survivor of slavery. Challenging Heights has always been a grassroots organisation, with blurred boundaries between staff and community. With consciousness raised, communities started to resist the trafficking of children to Lake Volta, and those with family members involved in trafficking started to question the practice. Through engaging community members in dialogue and persuasion, James was eventually able to recruit former traffickers and slave masters as Challenging Heights staff members, and some went on to become valuable informants and boat crew for rescues.

Education

Nobel Peace Laureate Archbishop Desmond Tutu said: "There comes a point when we need to stop just pulling people out of the river. We need to go upstream and find out why they're falling in." Inspired perhaps by thinkers such as Tutu, James' early actions focussed on prevention of trafficking, rather than directly rescuing children from conditions of slavery. He judged that his own experience of being denied access to education due to extreme poverty, a common problem for families in the region (Roelen & Chetti, 2014), was a key factor in his family's decision to send him to Lake Volta.

In poor coastal communities in Ghana, it is often difficult for families to trust that there will be an improved economic future to be gained from educating their children but once the decision to invest in the education of a child has been made, that child is more likely to be protected from family separation than those not in education (Schley et al., 2015). James began by personally sponsoring children from the poorest families to go to school, and supported promising students through University education. He was later able to persuade his extended family to donate their land and set up a school right in the heart of Winneba's source community for trafficking, which provided free or heavily subsidised education to children who otherwise would have been out of school.

Speaking Out as a Survivor

James used his own experience to raise consciousness in his community about the conditions on Lake Volta, and encouraged children to speak out about their rights and wishes to be educated. He began writing articles for national newspapers telling his story, and advocating for children's rights. Later, he played a lead role in changing the language used in public discourse in Ghana, as his articles and public speeches, as well as Challenging Heights' official language, helped shift the descriptions of the fishing industry from a focus on "child labour" (widely accepted in Ghana) to a process involving "hazardous labour" (which the government is committed to eliminating), "human rights abuses", "trafficking", "slavery" and "torture" (Annan, 2009; Editorial, 2010; Okyere, 2017).

James was conscious of the power of language to socially construct concepts (Berger & Luckmann, 1966), in a way that can obscure and legitimise power inequalities (Foucault, 1991). Many theoretical approaches to social change, such as liberation psychology (Martín-Baró, 1994), feminism (Moane, 2014), community psychology (Nelson & Prilleltensky, 2010) and participatory approaches to international development (Chambers, 1997) centralise the concept of "voice"—ensuring the views, desires and experiences of the oppressed are heard by those in power. James instinctively knew "voice" would be important in developing his organisation: the power of hearing first hand his experiences of slavery has since led to multiple donations and grants awarded to Challenging Heights, although the personal cost to James in sharing his story should never be underestimated.

Developing a Theory of Change and Going Further "Upstream"

From early beginnings, James developed Challenging Heights into a growing child rights charity. In common with community psychology approaches (Nelson & Prilleltensky, 2010), Challenging Heights' model of change sees human problems in the context of their local community and wider social and political context (see Fig. 23.2).

As Challenging Heights developed, using participatory practice (e.g. Ledwith & Springett, 2010) and listening to the voices of community members was key in understanding the root causes of the problem of trafficking. Drivers for trafficking identified by Challenging Heights include lack of access to education, poverty, cultural beliefs (such as those encouraging large family size, discouraging women's economic empowerment and devaluing children) and the government's inaction on upholding Ghana's existing anti-slavery laws (e.g. Schley et al., 2015). As Challenging Heights grew and became more successful at winning grants, it was able to create a number of projects focussed on the "upstream" causes of trafficking (Fig. 23.4).

Expanding Educational Provision

Anecdotal evidence suggests that having some financially successful extended family members reduces the chances of trafficking children, as they may

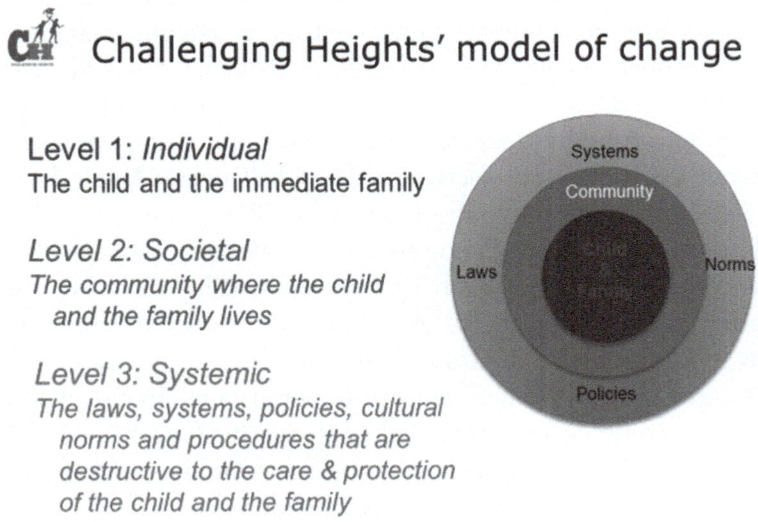

Fig. 23.2 Challenging Heights model of change

support the education of not only their own children but also their siblings, nieces, nephews and cousins. As well as Challenging Heights school, which provides free or heavily subsidised education for children who may otherwise have been trafficked into slavery, Challenging Heights provided business and entrepreneurial skills training to unemployed youth in the area.

Educational efforts also concentrated on women, including the provision of employment-related skills training, such as soap making and agriculture. In doing so, there was often a tension between the skills identified by Ghanaians as necessary in the local employment market and the type of skills Western donors were willing to fund. Structural inequalities at the level of international economic agreements mean that trade is inherently unfair (Black, 2002) and Ghana lacks key manufacturing industries—our experience of Western grant-giving bodies was that they failed to critique these wider injustices, and instead promoted a false narrative that suggests that individual entrepreneurial activity can, and indeed should, drive development. This leaves structural inequalities unchallenged and puts an unjust responsibility on the poor for alleviating their own poverty.

Women's Economic Empowerment and Business Infrastructure

From its early days, Challenging Heights offered micro-loans to women wishing to start small businesses and made cash grants available to those families willing to commit to not re-trafficking their rescued children. Research carried out by Challenging Heights in our local communities showed that ensuring women have more money directly contributes to reduced family separation and thus reduces the likelihood of trafficking (Roelen & Chetti, 2014).

Challenging Heights has been active in advocating to encourage the government to expand its provision of social protection cash payments to vulnerable families. The latest projects created by Challenging Heights have focussed on large-scale community infrastructure: in 2016, for example, Challenging Heights opened a women's co-operative community smokehouse and cold store, which protects families from financial hardship caused by the seasonal variation in coastal fish stocks, and allows women without their own smoke ovens to keep more of the fruits of their labour without being beholden to smoke oven owners. Women's empowerment in an international development context is a complex interplay of culturally specific factors (Grabe, 2012) and in Ghana, Challenging Heights sees women's economic empowerment as key to achieving many development goals for children.

Advocacy

As Challenging Heights grew, and its ability to win grants from aid-giving organisations and donations from private individuals increased, so did its power to raise the voice of enslaved children. James continues to write newspaper articles, organise public demonstrations and invite important people to bear witness to his story, and the stories of children Challenging Heights has rescued.

Personal advocacy has sometimes been at great cost: in focussing on the need for Ghana to implement and properly uphold its anti-trafficking legislation, James and Challenging Heights have come into conflict with powerful officials as they hold the government to account, by criticising existing provisions and advocating for change. Locally too, James' anti-slavery message has not always been well received, and he has been intimidated and threatened for speaking out.

In recent years, James and Challenging Heights have been able to draw on the power of the international community. By joining with international organisations focussed on fighting modern slavery, such as the Walk Free Foundation (www.walkfreefoundation.org), and being open to welcoming Western visitors to Challenging Heights, James has enabled Challenging Heights to become part of a global social justice movement that mobilises those with higher resources in the service of those with fewer (Gaventa, 2001). For example, in 2014 James was invited to read the International Declaration Against Modern Slavery signed by world faith leaders at The Vatican, an invitation which James was able to use to increase his status with Ghanaian faith leaders to bring about change at home.

Challenging Heights has developed its international social media presence, and welcomed students on study learning trips to Winneba, enabling Challenging Heights to harness the power of global citizen activism (Gaventa, 2001). For example, changing our interactions with foreign visitors to a model based on Fair-Trade Learning (Hartman et al., 2014) has led to successful partnerships with US Universities where visiting students remain engaged with Challenging Heights on their return to the US and commit to actions in the global movement against modern slavery. These international links not only help Challenging Heights to advocate and fund raise more effectively but also keep James and other Ghanaian staff safer from threats and intimidation.

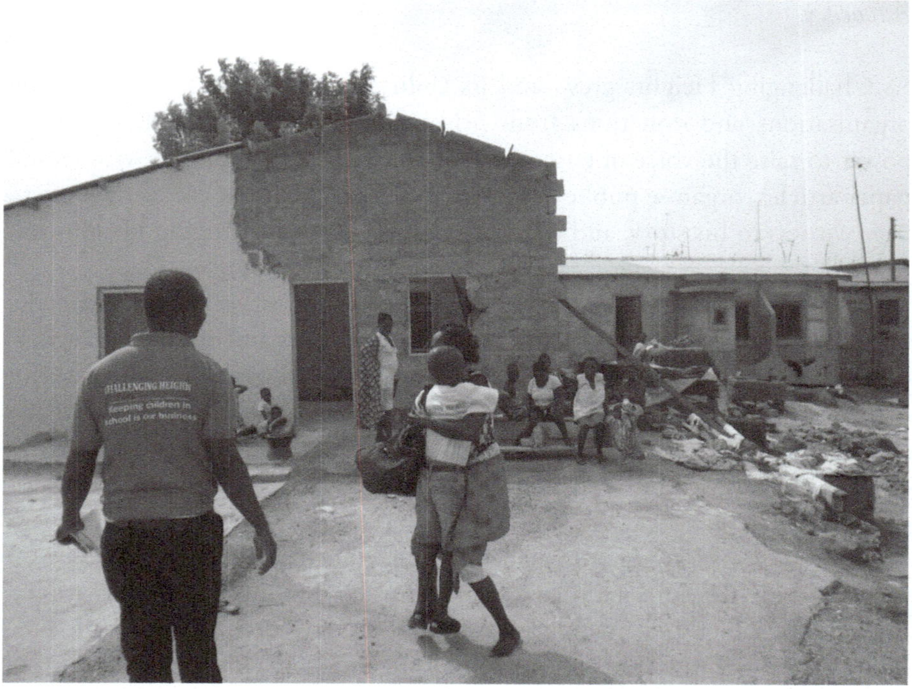

Fig. 23.3 Challenging Heights staff help to reunite a family in Winneba

Rights-Focussed Rescue, Rehabilitation and Reintegration

Rescuing children from trafficking is just one part of Challenging Heights' holistic approach to tackling modern slavery, and as such, it exemplifies the community psychology and liberation psychology approach of focussing not just on amelioration of suffering but also creating transformative social change (Lykes & Moane, 2009; Nelson & Prilleltensky, 2010). However, in the absence of immediate radical structural change, there is also a role for amelioration: James' core motivation has always been rooted in his survivor status, and needing to act to prevent harm to those children currently enslaved (Fig. 23.3 and 23.4).

Building on the prevention activities described above, today, part of Challenging Heights' work is direct rescue of children from Lake Volta. Rescue begins with community sensitisation activities, where child rights clubs and community child protection committees engage locals in talks, video presentations and demonstrations that raise consciousness about conditions on the Lake. Community members are encouraged to approach Challenging Heights staff if they know of a child who is working on the Lake, whom they would like to have returned to their care.

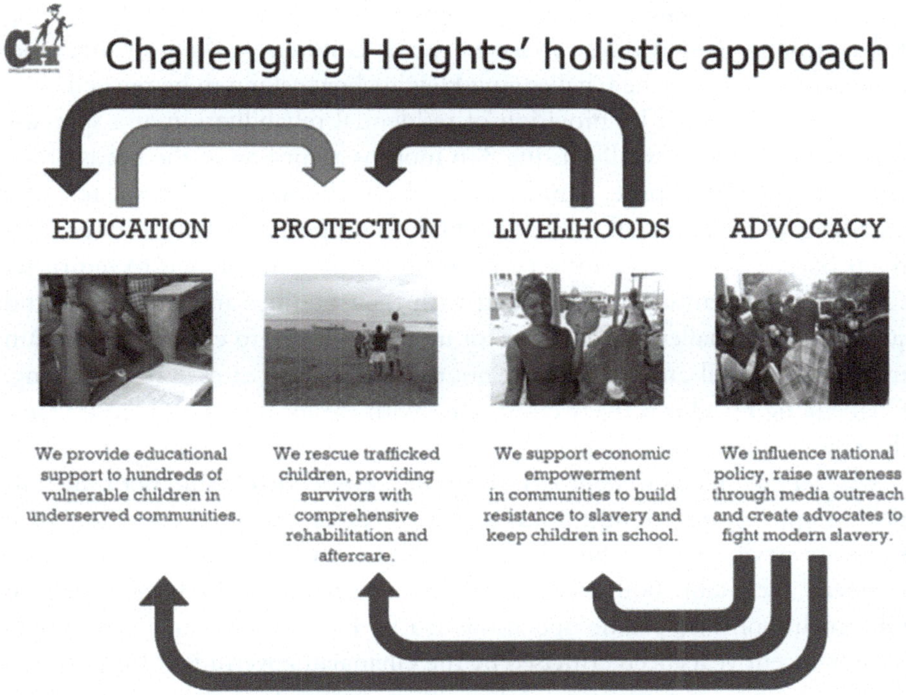

Fig. 23.4 The holistic approach

Challenging Heights staff collect information, such as the age and names of the children, description of the trafficker, name of the Lakeside community where the child is believed to be, as well as ensuring the family is committed to accepting the child on return. Information is passed to staff and informants on the Lake, who start asking around to try to locate the children. Information is also gathered from previously rescued children at the rehabilitation shelter, who are always keen to help their friends get rescued.

Over a period of months, a list of children and their possible locations is created, and the rescue trip is planned. Rescues involve travelling on the Lake from community to community for up to ten days. Staff members endure the same unsanitary conditions and dangerous weather as children working on the Lake, but experienced boat crew ensure safety of the staff and children rescued.

On arrival at a Lake community, staff members meet with village elders and persuade them to support them in insisting the traffickers and slave masters let the children go. Usually reminding elders of the laws against trafficking is enough to ensure community co-operation, but this can be backed up by returning with police if communities are resistant to handing over enslaved children. As Challenging Heights is now well known on the Lake, having been running their rescues for several years, children working on the Lake sometimes approach the Challenging Heights boat asking to be rescued.

Rescue is followed by provision of residential rehabilitation at a specially constructed shelter, usually lasting 3–6 months according to the needs of the child. During this time, families visit their children at the shelter, and Challenging Heights staff provide livelihoods support and work with government Social Services to ensure families' homes are safe enough to return to. Children are eventually reintegrated with their families and monitored and supported by Challenging Heights for up to two years, to ensure they remain in education, well cared for and are not re-trafficked. In cases of re-trafficking, Challenging Heights actively co-operates with the local police to ensure family members are prosecuted.

Challenging Heights' approach to rescue is embedded within both the trafficking and source communities, and involves extensive co-operation with statutory services (Police, Social Services and Health). This means it is sustainable, and acceptable both to the local population and to the Government of Ghana. In contrast, rescue operations led by high-profile American NGOs have in recent years been criticised by the Ghanaian government for misidentifying children as trafficked (and in effect, kidnapping them during "rescues") because the organisation "*never consulted with stakeholders, traditional rulers or opinion leaders to really understand the cultural setting*" (MP Betty Nana Efua Crosby Mensah speaking in June 2017, quoted in Okyere, 2017, p. 97).

Challenging Narratives of Trauma

As a psychologist trained in a Western tradition, the core difference I see between Challenging Heights' approach to "rescue" and a conventional psychological approach is that Challenging Heights takes a firm rights-oriented stance to the provision of care (Farmer, 2005), rather than a trauma- or victim-oriented stance. Fassin (2012) has argued that in recent years, there has been a shift away from rights-focussed action and a concern for social justice and reducing inequality, towards "humanitarian reason", a concern for alleviating suffering, trauma and exclusion. In this way, anger has been replaced by compassion, and the urge to fight has been replaced by the urge to rescue (Fassin, 2012). Consequently, survivors of rights abuses have come to be routinely viewed as traumatised or psychologically damaged (Fassin & D'Halluin, 2005): this elicits compassion in others, but such compassion relies on consistently performing a "victim" role (Good, 2012).

Western psychology has played into this age of humanitarian reason, in its development of individualised trauma-focussed psychological interventions and focus on alleviating suffering, in the absence of political action and thought (e.g. Ehlers & Clark, 2000). In contrast, in Challenging Heights' established approach to "rehabilitation", I observed a primary focus on providing reparations for rights abuses: children without education were given top-up classes; children with malnutrition, injuries and water-borne diseases were provided with medical attention; housework training was given to children who had missed out on normal routines of home life; slave masters and traffickers were chased through traditional and legal processes to provide cash compensation to children; and practical assistance was provided in the form of clothes, books and shoes.

As James puts it, Challenging Heights focusses on "correcting the injustice" done to these children. The focus was on maximising children's potential after reintegration to "fit in" with their families and communities, and access opportunities for education and future growth.

The possibility of psychological trauma was acknowledged, but not given central prominence in Challenging Heights' approach to rehabilitation. For example, in a Western psychological tradition, survivors of trauma might be carefully protected from intrusive questioning for fear of triggering psychological "symptoms": at Challenging Heights, children were asked publicly and in detail about their experiences and injuries, and freely encouraged to express anger and tell their stories through play, drama and art.

In line with recent developments in UK Clinical Psychology, the stance of Challenging Heights is firmly on "what's happened to you?" rather than "what's wrong with you?" (Johnstone & Boyle, 2018), and in this way, at Challenging Heights, the possibility of permanent psychological harm from trafficking is never given credence, and hence internalised shame and guilt (which I see so commonly in my therapeutic practice in the UK) is reduced through community fellow-feeling. To me it was refreshing to see that the staff at Challenging Heights appeared to be angry about what has happened to their children, rather than sad for their suffering.

Integrating Western and Local Psychologies

Bringing traditional Western psychology skills into this environment was a challenge for me: my choice to work for Challenging Heights centred on a wish to be part of an organisation bringing about transformative change, rather than just ameliorative change. But in their interest in my expertise in trauma-informed (e.g. NES, 2017) and trauma-focussed psychological interventions (e.g. Grey, 2009), Challenging Heights staff were asking me to help them improve their ameliorative skills, and my concern was I would inadvertently reinforce a problematic "psychologisation" of distress (Rapley et al., 2011) and thus be part of the long line of Westerners in international development causing harm through "unintended consequences" (Black, 2002).

I was lucky to partner with and learn from Linda Osabutey, a talented Social Worker and Challenging Heights' rehabilitation manager, whose professional identity I saw to be firmly rooted in human rights advocacy. Together, we negotiated a way through this potential conflict by maintaining rights-focussed discussion about our children, which prioritised practical and communal needs above or alongside psychological needs, always assuming recovery is possible, and basing our interventions on the premise that not all "traumatic" events cause "psychological traumatisation". For me, it was important to "give away" my professional knowledge and power (Miller, 1969; Burton, 2007) and allow decisions to be made by the local staff, who knew the children best.

For the minority of children where we judged some psychological intervention might be necessary, we framed the communal activities of art, drama and play (already in place in the rehabilitation centre, and aimed at raising "voice"), and the behavioural boundaries and basic nurture provided in the rehabilitation environment, as our primary psychological intervention. We created monitoring systems to review how children responded to these interventions, and only for a very few did we provide individual psychological therapy, in which case we chose to use Narrative Exposure Therapy (NET; Schauer et al., 2011).

NET is an approach based on Cognitive Behavioural Therapy (e.g. Ehlers & Clark, 2000) and the Chilean tradition of Testimony therapy (Van Dijk et al., 2003), where survivors of political torture tell their stories as a way to bear witness and hold accountable human rights violators. NET has been successfully used in refugee camps to reduce psychological distress and common post-traumatic experiences: refugees have been trained as peer therapists and the stories collected as part of therapy have been used as evidence in war crimes prosecutions (Schauer et al., 2011). NET fits well with Challenging Heights' approach, as it is an approach centred on upholding human rights and empowering community members to help each other reduce distress. NET also gives a structured and safe way for some child survivors to contribute to Challenging Heights' broader advocacy aims: they can be supported to become "survivor activists" if they choose to allow some or all of their stories to be shared outside of the therapy setting. In this way we were able to integrate individual therapy with the broader transformative remit of the organisation.

Survivors, Not Victims

Challenging Heights did show some signs of succumbing to humanitarian reason, primarily to fulfil its need to source donations from wealthy Western philanthropists and grant-giving bodies. Whilst the Ghanaian focus might be on pragmatic correction of injustice, Challenging Heights also had to interact with powerful Western agencies and individuals who prioritised a narrative of "deserving victims" common to Western discourses of international development (Lindorfer, 2009). For example, Challenging Heights partnered with American anti-slavery charities, some of which demanded intimate details of individual rescued children's stories to use in promotional fundraising material, including their photographs and details of violence they had endured. Others provided donations contingent on children personally writing "thank you" letters.

These demands caused children's confidentiality and rights to privacy to be breached in a way that would never be sanctioned for fundraising initiatives in the Western world (e.g. UK Fundraising Regulator, 2017), and required Challenging Heights to produce "performing victims" (Lindorfer, 2009) in order to access the resources their beneficiaries should be entitled to. Challenging Heights' internal beliefs about survivor agency were thus compromised by the demands of the Western funders: as Lindorfer (2009) points out, "*any idea of 'self-determined empowerment' becomes [difficult] in an environment where powerlessness pays more*" (p. 362, Lindorfer, 2009).

Working together with local and international colleagues at Challenging Heights, we began to have conversations about these practices, and local staff became empowered to challenge Western donors and question whether they would make the same demands of children from their own communities who had endured abuses. This led to an end to the use of "victim stories" at Challenging Heights, and the establishment of a code of practice which respected survivors' and beneficiaries' rights to privacy, including anonymising photographs used in promotional material and requiring informed consent before using details of survivors' stories in fundraising. Donors were required to comply with Challenging Heights' controls and protections of their beneficiaries' privacy, and the local staff group were pleased to find they did not lose valuable donors as a result of insisting on these standards.

How Can We Stand with Organisations Like Challenging Heights?

Whilst Challenging Heights is a great example of a grassroots, human rights-focussed project in keeping with community psychology principles, it is of course not perfect. Despite the integration of advocacy into Challenging Heights' holistic intervention model, there are limits to how far "upstream" a single organisation is able to go. During my time at Challenging Heights, the team achieved key advocacy aims, such as changing Ghanaian police policy on vehicle checks for trafficked children and getting Ghanaian religious leaders to sign up to an anti-trafficking commitment. However, it remained difficult for the organisation to comment on, or influence those policies even further "upstream", such as the inequalities between nations that lead to powerful governments dictating economic and social policies in "developing" countries.

These power dynamics were clearly played out in the paternalistic approaches of Western donor agencies, which often preferred to allocate money to agencies based in the West, despite their lack of local knowledge and understanding. As long as Challenging Heights remained largely reliant on Western grants and donations, we were forced to walk a fine line between criticising and pleasing our Western benefactors, limiting the extent to which we could be truly participatory and community led in our approach.

As community psychologists, when we work outside our own communities, I believe we can only be helpful through staying true to principles of accompaniment (e.g. Edge et al., 2003). This means listening to those with first-hand experience, bearing witness, giving our professional knowledge away and using our professional power strategically in the service of others. Whilst working for Challenging Heights inevitably became an all-encompassing obsession for the two years of my commitment, I was always conscious that this project belonged to James, his staff and his community. Given the historical and inherent power dynamics in international development work (Lykes, 2010), it was important for me to have been invited to Challenging Heights and to constantly reflect to ensure my actions were oriented towards local staff members' goals.

Working closely with James allowed me to see the personal toll he paid for telling his story so publicly—perhaps Challenging Heights would have achieved nothing at all without James' willingness to identify as a survivor and share his story, but at times it was shocking to witness the insatiable thirst from Western donors to pry into the details of his experience. When we aim as community psychologists to amplify the voices of the oppressed in order to help them "speak truth to power" (first use attributed to Bayard Rustin, 1942) we must also attend to the cost of raising voices. There is a limit to what the world can expect from survivor activists: we must all join as allies to share their burden where we can, and accept joint responsibility for achieving change.

Living Community Psychology Values in the NHS

It has been a privilege to work alongside and learn from James and the staff of "challenging, Challenging Heights". I will continue to personally reflect on James' view that by rescuing others we are rescuing ourselves, and hope that I will always have just a fraction of James' energy to correct injustice.

I now work in a Child and Adolescent Mental Health Service (CAMHS) with a speciality in working with looked after children. Returning to the NHS means again getting used to a relentless workload and the disciplines of clinical governance and key performance indicators, and it is difficult to practice in the same "free" way as our team in Ghana. But I do believe that, despite the constraints of our roles, there are opportunities for psychologists such as myself to live the social justice values and community psychology principles of organisations such as Challenging Heights. It's not always easy, but I strive for the following in and outside of my job:

- Taking an attitude to work which centres accompaniment and strives to maximise participatory practice and minimise a medical model of distress;
- Lending professional and positional power to help correct injustice, by speaking out as psychologists, writing letters on behalf of families and young people and being respectful critics of the systems within which we work;
- Staying active and engaged as a citizen in our own local political processes and social movements;
- Linking with other clinical psychologists using community psychology approaches in NHS settings or in partnership with charities, for example, through networks such as the BPS Community Psychology section, or Psychologists for Social Change;
- Bringing ideas such as rights-focussed practice and community psychology values into mainstream settings through training and advocacy.

Acknowledgements This chapter could not have been written without all I have learned from James Kofi Annan and the staff and beneficiaries of Challenging Heights. To find out more about their work, please visit www.challengingheights.org.

References

Annan, J. K. (2009, May). Difficulties in fighting child trafficking. *Daily Graphic*.

Berger, P. L., & Luckmann, T. (1966). *The social construction of reality: A treatise in the sociology of knowledge*. Penguin Books.

Black, M. (2002). *The no-nonsense guide to international development*. Verso.

Brecher, J., Costello, T., & Smith, B. (2000). *Globalization from below: The power of solidarity*. South End Press.

Burton, M. (2007). Address to the UK community psychology conference. UK Community psychology practice development day. Birmingham, UK.

Chambers, R. (1997). *Whose reality counts? Putting the first last*. Intermediate Technology Publications.

Danvers, K., & Osabutey, L. (2016). *Data analysis of the experiences of Challenging Heights' children rescued from slavery 2013–2015*. Unpublished.

Danvers, K. & Schley, D. (2016). Better discipline for Ghana's children: A comparative thematic analysis of attitudes to, and experiences of, corporal punishment in Ghana to inform advocacy on ending violence against children. Challenging Heights/family for every child. Retrieved February 1, 2018, from http://challengingheights.org/wp-content/uploads/2014/11/Better-Discipline-for-Ghanas-Children.pdf

Edge, I., Kagan, C., & Stewart, A. (2003). Living poverty in the UK: Community psychology as accompaniment. Retrieved November 14, 2011, from http://www.compsy.org.uk/LivingPoverty5b.pdf

Editorial: Challenging Heights inaugurates boat on Lake Volta (2010, March 11). Editorial. *Daily Graphic*, p. 11.

Ehlers, A., & Clark, D. M. (2000). A cognitive model of posttraumatic stress disorder. *Behaviour Research and Therapy, 38*(4), 319–345.

Farmer, P. (2005). *Pathologies of power: Health, human rights, and the new war on the poor*. University of California Press.

Fassin, D. (2012). *Humanitarian reason: A moral history of the present*. University of California Press.

Fassin, D., & D'Halluin, E. (2005). The truth from the body: Medical certificates as ultimate evidence for asylum seekers. *American Anthropologist, 107*, 597–608.

Foucault, M. (1991). *Discipline and punish: The birth of the prison*. Penguin Social Sciences.

Freire, P. (1972). *Pedagogy of the oppressed*. Penguin.

Fundraising Regulator. (2017). Code of fundraising practice, version 1.5. Retrieved February 26, 2018, from https://www.fundraisingregulator.org.uk/wp-content/uploads/2016/06/Code-of-Fundraising-Practice-v1.5–18102017.pdf

Gaventa, J. (2001). Global citizen action: Lessons and challenges. In M. Edwards & J. Gaventa (Eds.), *Global citizen action*. Earthscan Publications.

Ghana Statistical Services. (2010). *Ghana population and housing census*. Government of Ghana.

Good, B. J. (2012). Theorizing the 'subject' of medical and psychiatric anthropology. *Journal of the Royal Anthropological Institute, 18*, 515–535.

Grabe, S. (2012). An empirical examination of women's empowerment and transformative change in the context of international development. *American Journal of Community Psychology, 49*, 233–245.

Grey, N. (2009). *A casebook of cognitive behavioural therapy for traumatic stress reactions*. Routledge.

Hartman, E., Moris Paris, C., & Blache-Cohen, B. (2014). Fair trade learning: Ethical standards for community-engaged international volunteer tourism. *Tourism and Hospitality Research, 14*(1–2), 108–116.

Hope for Children (2014). Global slavery index. Retrieved June 2015, from http://www.globalslaveryindex.org/

International Labour Organisation/Ghana Statistical Services. (2003). *Child labour survey*. ILO/GSS.

Johnstone, L., & Boyle, M. with Cromby, J., Dillon, J., Harper, D., Kinderman, P., Longden, E., Pilgrim, D., & Read, J. (2018). *The power threat meaning framework: Towards the identification of patterns in emotional distress, unusual experiences and troubled or troubling behaviour, as an alternative to functional psychiatric diagnosis*. British Psychological Society.

Kinderman, P. (2007). Human rights and applied psychology. *Journal of Community and Applied Social Psychology, 17*, 218–228.

Kukwaw, P. A. (2013). Analytical study on child labour in Lake Volta fishing in Ghana. The International Labour Organisation. Retrieved February 1, 2017, from http://challengingheights.org/wp-content/uploads/2014/11/ILO_Analytical_Study_CL_in_Volta_Lake_Fishing_Ghana.Pdf

Ledwith, M., & Springett, J. (2010). *Participatory practice: Community-based action for transformative change*. The Policy Press.

Lindorfer, S. (2009). In whose interest do we work? Critical comments of a practitioner at the fringes of the liberation paradigm. *Feminism & Psychology, 19*, 354–367.

Lykes, M. B. (2010). Commentary on an overview of community psychology interventions. In G. Nelson & I. Prilleltnesky (Eds.), *Community psychology—In pursuit of liberation and well-being* (2nd ed.). Palgrave Macmillan.

Lykes, M. B., & Moane, G. (2009). Editors' introduction: Whither feminist liberation psychology? Critical explorations of feminist and liberation psychologies for a globalizing world. *Feminism & Psychology, 19*, 283–297.

Martín-Baró, I. (1994). *Writings for a liberation psychology*. Harvard University Press.

Maslow, A. H. (1943). A theory of human motivation. *Psychological Review, 50*(4), 370–396.

Miller, G. (1969). Psychology as a means of promoting human welfare. *American Psychologist, 24*, 1063–1075.

Moane, G. (2014). Liberation psychology, feminism and social justice psychology. In C. V. Johnson & H. L. Friedman (Eds.), *The Praeger handbook of social justice and psychology* (Fundamental issues and special populations) (Vol. 1, pp. 115–132). Prager.

Nelson, G., & Prilleltensky, I. (2010). *Community psychology: In pursuit of liberation and well-being*. Palgrave Macmillan.

NES. (2017). *Transforming psychological trauma: A knowledge and skills framework for the Scottish workforce*. National Health Service Education for Scotland.

Okyere, S. (2017). 'Shock and awe': A critique of the Ghana-centric child trafficking discourse. *Anti-Trafficking Review, 9*, 92–105. www.antitraffickingreview.org

Osabutey, L. A. (2015). *Rehabilitating victims of child trafficking: The role of Challenging Heights, an NGO in the Effutu municipal assembly of the central region of Ghana*. MA thesis. Winneba: University of Education, Winneba.

Perkins, D. D. (2009). International community psychology: Development and challenges. *American Journal of Community Psychology, 44*, 76–79.

Rapley, M., Moncrieff, J., & Dillon, J. (2011). *De-medicalizing misery*. Palgrave Macmillan.

Roelen, K., & Chetti, H. K. (2014). *Researching the linkages between social protection and children's care in Ghana: LEAP and its effects on child well-being, care and family cohesion*. Report by family for every child / Centre for Social Protection at the Institute for Development Studies, UK / Challenging Heights, Ghana. Retrieved February 15, 2018, from https://familyforeverychild.org/wp-content/uploads/2014/10/Social_protection_Ghana_report.pdf

Schauer, M., Neuner, F., & Elbert, T. (2011). *Narrative exposure therapy: A short-term treatment for traumatic stress disorders* (2nd ed.). Hogrefe Publishing.

Schley, D., Danvers, K., & Annan, J. K. (2015). Making economic strengthening work: A holistic approach to child trafficking in Ghana. In Symposium report: Keeping children and families together with economic strengthening. Supporting transformation by reducing insecurity and vulnerability with economic strengthening (STRIVE) Programme: USAID/FHI360.

Singh, K. (2001). Handing over the stick: The global spread of participatory approaches to development. In M. Edwards & J. Gaventa (Eds.), *Global citizen action*. Earthscan Publications.

Sloan, T. (2010). Globalization, poverty and social justice. In G. Nelson & I. Prilleltensky (Eds.), *Community psychology: In pursuit of liberation and well-being* (2nd ed.). Palgrave Macmillan.

Somasundaram, D. (1998). *Scarred minds: The psychological impact of war on Sri Lankan Tamils*. Sage.

Teo, T. (2009). Philosophical Concerns in Critical Psychology. In D. Fox, I. Prilleltensky, & S. Austin, (Eds.), Critical Psychology: An Introduction (2nd ed.). London:SAGE.

United States State Department. (2014). 2014 Trafficking in persons report. Retrieved June 2015, from http://www.state.gov/j/tip/rls/tiprpt/

Van Dijk, J. A., Schoutrop, M. J., & Spinhoven, P. (2003). Testimony therapy: Treatment method for traumatized victims of organized violence. *American Journal of Psychotherapy, 57*(3), 361–373.

24

Community-Based Participatory Research (CBPR) as an Emancipatory Modality Promoting Social Transformation, Empowerment, Agency, and Activism

Naiema Taliep, Samed Bulbulia, Sandy Lazarus, Mohamed Seedat, and Building Bridges Team

Writing this chapter was a participatory and engaging initiative with activist researchers from the Institute for Social and Health Sciences (ISHS), University of South Africa (Unisa) and the Macsulinity and Health Research Unit (MaHRU), South African Medical Research Council-University of South Africa (SAMRC-Unisa) and colleagues from the community. The chapter found collective expression in articulating the narratives of local and indigenous voices that reflect the critical imperative of redressing and disrupting colonised and hegemonic epistemes of research into transformative social justice research and praxis. The collective writing team endeavoured to creatively pen the often dismissal and marginalisation of community voices and experiences in academic peer-reviewed publications. Often these scholarly writings merely acknowledge community participation. The book and its editorial team provided a unique opportunity to the authors to be creative and innovative, and this allowed us to reimagine and write about what and for whom it really matters when conducting research and publishing articles. Therefore, we hope the chapter entitled "Community-Based Participatory Research (CBPR) as an Emancipatory Modality Promoting Social Transformation, Empowerment, Agency, and Activism" provides an easy but stimulating read of the rich tapestry and collage of voices in this journey of epistemic activism.

N. Taliep (✉) • S. Bulbulia • M. Seedat
Institute for Social and Health Sciences (ISHS), University of South Africa (Unisa), Johannesburg, South Africa
e-mail: Naiema.Taliep@mrc.ac.za; samed.bulbulia@mrc.ac.za; seedama@unisa.ac.za

Masculinity and Health Research Unit (MaHRU), South African Medical Research Council-University of South Africa (SAMRC-Unisa), Cape Town, South Africa
e-mail: seedama@unisa.ac.za

S. Lazarus • Building Bridges Team
Cape Town, South Africa

Institute for Social and Health Sciences (ISHS), University of South Africa (Unisa), Johannesburg, South Africa

C. Walker et al. (eds.), *The Palgrave Handbook of Innovative Community and Clinical Psychologies*, https://doi.org/10.1007/978-3-030-71190-0_24

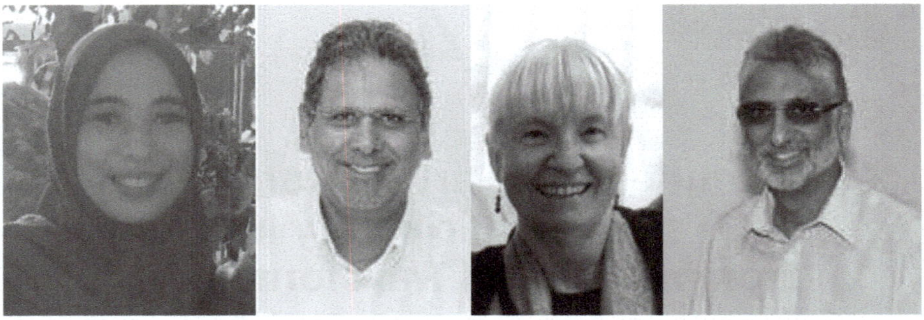

Introduction

Over the last decade, the field of public health has witnessed an increase in the use of Community-Based Participatory Research (CBPR) as an approach for addressing public health priorities (D'Alonzo, 2010; Israel et al., 2005; Wallerstein & Duran, 2008; Lazarus et al., 2015). This includes developing culturally and contextually focused interventions through a community-engaged research process that centrally involves communities in the planning, development, implementation, and evaluation of such interventions (Minkler & Wallerstein, 2008; Sandoval et al., 2012; Lazarus et al., 2015).

It could be argued that the increase in the use of CBPR emerged from a mistrust of academic researchers and scientific institutions accused of conducting research that is manipulative, does not benefit the community, and serves researchers' own selfish interests (Ahmed et al., 2004; Freudenberg, 2001; Higgins & Metzler, 2001). As social scientists, we tend to apply conventional 'top-down' approaches where academics exercise full control over the study from its formulation, research methods, and the outcomes produced, with limited opportunities for reflexivity, and exclusion of communities in decision-making processes. Achille Mbembe (2015) notes that this way of knowledge production has not only become hegemonic, but it also actively subjugates anything that is articulated, thought of, and envisioned outside these frames. This history of knowledge production and ownership, with its tendency to disregard and pathologise the vast majority of the people, as well as commodify research, has resulted in feelings of marginalisation, suspicion, distrust, and anger among community members towards academia and researchers (Adams et al., 2015; Eisinger & Senturia, 2001; Morrel-Samuels, Bower, Bacallao, & Zimmerman, 2016).

Another contention centring on knowledge production and marginalisation has emerged from scholars of the Global South. These scholars have challenged colonised epistemic knowledge and asymmetric powers in research paradigms that position Western male elites as the only legitimate producers of knowledge and the only ones "with access to 'universality', 'rationality' and 'truth', excluding women, 'non-Western' philosophies and social scientists, and even less community voices" (Grosfoguel 2013, p. 29). Maldonado-Torres (2007) notes that coloniality is kept alive in publications, academic performance measures, traditional patterns, common sense, and people's self-image and aspirations, amongst others. Scholars of the Global South thus call for the decolonisation of research and knowledge production. Maldonado-Torres (2007) explains that decoloniality means deconstructing relations of power and understandings of knowledge that stimulate the reproduction of gender, racial, and geopolitical hierarchies that arose or uncovered novel and more powerful methods of expression in the contemporary/colonial world. Smith (1999) posits that decolonising research requires a decisive and focused approach to transforming the institutions and structures involved in research, the conventional ways of organising and conducting research, and the dissemination of knowledge.

In this regard, Hussein Bulhan (2015) suggests that our focus is transformed from remedies for change to support for empowerment, from the treatment of inactive victims to formation of self-determining actors, and from globalised, top-down approaches to contextually relevant, bottom-up approaches. Top-down solution-focused research that endeavours to advance insight into understanding social transformation processes is not likely to have a significant impact on real-world circumstances if it is carried out in the traditional academic way (Moser, 2016). A bottom-up approach, which is congruent with the principles of CBPR, forces academics to examine motivations, interrogate and challenge dominant theories, and be amenable to learn the experiences, perceptions, knowledges, practices, and traditions of the recipients they seek to help, and it also compels researchers to recognise indigenous or local knowledges as valid academic knowledge (Watkins, 2015; Zavala 2013). This approach requires researchers to account for their positionality with respect to the field, the people they engage with, as well as the "geopolitics of knowledge" (Mignolo, 2009) more broadly. This approach also confirms that the supposed 'receivers of help' own the process and outcome of change or transformation (Watkins, 2015).

CBPR as a critically engaged and liberatory approach emphasises praxis over sterile theory (see Adams et al., 2015) and presents a viable alternative to conventional research methods, especially in low-income communities characterised by socio-economic marginalisation, high levels of poverty, and lack of resources. CBPR is conducive to liberatory action as it intentionally strives and adopts a critical and reflexive lens to comprehend and value reality from the viewpoint of the marginalised. Impelled by a need to redress health disparities, critical scholarship and communities are increasingly advocating the use of alternative and liberatory methodologies that focus on psycho-social health disparities, inequities, social justice, and transformation (D'Alonzo, 2010; Lazarus, in press).

There is a need to understand pathways, or agents of change, practices, and capacity building for transformative change (Moser, 2016). Understanding the process of social transformation, which is embedded in personal and collective empowerment, agency, and activism, is important to foster local ownership and enhance the sustainability of local initiatives (Foundation for Sustainable Development [FSD], 2016; Lazarus, Duran, Caldwell, & Bulbulia, 2012a). An analysis of social transformation thus requires an analysis of macro-social forces, local customs, experiences, and identities—the structure that changes, the elements of change, and their mutual relations (Khondker & Schuerkens, 2014; UNESCO, 2017).

The following section positions social transformation, empowerment, agency, and activism within a critical framework of CBPR followed by a summary of CBPR as a transformative approach to research. Drawing from practical experience, the authors then focus on a particular case study, that is, the Spiritual Capacity and Religious Assets for Transforming Community Health by Mobilising Males for Peace and Safety (SCRATCHMAPS) project conducted in a low-income community in the Western Cape, South Africa, reflecting on how CBPR served as an emancipatory framework for promoting social transformation, empowerment, agency, and activism. The chapter concludes with our collective reflections on what really matters when conducting research using a decolonising transformatory CBPR approach.

Social Transformation, Empowerment, Agency, and Activism

Social transformation generally implies a fundamental shift in how a society is organised (Hettige, Amaratunga, Haigh, & Weerasena, 2017). Some scholars regard social transformation studies as a domain of research that can set in motion positive efforts towards social and political action, to safeguard local and national communities against deleterious consequences of global change (UNESCO, 2017). Schutt (2001) suggests that a comprehensive social transformation strategy should include raising critical consciousness, empowering work for social change, mobilising agency and activism, bringing people together to work towards a common goal, developing alternatives, and social justice through challenging the status quo.

Empowerment is defined as an awareness-raising process, whereby individuals can assume control of their lives and subsequently become agents of their own lives, signifying the surfacing of agency (Lazarus, in press). Empowerment is a developmental, ongoing, democratic, and continuous participatory process, by means of which marginalised persons and groups attain better control over their lives and their environment, are involved in decision making at different levels, and acquire access to equitable and valued resources (Kanji and Greenwood, 2001; Maton, 2008).

Agency denotes the power or capacity to act, in particular, the ability to act as a person, directly and with choice, with freedom (Gough, 2009). Cerulli and Kossak (2009) expand the notion of agency from being active and 'transformative' to activities that not only create but also respond to shifting conditions. Agency is constituted by people's sense of purpose (conviction that a particular practice is valuable for achieving a specific outcome), competence (being aware of how to influence an anticipated outcome in reality), scope of autonomy (capacity to make a difference in a given structural environment), and reflexivity (an ability to monitor and appraise one's actions and structural contexts) (Pantić, 2017).

Activism relates to attitude made visible by means of actions and behaviour (Gough, 2009). The goals of social change activity are to protect traditional everyday life from novel, outside oppression, and restore things to normal (resistance), to overcome ongoing, long-established oppression; attain the total extent of everyday rights and opportunities (liberation, empowerment, social justice); spread power to make decisions and act more equally to every person affected by those decisions (enfranchisement, democratisation); and ensure that society will support and protect the rights of all citizens, especially the marginalised and disenfranchised (Humane-isation) (Schutt, 2001). It has been argued that conducting indigenous or community-based research in itself is a highly political social change activity, primarily because it regards the negotiation and transformation of institutional practices and research frameworks, and structures, as important as the actual carrying out of a research agenda (Smith, 1999).

CBPR as Emancipatory Praxis

CBPR falls within the ambit of participatory approaches to research, which are embedded in an epistemology[1] of participative and experiential knowing, guided by critical subjectivity and participatory processes (Holkup, Tripp-Reimer, Salois, & Weinert, 2004). The guiding principles of a CBPR approach include research that is culturally and contextually congruent and addresses the felt needs of a community; facilitates a collaborative and equitable partnership characterised by reciprocity, impartiality, and social justice throughout the lifespan of the research; is characterised by empowerment and symmetrical power-sharing, consciously attending to social inequalities; is committed to action, emphasising the dynamic correlation between theory and practice (praxis) that equally benefits both research institutions and the community; mobilises agency and active citizenship; focuses on strengths and resources (assets); challenges the hegemony[2] of knowledge production, and knowledge economy, and fosters a critical co-learning and co-creation approach to knowledge production; promotes capacity building among all partners; involves systems development by means of repeated, cyclical, and reflexive processes; and is committed to sharing outcomes and knowledge products and, more importantly, humanising research; and finally, CBPR is dedicated to a long-term research process fostering sustainability and engendering community building and transformation (Israel et al., 2003; Lazarus, Taliep, Bulbulia, Philips, & Seedat, 2012b; Lazarus, Bulbulia, Taliep, & Naidoo, 2015; Minkler & Wallerstein, 2008).

CBPR exemplifies participatory engagement, which "reflects a particular worldview that seeks to shape engaged research practices, embodying a holistic, critical, systemic, and relational approach to knowledge construction and research" (Lazarus et al., 2015, p. 88). A critical stance to research is characterised by a view of reality, and people, as being shaped by social, political, cultural, and economic values and ideologies, with socio-economic and political forces of society being emphasised, and further sheds light on matters of equity, power, domination, hegemony, privilege, and social justice (White, 2015). This perspective emphasises the need to understand and address power relations, with a particular focus on oppression, privilege, and inequities, for the purposes of promoting liberation and just social transformation. As a critical approach, CBPR necessitates reflexivity through deliberate mindfulness

[1] The theory of knowledge, especially with regard to its methods, validity, and scope, and the distinction between justified belief and opinion.

[2] Leadership, power, mastery, control, or dominance, especially by one state or social group over others.

of one's own social position as a researcher within the relations of power and values, and it engages with and embraces marginalised voices, including indigenous and community-embedded knowledges.

Case Study: SCRATCHMAPS

The SCRATCHMAPS project is nested in a broader safety, peace, and health promotion programme, the Ukuphepha Initiative: Demonstrating African Safety in the Masculinity and Health Research Unit of the South African Medical Research Council–University of South Africa (SAMRC–UNISA). The primary focus of this project, which was initiated from 2011 until 2016, was to establish how the mobilisation and leveraging of community assets, with a particular focus on spiritual capacity and religious assets, could promote safety and peace, specifically through the promotion of generative or positive forms of masculinity. The objectives of the study included developing conceptual and theoretical frameworks; mapping the dynamics underlying spiritual capacity and religious assets in one community; developing, implementing, and evaluating an intervention that mobilises community assets, including spiritual capacity and religious assets, to promote generative forms of masculinity; and contributing to the knowledge base of community engagement as it is expressed through a CBPR approach. The SCRATCHMAPS research design included a phased approach comprising: (1) preparation, (2) community asset mapping and action planning, (3) development, implementation, and evaluation of the main intervention, and (4) sustainability.

The participant community is located in Strand, a middle- and low-income coastal area, in the province of the Western Cape, South Africa. There are currently around 250 households in this low-income community. The primary lingua franca of the community is Afrikaans and the people were previously classified as 'coloured'[3] during the Apartheid era. The vast majority of the residents are below the age of 40; many have low to limited educational levels (45%), and close to half of the residents earn an income below the poverty line (Development Action Group, 1997). Social service interventions in this community are fragmented, and community advancement is limited.

[3] Coloured is the name given by the previous South African dispensation to an ethnic group of people who are of mixed race ancestry.

Two community structures (Advisory Committee and Community Activist Research Team[4]) were established to manage and conduct the SCRATCHMAPS research, alongside the academic partners. The Advisory Committee comprising of local residents with an array of experience was attended regularly by a core group of at least 10–15 members throughout the lifespan of the project. The meetings were chaired by a local male and female chair and co-chair. The community Research Team comprised ten members from the local community and reflected a combination of young and older adults.

In the following section, we reflect on the case study as an illustration of how CBPR as an emancipatory approach enacted social transformation and Schutt's (2001) framework for a comprehensive transformation strategy. The ensuing narrative will draw on both process evaluation data obtained from the case study and our own insights and experiences as research activists' team members.

Reflective Narrative: Raising Critical Consciousness

Proponents of participatory research generally commit to promoting critical consciousness, social justice, and emancipation as they confront and question their individual roles in communities within a political ideology (Wallerstein & Duran, 2008). Social transformation endeavours to point out conditions and factors that bring about the change of a society from one particular set of circumstances to another (Khondker & Schuerkens, 2014). Raising critical consciousness comprises of making people aware of and informing them about injustices and oppression so that they can develop an alternative vision. Strategies include several diverse campaigns for change that focus on a variety of important issues and affect a broad range of people (Schutt, 2001).

In the SCRATCHMAPS project, critical consciousness was raised by engaging in conversations about how our colonised past has impacted our histories, language, culture, ways of learning, unlearning, and knowing, and its impact on our being and communities. Active participation is liberating and empowering because it creates awareness of community members' innate power to transform their own lives as indicated by a participant who said that it made them realise "*that they (sic) can change things and they (sic) can reap the fruits from these changes*". Using the precepts of CBPR, and applying the

[4] This is used interchangeably with 'research team'.

teachings of Freirian, Fanonian and decolonial scholars created awareness and conscientisation amongst the group. We constantly reminded ourselves to be conscious and critical in how we construct and deconstruct our thoughts, writing, doing, and listening throughout the research process. A telling experience was when we were conducting a timeline workshop in which the community had to reflect on their apartheid past and highlight all the moments of resistance and protests until 1994. The emotional outpouring and voices of resistance were profound and left lasting imprints in our memories. In this exercise, we had a large white canvas which reflected a timeline spanning about 50 years. Participants engaged with their dehumanising and colonial past and came forward to document what events impacted their lives. Participants were encouraged to provide as much detail as possible, and there were not any noticeable differences in opinions since those present alluded to the same, if not similar traumatic experiences.

> On this day it was very touching because during the timeline exercise, the whole history of the [community]..., came out. People were telling historical stories ... that was [sic] moving. I was heartbroken to hear what the people of Erijaville went through in Apartheid. (Community Activist Researcher)

Differences in opinions and views are respected and encouraged because they stimulate discourse and dialogue. Differences are addressed in an amicable, sensitive, safe space, and manner, by starting and closing every meeting with a check-in and reflexive process, and are resolved in a participatory process by ensuring that all voices are affirmed and acknowledged by colleagues. Also, an Advisory Committee was formed, consisting of community-based members, who provided guidance and advice. The Advisory Committee met quarterly and was provided with all the relevant documents to review. All project decisions required their approval and consent before implementation.

A further illustration of raising critical consciousness was the sharing of literature from critical and decolonial scholars amongst ourselves so that we sharpened our thinking, analysis, and writings during the duration of the project and beyond. The community research team were enthralled when various 'academic constructs' were alluded too, and this was evident as expressed by a community research team member, "*we would like to hear and learn more about these constructs, and it should not be only for academics*". Ndlovu (2017) reminds us that though CBPR engenders emancipatory values, it must be contextualised and practised within a critical epistemic decolonial approach, which operates at epistemic, political, and methodological levels. We should not be afraid of *epistemic disobedience*, as Mignolo (2009) states. We need to design methods that speak to our realities—methods that are participative, interactive, and emancipatory, and of course ethical. In the SCRATCHMAPS study, this has been distilled into how the community research activists have planned campaigns, for example, Mandela Day, International Peace Day, poverty alleviation initiatives, such as food sovereignty (community gardens), and job creation opportunities by networking with other NGOs and social actors and hosting compassionate grassroots community conversations which addressed issues such as generative masculinities and femininities, and racism, amongst others.

The hosting of these compassionate grassroots conversations speaks to our mission of conducting compassionate research with and in the service of communities. Since communities are generally on the margins, and/or on the periphery of dialogue connected with research and praxis, one avenue of engaging and ensuring communities become part of the co-learning and co-sharing ethos was hosting these talks and engaging with communities on themes and issues which matter to them. We must begin to demystify knowledge, and dialogue on how and who produces knowledge, and give voice to indigenous embedded knowledge. Speakers invited represent academics, social actors, and community activists. These talks are energising, and the intention is to generate some action post conversations, that is, walk the talk. For example, after a conversation led by a community activist from the Bonteheuwel Walking Ladies, women in the broader area mobilised to form a similar group.

Empowerment

Empowerment constitutes both a developmental, ongoing, continuous participatory process and an outcome goal of CBPR. Lazarus (in press) points out that if the goal is broader social transformation and political action, the process of personal empowerment provides the stimulus to take action—either as an individual or as a collective. It is a process by means of which marginalised persons and groups attain better control over their lives, and their environment, and acquire valued resources (Maton, 2008). An empowerment approach values power-sharing and capacity building, through learning exchanges and mentoring, emphasising democratic participation in all phases of the research within a social justice framework, and fostering community ownership of the project, and in decision-making at different levels

(Kanji and Greenwood, 2001; Lazarus, Duran, Caldwell, & Bulbulia, 2012a; Schulz, Israel, Selig, & Bayer, 1998).

> I think the evidence of empowerment is for e.g. [Name] applying for ECD [Early Childhood Development training]. That is a direct thing. She did training; she was part of this process and on her own, nobody assisted her from this side. She wanted to do ECD. She got the information and registered. That is a symbol of empowerment, because now she is a powerful part of the community. (Community Activist Researcher)

Empowerment, that is, power-sharing, accountability, and transparency, was achieved through the establishment of a community advisory committee that provided "*ongoing oversight... guidance on all 'whole community' engagement processes, including meetings and other forms of communication with [the] community*" (meeting minutes). Capacity building in the SCRATCHMAPS project was pursued in various ways, including formal training workshops, and hands-on mentoring amongst academic and community research members (see Lazarus et al., 2012b). Workshops were aligned to the community research team's aspirations and the project requirements, such as understanding the basics of research, writing, leadership and management skills, conflict mediation, and asset mapping workshops, amongst others. It should be noted that in the empowerment process, academic members initially played a more central role in skills development and training relating to research. However, during the latter stage of the project, community research team members and academics began co-facilitating workshops, and ultimately, different aspects of the research process were conducted by the community researchers, while the academics provided an advisory and supportive role.

Research as Praxis: Agency and Activism

One of the most significant strengths of CBPR is praxis-oriented research, which is inextricably linked to the central involvement of participants in the research process and outcomes, to generate social transformation. Praxis denotes the relationship between reflection and action, between knowing and doing, and employing the action of doing research as a vehicle to alter stereotypes, habits of mind, and entrenched meanings that direct people's assumptions and thoughts regarding political and social matters, as well as promote actions that make evident these transformations in theories or worldviews underlining the ways people live in society (Given, 2008).

According to Rahman (1991) and Pantić (2017), self-conscious individuals, especially those who are poor, disenfranchised and oppressed, can progressively change their environment by their own praxis. The following quote lends credence to this claim: "*Participants [wanted] to improve themselves and thereby improve their community, to enhance their skills, improve and refine their … knowledge to help youth …*" One of the aspirations of the community activist research team was sustainable community building. An illustration of agency was the collective decision by the community activist research team members to start an afterschool programme, a local informal library, and Youth Café, reflecting the essence of individual and collective agency and praxis. One of the community activist researchers stated:

> We sat with a lot of pain from apartheid years … so we as parents were forced to work and our children were left alone to grow up on their own, so we are now we have the problem that our children are easy targets for group pressure, negative influences, violence, drugs, teenage pregnancy, sexual abuse, and child maltreatment. These were the challenges we faced, but we did not know how to handle it, but when we became involved in SCRATCHMAPS and the research, we learned how to deal with these problems.

Pantić (2017) alludes that agency is constituted by people's sense of purpose, competence, the scope of autonomy, and reflexivity. As research activists, working within the framework of CBPR, we remain critically mindful and intentionally reflexive of our roles in the research process.

A key challenge relating to research and action was a disparity between the time dedicated to the research process and community expectations for action. Community members often complained that we were too research-focused and that there was a lack of 'action' on our part in addressing the challenges they faced. *It is thus important to engage communities in the planning and action processes so that they understand the* action research imperative. During our reflexive sessions, we discussed that certain community priorities are achievable in the short term through community agency and activism, such as access to basic essential services, for example, ensuring parents or single mothers have their identity documents in order, to access the child grant which can assist them in taking care of some of their children's needs and to enrol children in school. The macro challenges such as housing and unemployment which are also a priority may require data to substantiate the urgency of action. Part of the action learning process is to have a conversation, brainstorm, or workshop to prioritise short-, medium-, and long-term goals and, if necessary, generate data/evidence that can support achieving these decided priorities to present to local government to strengthen your application to address the macro issues, that is, using local evidence to motivate for local action.

> When I came into the programme, I thought action was important, but there I learnt, even though action is important, there is a process that you have to go through before you can take action because, action without planning is useless. (Community Activist Researcher)

Developing Alternatives: Structural and Humanising Research

When we started to engage with this community and shared our enthusiasm in partnering with them on a community-based participatory action research project, we discovered that this community, like many of the disenfranchised communities in South Africa, was beset with the vestiges of apartheid and colonisation, compounded by unemployment, poverty, inequality, and violence, with minimum infrastructure, limited resources, and no evidence of formal or informal community initiatives. This was the beginning of a joint six-year partnership with us, the SAMRC–UNISA Violence, Injury, and Peace Research Unit.

Smith (1999) alludes to 'intervening', which takes action research to mean literally the process of being proactive, and becoming involved in and designing actions that produce structural and cultural changes. This was evident in SCRATCHMAPS, where community members actively started engaging with local politicians to transform a sports space, previously riddled with potholes, into a functioning sports and recreational space, where children and adults now enjoy playing various indigenous games, netball, and touch rugby (Fig. 24.1).

Another example is the building of a multipurpose community hall after 25 years of waiting and struggle. This was activated by a dynamic local committee, comprising young adults who mobilised the residents to take action and submitted an application to the local municipality. The resistance of the community to design alternatives resonates with Smith's (1999) account of the Maori peoples intervening, which is directed at changing institutions which deal with indigenous peoples and not at changing indigenous peoples to fit the structures, and the confidence of knowing that we have survived and progressed provides some impetus to a process of envisioning. This power of communities and indigenous peoples to transform their own lives, and set

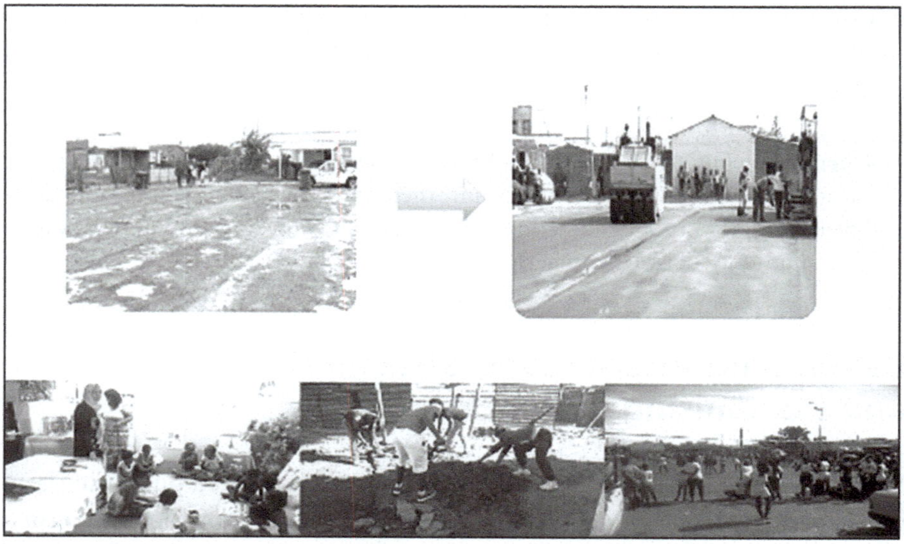

Fig. 24.1 Transforming spaces and places: Illustrations of community activism in Erijaville

new directions despite their impoverished and oppressed conditions, speaks to the politics of resistance.

Addressing poverty, unemployment, and inequalities—through the formation of a local network of care—and developing sustainable community building initiatives were another promising initiatives that evolved through SCRATCHMAPS. Networking is a process which indigenous peoples have used effectively to build relationships and disseminate knowledge and information. Smith (1999) calls this 'reframing', and it is about them taking much greater control over the ways in which indigenous issues and social problems are discussed and handled.

The study with community activist researchers also demonstrated that CBPR is a reflection of developing alternatives in how research is conducted, particularly in community settings and with indigenous peoples. This included decoloniality and resistance being synonymous with developing alternatives to existing colonised epistemologies and oppressive systems of knowledge production. The study, true to its research purpose, ensured that there was a decolonial shift in the producers and developers of knowledge systems—co-sharing and co-creation of the knowledge economy was pertinent by affirming that indigenous experiences, narratives, and storytelling and lives matter. Resisting bureaucracy and hierarchical systems, and replacing them with participatory modes of engagement, was another facet of the partnership and research process, that is, ensuring that the principles of CBPR underpin the community engagement research processes, taking cues from the advisory committee, and exercising reflexivity.

We were aware that since the unit was more resourced, the issue of power differentials to some degree became evident. However, we remained vigilant of this dynamic and did not allow it to impede our initiatives. The study also ensured that the present system of criteria for publications in institutions had to be disrupted by a form of insurgent community scholarship. This was achieved by ensuring that previously marginalised and indigenous voices of community activists were recognised and affirmed as co-authors in accredited journals. An honorarium was also provided for their co-authorship. The general practice is that community researchers are only acknowledged in accredited publications, and as SCRATCHMAPS, we wanted to disrupt this process, and find a mechanism whereby we could compensate community-based researchers as co-authors in our publications, and therefore the idea of an honorarium was discussed, integrated into the budget, and implemented. The process of writing for journals was an ongoing process of capacitation and included conducting of writing workshops as part of the research process. Prior to writing this chapter, we discussed the paper with the community activist research team, jotted down their ideas and input. These were integrated into the paper and reviewed by all the authors, including the community research team. Community activist researchers also shared their experiences and their participation in the study in various fora such as at national conferences and universities to masters and honours psychology students, and they co-facilitated workshops with academics. These initiatives affirm community-based activist researchers, their contributions to knowledge production and the knowledge economy, and also strengthen the assets and capacity of their community (Fig. 24.2).

Communities previously understood as 'recipients of research' were now innovators, producers, owners, and dignified scholars—humanising research. To assume in advance that people will not be interested in, or will not understand the deeper issues, or do not have views on the matter is arrogant. The challenge always is to demystify, to decolonise, and to remind ourselves, that sharing knowledge is a long-term commitment (Smith, 1999). Our study exemplifies how community activist researchers have transitioned from a context of risk and pathology to embracing an assets- or strengths-based perspective and resiliency. This disruption of mainstream authoring in publications was welcomed as an innovative, creative, and socially just approach to acknowledging and affirming contributions made by community-based activist researchers in publications.

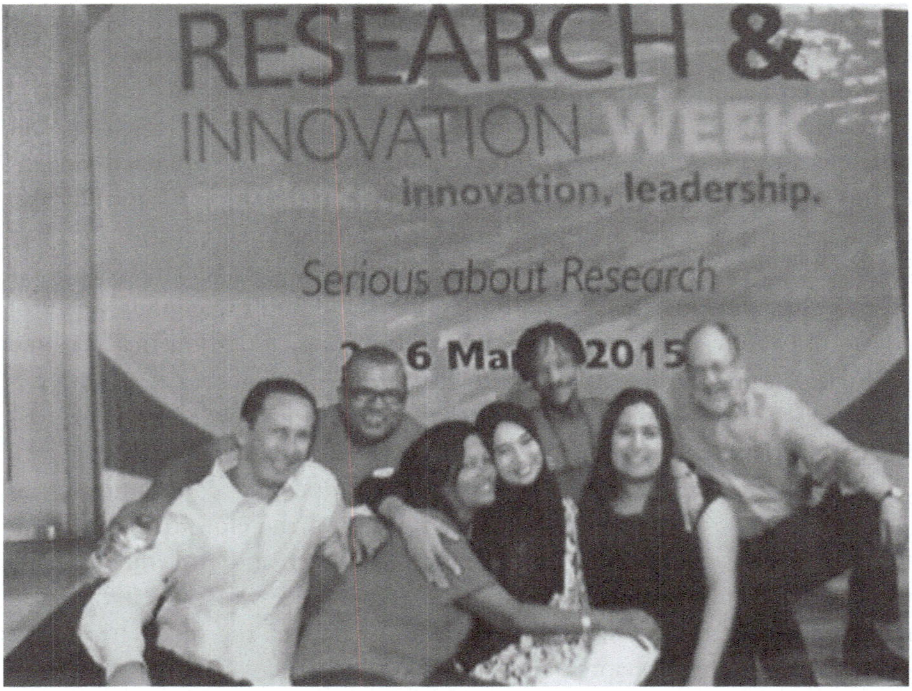

Fig. 24.2 Community activist researchers participating in the University of South Africa Research & Innovation Week

Social Justice: Challenging the Status Quo

The ultimate goal of CBPR is social transformation aimed at promoting social justice. Freire (1970) notes that a pledge to social justice necessitates an ethical attitude towards fairness and equality and a firm belief in the ability of people as agents who are capable of transforming their world. In CBPR, knowledge, policy, and practice are created jointly by means of a nascent process of action and learning, frequently involving some form of critical reflection, and re-evaluation of the norms, values, and beliefs through which we make sense of things, and a grasping of how power shapes these processes (Pettit, 2010). A poignant quote by a community research team member reflects our collective pledge to social transformation within the broader context of hegemonic knowledge and academic dominance:

> Big words, small words. In this research, I learned something which I had struggle with all these years. I used to think that the academic people knew everything. In the past, I had a lot of problems [with] … academic people [who]

> came and said that they wouldn't betray the people … but they did … but in this project, I learned that I am being asked something and they walk a path with you.

Thus, the process of social change, and advocating for social justice, has to begin with a self-reflective process that evaluates the inconsistencies between our adopted values, our everyday lived experience, and our actions (Freire, 1970). Reflective practice through journaling enable researchers to reflect on how their "own experiences, values, and positions of privilege in various hierarchies have influenced their research interest, the way they choose to do their research, and the ways they choose to represent their research findings" (Harrison, MacGibbon, & Morton, 2001, p. 325). In SCRATCHMAPS, advocating humanising research, and consciously using various reflexive strategies to contemplate our positionality in the research process, included journaling, a 'check-in' process, and debriefing sessions.

> My second family [the entire SCRATCHMAPS team] makes me feel like I'm worth something. You motivate me, encourage me and give me daily knowledge because we always learn from each other. (Community Activist Researcher)

SCRATCHMAPS was guided by the co-learning and co-construction of knowledge, where local traditional knowledge and experiences were shared, valued, and given equal importance to academic knowledge in the quest for social transformation. Such collaborative learning processes over time "give equal importance to what researchers and decision makers can learn from each other, can produce cultural shifts that facilitate the ongoing use of research knowledge in decision making" (Morgan et al., 2015, p. 7). Sharing the knowledge and methods, and the process of conducting research, is time-consuming and requires a long-term commitment and a passion for continuous learning and unlearning.

> I think we created a space where people could learn from each other, even as facilitators. Exercises and discussions were not just linked to theory, it was made real and linked to … assets and peace and safety… Some participants … stated that this training has provided them with a springboard to make a difference in their community. (Academic Activist Researcher)

Researchers should be dedicated to a course of action for social change in which the inequity of power in society is transformed or rectified and where the role of participants are transformed from passive 'subjects' of research to actors for change (Fernandes, 1992; Pettit, 2010). Guided by a CBPR approach, SCRATCHMAPS thus contested dominant knowledge influences by promoting social justice, reflexivity, co-sharing and co-construction of knowledge, mobilising agency, and active participation of community members to enhance transformation within a collaborative partnership framework.

Reflections: What Really Matters

Smith's (1999) exposition of her research experiences mirrors ours as co-researchers in this study. We observed the fortitude and resilience of our ten community activist researchers brimming with enthusiasm and excitement when the project began six years ago. As time passed, their passion and commitment became more visible, and in the process of co-learning and co-sharing, they were able to deconstruct academic talk with ease.

Be mindful that these colleagues of ours had no prior experience and exposure to CBPR. It was refreshing to see how their continuing belief in themselves grew with each passing day, and their optimism, hope, and also moments of anxiety would maybe one day transform their lives. Smith (1999) captures some defining moments when talking with people in the community when she became interested in the questions which researchers were asking of health, but were not being addressed by the research. This is what someone said, "We know we are dying", "but tell me why we are living?" "Our health will not improve unless we address the fact that we have no sovereignty", "We're sick of hearing what's wrong with us, tell us something good for a change", or "Why do they always think by looking at us they will find the answers to our problems, why don't they look at themselves?" The same questions were being asked of education and of justice.

> Freire's writings reinforce a deep belief in humanity and people's role in making change, and as such have critical importance to CBPR: To be a good [participatory researcher] means above all to have faith in people; to believe in the possibility that they can create and change things. You need to love … to be convinced that the fundamental effort of community … education is the liberation of people, never their "domestication." This liberation begins to the extent that men [and women] reflect on themselves and their condition in the world—the world in which and with which they find themselves. To the extent that they are more conscientized, they insert themselves as social actors' into their own history. (Adapted from Freire 1970, p. 61)

This resonates with our own inadequacies as co-researchers, and so, in this study, we also wanted to know why it was that community concerns tend to be always framed around conventional research problems. Through a critical decolonial CBPR lens, how could we collectively reframe and address such concerns from the ground up by working with the assets and strengths, and the needs of the community to develop initiatives that matter? The outcome of this process was that the community decided on a future programme of action. Building trust, bonding, and nurturing our relationships were central to our collective well-being. Power dynamics and differences were dealt with by creating, inventing, and inviting a safe space for us all, by doing a check-in whenever we met, whereby all of us spoke truth to unspoken silences and say what really matters—be it project related and/or personal.

Summary

As researchers, we have to consciously engage when we partner and conduct research with communities. Questions posed by indigenous peoples such as "how can research ever address our needs as indigenous peoples if our questions are never taken seriously, or remain unanswered?" are heard, and not simply passed over, or silenced, or become disconnected from their realities, and collectively appraised and addressed. These community activist researchers have taken ownership of the project and are implementing a youth mentoring project and continuing their efforts towards community building. We are privileged to be allowed into their lives, and we continue to grow together while journeying with them through our partnering in research.

Concluding Thoughts

The chapter, first, contextualised CBPR within the broader framework of public health research. Second, it emphasises the importance of using a critical social justice and decolonial perspective in conducting public health and community-engaged research. Third, this approach focuses on CBPR as an emancipatory praxis that engenders social transformation, empowerment, agency, and activism. Fourth, it imparts insights into our experiences of doing research within the CBPR paradigm.

CBPR and critical scholarship disrupts and transforms conventional ways of learning, thinking, and knowing by disentangling epistemic and ontological biases through 'un-silencing' marginalised voices, validating local knowledges, mindfulness, and critical reflexivity of our role as academics and institutional representatives, and remaining cognisant of the power dynamics, and hegemony of knowledge production. This approach affirms that community members not only are understood as key resources and social actors in the research process but are equal co-producers of knowledge and research outputs that can lead to just social transformation.

CBPR, through empowerment, can create awareness of personal agency and mobilise community members to take action. CBPR, understood as a decolonial transformative approach, ensures optimal participation by community members, seeks to find collective solutions through co-learning and co-sharing, fosters empowerment and ownership, promotes social justice, and, importantly, encourages activist researchers to be guided by the community's agenda to find bottom-up sustainable solutions. Decolonised CBPR is humanising and emancipatory.

References

Adams, G., Dobles, I., Gómez, L. I., Kurtiş, T., & Molina, L. E. (2015). Decolonizing psychological science: Introduction to the special thematic section. *Journal of Social and Political Psychology, 3*(1), 213–238. https://doi.org/10.5964/jspp.v3i1.564

Ahmed, S. M., Beck, B., Maurana, C. A., & Newton, G. (2004). Overcoming barriers to effective community-based participatory research in US medical schools. *Education and Health, 17*(2), 141–151. https://doi.org/10.1080/13576280410001710969

Bulhan, H. (2015). Stages of Colonialism in Africa: From occupation of land to occupation of being. *Journal of Social and Political Psychology, 3*(1), 239–256. https://doi.org/10.5964/jspp.v3i1.143

Cerulli, C., & Kossak, F. (2009). Agency and the praxis of activism editorial. *Agency and the Praxis of Activism, 3*(1), 1–4. http://field-journal.org/wp-content/uploads/2016/07/field_2009_Volume_3_web.pdf

D'Alonzo, K. T. (2010). Getting started in CBPR: Lessons in building community partnerships for new researchers. *Nursing Inquiry, 7*(4), 282–288.

Development Action Group. (1997). *Homes for all: A Development Action Group case study of the housing programme in Casablanca and Erijaville.* Development Action Group.

Eisinger, A., & Senturia, K. (2001). Doing community-driven research: A description of Seattle Partners for healthy communities. *Journal of Urban Health: Bulletin of the New York Academy of Medicine, 78*(3), 519–534.

Fernandes, K. (1992). *Conventional and Participatory Research Methodologies*. Working Paper Series # 6 1993. Sustainable Development Policy Institute. https://sdpi.org/publications/files/W6Conventional%20and%20Participatory%20Research.pdf

Foundation for Sustainable Development. (2016). *Our Approach*. https://www.fsd.org/our-approach/

Freire, P. (1970). *Pedagogy of the oppressed*. Herder & Herder.

Freudenberg, N. (2001). Case history of the Center for Urban Epidemiologic Studies in New York. *Journal of Urban Health: Bulletin of the New York Academy of Medicine, 78*(3), 508–518.

Given, L. M. (Ed.). (2008). *The SAGE encyclopedia of qualitative research methods*. Sage Publications.

Gough, T. (2009). Agency and gift of architecture. In C. Cerulli, & F. Kossak (Eds). Agency and the praxis of activism (pp. 143–150). *Field: A Free Journal for Architecture, 3*(1). http://field-journal.org/wp-content/uploads/2016/07/field_2009_Volume_3_web.pdf

Grosfoguel, R. (2013). Decolonizing Post-Colonial studies and paradigms of political economy: Transmodernity, Decolonial thinking, and global coloniality. *TRANSMODERNITY: Journal of Peripheral Cultural Production of the Luso-Hispanic World, 1*(1). http://escholarship.org/uc/item/21k6t3fq

Harrison, J., MacGibbon, L., & Morton, M. (2001). Regimes of trustworthiness in qualitative research: The rigors of reciprocity. *Qualitative Inquiry, 7*(3), 323–345.

Hettige, S., Amaratunga, D., Haigh, R., & Weerasena, N. (2017). Mainstreaming social transformation in recovery and development projects: Case of Sri Lanka. *Procedia Engineering, 212*, 387–394. https://doi.org/10.1016/j.proeng.2018.01.050

Higgins, D. L., & Metzler, M. (2001). Implementing community-based participatory research centers in diverse urban settings. *Journal of Urban Health: Bulletin of the New York Academy of Medicine, 78*(3), 488–494.

Holkup, P. A., Tripp-Reimer, T., Salois, E. M., & Weinert, C. (2004). Community-based participatory research: An approach to intervention research with a native American community. *Advances in Nursing Science, 27*, 162–175.

Israel, B. A., Eng, E., Schulz, J. A., & Parker, E. A. (2005). *Methods in community-based participatory research for health*. Jossey-Bass.

Israel, B. A., Schulz, A. J., Parker, E. A., Becker, A. B., Allen, A. J., & Guzman, R. (2003). Critical issues in developing and following community based participatory research principles. In M. Minkler & N. Wallerstein (Eds.), *Community based participatory research for health* (1st ed., pp. 53–76). Jossey-Bass.

Kanji, N., & Greenwood, L. (2001). *Participatory approaches to research and development in IIED: Learning from experience*. International Institute for Environment and Development (IIED).

Khondker, H. H., & Schuerkens, U. (2014). Social transformation, development and globalization. *Sociopedia.isa*. https://doi.org/10.1177/205684601423. http://www.sagepub.net/isa/resources/pdf/SocialTransformation.pdf

Lazarus, S. (in press). *Power and identity in the struggle for social justice: An autoethnographic study of community practice.* Springer Community Psychology Series.

Lazarus, S., Bulbulia, S., Taliep, N., & Naidoo, A. V. (2015). Community based participatory research as a critical enactment of community psychology. *Journal of Community Psychology, 43*(1), 87–98. https://doi.org/10.1002/jcop.21689

Lazarus, S., Duran, B., Caldwell, L., & Bulbulia, S. (2012a). Public health research and action: Reflections on challenges and possibilities of Community-Based Participatory Research. In J. Maddock (Ed.), *Public health – Social and behavioral health* (pp. 309–324). IntechOpen.

Lazarus, S., Taliep, N., Bulbulia, S., Phillips, S., & Seedat, M. (2012b). Community-based participatory research: An illustrative case of community engagement in one low income community. *Journal of Psychology in Africa, 22*(4), 511–519.

Maldonado-Torres, N. (2007). On the Coloniality of being: Contributions to the development of a concept. *Cultural Studies, 21*(2–3), 240–270.

Maton, K. I. (2008). Empowering community settings: Agents of individual development, community betterment, and positive social change. *American Journal of Community Psychology, 41*(1–2), 4–21. https://doi.org/10.1007/s10464-007-9148-6

Mbembe, A. (2015). Decolonizing knowledge and the question of the archive. In *Wits Institute for Social and Economic Research (WISER).* [Online]. Johannesburg: University of Witwatersrand. http://wiser.wits.ac.za/system/files/Achille%20Mbembe%20-%20Decolonizing%20Knowledge%20and%20the%20Question%20of%20the%20Archive.pdf

Mignolo, W. D. (2009). Epistemic disobedience, independent thought and De-Colonial freedom. *Theory, Culture and Society, 26*(7–8), 1–23. https://doi.org/10.1177/0263276409349275

Minkler, M., & Wallerstein, N. (2008). *Community-based participatory research for health: From process to outcomes* (2nd ed.). Jossey-Bass.

Morgan, D., Crossley, M., Stewart, N., Kirk, A., Forbes, D., D'Arcy, C., … Cammer, A. (2015). Evolution of a community-based participatory approach in a rural and remote dementia care research program. *Progress in Community Health Partnerships, 8*(3), 337–345.

Morrel-Samuels, S., Brown, S., Bower, M., Bacallao, M., & Zimmerman, M. (2016). Community engagement in youth violence prevention: Crafting methods to context. *Journal of Primary Prevention, 37*, 189–207.

Moser, S. C. (2016). Editorial overview: Transformations and co-design: Co-designing research projects on social transformations to sustainability. *Current Opinion in Environmental Sustainability, 20*, v–viii.

Ndlovu, M. (2017). Coloniality of knowledge and the challenge of creating African futures. *Ufahamu: A Journal of African Studies, 40*(3), 1–15.

Pantić, N. (2017). An exploratory study of teacher agency for social justice. *Teaching and Teacher Education, 66*, 219–230.

Pettit, J. (2010). Learning to do action research for social change. *International Journal of Communication, 4*, 820–827.

Rahman, M. A. (1991). Glimpses of the "Other Africa". In O. Fals-Borda & M. A. Rahman (Eds.), *Action and knowledge: Breaking the monopoly with participatory action research*. Intermediate Technology Pubs/Apex Press.

Sandoval, J. A., Lucero, J., Oetzel, J., Avila, M., Belone, L., Mau, M., ... Wallerstein, N. (2012). Process and outcome constructs for evaluating community-based participatory research projects: A matrix of existing measures. *Health Education Research, 27*(4), 680–690.

Schulz, A. J., Israel, B. A., Selig, S. M., & Bayer, I. S. (1998). Development and implementation of principles for community-based research in Public Health. In R. H. MacNair (Ed.), *Research strategies for community practice* (pp. 83–110). The Haworth Press, Inc.

Schutt, R. (2001). *Inciting democracy: A practical proposal for creating a good society*. Spring Forward Press.

Smith, L. T. (1999). *Decolonizing methodologies: Research and indigenous peoples*. ZED Books Ltd.

United Nations Educational, Scientific and Cultural Organisation (UNESCO). (2017). *Social transformations and intercultural dialogues*. http://www.unesco.org/new/en/social-and-human-sciences/themes/international-migration/glossary/social-transformation/

Wallerstein, N., & Duran, B. (2008). The theoretical, historical and practice roots of CBPR. In M. Minkler & N. Wallerstein (Eds.), *Community-based participatory research for health: From process to outcomes* (2nd ed., pp. 25–46). Jossey-Bass.

Watkins, M. (2015). Psychosocial accompaniment. *Journal of Social and Political Psychology, 3*, 324–341. https://doi.org/10.5964/jspp.v3i1.103

White, C. (2015). Internationalizing education: Critical qualitative case studies in Social Education. *American Journal of Educational Research, 3*(2), 211–219.

Zavala, M. (2013). What do we mean by decolonizing research strategies? Lessons from decolonizing, Indigenous research projects in New Zealand and Latin America. *Decolonization: Indigeneity, Education, and Society, 2*(1), 55–71.

Part IV

Creativity and Social Change

> It is more than likely that men, if they were ever to lose the appetite for meaning we call thinking and cease to ask unanswerable questions, would lose not only the ability to produce those thought-things that we call work of art but also the capacity to ask all the answerable questions upon which every civilisation is founded. (Hannah Arendt, *The Life of the Mind*)

This section provides a number of contributions that use arts and creativity as tools to change how *psy* professionals, students, service users, and trainees can be in touch with their humanness at the personal, interpersonal, and community level. In doing so, they all share the epistemological assumption that creative methods are fundamental to psychological praxis as they allow for the most basic and important activity for the human mind: meaning-making.

In line with the words from Arendt, the authors argue that co-producing meaning with participants is necessary in order to enact social change within communities and for the people. In Chap. 25, Price et al. reflect on their experience of UK Doctoral Trainees in Malawi and how the Malawian concept of 'umoza' (togetherness, oneness) can be incorporated in culturally sensitive community-based work using arts to tackle the sense of isolation and disconnection. Together with cultural sensitivity, in Chap. 26 Fisher et al. analyse how a fluid concept of space is pivotal to different modes of participation and co-production presenting projects from Guatemala, the UK, and Brazil. The results of such processes, facilitated through creative approaches, are both materialistic outputs (artefacts) and intangible outcomes (relational wellbeing) which contribute to place-making. Continuing a thread of contributions to the relevance of togetherness and space, in Chap. 27, Higson et al.

highlight the importance of safe and warm places as a community-shared resource which is necessary to ground more formal projects. Here the authors present the co-produced project and space 'Life Rooms' in Liverpool (UK) as a contextual response to the impact of neoliberal ideologies and austerity measures on the helpers, resulting in increased lack of compassion for the vulnerable and the marginalised amongst the *psy* professionals.

In Chap. 28 Wood and Sools merge their experience as clinical and narrative psychologists with the creative and powerful tool of writing sci-fiction. In doing so, they reclaim writing stories of and from the future as a 'psychologically fundamental practice' of meaning-making and resistance for individuals, groups, and communities. Along the line, in Chap. 29 Sagan uses a psychoanalytic phenomenological lens to outline how people enduring mental distress creatively engage in making sense of their humanness and 'being-in-the world' through arts. The restitution of agency to people who fall under the label of 'vulnerable population' is the focus of Chap. 30. Here Partridge and the Elder Care Alliance present an art-based study and subsequent work in which older adults, traditionally excluded in the name of 'protection', act as co-researchers and speak directly to the decision-makers.

The section concludes with Chap. 31 by Ahmed et al. who work with communities living in temporary residence areas (TRAs) in Blikkiesdorp, South Africa. As scholars who acknowledge the distance between academia and the 'outside world', the authors reflect on their interventions with such disadvantaged communities and on the barriers that continue to distance psychological practice from the very same communities they aim to 'help'. However, as for all the chapters of this book, recognising the obstacles and the difficulties in creatively working towards social change is not detrimental to the validity and value of the contributions. On the contrary, as the quote from Arendt reminds us, the faculty of thinking expressed through the reason (*Vernuft*) is a fundamental human activity, and represents a lifetime process of 'quest for meaning' detached from any utilitarian or functionalist goal (Arendt, 1971). The chapters in this section contain a number of creative projects that, in different contexts, provide physical and psychological spaces for people to think, and searching for meaning as individuals, groups, and communities.

25

The Value of Togetherness Across Cultures

Kelly Price, Hayley Higson,
and Ndumanene Devlin Silungwe

Consideration of alternative ways of workings is necessary for inclusion and our aim of achieving greater collaboration across communities. This is something we feel passionately about—developing a shared vision of what services could or should look like through stronger partnerships and integration. For us, this means being creative about how we approach our work and considering alternatives, beyond the evidence base. This often leads to inventive ideas, drawing on some excellent examples of how other cultures engage with people, beyond the therapy room. Working in this 'innovative' way helps us to challenge the status quo and ask those accessing services what they want, what they need and what ideas they have for how psychological support (in any guise) could be different, or better. Who wouldn't want to work in this way?! New ideas and ways of working involve developing aptitude to be sensitive, and listening and responding to the silent voices in society.

K. Price (✉)
Enumclaw, WA, USA

H. Higson
Ormskirk, UK

N. D. Silungwe
Saint John of God Hospitaller Services, Lilongwe, Malawi
e-mail: ndumanene.silungwe@sjog.mw

C. Walker et al. (eds.), *The Palgrave Handbook of Innovative Community and Clinical Psychologies*, https://doi.org/10.1007/978-3-030-71190-0_25

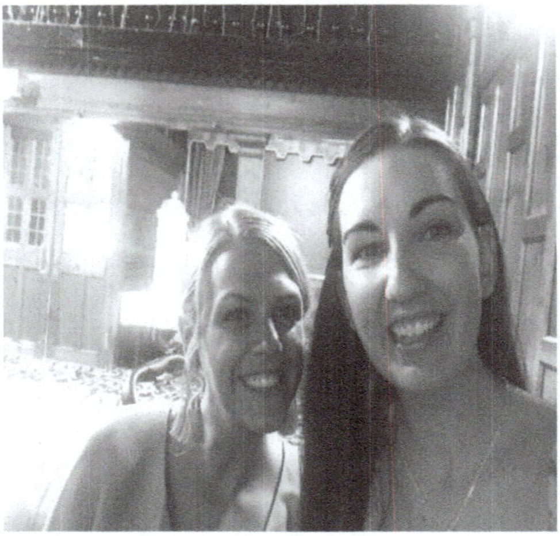
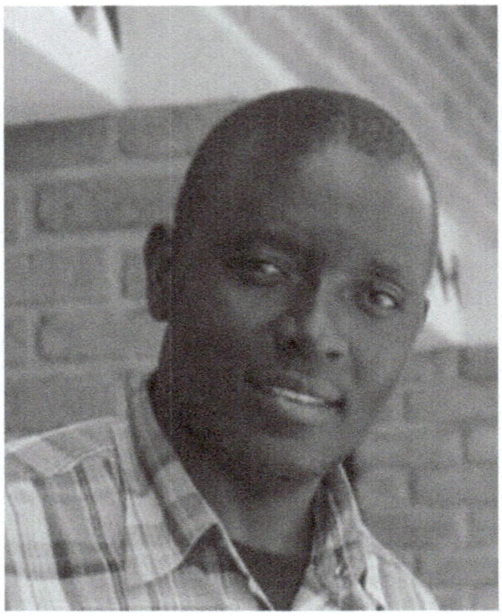

In June 2016, as part of our doctoral training at Lancaster University, we undertook an innovative[1] placement in Malawi, a country located in the South Eastern region of Africa. This placement was facilitated in collaboration with St John of God Hospitaller Services and the Umoza Trust Charity.

This placement had a profound effect on our learning and development in both a professional and a personal capacity. Specifically, we began to consider cultural influences on the ways in which we conceptualise mental health and how families and communities form part of these conceptualisations. Furthermore, this placement provided us with first-hand observations of how mental health services can excel in spite of the limited financial resources.

Wealthy countries generally have more services to combat mental health problems in comparison to lower-income countries. McKenzie et al. (2004) reported that there are limited number of mental health resources, medications and practitioners working throughout lower-income countries. Given this disparity, it is easy to conclude that there is little that can be learned from lower income countries in relation to mental health service provision, but this is not the case (McKenzie et al., 2004). While greatly under-resourced, our placement taught us that there is a lot to learn, born from the ingenuity of necessity and cultural knowledge. This chapter aims to share some of these observations and learning points, drawing on our reflections and considerations of how mental health services can utilise creativity, community-centred approaches and togetherness in a way that supports people experiencing psychological distress.

[1] 'Innovative' in the sense that this placement was outside the traditional parameters of working within the National Health Service in the UK. Rather, this placement was organised in collaboration with a charity, Lancaster University and a local organisation supporting mental health in Malawi.

Setting the Scene

Malawi has a population of approximately 17 million, and currently there are just two clinical psychologists working throughout the country. According to the World Bank (2017), at least 50% of Malawi's population live in poverty, and as such, it is regarded as one of the poorest countries in the world. In 2005, the World Health Organization (WHO) reported that 70% of African countries contributed less than 1% of their health expenditure to mental health resources. From our observations, we learnt that there are limited services in the country generally, but there appeared to be a good structure around what was offered via St John of God (SJOG).[2]

SJOG is an international Catholic-based organisation which endeavours to provide support to vulnerable people, namely those experiencing physical and mental health difficulties. SJOG currently provides support to people in over 50 countries. The order in Malawi was initially established in the northern city of Mzuzu, in 1993. The organisation in Mzuzu provides a number of services to local people including mental health inpatient wards, a drug and alcohol rehabilitation unit, a child development centre (for children with physical and learning disabilities), a street children programme, older people's community centres, women's groups, vocational colleges, community outreach, drop-in centres and in-reach services for those detained in prison. In 2016, SJOG extended its strategic plan to begin to offer support to other people within the country, and as a result, a further inpatient unit was built in Lilongwe, the capital of Malawi, with the vision to replicate the services in Mzuzu. During our placement, we were based in Mzuzu and had regular input into the SJOG mental health inpatient wards, older adult services and the child development centre.

SJOG has developed an infrastructure for primarily supporting mental health needs. SJOG endeavours to do this through the promotion of specific values, namely hospitality, respect, compassion, justice and excellence, which are noticeably aligned with core values of the UK National Health Service.[3] These SJOG values were certainly apparent throughout our placement; we were made to feel extremely welcome and the hospitality, compassion and

[2] It is important to note that while SJOG is a Catholic-based organisation, there is no expectation that employees, clients or volunteers identify as Christian. Further, individuals who do not identify with the Christian faith are not excluded from services. Furthermore, SJOG services are not run by Catholic priests or Brothers. Lay people or co-workers of SJOG are fully in-charge of the operation of the organisation, with its mission being to continue the work of hospitality and compassion John Ciudad started in the 1400s.

[3] The NHS core values centre upon working together for patients, doing so with respect and dignity, being committed to providing quality of care, demonstrating compassion and valuing each individual.

respect shown to us by people of the organisation and further afield were heart-warming. Indeed, Malawi is known as 'the warm heart of Africa' and many residents expressed their pride towards this sobriquet and were eager to demonstrate this aspect of their cultural identity. Many local people made contact with us and were enthusiastic to make friends.

While we were extremely grateful to receive such warm and welcoming greetings, we could not help but compare our experiences to those who may visit the West, and we were hit with a sense of humility at how their experiences are likely to have been very different to our own, particularly in the wake of momentous political shifts to the right. We were therefore struck with how the values of SJOG, as an organisation, were united with the values which seemed to be embedded within Malawian culture. 'Umoza' is a word used in Malawi meaning 'togetherness' or 'oneness'. During our placement, we quickly came to learn that 'umoza' is more than just a word; it is a felt sense of connection, community and belonging underpinned by acceptance and genuine compassion. Trying to convey the power of this felt sense is, however, extremely difficult to achieve via written format, but it is safe to say that we felt included and part of a community, and regardless of how temporary this was, it felt genuine and honest. By 'community', we mean we felt a strong sense of shared motivation and ethos to support one another, as part of a society that believed it should take responsibility for caring for others.

As psychologists, we were interested in how we both shared this profound connection with a culture that felt very different to our own. We spent time reflecting and questioning each other about the mechanisms at play. We considered the role of our demographics in this experience, yet similar discussions with other visitors, in particular, left us to conclude that there was a very real and powerful hospitable nature to the culture, which meant that adjusting to life back home in the UK was extremely challenging.

From returning home it became quickly apparent that a sense of disconnection and isolation were commonplace in our familiar society. Furthermore, we were struck by the emotional impact that this had on us both. We considered how societal influences can have a significant impact upon one's psychological well-being and, as relatively healthy individuals, it highlighted to us just how much society can influence well-being and how this influence may be much more profound for vulnerable people living in this context. Indeed, the milieu of austerity, neo-liberalism and social inequality brings with it a sense of dividedness and segregation. Our aim for this chapter is to, therefore, explore the ways in which 'umoza' may be integrated within services that are set up to support vulnerable citizens. Furthermore, we hope to draw upon the values of community psychology to consider issues related to social justice around the experience of distress and provision of mental health services.

Service Provision in Malawi

The sense of community, connection and togetherness featured strongly throughout SJOG service provision and development. As outlined earlier, SJOG offers a range of services that were set up in an attempt to support the needs of people in the local area. One of its most recent initiatives involved the development of an older adult service, which was initiated when programme managers became aware of loneliness affecting this population. The loneliness and isolation experienced by many older adults has been suggested to be a result of the HIV epidemic, where there was said to be a 'lost generation' following the deaths of many citizens in the 1990s. As a result, many of the older adults lost their children and are now experiencing isolation due to diminished family networks. It is worthwhile reflecting that stigma surrounding HIV in congregational settings remains an issue for many across the world, bringing shame and casting blame. Derose et al. (2016) discuss this as being associated with religious taboos surrounding homosexual contact between men, perceptions of individuals having multiple sex partners and drug use, which are likely to be viewed through a moral lens. While the role of religion is an important factor to consider with regard to context, empathy and provision of care, we experienced of SJOG as holding high levels of compassion for those affected by HIV and/or AIDS.

The older people's services operate from within the same grounds as local schools and within village centres; this was done to make use of available resources that were cheap whilst simultaneously integrating older people within their communities, aiming to reduce isolation. Integration within communities is further enhanced via community awareness events coordinated by SJOG and service users, which aim to educate communities on the needs of older people and challenge stereotypes and stigma. This is often done via the media of song, dance and drama as a way of engaging people in accessible and creative ways, drawing on personal interests, strengths and talents. We witnessed a community event, whereby service users wrote and performed a play that challenged historical narratives disseminated by witchdoctors, suggesting that older people were witches and wizards, which had a residual stigmatising effect for some older people. The aim of the play was to relieve the burden experienced by older people and provide alternative accounts of their experiences that stepped away from narratives that may increase fear. It is noteworthy that our observations of this run alongside acknowledgement that 'witchdoctors' may be regarded as healers, and it is not our intention to demonise traditional cultures, but recognise some of the stigmatising impact historical narratives had on the older people we met. Individuals working with SJOG supported local communities to challenge deep-rooted assumptions around causes of dementia being related to witchcraft (ActionAid, 2013), with a view to reducing fear, discrimination and social isolation (Mkhonto & Hanssen, 2018).

The emphasis on improving community connections features prominently within SJOG and as such they facilitate a programme, called Self-Help, which aims to empower women, many of whom are parents/guardians of service users across the services and formerly depended on unsustainable handouts from the Saint John of God Brothers[4] and Social Work department. This project enables small groups of women to come together to share financial resources in a means tested way, in order to invest and stimulate economic growth within the group. Any profits are then shared equally amongst the group and the process is repeated, with all members benefitting as the investments and profits gradually increase. The results of Self-Help have been further shown to have significant benefits for the wider communities as many women in the group choose to invest in more community-based projects.

Simultaneously, this mobilisation of women challenges gender-biased discourses and gives women the influence to make positive changes for themselves, their families and, as has been found, their communities. Similarly, people residing within the SJOG inpatient facility are provided with opportunities to learn and develop skills, and the vocational programmes offered by SJOG are also done to provide people with the necessary skills and knowledge to achieve financial independence. This is pertinent given historic models of aid have only served to magnify many people's dependency.

SJOG therefore works in a way that is congruent with the Chinese proverb, 'You give a poor man a fish and you feed him for a day. You teach him to fish and you give him an occupation that will feed him for a lifetime'. (The irony that this proverb uses a masculine object is not lost on us, but we hope that it offers an example of the motives behind such programmes.) Nevertheless, it remains important for communities to challenge the discourse that donations are the best way to help those experiencing poverty; instead it is the provision of opportunities to help people acquire skills and knowledge that will help communities to thrive. Indeed, while in Malawi we were introduced to a film (*Poverty, Inc.*) that reflected on how non-governmental organisation donations and charities can have a negative impact on the local economy. The

[4] Throughout Malawi, there are also God Sisters within the Catholic community. The basis for supporting individuals to increase their financial independence was described to us as being related to the teaching, 'teach them how to fish rather than giving them the fish'. This is also fuelled by a wider context that requires individuals to be self-sufficient to some extent since no financial support is provided by the State.

filmmakers argued that while 'free handouts' are well intentioned, they have a damaging effect on long-term development. As we witnessed locally, partnerships can better support empowerment through providing small financial relief initially that enables individuals to take ownership and develop their own business through their unique skills. Of course, this remains a strong area of debate, with organisations such as GiveDirectly presenting strong evidence to indicate the positive longer-term impact of direct cash transfers in supporting health, future income generation, food security and mental well-being. Perhaps wider reflection on structural inequalities and Western influences of models of economic growth are required to challenge the factors maintaining poverty (such as structural adjustment programmes by the World Bank and International Monetary Fund), rather than the notion of 'handouts' to support communities.

In the UK, in particular, it seems that opportunities for development are significantly decreasing. This may be as a result of the so-called austerity measures, whereby reductions to welfare spending are made whilst also increasing taxes. As a result of the austerity measures, there have been reports of increased job cuts and thus financial insecurity due to more people being employed with 'zero-hours' contracts, alongside increases in people working in roles which require a lower skill set (Trade Union Centre, 2015). Due to financial pressures and increased job insecurity, alongside the rise in university tuition fees and abandonment of bursaries (e.g. nursing), more people are now facing marked barriers to developing their skill set, ultimately reducing the career prospects for specific groups of people (Trade Union Centre, 2015). It was interesting to note that in spite of the financial constraints encountered by the people of Malawi, the importance of skill development remains to be viewed as a priority.

Conceptualisations of Mental Health in Malawi

Throughout Malawi we learned that there is a wide range of cultural beliefs surrounding mental health, both traditional and emerging. Historical and spiritual beliefs often featured in formulations of people's mental health difficulties. Chilale et al. (2017) found that individuals in Malawi attributed their poor mental health to sociocultural factors including witchcraft, spirit possession and curses as being important factors and that individuals still show a high preference for traditional healers. Assad et al. (2015) suggest that within developed nations, there is a higher prevalence of individuals attributing their experiences to biological and psychological cause, while in developing and collective cultures, individuals are more likely to attribute this to supernatural and sociocultural causes.

While our experiences of compassion were commonplace, we heard accounts that some people were subjected to abuse and torture as a result of their distress, with people chained to trees. Certain people within local communities held onto historical beliefs that the experience of mental health difficulties may be as a result of witchcraft or was a form of punishment from God or ancestors. Indeed, we witnessed a protest against the killing of albino people, which is a story very often featured in the Western news. It is not our role as psychologists to determine the 'truth' of these beliefs but merely to acknowledge their presence in people's cultural contexts and the further impact this may have upon psychological well-being. If people are struggling with their mental health and subsequently internalise beliefs that they are in some way to blame, this could exacerbate experiences of distress. While religion and spiritual beliefs are rarely explored within Western clinical contexts (Bracken & Thomas, 2005; Gilbert & Parkes, 2011), giving us scope for development, the role of 'blame' throughout conceptualisations of mental health seems somewhat significant across the contexts.

In the West, methods of labelling, diagnosing and 'treating' mental health problems often infer individual responsibility for the experiences of distress, concurrently neglecting wider systemic influences. Indeed, many people in the West are subject to stigma in relation to their mental health problems, which may be as a result of the tendency to individualise and therefore covertly 'blame' people for their difficulties. These negative social attitudes are therefore significant factors to consider, across cultures, given that many people often internalise negative social attitudes which again holds the potential for psychological distress to be exacerbated (e.g. Pemberton et al., 2015).

The Western influence of the dominant biological model was further apparent in aspects of mental health care in Malawi, and there was a sense that this may increase over time as technology and access to Western influences prevail. While the roots of care in Malawi may be linked with genuine compassion and an understanding of wider contexts, there does appear to be a danger that these Western influences may serve to create an added perspective which continues to individualise mental health problems. Timimi (2010) has suggested that a failure to engage with alternative non-Western perspectives has resulted in 'Western' narratives about mental illness dominating over local understanding in low- and middle-income countries (LMIC).

Within high-income countries, there is a prevalence of the 'biopsychosocial' model in addressing difficulties related to mental health; however, this has been criticised by many as neglecting psychological and social factors

(Read et al., 2009). There are calls for broader conceptualisations and the acknowledgement of the role that sociocultural factors play in the experience of distress (White et al., 2014). Moreover, they highlight that allopathic medicine is only one approach that exists in a broad spectrum of other therapeutic approaches including various forms of indigenous medicine and traditional healing. Generally speaking, these systems seek to 'restore harmony, balance and equilibrium, not only by alleviating physical symptoms, but also by re-integrating the person with his or her community, the earth and the spiritual world' (Ross, 2010, p. 45).

The differences between our approaches to discussions around mental health were also noticed at the very outset of our placement. There was a sense that discussions around mental health in Malawi were more direct and steadfast. One observation which struck us was that explicit and emotive pictures were painted onto the walls of therapeutic rooms, which were accessed by children. These pictures included a woman and child being beaten by a male figure, a road traffic accident and a depiction of suicide as someone hanged from a tree, amongst others. Strikingly, all of the pictures were of specific situations or events. While the pictures were primarily considered as an aid to help children and vulnerable people articulate sensitive topics they may have encountered, we also considered how they implicitly offered an external rationale or narrative behind the emotions that people may experience. Within a biological framework of mental health, which continues to be highly regarded in the West, there is often a sense that mental health difficulties are a result of biological malfunctions within the brain that need to be altered with medication. The underlying connotations of having these pictures displayed therefore helped to introduce the role of external difficulties, which is likely to provide people with a sense of validation and togetherness, which is often overlooked in Western cultures.

What We Can Learn

From our observations and experiences, it was clear that key themes emerged which may be incorporated into Western mental health service provision to bring about a sense of community and 'umoza'.

1. **Co-production**: Within the female empowerment groups and the older adult's service, in particular, we were struck with the level of co-production. The older people accessing the services were heavily involved in the organisation of community events, which seemed to provide people with a sense

of purpose and occupation. The need for rehabilitation, including opportunities for skill (re)acquisition, has been highly valued by older adults in LMIC (Modie-Moroka, 2014) and fosters increased financial security through employment, greater independence and promoting involvement in the wider community (Skeen et al., 2010). Indeed, SJOG took a step back when encouraging women to come together to enhance their finances. While co-production is often advocated in Western cultures, we have yet to see it thrive in the way we saw in Malawi. SJOG, by virtue of its existence and prominence in the local area, held a level of power, but what was interesting was that the service as a whole did not seem overly eager to hold onto this power and instead worked in a way which appeared to communicate trust and acceptance towards service users, giving them the freedom and opportunities to use their skill set and to come together to deliver awareness-raising events.

2. **Creativity and flexibility**: As SJOG is a charity, there was a need to ensure that services offered remain 'efficient'. The drive to work in efficient ways did not however hold the same implication as it seemingly does in the UK, and instead it seemed that creativity and the need to be flexible with services was key. Offering outreach services to those who needed it, using cheap but easily accessible buildings and volunteers, all seemed to ensure that the services continued to thrive in spite of economic hardship. With this, rooms were used for older adults' services in local schools which inadvertently gave way to intergenerational working which seems to be gaining more attention in the West. One such example is a research project bringing together younger and older adults to create and develop play, which was found to increase confidence, increase generative learning, reduce ageism/fear of ageing and increase social networks (Anderson et al., 2017). Importantly, the researchers reported a shift in attitudes by participants about the other generation and increased perception of their own tolerance of diversity.
3. **Community-based work**: A theme throughout services in Malawi, and indeed their culture, was one of togetherness, which featured prominently throughout services. Services worked to prevent more people requiring services by offering awareness projects, for example, events were held to address societal problems including excessive drinking and drug use. The community awareness projects created another reason to bring people together, to make links, ultimately reducing isolation and loneliness, which has been found to contribute to low mood (Cacioppo et al., 2011).

Additionally, SJOG conducted a broad range of outreach work to promote its services in hard to reach areas. This included obtaining buy-in from those in a position of power (usually the village chief) to increase awareness around mental well-being and was usually accompanied by opportunities for those already accessing the service to share their experiences through the medium of dance, drama and art. Similarly, SJOG operates an Umoza Street Children Project that offers a variety of centre- and community-based support services to children and their families, including offering material support and scholarships to enable children to start or return to school (Silungwe & Bandawe, 2011).

4. **The use of the arts**: The use of art, drama, music and in particular dance featured prominently throughout the entirety of our visit. We regularly ensured we were around the SJOG campus on Thursday afternoon to watch children from the Umoza project practise their dance routines. Dance was a regular activity within the inpatient ward and throughout the older people's services. It was clear to see the power of dance in psychological well-being and the connections this created between the staff and service users who danced together. Research has found that the benefits of dancing help with mental health (Froggett & Little, 2012). Within the West, individualised therapy has been shown to be difficult to access for people from lower socio-economic status and is deemed to be middle-class concept (Appio et al., 2013; Kim & Cardemil, 2012; Levy & O'Hara, 2010). However, it seems that using the arts as a way of creating connections and delivering powerful messages about well-being may be a useful strategy in creatively ensuring services are accessible to all citizens.

   Within the West, art and creativity often feature in anecdotal and individual recovery journeys (Spandler et al., 2007) despite research suggesting that participatory art has a broad spectrum of positive therapeutic benefits for people with mental health needs (Heenan, 2006) across all age groups (Anderson et al., 2017). While events such as the DCP Fringe Festival and #Psygrafitti have begun to work in this way, it seems that the West can learn a great deal from Malawian culture to shift power differentials, create connections and engage in fun and meaningful activities to educate and inspire others as a means of bringing about psychological wellness.

Overall, in Malawi, a lot of the services which were offered were done from a sense of compassion, genuineness and common sense. While we can easily relate their services to an evidence base to potentially explain their success, it was interesting to note that instead of coming from the evidence base to the service, the opposite was done. People's needs were thought about in a direct way and addressed with practical solutions. In Western cultures we can be overly focused on the risks, the potential for harm and problems. This is understandable in an age of compensation claims, but how do we move forward if we continue to think about service delivery and innovation from a place of fear and rigidity? We must consider new ways of working to ensure that the ever-changing needs of our citizens are met in a compassionate, creative and person-centred way.

How Can We Get There?

For us, a key step is to broaden our approaches to mental health and to engage in wider discussions about 'what works' or has the potential to. Anecdotally, we experienced the power of the arts and suggest that a recovery approach to mental health must recognise the potential contribution of arts and creativity within social care and mental health provision. Winnicott (1971) argued that creativity has the potential to increase agency and hope through instilling a sense of meaning in one's life. This recognises individuals' cultural experiences and promotes transgressions from personal boundaries to a shared and felt connectedness with others. Ventevogel (2014) highlights the need to promote community-based recovery-oriented interventions within mental health. Indeed, it is important that while the wider social inclusion agenda prioritises participation in 'mainstream' settings, we look to expand these other ways of working and seek out opportunities to work alongside community settings that offer mutual support in less formal settings. One such novel example is the use of the 'friendship bench' whereby a trusted and respected member of the community is utilised as a lay person to open discussions about distress with the local community, whilst also offering opportunities for individuals to discuss their struggles as they await access to routine primary health care (Abas et al., 2016). A similar concept to the idea of mutual aid has recently been piloted and adopted in London for mental health awareness week by the OWLS social enterprise. During this initiative, make-shift 'problem solving booths' were set up to encourage members of the local community to come together and talk about difficulties and help normalise problems whilst offering support to each other (Tavistock and Portman NHS, 2017). In an age where we as a society are more inclined to 'watch friends and neighbours over making friends with our neighbours' (Russell, 2018), it is schemes like this which may be imperative in re-building communities and enhancing wellbeing. Attempts to include members of the community to support one another, listening and offering solutions, would also aim to increase accessibility to support across cultures and/or religious/spiritual beliefs. Developing ways in which to build connections and increase dialogue around mental health would hope to strike a balance between curative interventions and preventative actions to address the social determinants of mental health problems.

There is a growing body of research to support the use of arts, drama, dance and meaningful activity being integrated into 'therapy' and recovery (Van Lith, 2015). For us, this is a significant aspect of our learning from Malawi that we try to integrate into our work and feel strongly that broadening our ideas of 'therapy' to something beyond the therapy room and more traditional talking therapies may be beneficial in aiding communication, coping and connection. For example, Ørjasæter et al. (2017) report how the use of a music and theatre workshop in an inpatient hospital fostered opportunities for individuals to gain a sense of belonging and expanded their identity. These creative ways of engaging those in distress through less formal settings are, in our view, a helpful way of also reducing the idea of 'us and them', as professionals are encouraged to take part and share in the activity. We have heard anecdotal stories of psychologists knitting, engaging in yoga or cooking with those they support and the positive impact this has had on not only the therapeutic relationship, but increasing their capacity to engage in wider social, community groups. A recent systematic literature review however reported that the quality of trials for studies examining the impact of creative arts therapy in PTSD was poor (Baker et al., 2018). It is postulated that difficulties in gaining funding to support the research may be hampered by a lack of buy-in, knowledge about the use of creative arts therapy and interdisciplinary working. Thus, perhaps a significant role for psychologists is to support the development of robust proposals to aid further research as a way of evidencing this work and extending the parameters of what it means to engage in 'therapy'. However, this also reflects wider issues of epistemic injustice—that greater value is given to Randomised Controlled Trial (RCT's), and power over what is deemed more 'valid' as an area of therapeutic intervention, warranting research funding or investment. Within, we must also question and reflect upon issues relating to co-production and structural barriers to this, which means the involvement of citizens in public services may be idealised. There is a challenge for us to ensure that coproduction *means* co-production and that patients and experts by experience do not occupy a passive recipient role or, importantly, are not excluded from opportunities, due to system factors (e.g. ideas that it is too time-intensive or other organisational barriers) and that we question where the power lies in deciding who is involved in voicing their thoughts/ideas (Vennik et al., 2016). Both the Psychologists for Social Change (2018) and Community Psychology movement aim to draw attention to the idea of mental health and well-being services being 'too individualised' in UK society and aim to enhance a community-led approach that incorporates collective responses to an individual's needs, appreciating their social, political, economic and cultural influences.

Additionally, an approach we strongly value is the Tree of Life (ToL), within narrative therapy, which might be a useful approach for sharing stories and fostering connections across communities. Pioneered by Ncube-Mlilo and Denborough (2006), ToL is a tool that uses different parts of a tree as metaphors to represent the different aspects of our lives and aims to give language to people who may otherwise struggle. The approach aims to enhance social inclusion and community cohesion (White & Epston, 1990; Billington, 2000; White & Morgan, 2006) and facilitates discussions of strength, peace, solidarity and determination. ToL has been used worldwide with different groups of children (Woods, 2010), adolescents (Yuen, 2009) and adults (Denborough, 2014). There have also been extensions of this idea, supporting Muslim women (Elhassan & Yassine, 2017), in London Hackney community projects with adults with HIV (Iliopoulou et al., 2009) and with African and Caribbean men who have experienced mental distress (Byrne et al., 2011). Importantly, the tool has also been used powerfully in exploring inequalities including racism (German, 2013). Western psychology is often critiqued for its lack of recognition and acknowledgement of culture, and our connections and heritage that are central to psychological well-being (Crooks, 2008). Consequently, ToL might facilitate explorations of these factors and increase discussions around mental health, whilst also enabling individuals to make connections in a group or collection (Denborough, 2008).

In order to better support those in distress, we need to recognise the limitations of our current ways of understanding this and the social, political, cultural context within which we work. Our current mechanism of focusing on the individual acts to perpetuate isolation and despair, rather than, as Verhaeghe (2014) argues, focusing on fostering bonds and belonging. This can be achieved by supporting communities to respond to their own needs (Nelson & Prilleltensky, 2005). One such approach is Open Dialogue that provides a safe space for families, carers and communities to support individuals experiencing distress, embracing the view that they can bear the emotional pain of a loved one and are best equipped to support them. Similarly, the Hearing Voices Network serves as an indicator that communities and services led by experts by experience can be extremely empowering, supportive and healing. Thus, while much of our traditional approaches for responding to mental distress are influenced by Western, individualised models, we propose that a greater focus on the community, and drawing upon the knowledge and experience of those in distress, is perhaps the best starting point for any intervention(s). By adopting the view that communities are most likely to know what they need, what will be helpful and/or what changes are required, we believe psychologists are perfectly placed to begin this dialogue and draw upon the resources in the communities we serve, to support projects that take a community-based approach to mental health. Herein lies the challenge; the conflict between collective community responsibility taking to accept shared accountability for distress, whilst working and existing within a Western paradigm that pushes for 'fault' lying with the individual. Summerfield (2008) calls for the decolonisation of the global mental health movement, arguing a fundamental opposition to the medicalisation of human distress and universality of Western diagnostic categories, viewing this 'as a kind of cultural imperialism' (Summerfield, 2012). Rather, Summerfield posits that distress can be understood as a 'normal' response to difficult, harsh living conditions and highlights the importance of social connectedness as a way of increasing well-being and resilience. Of course, this also brings to question wider issues that have seen the gradual decline in community infrastructures and spaces, including privatisation of community spaces and hospitals. Austerity and social inequalities have seen structural changes that increase isolation and have the potential to decrease well-being. Webb (2013) calls for strategies to 'counter individualisation with social understanding' (p. 646) and those in positions of power to challenge the status quo of social injutsice, through a shared vision and commitment.

In the West, we are arguably able to draw upon an array of mental health approaches, at times, at the expense of giving consideration to traditional methods of care that could be used alongside these approaches. As such, reciprocal learning is paramount between organisations and countries and facilitating this between the Global North and the Global South will be essential to moving forward (White et al., 2017). For example, Swancott et al. (2014) discuss how an NHS trust is working jointly with local charities and universities in Ethiopia to engage in knowledge exchange to promote shared approaches to mental health and increase dialogue, without privileging one perspective or position. It is this shared learning opportunity that will enable us to integrate traditional approaches with more recent developments, in a way that promotes HIC (High Income Countries) in critically reflecting on health and the further acknowledgement of the cultural context and impact (and protective role) on well-being.

Perhaps an important way forward is to look to our clinical psychological doctorate training programmes (and other advanced training for professionals), urging them to be more inclusive of this paradigm and encouraging greater opportunities outside of the traditional NHS placements. Rhodes and

Langtiw (2018) propose that increasing diversity in training programmes and teaching on the philosophy of community psychology is fundamental, requiring a collective address of structural issues. This not only will serve to enrich understanding and experiences but may foster thinking around the scope of our professional roles and broaden opportunities for social justice and social inclusion to be a focus. Additionally, focus on doctoral programme towards empowering marginalised individuals and communities through co-production and training opportunities to promote diversity may also be of benefit, in keeping with the values and ethos of community psychology.

Potential Challenges

While there is increasing interest in the concept of 'recovery', by both the service user movement and policy drivers (NIMHE, 2005), Spandler et al. (2007) highlight the difficulties of an agreed-on conceptual model and clarity on the process of recovery or indeed what the outcomes of recovery should be (Ralph & Corrigan, 2005). In an age of increased pressure to demonstrate clinical outcomes within the NHS and Payment by Results, opportunities to implement some of the practices from other cultures may be hindered. Similarly, in a culture where there is a strong drive to 'get people back to work', the recovery journey of individuals may not be prioritised. Moreover, the drive for cost-effectiveness has increased demand by policy drivers for researchers/organisations to demonstrate the successes of interventions within given time periods (Staricoff, 2006). Consequently, while practitioners may intuitively recognise the benefits of working creativity and flexibility, funders want empirical results to demonstrate programme benefits to individuals and communities (Currie, 2010; De Medeiros & Basting, 2014; Hancock, 2007). Thus, since interventions are primarily appraised according to clinical outcomes (Froggett & Little, 2012), without initial support from those in positions of power, these initiatives may never get off the ground. Despite these challenges, there are opportunities to think outside of the box and perhaps develop novel approaches to supporting those who experience mental distress. As Ventevogel points out, 'in order to build holistic primary mental health-care systems, policy-makers and health workers need to embrace a public mental health approach' (p. 676).

Acknowledgements Thank you to the wonderful people of Malawi and SJOG who embraced us with open arms and showed such care and compassion. You have provided us with many examples of what is possible and have truly shaped our ways of thinking.

References

Abas, M., Bowers, T., Manda, E., Cooper, S., Machando, D., Verhey, R., Lamech, N., Araya, R., & Chibanda, D. (2016). 'Opening up the mind': Problem solving therapy delivered by female lay health workers to improve access to evidence based care for depression and other common mental disorders through the Friendship Bench Project in Zimbabwe. *International Journal of Mental Health Systems, 10*(39), 1–8. https://doi.org/10.1186/s13033-016-0071-9

ActionAid. (2013). Condemned without trial: Women and witchcraft in Ghana. https://www.actionaid.org.uk/sites/default/files/doc_lib/ghana_report_single_pages.pdf

Anderson, S., Fast, J., Keating, N., Eales, J., Chivers, S., & Barnet, D. (2017). Translating knowledge: Promoting health through intergenerational community arts programming. *Health Promotion Practice, 18*(1), 15–25. https://doi.org/10.1177/1524839915625037

Appio, L., Chambers, D. A., & Mao, S. (2013). Listening to the voices of the poor and disrupting the silence about class issues in psychotherapy. *Journal of Clinical Psychology, 69*(2), 152–161.

Assad, T., Okasha, T., Ramy, H., Goueli, T., El-Shinnawy, H., Nasr, M., & Shorab, I. (2015). Role of traditional healers in the pathway to care of patients with bipolar disorder in Egypt. *International Journal of Social Psychiatry, 61*, 583–590.

Baker, F. A., Metcalf, O., Varker, T., & O'Donnell, M. (2018). A systematic review of the efficacy of creative arts therapies in the treatment of adults with PTSD. *Psychological Trauma Theory Research Practice and Policy, 10*(6), 643–651.

Billington, T. (2000). *Separating, losing and excluding children: Narratives of difference.* Routledge Falmer.

Bracken, P., & Thomas, P. (2005). *Postpsychiatry: Mental health in a post modern world.* Oxford University Press.

Byrne, A., Warren, A., Joof, B., Johnson, D., Casimir, L., Hinds, C., Mittee, S., Johnson, J., Ade, A., & Griffiths, S. (2011). 'A powerful piece of work': African and Caribbean men talking about the 'Tree of Life'. *Context: The Magazine for Family Therapy and Systemic Practice in the UK, 117*, 40–45.

Cacioppo, J. T., Hawkley, L. C., Norman, G. J., & Berntson, G. G. (2011). Social isolation. *Annals of the New York Academy of Sciences, 1231*, 17–22.

Chilale, H. K., Silungwe, N. D., Gondwe, S., & Masulani-Mwale, C. (2017). Clients and carers perception of mental illness and factors that influence help-seeking: Where they go first and why. *International Journal of Social Psychiatry, 63*(5), 418–425. https://doi.org/10.1177/0020764017709848

Crooks, P. (2008). *A tree without roots: The guide to tracing British, African and Asian Caribbean ancestry*. Arcadia.

Currie, C. T. (2010). Health and social care of older people: Could policy generalise good practice? *Journal of Integrated Care, 18*(6), 19–26.

De Medeiros, K., & Basting, A. (2014). Shall I compare thee to a dose of donepezil? Cultural arts interventions in dementia care research. *The Gerontologist, 54*, 344–353.

Denborough, D. (2008). *Collective Narrative Practice: Responding to individuals, groups and communities who have experienced trauma*. Dulwich Centre Publications.

Denborough, D. (2014). *Retelling the stories of our lives: Everyday narrative therapy to draw inspiration and transform experience*. Norton & Company.

Derose, K. P., Kanouse, D. E., Bogart, L. M., Griffin, B. A., Haas, A., Stucky, B. D., Williams, M. V., & Flórez, K. R. (2016). Predictors of HIV-related stigmas among African American and Latino religious congregants. *Cultural Diversity and Ethnic Minority Psychology, 22*(2), 185–195. https://doi-org.ezproxy.lancs.ac.uk/10.1037/cdp0000062

Elhassan, O., & Yassine, L. (2017). Tree of life with young Muslim women in Australia. *International Journal of Narrative Therapy & Community Work, 3*, 27–45.

Froggett, L., & Little, R. (2012). Dance as a complex intervention in an acute mental health setting: A place 'in between'. *British Journal of Occupational Therapy, 75*(2).

German, M. (2013). Developing our cultural strengths: Using the "tree of life" strength-based narrative therapy intervention in schools to enhance self-esteem, cultural understanding, and to challenge racism. *Educational and Child Psychology, 30*(4), 75–99.

Gilbert, P., & Parkes, M. (2011). Faith in one city: Exploring religion, spirituality and mental wellbeing in urban UK. *Ethnicity and Inequalities in Health and Social Care, 4*(1), 16–27. https://doi.org/10.1108/17570981111189551

Hancock, T. (2007). Creating environments for health—20 years on. *Global Health Promotion, 14*, 7–8.

Heenan, D. (2006). Art as therapy: An effective way of promoting positive mental health? *Disability and Society, 21*, 179–191.

Iliopoulou, G., Jovia, K., & Lucy & Sandra. (2009). The 'Tree of Life' in a community context. *Context: The Magazine for Family Therapy and Systemic Practice in the UK, 105*, 50–54.

Kim, S., & Cardemil, E. (2012). Effective Psychotherapy With Low-income Clients: The Importance of Attending to Social Class. *J Contemp Psychother, 42*, 27–35.

Levy, L. B., & O'Hara, M. W. (2010). Psychotherapeutic interventions for depressed, low-income women: A review of the literature. *Clinical Psychology Review, 30*(8), 934–950.

McKenzie, K., Patel, V., & Araya, R. (2004). Learning from low income countries: Mental health. *British Medical Journal, 329*, 1138–1140. http://www.jstor.org/stable/25469417

Mkhonto, F., & Hanssen, I. (2018). When people with dementia are perceived as witches. Consequences for patients and nurse education in South Africa. *Journal of Clinical Nursing, 27*(1–2), 169–176. https://doi-org.ezproxy.lancs.ac.uk/10.1111/jocn.13909

Modie-Moroka, T. (2014). Stress, social relationships and health outcomes in low-income Francistown, Botswana. *Social Psychiatry and Psychiatric Epidemiology, 49*, 1269–1277. https://doi.org/10.1007/s00127-013-0806-8

Ncube-Mlilo, N., & Denborough, D. (2006). *Mainstreaming psychosocial care and support: A manual for facilitators*. REPSSI.

Nelson, G., & Prilleltensky, I. (Eds.). (2005). *Community psychology in pursuit of liberation and well-being*. Palgrave Macmillan.

NIMHE. (2005). *National Institute for Mental Health in England Guiding Statement on Recovery*. London: Department of Health.

Ørjasæter, K. B., Stickley, T., Hedlund, M., & Ness, O. (2017). Transforming identity through participation in music and theatre: Exploring narratives of people with mental health problems. *International Journal of Qualitative Studies on Health and Well-Being, 12*. https://doi-org.ezproxy.lancs.ac.uk/10.1080/17482631.2017.1379339

Pemberton, S., Fahmy, E., Sutton, E., & Bell, K. (2015). Navigating the stigmatised identities of poverty in austere times: Resisting and responding to narratives of personal failure. *Critical Social Policy, 36*(1), 1–17. https://doi.org/10.1177/0261018315601799

Psychologists for Social Change. (2018). How do we create a more equitable and psychologically healthier society?. http://www.psychchange.org/blog/category/psychologically-healthy

Ralph, R. O., & Corrigan, P. W. (Eds.). (2005). *Recovery in mental illness: Broadening our understanding of wellness*. American Psychological Association.

Read, J., Bentall, R. P., & Fosse, R. (2009). Time to abandon the bio-bio-bio model of psychosis: Exploring the epigenetic and psychological mechanisms by which adverse life events lead to psychotic symptoms. *Epidemiologia e Psichiatria Sociale, 18*, 299–310.

Rhodes, P., & Langtiw, C. (2018). Why clinical psychology needs to engage in community-based approaches to mental health. *Australian Psychologist*. https://doi-org.ezproxy.lancs.ac.uk/10.1111/ap.12347

Ross, E. (2010). Inaugural lecture: African spirituality, ethics and traditional healing – Implications for indigenous South African social work education and practice. *South African Journal of Bioethics and Law, 3*(44), 51.

Russell, C. (2018). *Communities and assets: Food for thought*. Online presentation. https://memoryfriendly.org.uk/programmes/shifting-paradigms-in-dementia/community-empowerment-and-dementia/cormac-russell-communities-and-assets-food-for-thought/

Silungwe, N., & Bandawe, C. (2011). Implementing a dynamic street-children's program: Successes and challenges. *Malawi Medical Journal, 23*(3), 78–840.

Skeen, S., Kleintjes, S., Lund, C., Petersen, I., Bhana, A., Flisher, A. J., & The Mental Health and Poverty Research Programme Consortium. (2010). 'Mental health is everybody's business': Roles for an intersectoral approach in South Africa.

International Review of Psychiatry, 22(6), 611–623. https://doi.org/10.3109/09540261.2010.535510

Spandler, H., Secker, J., Kent, L., Hacking, S., & Shenton, J. (2007). Catching life: The contribution of arts initiatives to recovery approaches in mental health. *Journal of Psychiatric And Mental Health Nursing, 14*(8), 791–799. https://doi.org/10.1111/j.1365-2850.2007.01174.x

Staricoff, R. L. (2006). Arts in health: The value of evaluation. *Journal of the Royal Society for the Promotion of Health, 126*(3), 116–120.

Summerfield, D. (2008). How scientifically valid is the knowledge base of global mental health? *British Medical Journal, 336*(7651), 992–994. https://doi.org/10.1136/bmj.39513.441030.AD

Summerfield, D. (2012). Afterword: against 'global mental health'. *Transcult Psychiatry, 49*, 1–12.

Swancott, R., Uppal, G., & Crossley, J. (2014). Globalization of psychology: Implications for the development of psychology in Ethiopia. *International Review of Psychiatry, 26*(5), 579–584. https://doi.org/10.3109/09540261.2014.917610

Tavistock and Portman NHS. (2017). *A problem-solving booth for Mental Health Awareness Week 2017*. UK. https://tavistockandportman.nhs.uk/about-us/news/stories/problem-solving-booth-mental-health-awareness-week-2017/

Timimi, S. (2010). The McDonaldization of childhood: Children's mental health in neo-liberal market cultures. *Transcultural Psychiatry, 47*, 686–706.

Trade Union Centre. (2015). TUC young worker issues: Policy briefing. UK. https://www.tuc.org.uk/sites/default/files/TUCYoungWorkerIssues.pdf

Van Lith, T. (2015). Art making as a mental health recovery tool for change and coping. *Art Therapy, 32*(1), 5–12. https://doi-org.ezproxy.lancs.ac.uk/10.1080/07421656.2015.992826

Vennik, F. D., van de Bovenkamp, H. M., Putters, K., & Grit, K. J. (2016). Co-production in healthcare: Rhetoric and practice. *International Review of Administrative Sciences, 82*(1), 150–168. https://doi.org/10.1177/0020852315570553

Ventevogel, P. (2014). Integration of mental health into primary healthcare in low-income countries: Avoiding medicalisation. *International Review of Psychiatry, 26*, 669–679. https://doi.org/10.3109/09540261.2014.9660674

Verhaeghe, P. (2014). *What about me? The struggle for identity in a market-based society*. Scribe.

Webb, J. (2013). Austerity psychology. *The Psychologist: British Psychological Society, 26*, 646–666. https://thepsychologist.bps.org.uk/volume-26/edition-9/austerity-psychology

White, M., & Epston, D. (1990). *Narrative means to therapeutic ends*. W.W. Norton.

White, M., & Morgan, A. (2006). *Narrative therapy with children and their families*. Dulwich Centre Publications.

White, R., Jain, S., & Guirgi-Oncu, C. (2014). Counterflows for mental well-being: What high-income countries can learn from low and middle-income countries. *International Review of Psychiatry, 26*(5), 602–606.

White, R. G., Gregg, J., Batten, S., Hayes, L. L., & Kasujja, R. (2017). Contextual Behavioral Science and Global Mental Health: Synergies and opportunities. *Journal of Contextual Behavioral Science, 6*(3), 245–251. https://doi.org/10.1016/j.jcbs.2017.07.001

Winnicott, D. (1971). *Playing and Reality*. New York: Brunner-Routledge.

Woods, K. (2010). *The Tree of Life growing in Nepal*. Retrieved June 6, 2013, from http://www.dulwichcentre.com.au/tree-of-life-nepal.pdf

World Bank. (2017). Malawi. Retrieved January 4, 2018, from https://data.worldbank.org/country/malawi?view=chart

Yuen, A. (2009). *Getting through the storms*. TDSB. Retrieved February 24, 2018, from https://www.dulwichcentre.com.au/getting-through-the-storms.pdf

26

Linking Space, Place, and Relational Well-being in Co-productive Ways

Jenny Fisher, Rebecca Lawthom, Leanne Rimmer, Andrew Stevenson, and The Manchester Street Poem Collective

The writers of this chapter very much work in engaged ways with people. Despite being housed in academic departments and institutions, which tend to imagine research in particular ways, we bend and shape the agenda to work on problems identified in and by communities. The spaces we are writing about presume that people within contexts are expert knowers of issues facing us in communities, housing, and education. We embrace an approach to working which fuses creative ways of making sense with humans alongside understanding how systems position us as researchers/people/marginalised. Working in these ways engages and stretches institutional boundaries as well as reinforcing collective solutions to issues. Curating knowledge and creating innovative ways to share knowledge is a practice we hold dear.

The Manchester Street Poem Collective are Nigel Allmark, Mooch Ashley, Danny Collins, Jez Green, Sarah Hiscock, Karl Hyde, Beth Knowles, Simon Leroux, Tommy O'Donnell, John Organ, and Jo Wilson.

A. Stevenson
The Manchester Street Poem Collective

J. Fisher • L. Rimmer
Manchester Metropolitan University, Manchester, UK

R. Lawthom (✉)
University of Sheffield, Sheffield, UK
e-mail: R.Lawthom@mmu.ac.uk

C. Walker et al. (eds.), *The Palgrave Handbook of Innovative Community and Clinical Psychologies*, https://doi.org/10.1007/978-3-030-71190-0_26

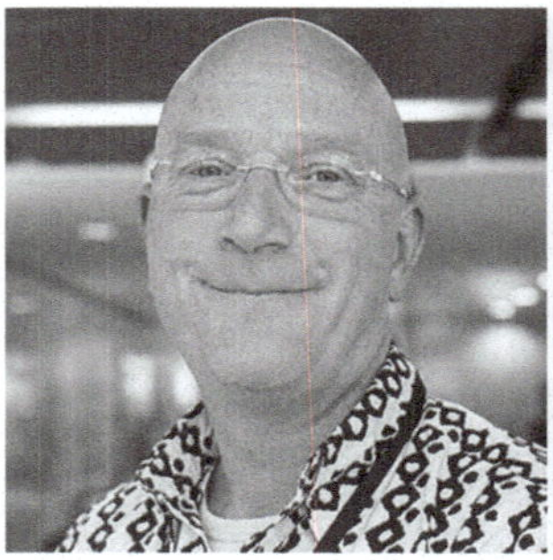

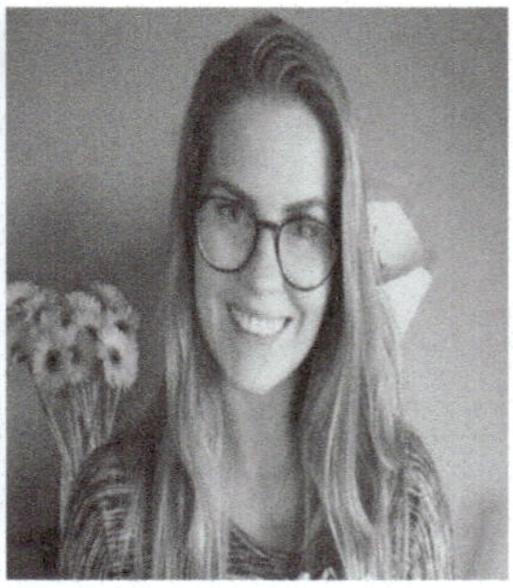

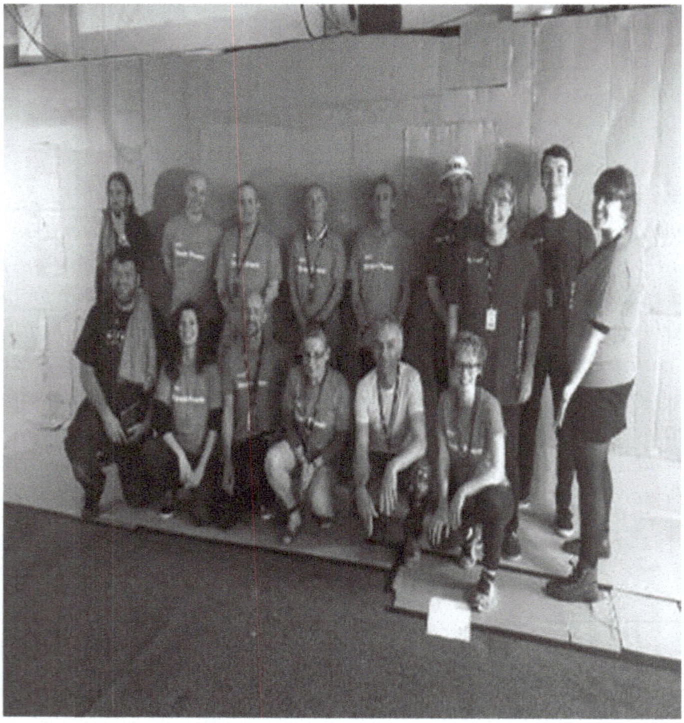

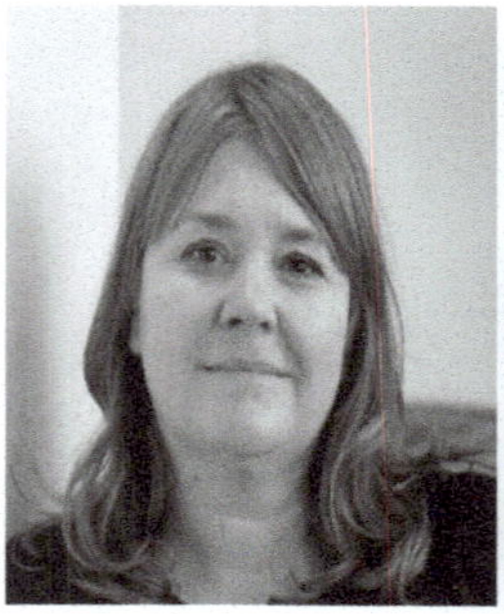

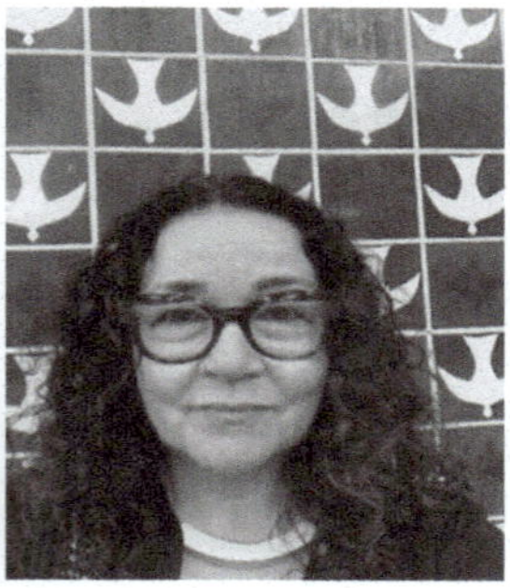

Community psychology takes context seriously. By this we mean, the material context of the world we are embedded in but also political, psychosocial, and cultural realities of existence. This attention to 'the social context of people's lives' (Orford, 2008: 3) also engenders a commitment to theorising this context and finding ways to explore context when working with people. People do not operate within a social vacuum, and experiences are linked to the environment(s) in which we are embedded. Therefore, how people negotiate and create meaning from 'space(s)' and the experience of 'place' should be considered, and research should not solely concern the evaluation of individual or group attributes. In work firmly embedded within the North West of England, Kagan et al. make the point that it is Manchester as a place that binds the authors together in place and time. Bauman (2007) notes:

> *It is around place that human experience tends to be formed and gleaned, that life sharing is attempting to be managed, that life meanings are conceived, absorbed and negotiated. And it is in places that human urges and desires are gestated and incubated, that they live in the hope of fulfilment, run the risk of frustration—and are indeed, more often than not, frustrated and strangled.* (p. 81)

The work in this chapter articulates some of this tension in exploring a number of projects in which local and global contexts are made sense of, always alongside those who are local experts or those with lived experience ('co-productive'). In anticipating this exploration of projects, well-being is seen as more than an individual project; it is relational not only to others but to place and space. To enable this way of working, we argue that Community Psychology offers a 'framework for working with those marginalised by the social system that leads to self-aware social change with an emphasis on value based, participatory work and the forging of alliances' (Burton et al. 2011: 219). By this, we mean that engagement with others and partnership working creates a rather different approach to practice. Here, community is conceived of as a level of analysis which is required to be beyond the individual. Similarly, in exploring the setting, community psychology resists the concept of intervention which targets the individual, focussing on joint action. Whilst the projects themselves could be considered interventions, the orientation of the research is aligned to social justice.

A shift in psychological focus away from a dominant psycho-medical model with individual attribution emphasises the importance of systems and how scene-setting should be integral to the research process. A nested ecological level of analysis is a useful framework to evaluate space and place, as it captures the interaction between 'individuals and the multiple systems in which they are embedded' (Nelson & Prilleltensky, 2010: 71). A simplified visual representation of an ecological framework can be found in Fig. 26.1.

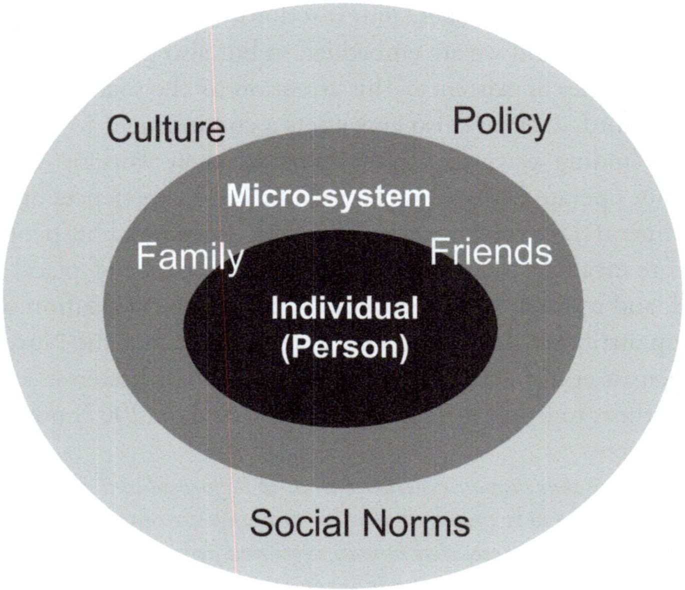

Fig. 26.1 Ecological metaphor of multiple systems of analysis

In order to understand something of the dynamic nature of the context, as community psychologists, we need to engage in place and reflect upon that engagement. We do this engagement through grounding ourselves in experience and not presuming that we can study or know things from afar. How we engage in other places, and how we approach working alongside others, is not straightforward or methodologically near. Rather, the co-productive element requires different skills and a more generous reading of people as co-researchers and participants with a set of skills and capacities. In a discipline where relatedness is important, the issue is not about individuals in society, but the relations between individual, community, and society.

Analysis of person-environment interactions/fit enables further understanding of how different contexts affect diverse individuals in distinctive ways. This includes intersubjectivities, including beliefs, values, and experiences that are shared by participants.

One element which contributes to participant experience in place is sense of community. This involves shared identity and emotional bonds, mutual trust, and caring and commitment amongst participants (Kloos et al., 2012). Sense of community is contextually bound, and the projects below explore in very different ways how people see themselves, in relation to others and in relation to local places/communities. And this chapter embraces a global perspective, drawing from case studies in Guatemala, Manchester (UK), and Brazil. Each represents a different participatory project which aims for further understanding of the relationship between space, place, and well-being.

Co-producing and Capturing Experience?

Quality criteria in Community Psychology research include promoting empowerment and giving voice to traditionally under-represented populations (Barker & Pistrang, 2005). These principles are integral to participatory approaches and ways of working. Participatory Action Research (PAR) is a particular form of this where even research questions are designed *with* communities, rather than research done 'on' them. A commitment to work in ethical and participative ways informed our drive to produce records of place using media and methodologies that were most comfortable to participants. As each of the projects involved obtaining funding (prior to beginning the work), it would have been difficult to engage in participatory action research in its purest form. Rather, each project was designed in order to engage in co-production of methods, analysis, and/or dissemination. Working in collaboration and in partnership disrupts many of the traditional approaches associated with dominant, 'outsider' style research. Partnership working requires a reframing of whose knowledge counts and whose research is this. To establish within a community what the focus of the research is and how to subsequently explore it requires a commitment to co-production and collaboration with 'experts by experience'. The recognition of lived experience can be and often is linked to place. Co-production requires a strength-based approach and involves a process of engagement to facilitate the construction of place. Strength-based approaches provide an opportunity to use creative methods, where traditional approaches to research may not suit participants or serve as a barrier to engagement. Being creative around method choice can elicit different outputs as well as engaging participants in different methods. In previous work, we have used ethnographic filmmaking (Stevenson and Lawthom, 2017), mobile interviews, diary methods (Siddiquee et al., 2016), and participatory narratives.

Each of the participatory projects is presented in turn as case studies, where we show the development of the project, the approach to research, and the inclusion of place. These places, whether urban, rural, or located in the Global North or South, make a difference to what and how we work. Box 26.1 outlines the project '"Streets of Resilience": Exploring Resilience in Street-Connected Young People in Guatemala City'; Box 26.2 outlines the project 'Co-production Research in Action: A Case Study in Homelessness'; and Box 26.3 outlines the project 'Place-Making with Older Adults'. This is followed by the presentation of a set of themes which encapsulate space, place, and relational well-being in co-productive ways.

Box 26.1 'Streets of Resilience': Exploring Resilience in Street-Connected Young People in Guatemala City

During 2016 and 2017 three researchers (one who is based in Guatemala, the other two from a UK university) worked alongside two Guatemalan charities, *Puertas de Esperanza|Doors of Hope* and *Resplandece|Radiance*, on a research project exploring resilience with Street-Connected Young People in Guatemala City. These two charities were selected as two of the researchers had established connections with them and had volunteered for them in the past. Both charities are run by volunteers and provide additional educational support for young people in Guatemala City. We say someone is resilient when they show better than expected levels of achievement and well-being despite experiencing adversity or hardship (Ungar et al., 2013). For the young people in our study, hardship arises in the form of poverty and the need to work at a place called 'The Terminal', in Guatemala City.

Our project was carried out in three locations in Guatemala City: first, 'The Terminal', an extensive wholesale/retail market, bus station, dump, housing blocks where hundreds of families live, work, and sell recycling waste; second, a residential house, which is used by an educational outreach charity project called *Puertas de Esperanza*; and third, a church building, used by another outreach project, *Resplandece*. The participants and collaborators in our study were volunteers and project leaders at *Puertas de Esperanza* and *Resplandece* and eight young people who agreed to be interviewed for this project. All of these people shared with us their experiences of living, working, learning, and teaching in and around The Terminal, in Guatemala City.

As interviewing project leaders and volunteers about their work, the young people walked us around The Terminal, talking with us, making drawings and photographs along the way, in order to share their experiences with us. We used creative methods such as participatory photography (Wang, 2007) and participatory drawing (Literat, 2013), so that we could explore young peoples' perspectives on living, working, and studying in The Terminal. We also made a 30-minute documentary about the lives of these young people, entitled *Los Ninos De La Terminal* (trailer https://vimeo.com/231724416), which has since been screened in Guatemala for the families and young people involved, as well as for the public.

Our aims were threefold. First, to find out how young people who attend *Puertas de Esperanza* and *Resplandece* are protected against risk and become more resilient. Second, to find out how *Puertas de Esperanza* and *Resplandece* work with young peoples' families to help them become more resilient. Third, to see how young people respond to and reflect on the spaces where they study, live, and work.

Following a thematic analysis of interview material, a number of key themes emerged from our research. First, in terms of belongingness, we found that young people with a higher level of belongingness to *Puertas de Esperanza* and *Resplandece* projects were generally more resilient. However, young people with a higher level of belongingness to their peers were generally less resilient. In terms of space and place, we found that *Puertas de Esperanza* and *Resplandece* were very effective in adapting spaces such as houses, church buildings, and corridor spaces at The Terminal for use as places of teaching and learning. This provided great opportunities for learning for young people and, in some cases, their parents. Effectively, these adapted spaces became what Soja (1999) has termed 'third spaces' of possibility, wherein locations are re-imagined in a practical sense with alternate functions. We also found that locating educational opportunity in houses, in and around the corridors at The Terminal, and in church buildings enabled *Puertas de Esperanza* and *Resplandece* to address the needs of the whole young person, rather than just their educational needs. This involved fulfilling young peoples' pastoral needs, as well as teaching them life skills like cooking, as well as reading and writing, largely due to the plasticity and adaptability of the spaces being used.

(*continued*)

Box 26.1 (continued)

The creative and participatory methods employed for this project were a response to a need to engage young people in research. Enthusiasm for drawing and photography enabled the young people to create images of their environments which they themselves have ownership of. The process of making these images facilitated lively interview scenarios. We can see the value of conducting research which yields participant-led images in this montage (https://vimeo.com/249989168), which shows the young people, families, and volunteers responding to the images and the documentary from the project.

Box 26.2 Co-production Research in Action: A Case Study in Homelessness

The Manchester Homelessness Partnership (MHP) was formed in 2016 around a charter which aimed to bring together all the organisations working on homelessness in Manchester (https://charter.streetsupport.net). Manchester is amongst the five Local Authorities in England with the highest recorded figures of people sleeping rough in the Local Authority (DCLG, 2016). Official government figures estimate that the number of people in temporary accommodation or sleeping rough is 3511 (Shelter, 2017), yet this number is suggested as underrepresenting the true scale by at least two-thirds. The crisis of homelessness extends beyond rough sleeping; in 2015, Manchester City Council received 5000 approaches for assistance from members of the public and this includes people living in substandard or temporary accommodation. These issues came to the attention of the national media in the summer of 2015 following a public protest against austerity and a tent occupation in the city centre that lasted five months. It was through these events that the city began to consider how to conceptualise homelessness differently.

Nigel Allmark is undertaking a PhD which explores how the MHP works to enable co-production. After eight months of the Charter, the artist Karl Hyde and the Manchester International Festival (MIF) came to meet the Arts & Heritage Action Group. As part of the MHP, this Action Group is one of a series of specific groups working to co-produce solutions to specific issues around homelessness affecting people in our city. Each action group has a mix of representatives from across the board of traditional service provision but most importantly, including the equal involvement of 'experts by experience'. Our group had already been working on projects that helped to challenge stereotypes and increase the accessibility of art, so started to get excited as we found out that Karl Hyde and MIF shared our vision. He'd previously worked in Tokyo where he walked the streets, thinking and writing about homelessness, which he then used to transform a gallery, as artist in residence, by writing the stories up on cardboard covered walls for the duration of that exhibition. The Manchester Street Poem would be a collaboration; people sharing their own stories, in their own words, getting their message out there, as one of us said:

> *we're all the same, go through the same things and can have more in common than what divides us.... if we look to see it. (Jo)*

Planning and running the show:

> *The process of co-production was helped massively by having clear roles early doors and an end goal; all supported and facilitated by Sarah at MIF in her role as co-ordinator. So, funding is really important, co-production can't*

(*continued*)

Box 26.2 (continued)

be done "on-the-cheap" ... and it had that bit of glitz from someone new, which is needed to get people rallying round. (Simon)

Some of our team took the role of peer interviewers and what followed was a necessary negotiation about how to make the recordings as natural as possible whilst retaining high production quality. One issue was whether to record stories on the street or at a local day centre. We chose the latter option and in our own words:

As someone with experience of homelessness and in my role as a peer interviewer, I could tell those stories were genuine, people were opening up and had been treated badly by others and the system. (Tommy)

So, the ten-day exhibition happened in the summer of 2017, in a disused shoe shop in a vibrant area of the city centre. We were open every day, it was free, and more than 3000 people came, walked round, and read the stories—painted ceiling to floor, cardboard and paint covering every inch of wall space.

I must have been comfortable talking because I said things I didn't even remember saying. I was shocked hearing back how I talked about my sister's boyfriend introducing me to crack by saying, "here, here's a friend for you". But then, during the festival, it was a crazy ten days; we did this Q&A thing and the people from the talk all came to see my story which they knew was being written up afterwards. There were so many of them that we had to lock the doors and they were queuing down the road. People couldn't believe it was my story, they just thought it was some bloke. Karl put two handprints out below that quote. I decided that I wanted that piece of the art to take home and I'm going to put it on the wall. (Jo)

A bespoke soundscape was created by the band Underworld adding further emotion to our stories, which were varied but all real, describing invisibility, the violence of street life, and the strength of survival. The space enabled the visitors to meet some of the storytellers, co-producers, and the artist, who would greet with a smile and talk about anything, whether it be how the experience made the visitor feel, telling them how services are being redesigned in the city or even to:

funnel you into other great projects some of the people were doing in the city, like the Portrait Exhibition we did at the Central Library. (Danny)

But of course, the original Mr Streetwise sculpture was a clear favourite—developed by one of our co-producers. Mr Streetwise is a sculpture of a man, with a backpack adorned with poetry about his life, encouraging you to:

look at the person, not the sleeping bag. (Danny)

This was co-production, where traditional power dynamics between the researcher and the researched are dismissed. Here, the action group collaborates with a project enabling voices traditionally given little space to be heard. The creation of the exhibition space enabled the homeless co-researchers to act as hosts/artists. The usual position of visible homelessness in city centres renders homeless people as takers of space. Here using a different space, and through exhibition space, these artists cannot be overlooked by the dominant narrative in our society. In creating something transformational and attention grabbing, it gives exposure and plays with visibility using a creative medium.

https://www.youtube.com/watch?v=3DgtFXolzjc

Box 26.3 Place-Making with Older Adults

The final project that we consider is drawn from a three-year (2016–2019) cross-national study called 'Place-Making with Older Adults'. This research was awarded and is totally funded by the Economic and Social Research Council (ESRC) under its Urban Transformations in Brazil Research Programme. The overall project aims to improve understanding about what older adults want from their communities and cities in order to remain active, engaged, socially connected, and independent. The World Health Organization (2007) recognises the importance of designing age-friendly cities and communities to support older adults to age at home and in their communities. This project aimed to explore how older adults experience ageing in their communities and neighbourhoods, the challenges and opportunities to ageing in communities, and how communities and cities can be better designed to support older adults to age in place (Wiles et al., 2011). The overall project is informed by a participatory approach and works with older adults, community organisations, policy makers, and practitioners.

The key theoretical focus of the research is sense of place. Sense of place is defined as the social, psychological, and emotional connections that people have with their environment. For older adults, a lack of a sense of place or identity with a place can lead to feelings of social isolation and loneliness and impact negatively on well-being. The first phase of the research investigated how sense of place is experienced by older people from different social settings living in diverse neighbourhoods in Brazil and the UK. We used mixed methods and included questionnaires, go-along interviews, in place interviews, and photo diaries. The second phase (the focus in this chapter) was about translating the findings into designs for age-friendly communities that support sense of place.

Authors Fisher and Lawthom were the leads for this participatory mapping of sense of place with older adults across Brazil and the UK. Participatory mapping is a research method that allows for the creation of artefacts (maps) that can be owned by the people who developed them. It has been applied across a range of disciplines including community psychology with the process of making visual maps through discussion and giving precedence to the community. Thirty-six mapping workshops took place across 6 cities and 18 neighbourhoods between November 2017 and March 2018 with older adults, professionals working with older adults, and the researchers. As with the previous case studies, this project is underpinned by a creative and strength-based approach to construct place that prioritises the fluid, lived experiences, and knowledge of older adults. In designing the participatory mapping workshops, we wanted to ensure that older adults' voices and their embodied lived experiences of their neighbourhoods were the focus and were aware that professionals can often dominate work with community residents (Dobbs & Moore, 2002). Hence, we devised two workshops for each neighbourhood to be run sequentially, the second workshop two months after the first to allow for analysis. The first workshop (Workshop A) was for older adults only and professionals were invited to attend the second workshop (B) with older adults. At Workshop A older adults worked in small groups around a large size aerial, colour map of the neighbourhood to construct their interpretation of the community. Post-it notes, model houses and cars, stickers denoting hazards, and age-friendly points were provided to support the construction of the sense of place maps. Each group had a facilitator and the discussions were audio-recorded, and photographs taken during the workshops of the maps as they developed.

The case studies provide three examples of how co-productive approaches in participatory research can explore space and place in relation to well-being. We note three themes that are apparent throughout all three cases:

1. Place as a fluid concept
2. Co-produced artefacts as records of place-making
3. Techniques of engagement

Place as a Fluid Concept

Recognising that place is suffused with meaning is core to the three projects. With the street-connected project, the mobile and creative methods allow the children themselves to orient the city through a different lens. The documentary film shows how places, which appear to have a negative meaning (of litter and rubbish) can be captured by those with lived experience, the children who navigate this urban landscape. Showing how spaces can be places, in which the children learn, shows the fluidity of place. In the exhibition project around homelessness there is power in creating a transient/temporal display. By occupying a prior consumerist space, a shop, the exhibition, proudly narrating the lives of homeless artists, the space itself is symbolic of homelessness and lack of permanent 'space'. Indeed, the way in which space can be transformed and redesigned for other purposes (here, a living exhibition) provides a resistance to the taken-for-granted invisibility of homelessness in urban spaces. In the older adult project, the idea of age-friendly cities is explored. Here whilst cities may be badging themselves as being considerate to age, and adhering to the World Health Organization's principles, the reality for older people can be quite different. Recognising that experience of place and one's relationship to a city is often more clearly articulated at a local level, the data gathering occurs always in a neighbourhood place. Here, workshops where older people are knowers of their communities allow a re/imagining of place through mapmaking. In the first workshop, older adults redraw the local map in terms of their sense of place. In the second workshops, again in neighbourhood, local stakeholders are joined by decision makers to make the place differently. Soja's (1996) 'thirdspaces' of possibility are richly evident in the cities of Guatemala, Manchester, and Brazil. In each of these projects, place is seen as central to understanding and not as a static research setting or backdrop against which research encounters happen. Rather, the construction of place, and the rich sense of it, becomes central to understanding how the actors within it live, work, and exist. Recognising that places and contexts can be made differently is reinforced in the projects. For the street-connected children, the places present opportunities for support, wherein locations are re-imagined in a practical sense with alternate functions. For older people, the community they inhabit provides or hinders support for them to remain at home, travel around, and connect with others.

Techniques of Engagement

If a recognition of context, of place, is often poorly articulated in many other forms of psychology, then participatory approaches, which require expert knowledge, underpin community psychology. Making sense of the context with others is linked to the values of community psychology, where power is explicit. Understanding that knowledge can be co-created can engage in participants being co-researchers. In the older adult place-making project, the interrogation of space and sense of this is done through combining the local knowledge with disciplinary knowledge. Here, working with architects, we draw on participatory mapping to engage older people and produce maps which represent for them, their local neighbourhood. Using creative methods modelled on local knowledge to explore places and place-making enables the project team to de-expertise knowledge. Alongside participatory mapping, the street-connected children are invited to engage in participatory drawing and photography. Seeing their representations of place, and delight with photography as a resource, creates new opportunities for the children and has legacy value. Using mobile interviews engages children as hosts for the area, enabling knowledge and know-how to be amply demonstrated. In the street art project, the action group members become peer researchers, collecting stories and using them to make art. In all of the projects, the engagement is a value-driven process, a recognition of knowledge and instrumental to outcomes which are produced. We shall turn to these next.

Co-produced Artefacts as Records of Place-Making

Working with others in collaboration to interrogate place is a creative venture. Places are constructed through practices and processes in research which are participatory and yield varied outputs. Working with older people in exploring neighbourhood maps are physical artefacts to be displayed. An exhibition in each of the six UK and Brazilian cities allows the older adults to be recognised as 'architects' and experts. The team is also publishing a book of photos and maps across the neighbourhoods. In the street-connected project, the photos taken by children feature in the documentary film, *El Terminal*, which has been shown in the neighbourhood, in Manchester, and at documentary film festivals. The recording of life and dissemination beyond Guatemala reaches diverse audiences, again mobilising the children's agency. In the street Poem, the word art and the pop-up exhibition are testimonies of the action group members working with artists. The exhibition which formed part of an international festival received media attention and visibility around the homelessness issue. All of these artefacts are jointly made and produce outputs more meaningful to the participant co-researchers than traditional methods. In foregrounding place, the artefacts give a vibrancy to research which can engage beyond academia.

In this chapter, we have emplaced ourselves within research through the showcasing of three ongoing collaborative projects. Through this, we have demonstrated the potential for community psychologically inspired research to engage with place as meaningful context.

References

Barker, C., & Pistrang, N. (2005). Quality criteria under methodological pluralism: Implications for conducting and evaluating research. *American Journal of Community Psychology, 35*(3–4), 201–212.

Bauman, Z. (2007). *2007: Consuming Life*. Cambridge: Polity. ISBN 0-7456-4002-8.

Burton, M., Kagan, C., Duckett, P. S., Lawthom, R., & Siddiquee, A. (2011). *Critical community psychology*. London: Wiley.

Department for Communities and Local Government. (2016). Rough sleeping statistics: Autumn 2016. England.

Dobbs, L., & Moore, C. (2002). Engaging communities in area-based regeneration: The role of participatory evaluation. *Policy Studies, 23*(3), 157–171. https://doi.org/10.1080/0144287022000045966

Kloos, B., Hill, J., Thomas, E., Wandersman, A., Elias, M. J., & Dalton, J. H. (2012). *Community psychology: Linking individuals and communities* (3rd ed.). Wadsworth Cengage.

Literat, I. (2013). A pencil for your thoughts: Participatory drawing as a visual research method with children and youth. *International Journal of Qualitative Methods, 12*, 85–98.

Nelson, G., & Prilleltensky, I. (2010). *Community psychology: In pursuit of liberation and well-being*. Palgrave.

Orford, J. (2008). *Community psychology: Challenges, controversies and emerging consensus*. John Wiley and Sons.

Shelter. (2017). *Far from alone: Homelessness in Britain in 2017*. Shelter.

Siddiquee, A., Sixsmith, J., Lawthom, R., & Haworth, J. (2016). Paid work, life-work and leisure: A study of wellbeing in the context of academic lives in higher education. *Leisure Studies, 35*(1), 36–45.

Soja, E. (1996). Thirdspace: Journey to Los Angeles and other real and imagined places. Malden, MA: Blackwell.

Stevenson, A. & Lawthom, R. (2017). How We Know Each Other: Exploring the Bonds of Friendship Using Friendship Ethnography and Visual Ethnography. Anthrovision. https://doi.org/10.4000/anthrovision.2525.

Ungar, M., et al. (2013). What is resilience within the social ecology of human development? *American Journal Orthopsychiatry, 81*(1), 1–17.

Wang, C. (2007). Youth participation in photovoice as a strategy for community change. *Journal of Community Practice, 14*(1), 147–161.

27

Mediating the Effects of Austerity with Creativity, Compassion and Community-Based Approaches

Hayley Higson, Ste Weatherhead, and Suzanne Hodge

Austerity in the UK

Austerity has arguably affected the most vulnerable people in society, namely those who were already in less privileged positions (Mattheys, 2015; O'Hara, 2014). Ultimately, the effects of austerity have reduced financial security, driving citizens into poverty (Hastings et al., 2015; Loopstra et al., 2015; The Centre for Local Economic Strategies, 2014). Consequently, more people are finding themselves in situations where they are unable to fund basic needs, such as food and shelter. According to Maslow's hierarchy of needs, as people encounter poverty and the related barriers to securing basic needs, they are also at risk of experiencing psychological distress (Maslow, 1957 cited in

H. Higson (✉)
Ormskirk, UK
e-mail: h.williams1@live.co.uk

S. Weatherhead
Wirral, UK
e-mail: ste@neurotriage.com

S. Hodge
Division of Health Research, Lancaster University, Lancaster, UK
e-mail: s.hodge@lancaster.ac.uk

C. Walker et al. (eds.), *The Palgrave Handbook of Innovative Community and Clinical Psychologies*, https://doi.org/10.1007/978-3-030-71190-0_27

McLeod, 2007). Although debate exists regarding the origins of psychological difficulties amongst individuals living in poverty (Patel & Kleinman, 2003), research clearly demonstrates the high prevalence of mental health problems throughout this population (Das et al., 2007; Patel et al., 1999).

Negative attitudes towards those experiencing poverty are often reinforced by unhelpful narratives about benefits claimants, and the resultant stigma further impacts people's psychological wellbeing (Baumberg et al., 2012). Pemberton et al. (2015) found that negative social attitudes were often internalised by people in poverty, thus shaping attributions of their situation and altering their self-perception. These negative self-perceptions may therefore contribute to feelings of shame, which has been associated with the experience of depression (Kim et al., 2011). Indeed, shame has been found to be a common experience amongst those relying on food banks (Van der Horst et al., 2014) and given the rising numbers of these operating throughout the UK since the implementation of austerity policies (Loopstra et al., 2015; Trussell Trust, 2016), it is logical to assume that many may encounter the associated psychological effects. Whilst poverty and the issues relating to this have consistently impacted people within the UK (Tomlinson et al., 2008), it seems that austerity has served to magnify these problems and consequently more people are now seeking support for their mental health via the National Health Service (NHS) (O'Hara, 2014; Spence et al., 2014). Although this could be a result of improved social dialogue surrounding mental health, the evidence reported above suggests that the psychological implications of austerity could play a key role.[1]

The Impact of Austerity on the Helpers

Look for the helpers, you will always find people who are helping
—Fred Rogers

As demand for services escalates at a time when services look to make 'efficiency savings', the emphasis on setting and meeting targets is prioritised (Department of Health, 2012) and scope for working in flexible and potentially more time-consuming ways with Service Users (SUs) is diminished. Hannigan and Allen (2011) found that mental health nurses perceived significant changes to their roles due to changing needs of service users, which

[1] For more information on the psychological ramifications of austerity, see: http://www.psychchange.org/psychologists-against-austerity.html

they postulated would exacerbate in the context of austerity. In our own research we set out to explore if the same could be said for psychologists and psychological therapists.

Our study, which was granted ethical approval via Lancaster University, aimed to explore the impact of funding cuts on the work conducted by accredited psychologists and psychological therapists who were currently providing 1:1 therapy within NHS adult mental health services. We collated qualitative data from semi-structured interviews with 12 participants, who were recruited via social media and professional mailing lists. The sample consisted of five cognitive behavioural therapists, six psychologists and one counsellor, working in primary care (Improving Access to Psychological Therapies [IAPT] services: n = 6), secondary care (n = 5) and inpatient services (n = 1). Participants were recruited from across the UK (Lancashire n = 3; Manchester n = 3; Yorkshire n = 1; Norfolk n = 1; Suffolk n = 1; London n = 1; Scotland n = 1; Wales n = 1). Interviews took place either face-to-face (n = 5), over the telephone (n = 4) or via Skype (n = 3). The data were transcribed verbatim and then analysed using the six-stage method developed by Braun and Clarke (2006).

The results of which led to the development of six inter-related themes (Fig. 27.1):

The research found that participants conceptualised austerity as 'cuts' to welfare expenditure, which created a sense of threat to their patients and themselves. These threats, alongside the perception of increased pressures and futility within their role, had implications for their emotional well-being leading therapists to manage this with a flight, fight or freeze response.

"There's a General Atmosphere of Threat"

It feels like everyone is threatened within the service. Everybody's scraping by, managing, trying to do their best to maintain the service to clients. (Joleen[2])

This theme encapsulates the sense of threat experienced by participants working in a context of austerity. When reflecting on his previous NHS work, Lewis stated: "Things [cuts] hadn't bitten, there wasn't the same sense that 'bloody hell everything is under threat'." Lewis therefore acknowledged existing threats in the NHS but felt these were more pronounced due to austerity. Lewis also perceived a threat that things were going to get worse, likening

[2] All names used are pseudonyms.

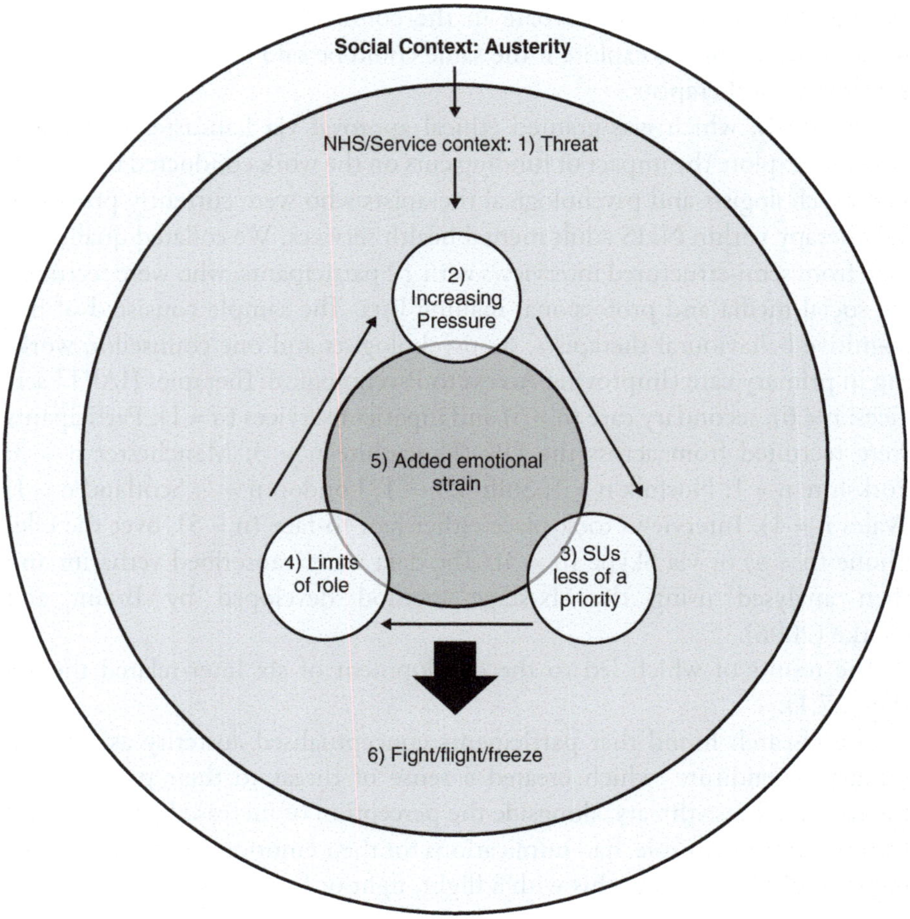

Fig. 27.1 Conceptual diagram of themes

austerity to a swamp: "It's a fucker of a swamp and I think it's gonna get deeper and nastier and more full of unpleasant things as we go forward."

The threat of NHS privatisation was reported by nine of the participants: "I really do fear for the privatisation of the NHS, I think we are dangerously close" (Paul). Acknowledging the enduring threats of privatisation, Martin felt that this threat was currently more pronounced due to austerity: "As long as the NHS has been standing there have been people trying to hack it to pieces … at the moment it feels like the most concerted effort."

These threats were actively induced in Mark's service via communication from management and both Mark and Jessica referred to explicit threats to their jobs and salaries: "There was talk of re-banding us all and us all having to re-apply for our jobs" (Jessica). While these threats created a sense of job insecurity, other participants considered fears that privatisation would provoke increasing levels of social inequality.

Although certain participants experienced threats, there was acknowledgement that these threats were more pertinent for SUs:

> The people I'm working with have a much more pronounced sense of threat in terms of their benefits, of what they might be able to claim or the sense of fear that things will be taken away from them. (Lewis)

Consequently, participants had fears regarding further cuts and the related financial implications for SUs, and there was an overall recognition that these threats impacted upon SUs' well-being: "It fills them with dread, and I've had people feeling suicidal" (Mary). Similarly: "They [SUs] feel hopeless, their environments are crap, no wonder their mental health's crap" (Christina).

"You're Squeezed": Increasing Pressure

> *Everybody's feeling pressure to some level ... [it] seems to be the way it is to ensure that the service doesn't lose funding. (Joleen)*

Due to threats of NHS privatisation and increased demand for their services at a time when NHS funding diminished, participants felt increasing pressures. The introduction of competitive practices in certain services intensified these pressures and participants employed terms such as feeling "squeezed" (Christina, Jessica, Joleen, Mark, Simone) or "stretched" (Joleen, Martha) in relation to their work. Highlighting the physical consequences of these pressures, Simone reported: "You're squeezed. They want every drop of blood from you (laughs)."

Christina, Jessica, Joleen and Simone, who all worked in IAPT services, expressed a common narrative within their workplace about needing to take work home due to the lack of capacity to meet necessary demands during their contracted hours. Although there was acknowledgement of the theoretical ability to take back time owed, participants felt unable to do that given the increasing pressures.

In an attempt to manage the time constraints Christina's service abandoned team meetings and participants overall acknowledged increasing levels of isolation within their work due to reductions in formal and informal peer support. It was further identified that there was generally less capacity to reflect on cases:

> You've not got time to sit down and think about that person and what might be best for them … you're doing it at night when you come home … because you've not had time to do it in the space you've been given. (Christina)

Paul explained that increasing pressures arose due to limited resources resulting from austerity and the related impacts on NHS budgets: "The lack of resources adds to the stress." Christina, Joleen, Mark and Simone concurred with this, acknowledging that problems with IT, estates and staffing all intensified the pressure.

"It's Just Maths": Service Users Are Becoming Less of a Priority

> *They've [services] lost contact with what we're about. We're about care aren't we? We are about caring for people and making things better. It's not anymore. It's about ticking boxes, that's what it's become. (Christina)*

Participants perceived a change in service ethos as a result of increasing pressures, with SUs becoming less of a priority. When considering the pressures placed upon her, Joleen stated: "It feels like it [clinical work] gets deprioritised quite a lot." Indeed, an emphasis on discharging SUs from services "getting them in and out" (Mark) was evident throughout the data. It transpired that while some services concentrated on statistics, others adjusted referral criteria in an attempt to mitigate the increasing pressures. For example, in Paul's service, SUs could not access psychology until basic needs, such as housing, were met. Similarly, Mary stated that in her area "each service has become quite restrictive", in terms of the referrals they would accept.

The increasing focus on targets (e.g. SU outcomes and waiting lists) was most prevalent amongst those working in IAPT services. Simone stated: "Austerity plus the IAPT model is a bit of a lethal combination." However, Tamara also spoke about the prioritisation of statistics in her non-IAPT, inpatient service and stated that some SUs were aware of this: "They come in and it's like, 'no one cares, we're just a number'." Moreover, problems in quantitatively evaluating intervention effectiveness were commonly reported, with participants describing the limitations of self-reported measures. Indeed, Simone highlighted the difficulties of evaluating statistics in this line of work:

> There's this model of X number of staff, you see X number of clients. No consideration of the emotional impact of the work we do, of the locations we are, the sessions we're in, the local need. It's just maths. X number of staff equals X number of clients.

This emphasis on statistics created further pressures for participants as there was the threat that if set targets were not met, they would be monitored: "If we don't meet those targets we would then be put under a performance review … I know of at least two people within our team that has happened to" (Jessica).

"You're Definitely More Limited in What You're Able to Do"

> *I've got a lot more skills but it feels like a waste. So, I'm being paid a certain salary and you can't really make the difference that you want to make in that context. (Martha)*

The level of inflexibility and restrictions, alongside a greater focus on targets and throughput, meant that participants felt frustrated and powerless that they could not effect meaningful change for SUs within the therapeutic context. It was recognised that socio-economic difficulties created barriers for SUs attending therapy and these broader issues further impacted on therapeutic outcomes.

Participants felt that it was the increasing pressures which led to limitations in their ability to effect change: "You're not given the right amount of, … time to … work with people" (Mary). Similarly, Mark and Jessica acknowledged that therapy had become "much more, fast pace" (Mark). Jessica spoke about the negative impact this change of pacing had on her ability to develop the therapeutic relationship and ultimately fulfil her role. Indeed, when discussing working with SUs with trauma histories, Martha stated:

> Unless you agree, okay they can come for 30 sessions or however many sessions they need, then that piece of work is never actually going to get done … So that's very frustrating, it feels futile. It feels silly really. *That* feels like a waste of money.

The efficacy of therapy was questioned by most participants and this was commonly triggered by SUs re-entering the system, exacerbating the pressures: "It makes no bloody sense because they're gonna relapse and that's going to cost them far more money in the long-term" (Tamara). However, for Lewis, Lola and Simone, this was less of an issue as they accepted that certain SUs may regularly re-enter services due to their level of need.

"It's Just so Upsetting": Added Emotional Strain

I didn't realise how emotional I was about it … I got upset 'cause I feel so bad for the patients and … I'm angry. I'm swearing a lot. (Tamara)

Working in the context of austerity entailed emotional implications for participants. Participants described how threats, pressures, perceived limitations of their role and the acknowledgement of the de-prioritisation of SUs within the systems, contributed to added emotional strain. Participants consequently described an underlying threat of burnout within their work.

There were times during the interviews when participants became emotional. Some cried, whilst others became angry: "It makes me feel sad. I feel emotional now thinking about it. It makes me feel like … (Cries) I'm crying now!" (Christina). Additionally, many questioned their role within the current system, with a sense of internal conflict about being part of something that could perpetuate or create difficulties for SUs: "You kind of get to the point where sometimes you're not quite sure if actually what's being delivered is almost unhelpful" (Joleen). Similarly, when talking about the potential for the system to exacerbate SUs' difficulties, Martha stated:

> I dunno, it taps into something about being a let-down or not cared about, you know? All of those things: rejected, ignored. These sort of like relational patterns that they've [SUs] experienced in childhood. It's being repeated again but on a huge scale.

Additionally:

> The messages people have received, not the messages as clinicians we tend to give, is that "I'm unhelp-able" and actually no! If you had a roof over your head and food in your belly and you weren't sick, you probably wouldn't be depressed or anxious. (Simone)

The combinations of emotions experienced in relation to the work and the threat of burnout were directly referred to by certain participants: "People can very quickly fall into feeling a bit more hopeless and that burnt out kind of feeling" (Martin). Equally, when considering burnout, Mark stated: "You're riding on a wave", explaining a fear that working in this context would inevitably lead to burnout.

A Fight, Flight or Freeze Response: The Mediating Role of Hope

How do you remain professional, but also fight for what you think your client deserves? I think it's difficult and ultimately that's why I'm going part-time. (Martha)

In response to austerity, and the related implications for their work, participants described a number of coping strategies. These strategies corresponded with a fight, flight or freeze response, yet were overlapped and guided by levels of hope.

Some participants would 'fight' against the system by working outside of their roles to offer practical support to SUs with issues such as housing and finances. Indeed, others talked about the need to draw on skills from historical roles and other therapeutic modalities to preserve their professional identity and support SUs. Interestingly, five of the participants were CBT therapists and all of these participants acknowledged the need to draw on additional skills, particularly third-wave CBT, to address SUs' needs: "I'm sure not many people are doing CBT to be honest if they're experienced therapists, or very little CBT. I'm guessing most people are … using lots of different skills … depending on their background" (Christina). Nevertheless stepping outside of their roles served to protect hope as the benefits could often be seen in the short-term, thus reinforcing this response.

Lewis and Martin considered the importance of influencing change via systemic means. There was a strong sense of hope amongst these participants specifically which served to enhance their 'fight' response:

> I'm not prepared to give up though. It's not gonna take me. I'm gonna keep … pushing back, keep … fighting what I can, 'cause actually nothing's gonna change if you just sit back and let it slide, you've gotta keep fighting, keep pushing forward, keep the hope alive. (Martin)

Others acknowledged that maintaining a 'fight' response becomes increasingly difficult due to increasing pressures which seem to diminish hope, thus activating 'freeze' or 'flight' responses. 'Freeze' responses accounted for ways in which participants remained in work, adhering to the pressures placed upon them without challenge and was related with acceptance: "It is just the way it is" (Jessica). Despondence, however, initiated a 'flight' response. When reflecting on the rationale for her career break and reduction in working hours Tamara stated: "Everything feels quite hopeless at times."

Indeed, a loss of hope in positive change contributed to some participants' reduction of working hours which could be regarded as an explicit 'flight' response. High rates of staff sickness was an issue discussed by many, while sickness could be the result of embracing a prolonged 'fight' response, it could also be perceived as an underlying 'flight' response. Mark explained that his own previous absence was a direct result of 'burnout'.

The Implications for Our Helpers

Direct clinical work is often regarded as the most valued component of a therapist's role (Southall, 2009) and many are prompted to pursue a career of this nature to 'help' vulnerable people (Norcross & Farber, 2005). Acknowledging the limitations to truly 'helping' SUs, as well as acknowledging that SUs are becoming less of a priority within the system, may detract the focus away from the most important aspect of therapists' roles and could therefore explain the emotional strain experienced.

Our results corroborate the findings from a UK survey conducted by the British Psychological Society and New Savoy (2016) exploring the well-being of psychological therapists. The findings of which suggested that stress and perceptions of failure were commonplace. Exhaustion and a perceived lack of accomplishment are key components of burnout (Maslach & Jackson, 1984), which has historically been viewed as a salient issue for mental health professionals due to the emotional demands of the role (Pines & Maslach, 1978). Hacker-Hughes et al. (2016) also reported on the increasing rates of sickness amongst mental health professionals, suggesting that greater pressures placed on staff, alongside increased rates of bullying within the workplace, may be to blame. Therefore, while mental health professionals may encounter a vulnerability to burnout due to the nature of their role, this risk is amplified with the added pressures of working in a context affected by austerity.

Overall, our research has found that in the midst of austerity, helpers are also being negatively affected due to changing roles and environments. Consequently, working in the NHS within adult mental health services at a time of austerity may be detrimental to our colleagues' well-being. While 'stress management' programmes are offered in some NHS trusts (e.g. Marx et al., 2014), staff may struggle to access these due to existing pressures. More significantly, however, focusing on stress management and mindfulness programmes as a solution continues to individualise the problems and strengthens the narrative that the difficulties encountered stem from therapists' lack of resilience and inability to manage stress, therefore neglecting the systemic issues which undoubtedly have a role.

The Power of Compassion

According to Gilbert's (2009) compassion-focused model of affect regulation emotion comprises three crucial states: (1) threat, (2) drive and (3) contentment. The practice of compassion is regarded as a means of helping people to establish a balance between the three systems thus enhancing psychological well-being (Gilbert, 2009). Compassion, namely systemic compassion, is largely absent. This was demonstrated in our research as we found that SU needs were becoming less of a priority, as services became more geared towards statistics.

The threat system is regarded as the survival system, alerting individuals to threats and inducing feelings such as anxiety and anger to incite change. People are believed to respond to this state via fight, flight or freeze responses (Gilbert, 2009). The drive state is regarded as a 'resource-seeking state' and as such is viewed as the motivating system. While all the states are inter-related, Gilbert suggests that the link between the threat and drive systems is especially intricate. At a basic level, if people encounter threats they may continually strive to safeguard against them, therefore initiating the drive state. Gilbert (2009) asserts that functioning predominantly between threat and drive states can diminish well-being. Furthermore, functioning solely between drive and threat states in work could lead to staff burnout (Patsiopoulos & Buchanan, 2011). Indeed, this was supported by the results from our research.

Our research highlighted that many of the challenges currently experienced within the NHS stem largely from higher-level societal and political influences. Dominant neo-liberalist ideology encourages us to maintain our position within the drive state, working hard to increase profits, which ultimately maintains the status quo and societal inequalities. These ideological norms are regularly reinforced by mainstream media, which has a significant role in promoting the pursuit of materialistic goals, further pushing people into a drive state (Gilbert, 2009). Compassion is largely neglected within this neo-liberal ideology (Fig. 27.2). This is evidenced as those who are unable to meet these social expectations, for example, those who cannot work or who are in receipt of benefits to supplement the income from low paid jobs are viewed less favourably as their role in creating profits for society is deemed negligible. These individuals are very often excluded from society and are further subject to criticism via media misrepresentation (Baumberg et al., 2012; Pemberton et al., 2015). Many people in these positions internalise these criticisms, reinforcing psychological distress (Pemberton et al., 2015). Simultaneously, the gap between the rich and the poor increases and compassion diminishes (Grewal, 2012; Wilkinson & Pickett, 2009).

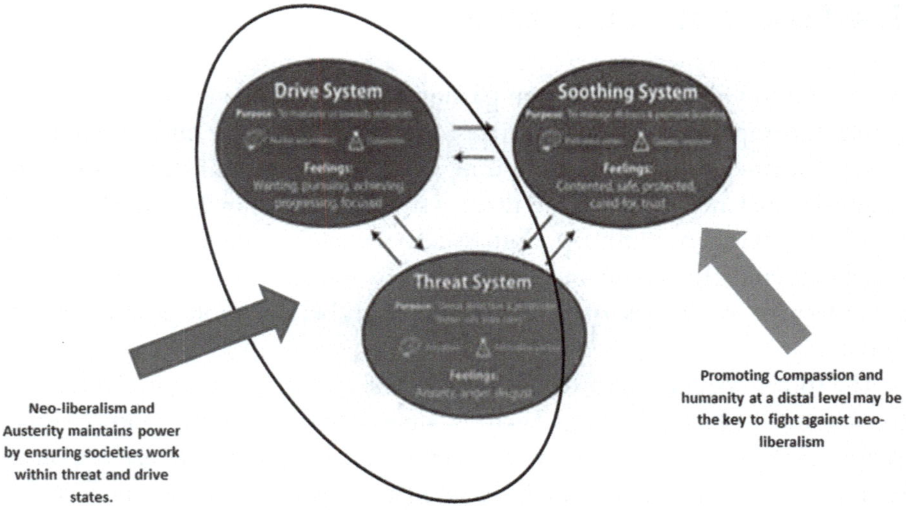

Fig. 27.2 Compassionate formulation and neo-liberal ideology

The Need for Community and Creativity

The lack of compassion throughout society has detrimental implications for both individuals and the systems operating to support such individuals. Smail (2005) encouraged conceptualisations of psychological well-being to encompass the role of distal powers. Smail pointed out that "being human entails suffering" (p. 93); however, he also asserted that while some may benefit from individual psychotherapy, more needs to be done to tackle the substantial issues originating from the distal powers. Similarly, Harper (2016) reported that despite the growing number of available psychotherapies, therapy predominantly seems to be 'reactive' as opposed to 'preventative'. Harper encouraged psychologists to work within the 'preventative' stages, calling for services to raise awareness of psychological well-being and intervene early.

While the argument for psychologists to use their skills to challenge the status quo and influence change at the macro-level is a well-supported argument (e.g. Thomas, 2016; Weatherhead, 2016; White, 2008), there do appear to be barriers in attaining this objective. Engaging with distal powers may therefore require additional skills, which may well suggest adjustments are needed for clinical psychology training and post-qualification Continuing Professional Development (CPD). The British Psychological Society accreditation processes could play a pivotal role in assuring that training courses effectively prepare future psychologists to engage within these relevant and necessary domains.

Furthermore, drawing on examples of excellence from services which have used creative approaches may inspire professionals to embrace the challenge of rejuvenating services. There are many examples of how services continue to truly support individuals in spite of economic hardship. One example is that of the community services for older people in Liverpool (Mersey Care NHS). This service specifically facilitates monthly 'making new memories' trips whereby people with a diagnosis of dementia and their carers visit local attractions. While there are a number of benefits to these trips, there are particular benefits to well-being through the reduction of isolation and the opportunities for people to enhance their networks (e.g. Cattan et al., 2005; Courtin & Knapp, 2015).

In East Lothian, communities within older people's care homes are promoted through the medium of yoga (Northrop, 2018). In an email discussing this group Northrop told us: "The practice of yoga is fundamentally about connection to self, others, the world and the spiritual. By focussing on a practice that builds relationships, we build community. So I talk about community, we have rituals and jokes, we have boundaries and we have practices we share. I work in ways that builds relationships not just exercises, limbs or lungs." While partaking in yoga, the community also connect before and after sessions so that networks are strengthened. Talking about and using the practice to manage specific difficulties encountered by group members further consolidate this connectedness and sense of community.

Examples of services utilising compassion, creativity and community are not exclusive to older people's services and the Mersey Care NHS Life Rooms project was set up in an attempt to offer a community hub to support people of all ages residing in Liverpool. Life Rooms was co-produced with SUs, carers and community members and offers a variety of opportunities and experiences, including a recovery college, pathways advice and volunteering opportunities. Clare Rotherham, a social worker working with the Life Rooms, writes: "The Life Rooms also functions as a community resource. There are IT, cafe and library facilities, which foster community access and support the use of the space beyond a formalised service. Events that celebrate the arts or promote family-friendly activities create a social, fun and celebratory space. The Life Rooms offers a safe and beautiful place to be; the environment is non-clinical, safe, and warm. There is a fundamental acknowledgement that simply 'being' in the right sort of environment can be the most humane response to distress. Anyone can access the Life Rooms and use any of the offerings. The Life Rooms is a place that offers support for those wanting to take the next steps in their life journey, whatever they may be. People that come to the

Life Rooms include service users and carers, people referred from primary care or third sector organisations, and the general public. No formal referral is required; many Life Rooms users simply 'drop-in'."

> *(It's) being able to touch base, lean on someone. (Life Rooms* user)
> *Here is sanctuary, peace and calm. (Life Rooms user)*

It is apparent that the examples presented lean towards community psychology principles. Indeed, the value of 'community spirit' (or 'Gemeinschaftsgefuhl'), for maintaining psychological well-being, was acknowledged as early as the early nineteenth century by Psychologist (and socialist) Albert Adler (Johnson-Migalski, 2013). While 'community teams' are, however, widely established throughout the NHS, they are often hidden by formalised clinical environments, segregated from communities (Holmes, 2010). While positive examples like the ones outlined exist, these approaches which seem to thrust "psychology into the real world" (see Holmes, 2010) remain to be the minority, with services often deferring to a business model.

This business model largely focuses on measuring intervention effectiveness via quantitative 'clustering tools' or 'self-report' questionnaires with arbitrary clinical scores. This practice therefore creates difficulties in evaluating the effectiveness of 'real world psychology' and true community-based approaches. Favouring positivist, epistemological approaches within CBT research, National Institute for Clinical Excellence (NICE) guidelines and IAPT services were identified by Williams (2015) and were considered a cumulative issue within mental health. Community-based approaches simply do not conform with these models and evaluative measures. Consequently, new ways of evaluating services ought to be considered and psychologists could innovate these practices, particularly as a means of incorporating valuable qualitative data offered by those in receipt of, and working into, those services.

In a context where numbers and 'targets' are prioritised through initiatives such as 'Payment by Results' (Department of Health, 2012), it remains imperative that as psychologists, we continue to apply knowledge and skills outside of the therapy room to facilitate a 'scientist-practitioner-advocate' model (Mallinckrodt et al., 2014), to influence policy and service development, and to continue to challenge current practices that serve to individualise psychological distress and oppress service users. For us to continue to develop new ways of working we therefore need to find our voices and speak up when we encounter issues of injustice.

Speak your mind even if your voice shakes.
—Maggie Kuhn

Conclusion

Rather than succumbing to the threat created by austerity, the current climate may provide us with an opportunity to rejuvenate services. For this objective to be reached, however, psychologists need to continue to apply valuable skills and knowledge outside of the therapy room to challenge the current rhetoric and create a space where preventative, community-based approaches can be incorporated into daily service provision. More support via CPD and teaching is further required to ensure that we enable the profession to feel confident and competent in achieving this goal.

Focusing on the micro-level, time is required to explore therapeutic approaches which adequately support service users whilst also meeting service requirements. Clinicians working within challenging contexts may find such opportunities in the development of group work. Particularly in systems where statistics are paramount, groups could serve to meet the requirements of a 'business model' whilst simultaneously meeting the specific mental health needs of service users. Further, groups held in local community settings and those which are co-produced, and co-delivered, offer additional opportunities for enhancing psychological well-being.

Additionally, direct clinical work which educates people on the wider systemic issues could allow people to acknowledge the role of distal powers and identify how these can influence psychological health. Specifically, therapeutic approaches which draw on external influences, such as narrative and compassionate focused models, could be used to enhance formulations and support the development of realistic care plans.

References

Baumberg, B., Bell, K., Gaffney, D., Deacon, R., Hood, C., & Sage, D. (2012). Benefits Stigma in Britain. *Turn 2 Us*. UK. https://wwwturn2us-2938.cdn.hybridcloudspan.com/T2UWebsite/media/Documents/Benefits-Stigma-in-Britain.pdf

Braun, V., & Clarke, V. (2006). Using thematic analysis in psychology. *Qualitative Research in Psychology, 3*(2), 77–101. https://doi.org/10.1191/1478088706qp063oa

Cattan, M., White, M., Bond, J., & Learnmouth, A. (2005). Preventing social isolation and loneliness among older people: A systematic review of health promotion interventions. *Ageing & Society, 25*, 41–67. https://doi.org/10.1017/S0144686X04002594

Courtin, E., & Knapp, M. (2015). Social isolation, loneliness and health in old age: A scoping review. *Health & Social Care in the Community*. Advance online publication. https://doi.org/10.1111/hsc.12311

Das, J., Do, Q. T., Freidman, J., MacKenzie, D., & Scott, K. (2007). Mental health and poverty in developing countries: Revisiting the relationship. *Social Science and Medicine, 65*(3), 467–480. http://dx.doi.org.ezproxy.lancs.ac.uk/10.1016/j.socscimed.2007.02.037

Department of Health. (2012). *Payment by Results Guidance for 2012–2013*. https://www.gov.uk/government/uploads/system/uploads/attachment_data/file/216212/dh_133585.pdf

Gilbert, P. (2009). Introducing compassion-focused therapy. *Advances in Psychiatric Treatment, 15*, 199–208. https://doi.org/10.1192/apt.bp.107.005284

Grewal, D. (2012, April 10). How wealth reduces compassion: As riches grow, empathy for others seems to decline. *Scientific American*. https://www.scientificamerican.com/article/how-wealth-reduces-compassion/

Hacker Hughes, J., Rao, A. S., Dosanjh, N., Cohen-Tovée, E., Clarke, J., & Bhutani, G. (2016). Physician heal thyself (Luke 4:23). *British Journal of Psychiatry, 209*, 447–448. https://doi.org/10.1192/bjp.bp.116.185355

Hannigan, B., & Allen, D. (2011). Giving a fig about roles, policy and context in mental health care. *Journal of Psychiatric and Mental Health Nursing, 33*(3), 20–21. https://doi.org/10.1111/j.1365-2850.2010.01631.x

Harper, D. (2016). Beyond individual therapy. *The Psychologist, 29*, 440–444. https://thepsychologist.bps.org.uk/volume-29/june/beyond-individual-therapy

Hastings, A., Bailey, N., Bramley, G., Gannon, M., & Watkins, D. (2015). A Joseph Rowntree Report: The cost of the cuts: The impact on local government and poorer communities. UK. https://www.jrf.org.uk/sites/default/files/jrf/migrated/files/CostofCuts-Full.pdf

Holmes, G. (2010). *Psychology in the real world: Community-based group work*. PCCS Books.

Johnson-Migalski, L. (2013). Transforming Practice: The significance of Alfred Adler's ideas today. *Gemeinschaftsgefuhl*, Summer, 8. https://www.adler.edu/resources/content/1/9/9/documents/2013_Gemein_LowRes.pdf

Kim, S., Thibodeau, R., & Jorgensen, R. S. (2011). Shame, guilt, and depressive symptoms: A meta-analytic review. *Psychological Bulletin, 137*(1), 68–96. https://doi.org/10.1037/a0021466

Loopstra, R., Reeves, A., Taylor-Robinson, D., Barr, B., McKee, M., & Stuckler, D. (2015). Austerity, sanctions, and the rise of food banks in the UK. *British Medical Journal, 350*, h1775. https://doi.org/10.1136/bmj.h1775

Mallinckrodt, B., Miles, J. R., & Levy, J. J. (2014). The scientist-practitioner-advocate model: Addressing contemporary training needs for social justice advocacy. *Training and Education in Professional Psychology, 8*(4), 303–311. https://doi.org/10.1037/tep0000045

Marx, R., Strauss, C., Williamson, C., Karunavira, & Taravajra. (2014). The eye of the storm: A feasibility study of an adapted Mindfulness-based Cognitive Therapy

(MBCT) group intervention to manage NHS staff stress. *Cognitive Behaviour Therapist*, 71–77. https://doi.org/10.1017/S1754470X14000300

Maslach, C., & Jackson, S. E. (1984). Patterns of burnout among a national sample of public contact workers. *Journal of Health and Human Resources Administration, 7*(2), 189–212. http://www.jstor.org.ezproxy.lancs.ac.uk/stable/25780192

Mattheys, K. (2015). The coalition, austerity and mental health. *Disability & Society, 30*(3), 475–478. https://doi.org/10.1080/09687599.2014.1000513

McLeod, S. (2007). *Maslow's hierarchy of needs*. Retrieved February 27, 2016, from http://scannedretina.com/2014/07/24/maslows-hierarchy-2/

Norcross, J. C., & Farber, B. A. (2005). Choosing psychotherapy as a career: Beyond "I want to help people". *Journal of Clinical Psychology, 61*(8), 939–943. https://doi.org/10.1002/jclp.20115

Northrop, S. (2018). Dementia friendly communities: Creating collective stories of hope. *Psychology of Older People: The FPOP Bulletin, 141*, 46–59. ISSN: 2052-8914.

O'Hara, M. (2014). *Austerity Bites: A journey to the sharp end of cuts in the UK*. Policy Press.

Patel, V., Araya, R., de Lima, M., Ludermir, A., & Todd, C. (1999). Women, poverty and common mental disorders in four restructuring societies. *Social Sciences & Medicine, 49*(11), 1461–1471. http://dx.doi.org.ezproxy.lancs.ac.uk/10.1016/S0277-9536(99)00208-7

Patel, V., & Kleinman, A. (2003). Poverty and common mental disorders in developing countries. *Bulletin of the World Health Organization, 81*(8), 609–615. http://web.b.ebscohost.com.ezproxy.lancs.ac.uk/ehost/pdfviewer/pdfviewer?sid=cd7e4078-37ad-48fa-8d8c-34e9d48800c8%40sessionmgr106&vid=1&hid=101

Patsiopoulos, A. T., & Buchanan, M. J. (2011). The practice of self-compassion in counseling: A narrative inquiry. *Professional Psychology: Research and Practice, 42*(4), 301–307. https://doi.org/10.1037/a0024482

Pemberton, S., Fahmy, E., Sutton, E., & Bell, K. (2015). Navigating the stigmatised identities of poverty in austere times: Resisting and responding to narratives of personal failure. *Critical Social Policy, 36*(1), 1–17. https://doi.org/10.1177/0261018315601799

Pines, A., & Maslach, C. (1978). Characteristics of staff burnout in mental health settings. *Hospital and Community Psychiatry, 29*(4), 233–237. https://www.researchgate.net/profile/Christina_Maslach/publication/22510052_Characteristics_of_staff_burnout_in_mental_health_settings/links/556b9e3708aeccd7773a1c57.pdf

Smail, D. (2005). *Power, interest and psychology: Elements of a social materialist understanding of distress*. PCCS Books.

Southall, A. (2009). Enough's enough: Conversations with myself and other practitioners. *Clinical Child Psychology and Psychiatry, 14*(4), 481–194. https://doi.org/10.1177/1359104509449053

Spence, R., Roberts, A., Ariti, C., & Bardsley, M. (2014). Focus on: Antidepressant prescribing trends in prescribing of antidepressants in primary care. Project Report. London: Nuffield Trust.

The British Psychological Society. (2016). Press Release: Psychological therapies staff in the NHS report alarming levels of depression and stress—their own. UK. http://www.bps.org.uk/system/files/Public%20files/Comms-media/press_release_and_charter.pdf

The Centre for Local Economic Strategies. (2014). Austerity uncovered: Final report. UK. http://www.cles.org.uk/wp-content/uploads/2015/01/TUC-Final-Report-Dec14.pdf

Thomas, P. (2016). *A prescription for clinical psychology* [Web Blog Post]. http://www.philipfthomas.com/index.php/2-uncategorised/44-a-prescription-for-clinical-psychology

Tomlinson, M., Walker, R., & Williams, G. (2008). Measuring poverty in Britain as a multi-dimensional concept, 1991 to 2003. *Journal of Social Policy, 37*, 597–620. https://doi.org/10.1017/S0047279408002237

Trussell Trust. (2016). *Press Release: Food bank use remains at record high as new data mapping tool gives fresh insight into UK hunger.* https://www.trusselltrust.org/2016/04/15/foodbank-use-remains-record-high/

Van der Horst, H., Pascucci, S., & Bol, W. (2014). The "dark side" of food banks? Exploring emotional responses of food bank receivers in the Netherlands. *British Food Journal, 116*(9), 1506–1520. http://search.proquest.com.ezproxy.lancs.ac.uk/docview/1650541107?accountid=11979

Weatherhead, S. (2016, May 23). *Psychologists and the benefits system: Time to get off the fence* [Web Blog Post]. http://www.neurofamilymatters.co.uk/news/2016/5/23/psychologists-and-the-benefits-system

White, J. (2008). Stepping up in primary care. *The Psychologist, 21*, 844–847. https://thepsychologist.bps.org.uk/volume-21/edition-10/stepping-primary-care

Wilkinson, R., & Pickett, K. (2009). *The spirit level: Why equality is better for everyone.* Penguin.

Williams, C. H. J. (2015). Improving access to psychological therapies (IAPT) and treatment outcomes: Epistemological assumptions and controversies. *Journal of Psychiatric and Mental Health Nursing, 22*, 344–351. https://doi.org/10.1111/jmp.12181

28

Writing Stories of and from the Future: Fostering Personal and Socio-Political Action

Nicholas Wood and Anneke Sools

Introduction

The chapter takes the shape of alternating viewpoints and considerations on using stories of and from the future as vehicle for personal and social change. Our respective views are illustrated by experiences of the two authors. Clinical psychologist and science fiction (SF) writer Nick/Nicholas Wood focuses on the writing of his debut novel *Azanian Bridges* and how he weaved in his experiences with a patient (the unfolding 'Sibusiso's' story). Narrative psychologist and SF enthusiast Anneke Sools draws on examples from her research on how personal narrations from the future (Letters from the Future) guide present thought and action. All in all, our respective viewpoints and experiences can scaffold ideas about changing the self and the future for individuals, and potentially larger groups, such as whole communities. Together, we propose ways forward for promoting the creation of stories that embrace the struggles

N. Wood (✉)
Department of Psychology, University of East London, London, UK
e-mail: nwood@uel.ac.uk

A. Sools
Department of Psychology, Health & Technology, University of Twente, Enschede, The Netherlands
e-mail: a.m.sools@utwente.nl

C. Walker et al. (eds.), *The Palgrave Handbook of Innovative Community and Clinical Psychologies*, https://doi.org/10.1007/978-3-030-71190-0_28

of now, but also potential ways of building alternative, hopefully more meaningful and communal futures.

Drawing on narrative theorists Brockmeier (2013), we argue that stories of and from the future (like all narrative) constitute "a psychologically fundamental practice of meaning construction, a practice which cuts across the putative divide between fiction and nonfiction" (Brockmeier, 2013, p. 7). In other words, the mind does not 'mind' whether a story is 'real' (i.e. happened in reality) or imagined (i.e. not yet happened); it perceives imagined story characters and situations as real (Schiff et al., 2017). In this ability lies the potential to create new experience to the extent that stories differ from the past; for as long as past experiences are repeated, newness cannot take effect (Sools et al., 2017; Squire, 2012).

From this view, psychology could benefit from a change in perspective from looking at what *is* (and at how current experience and behaviour came into being) to what *could* and *should be*. Such a psychology that is interested in "the possible as an emerging field of inquiry" (Glaveanu, 2018) changes focus from the question of factual truth of an imagined future (whether personal or collective) towards its psychological relevance, that is, how meaning of the "not yet" (Bloch, 1986) is constructed through stories (which can be more and less 'fictionalised') by both author and reader. We will contribute to this call for psychology as the inquiry of the possible by offering reflexive ways of writing of and from the future. Such writings not only enable "becoming aware of it [the future] and actively exploring it" (Glaveanu, 2018), but can also be used to "depict, rehearse, motivate, interpret and evaluate" (Sools, 2019) personal and socio-political action. To this end, we will focus on writing that is future facing as an act for both personal and socio-political change.

Why Write Science Fictional Differences?

(a) *Nick*: So, why do I write? And, even more specifically, why am I writing this? The short answer is because I want to both make sense of the world—and to try and write a better world into being. And this book—proposing 'new ideas for new times: a handbook of innovative community and clinical psychologies'—seems to me to be about stretching the boundaries of the psychological profession, to engender positive and progressive change.

I write genre fiction—and not just any genre, but science fiction (SF)—a form of fiction that has long been looked down on from more 'literary' circles. Growing up as a privileged white young male during apartheid in South Africa, however, reading science fiction offered an escape from a pending militarised future to reinforce the iniquitous status quo. Most importantly, though, science fiction is premised on a crucial question that needs constant asking, as it moves beyond the constraints of 'accepted reality': '*What if things were different*?' I knew—and from an early age—that there were alternatives to the grand narrative of apartheid—which was why the censors were such a powerful force within State officialdom at the time.

SF faces forward, proposing alternative models of the future—different ways of living, organising and being within the world. Because such models may function as a threat to the status quo, it was no accident that a number of SF novels were banned for periods in South Africa—such as Heinlein's *Stranger in a Strange Land*, Mary Shelley's *Frankenstein* and Anthony Burgess' *A Clockwork Orange*—alongside more overtly political novels challenging apartheid (McDonald, 2009).

Implicit within one of the central questions of SF is the realisation that things can be different from the prevailing system—and seeking this difference can be a worthwhile, if difficult, goal. This was the aim of the political Struggle during apartheid, or as Nelson Mandela eloquently put it, at the end of the 1964 Rivonia 'Treason' Trial:

> *I have cherished the ideal of a democratic and free society in which all persons live together in harmony and with equal opportunities. It is an ideal which I hope to live for and to achieve. But if needs be, it is an ideal for which I am prepared to die.* (Nelson Mandela Foundation, 2007)

(b) *Anneke*: I am interested in the transformative potential of the question *what if things were different?* For this purpose, I give research participants the instruction to imagine travelling with a time machine to a desired situation in the future. Consequently, they are asked to imagine this future situation as if already realised and to write a letter from that future back to the present (see Sools, 2020, for a more in-depth discussion of the theoretical and methodological landscapes in which this methodology is embedded). This *Letter from the Future* exercise originates from a life review course for older persons with mild depressive symptoms (Bohlmeijer, 2007). I modified the instruction for research purposes, and

> over the years I refined the instruction and tailored it to various contexts (health, education and upbringing, employment, politics), research questions (e.g. imagine a personal future with a universal basic income; a desired future with chronic illness; a desired future in the face of precarious working conditions), and settings (university, schools, psychiatric clinics, forensic care) and for both individual and group settings (Sools, 2020; Sools et al., 2015; Sools et al., 2017; Sools et al., 2018; Sools & Mooren, 2012).

The idea behind the *what-if* question is that it taps into desire—a desire for things to be different. This may appear superficially in keeping with the (Hollywood) notion that you start off with someone wanting something ('motivation')—and the story is about their muddled struggle to obtain that thing—with eventual success and/or failure (Booker, 2004). Desire is sometimes equated with appetite, or taste (Salvatore, 2016), and often linked to (problematic) sexuality and to addiction, a phenomenon associated with automatic responses luring us into (socially) undesired behaviour (Hofmann & Nordgren, 2016).

However, desire is something much more profound than mere motivation and can be constructive rather than destructive (as in the case of addiction). Abensour (1999) argues there is a need to learn how to desire and how to desire differently. Desires have been used by a media saturated with consumption ideals—you can become fulfilled, by what you buy. The point is not to assign 'true' or 'just' goals to desire but rather to 'educate desire', to stimulate it, to awaken it and to open a path for it. Abensour (1999) continues: "Desire must be taught to desire, to desire better, to desire more, and above all *to desire otherwise*."

Desiring differently requires the imagination. The prime example here is the pivotal role of women suffragettes imagining a future where women could vote. If we can't imagine things differently—which seems to be the imprisoning intent of the phrase 'there is no alternative'—then we are trapped to repeat and survive the present—something which the austerity agenda appears intent on engendering (Psychologists Against Austerity, 2015). For imagination requires the freedom to play and think—scarce resources indeed, when survival can be the sole and enervating focus of just meeting basic human needs.

An example of an economically scarce situation is Greece with historically high unemployment numbers. In a focus group study, we asked young unemployed adults with tertiary education who were participating in an employment programme to imagine and reflect on a desired future (Sools et al., 2017). We analysed how focus group participants construct together an inescapable reality where they either don't know what they want, are not educated on how to discover their own abilities or do not know how to pursue their desire even when they would know it. The only person in the focus group with a more positive view on the possibility to know and pursue one's desires is perceived by the others to be 'living in his own bubble'. In this bubble, he is thought to ignore the "standardized paths" provided by society that the others construct as inevitable (Sools et al., 2017, p. 328). These reflections on stories from the future show the intricacies of desire: the focus group participants both endorsed and perpetuated the enlightenment discourse of growth and self-enhancement while at the same time demonstrating a sense of loss and powerlessness of how to live up to that ideal in an economically truncated discourse of desire.

What Is the Ground, for the Seeds of Stories? The Importance of Context

(a) *Nick*: When I was training as a clinical psychologist, South African psychology at the time was a predominantly white and western affair, and the emphasis was on individual models of therapy; learning the Diagnostic and Statistical Manual of Mental Disorders—at that time, the third of what now feels like an endless iteration; and the emphasis was on writing case reports and research in 'objective scientific' fashion. It was with some relief I joined a nascent organisation called the Organisation for Appropriate Social Services in South Africa (OASSSA), as they recognised psychology in South Africa was, in fact, a tool to enforce an individualised status quo and that there could be no mental health without social justice (Hayes, 2000). What I had also learned from my earlier time as a community worker was that engagement within larger, collective communities—rather than individuals in sanitised clinic rooms—held the best key to maximise chances for lasting and positive change. Clinical psychology (CP) needs a community focus if it is going to challenge the socio-political context of mental ill health (Cain, 2018). And it also needs stories and books. Books of all sorts. *So where do the seeds of a story come from?*

From 'real' life: I met 'Sibusiso' (nom de plume) when I was a young intern psychologist (trainee) and he was brought to me, for 'therapy', during the State of Emergency in the mid-1980s in apartheid South Africa. Sibusiso was a significantly depressed young man struggling with his college course. I was initially told (by a white supervisor) to 'fix' him with the newly emerging Beckian CBT. I was loath to jump in with this, however, and argued I needed to immerse myself in Sibusiso's story first. Chimamanda Adichie (2009) has warned of the dangers of a single (African) story and who was I to colonise Sibusiso's experience with yet another western model? So, I read, on politics and amaZulu (e.g. the plural noun for the Zulu people) culture amongst other things.

As the years rolled by—after 'Sibusiso' had become well and left the hospital—I came to realise his story and struggles were still relevant for those facing racism and mental health issues in the west, when the austerity agenda and Donald Trump loomed large. I wrote my SF novel *Azanian Bridges* (2016) within this looming and impending shadow. Fiction is transforming what has been into what might be.

(b) *Anneke*: In what I have come to call 'FutureNowExperience' workshops (Sools et al., 2013) where people write and share a *Letter from the Future*, I found how difficult it can be for them to write differently about their unique experiences. Previous exposure to books, films and popular media provide templates to structure one's personal story. Ideas about what a 'good story' is play a role as well, as anticipations on what others expect and may validate. This became apparent in, for example, workshops I hosted with undergraduate students in a psychology programme. These students are crafting a self (Goffman, 1959) that is perceived as 'normal', 'logical', 'realistic' and 'coherent' while simultaneously demonstrating depth of character. Protecting the self by taking measures to minimise disclosure to peers (which may be highly relevant in students' phase of identity development) comes in conflict with the rewards of fuller disclosure and trying out alternative self-presentations. Such rewards include a sense of pride, courage and a desire to be known by others.

The creation of a safe space for the exploration of self beyond standardised cultural, social and narrative templates is of great importance in the pursuit of an education of desire. Recent political and societal changes (e.g. drop in student financial support, increase in achievement culture and less room to fail) find their way into student stories from the future as many of them showed distress and some envisioned much shorter time horizons than some years earlier (end of the course rather than end of their studies). These short time horizons reflect narrowed subjective space dominated by anxiety. In this context, a single workshop session has clear limits to the process of stretching the imagination. However, I noticed how the act of writing and reading aloud a letter to a supporting audience provides a means to imaginatively rehearse the future in a safe way before acting out this future in real life (Sools, 2020). In one of the workshops, a young man who portrayed himself as introvert surprised himself with the big dream he had written down of wanting to live his own life without bothering too much about what others thought of him.

Perhaps even more important for the education of desire is that writing may be the act of listening to the stories of others. The role of witness (i.e. listening *with* rather than hearing about) to the stories of others can open new perspectives on self, for example, fellow students telling about alternative ways of dealing with achievement anxiety. The very act of hearing some students stretching the time horizon further ahead to years after the study instead of to the end of the course was illuminating to many. Listening to others helped to foster empathy for struggles self and others experienced, hence growing awareness into our "common humanity" (Butler, 2004). By hearing the stories behind surface appearances helped students to (re)gain a new sense of respect for each other.

The Story Seeds Are Sharing What You Know—And Learning Too

(a) *Nick*: I decided to fictionalise 'Sibusiso's' story because his voice had stayed lingering within me over the years, along with the realisation that racism has remained pervasive but dangerously covert, despite the memory of apartheid dissipating from cultural memory (Wood & Patel, 2017). The other main character, Martin, was a clinical psychologist. Now that, I know. (For an overview of clinical psychologists in fiction, read Goodwin, 2017.)

(b) *Anneke*: The building blocks of fiction are life experiences and our experiences with others and the world around us—writers mix and match the best they can to disguise characters, but no character is ever a naked creation. And I had wanted to give voice to 'Sibusiso'—someone I met and came to know over weeks and, eventually, six months of talking and even playing together in 'therapy', someone who, it turned out eventually, had been badly damaged by a violent political system, for daring to try and make a difference.

I eventually asked 'Sibusiso' for his understanding of his difficulties. "I dropped a pencil," he told me gloomily, after a long hesitation: "A girl picked it up and gave it back. But I could tell from her look that she had bewitched the pencil—and me."

Amafufanyana. One word capturing the central theme in the small but illuminating story 'Sibusiso' told me—but only in our third sessions, after trust had been built to a degree. *Amafufanyana*—the isiZulu term for bewitchment or possession. A different story indeed from western psychopathology—and one that I was going to respect, not erase with 'cognitive restructuring'. This was the start of our 'building a bridge' across the existential chasm between black and white under apartheid. A bridge across the shared river of life—the Umgeni River in my book—also required a solid storied base to be established on both sides first.

I could tell Sibusiso was torn—his cultural heart believed he was 'bewitched', but his 'modern head'—his words, not mine—was both sceptical and afraid of my judgement. Knowing I had so much power to contest or validate his stories, I opted for validation of both 'organs'. He had clearly been split by the assertion of his own more indigenous voice—and why should 'heart' and 'head' be a choice, when they are so often in messy conflict anyhow?

I suggested a traditional healer might also be helpful. He was both relieved—and worried. It turns out he wanted to see us both. So, by month three, 'Sibusiso' was well set with a *sangoma* (traditional healer) and increasingly conversant with CBT. So, to *Azanian Bridges*:

> The bridge starts with just one young man.
>
> *Silence…*
>
> *Silence shrinks an already small room and I stare at the young man who will not talk, wondering how I reach out across the space between us, how to make his words flow. He stares across to the picture on the wall behind me: his eyes are hooded; his body is slumped. The room is a tight box of peeling institutional yellow, mould-flicking corners of the ceiling, the narrow walls groaning with a history of mad voices … or so I've been told. The young man's head is cocked: as if he's listening. Perhaps the voices in the wall have overwhelmed him. Me, I've never heard them, sitting as I am on the right side of this small square desk, panic button comfortably within range on the wall next to me.*
>
> *"What do you hear, Sibusiso?" I ask, normalising his experiences, just in case.*
>
> *He flicks a glance to my mouth, as if unsure that's where the voice has indeed come from, but his eyes scan back behind me.*
>
> *How indeed to build a link between us?*
>
> (Wood, 2016, p. 31)

(a) *Anneke*: In smaller workshop settings, with ten or less participants allowing plenary sharing of the letters, I always participate myself to create equal relationships between host and participants. This practice forces me to relate to participants and to engage personally with the topic of the group session. Where do I imagine finding common ground with participants? How can I relate? One particularly challenging context for me occurred when I was invited to host a FutureNowExperience workshop for parents in The Hague, who had trouble raising their children in a multicultural, digital, complex world. Not being a parent myself, I wondered how I could relate to their experience. The instruction for this particular workshop was to imagine a future where their child had grown up successfully (according to their own visions of 'success') and how they had contributed to a successful upbringing. I used guided meditation to help participants visualise their future life intuitively and spontaneously, rather than constructing a future in a purely mental, detached way. During meditation, the idea emerged to write a letter to my imagined future daughter and express my gratitude for her birth, after having lost her little brother in childbirth some years ago. Thus, weaving my past experience into my projection of the future made me simultaneously both profoundly sad and happy.

(b) This exercise greatly helped me to relate to the vulnerabilities and responsibilities of being a parent. However, sharing this intimate part of my life stretched the boundaries of what constituted my own hybrid professional-personal identity beyond, for example, career goals. Having shared my letter—*after* all other participants had shared their own letter—guaranteed that my letter would not dominate the workshop. Showing my vulnerability may have supported an ongoing empowerment process in this group. One of the mothers, who was initially hesitant to share her letter because of her (on her own account) lack of command of the Dutch language (she had migrated from Iran), was chosen by the group (and favoured over a highly verbal male participant) to summarise our workshop findings in the plenary meeting, where all parents from various workshops came together. She spoke with confidence and clarity and her courage was warmly welcomed.

What's the Water on the Ground? The Impetus for Developing an Idea

(a) *Nick*: The spark for writing *Azanian Bridges* came when I was living and working

in London at the time—the original anonymised case report now yellowed by the passing of a quarter of a century. Then the so-called Tottenham Riots happened, and I was reminded of the 'Soweto Riots' (Uprising) of 1976 in South Africa—'riots' echoing across decades and places as deliberate media discourse used to take away the agency and humanity of the participants, all searching for a way to express their own oppressed and marginalised stories.

Why Azania? This was a term for the new South Africa envisioned beyond liberation—the Dream Country that awaited. (And it was eventually discarded, in a less radical naming break with the past, in post-apartheid South Africa.) By 2011, with minimal structural shifts in wealth distribution and ongoing violence, the 'rainbow dream' of the 'New South Africa' was fading fast.

And then, 'Sibusiso's' long-lingering voice came back into my head. *'What about me?' he asked, 'What would I be doing right now?'* (There was no way of knowing, of course. His case report was anonymised, the past effectively untraceable.) But, over the twenty-five years living and working subsequently in South Africa; Aotearoa New Zealand and England, I had become aware of the subtle toxic pervasiveness of racism and institutionalised white patriarchy. Not an easy topic to broach with white people in particular—or to facilitate an open discussion around (DiAngelo, 2018; Eddo-Lodge, 2017; Sue, 2015; Wood & Patel, 2017).

What would Sibusiso say to this? Right here, right now, in the twenty-first century, in a parallel universe where apartheid remains, and we can sit and relax with the characters, safe in the knowledge that this is just a book—and set in another reality too.

But, in the reality of *Azanian Bridges*, Nelson Mandela fulfils his Rivonia Treason Trial Declaration and does die, alone, in solitary confinement for his ideals, on Robben Island—and there is a white-right coup. Not a million miles away from some countries right now, where cultural wars around refugees, immigration and 'national identity' are rife.

How Do We Learn to Recognise Our Common Humanity in Everyone?

Much has been written about how fictional worlds can build and hone our empathy (Dam & Siang, 2017)—but, just to make sure, I plonked an empathy device squarely into the book, as a central McGuffin.[1] A plot engine, driving change—because story is about change—both of our circumstances, and how we see ourselves and others.

(a) *Anneke*: I'm never short of inspiration about which context or topic could be central to my next study on imagining the future differently. The difficulty is rather one of choosing out of the infinite possibilities the future can hold. Sometimes it is not us who chose the topic, but the topic is choosing us. A recent example of a subject matter that presented itself to me confronted me with a context (psychiatry and psychopathology) I had been carefully avoiding for many years. After being invited to give lectures to various audiences about the role of the future in psychiatry, I looked up an MSc thesis I supervised some years ago about letters from the future written by psychiatric patients in a German clinic. I started reading about the importance of hopefulness for psychiatry (Nunn, 1996). I reread psychiatrist Melges' (1982) long-forgotten work on a temporal approach to 'psychiatric disorders'. I learned about the importance of opening a space of possibility, difference and desire for people struggling with severe and enduring mental health difficulties. They are often (although the recovery movement has affected change) perceived of—and treated as—'chronic patients', without a future. I also learned about the ways these people in severe distress imagine the future: mostly akin to imaginations in other studies with non-clinical samples, but sometimes differently, poetic at times, using powerful language I found difficult to understand. The following example comes from the MSc thesis mentioned above, where one participant with suicidal ideation writes rather poetically about a moment at an unspecified future time where he enacts his experience of fear:

That the fear one overpowers,
motionless inwardly shattered,
left behind, tortured, demoralized to the bone.
Scared as a sparrow flying from the cat.

[1] An object or device in a film or a book which serves merely as a trigger for the plot.

And yet no expression to be allowed, no fear no rage no horror…
pushes outwards…no not that all!!!!!!

These letters stretched my own imagination as these words almost viscerally communicate the embodiment of living in fear. Empathising with this experience requires me to go out of my comfort zone, to open up to difference (and simultaneously some hidden part of myself), again and again.

Whose Story Is This?

(a) *Nick:* I rewrote the ending many times before I decided on the 'right' one.

One of the pivotal decisions was around whose voice needed to linger most in the reader's mind. We know of the primacy and recency effect and I decided, in the end, that both belonged to Sibusiso. The start and end of the story, they are both his.

And, in a tribute to the realities of his traditional beliefs too, Sibusiso is released from *Amafufanyane*, his 'bewitchment', by the arrival of a benevolent ancestor, in a dream. (Dreams, in amaZulu society are often seen as ancestral messages, linked to the divine; Wood, 2006.)

How then can one write about a life of someone who has lived as if an 'existential chasm' away, from one's own story and lived experiences? (Such too, as those with severe mental health difficulties, referred to by Anneke previously.)

With due care, respect and seeking feedback from cultural 'insiders' to try and ensure there is some verisimilitude in the telling (Shawl & Ward, 2005). And you are bolstered by the realisation that, at the heart of all stories, everyone is human. What unites us is far bigger than what may divide us (Witherspoon et al., 2007).

And, if Sibusiso was around, we may well have tried co-writing this book. It certainly felt ethically dubious that a privileged white writer should be the sole financial beneficiary from a novel about apartheid. I asked for advice from other South African writers, and I eventually agreed, with my publisher and the relevant organisation, to split the authorial royalties with a body dedicated to encouraging and fostering 'black' writing in South Africa, *Long story SHORT* (Masilela, 2015). Who knows, perhaps Sibusiso himself is a member?

And then I let *Azanian Bridges* loose on the world.

(b) *Anneke*: My position towards the question whose story to tell as a researcher is inspired by Ruthellen Josselson's (2004) reframing of Ricoeur's distinction between two types of hermeneutics (i.e. the study of interpretation). The hermeneutics of restoration (faith) aims to give voice to participants and is closely aligned with empowerment movement and oral history ideals. The hermeneutics of demystification (suspicion) represents critically oriented researchers interested in exposing unconscious processes (psychoanalysis) and oppressive structures (post-structuralism and critical theory). Josselson's proposal, which I endorse, is to start from the hermeneutics of restoration before moving to a more critical stance. By grounding a demystifying analysis in the actual data, this procedure helps to avoid *ascriptivism*, for example, imposing researcher views that cannot be accounted for on the basis of the data. Applied to the Greek case study (Sools et al., 2017) mentioned earlier in this chapter, this procedure can be seen in that we first tried to understand all perspectives represented in the focus group (restoration), before taking a more critical stance in which we looked for alternative positionings. The aim was not to represent the dominant narrative per se (about the difficulty to desire and pursue one's desire), but to locate the space for negotiation and difference, however small.

More generally, my research stance is critical in the sense that my interest is in understanding how cultural, historical and societal patterns shape human creativity and potentiality. Therefore, I strive to cover the variety of ways in which culture affords and constrains human potentiality. This means that I give equal weight to exceptions and to common responses. I show how emerging seeds of change are fostered or neutralised (Sools, 2012). Examples are stories saturated with illness which have seeds of well-being (Sools, 2012), stories about unemployment futures saturated with scarcity discourse containing also seeds of freedom and connection (Sools et al., 2017), stories about paradoxes holding sway over potential voters in anticipation of the Greek Referendum in 2015 (Sools et al., 2017). The commonality in these studies is that attention to the future and to novelty opens new perspectives on a narrow, often anxiety-ridden present. The idea is not to negate the present problem, but to look at the problem with new eyes, from the perspective of a different future. My dialogue is not with one particular storyteller, but with the multiple perspectives in a community and the reality that is created by telling some stories and silencing others.

Which Stories Get Heard?

(a) *Nick*: It was a hard slog to get published. South African publishers did not want it—'too close to home' as it were, from the feedback. (If any are interested, there are more details in the online interview of me by Geoff Ryman, 2017.) But being 'close to home' was one of the whole points of writing *Azanian Bridges*! There is a need to focus on the realities of 'now', if we are to shape a new future.

Geoff Ryman (2013) himself spearheaded the 'Mundane' movement in science fiction—which maintains SF, that is Science or Speculative Fiction, should focus on the Earth-centred, more malleable near-future scenarios, rather than pursue flights of fantasy into a distant, space-faring and less certain future. That is, it should focus on imminent realities and crises, as a form of activist 'thought experiment', to address the critical—and proximal—issues of the age. Streeby (2018) collates SF 'climate fiction' or 'cli-fi', as an exemplar of this. Streeby goes on to detail writing workshops being run by black feminist activist adrienne maree brown—who, like bell hooks, prefers to use lower case for her names—focusing on building an indigenous and intersectional reclaiming of the climate future, that is, via giving voice to the dispossessed and the voiceless.

(b) *Anneke*: From a narrative perspective, the question of which stories get heard can be framed as a question of audience reception and of 'tellability'. Tellability in narrative research refers to which events are considered worth telling (Georgakopoulou, 2006; Ochs & Capps, 2001). Stories that in content or form breach what is expected to be tellable need more work to find a receptive audience. A few years ago, convincing a psychological academic audience that researching the future is indeed scientific was quite a challenge (e.g. see the way Seligman et al., 2013, take a lot of effort to establishing the scientific credibility in their call for a "science of prospection" by demarcating it from fortune-telling). Researching the future is here not about predicting the future, but about understanding how imagining the future affects present thought and action.

A more challenging task comes into view when the transformative potential of telling stories from the future becomes central as Gergen (2015) argued in his call for a future-forming science. Imagining the future inevitably sets in motion a process of meaning making, even more than is the case when telling stories about the past. As long as positivistic epistemology and methodology dominate psychology as a discipline, research on stories of and from the future will remain limited to explanatory research on their effects and underlying processes. My dream is that descriptive, interpretive and action research on practices of telling the future differently becomes a more widely accepted approach in psychology. Because if we want psychology to not only "mirror the past" (Gergen, 2015), but effectively contribute to more sustainable and meaningful futures, we need to imagine differently what research and methods psychology needs. Stories of and from the future provide a promising approach.

Feedback from Our Storying

(a) *Nick*: Out of the reviews I've seen on *Azanian Bridges*, one of the most interesting is by a reviewer on Amazon called Ken Arenson (2018). He liked it, referring to it as "a gripping read". But he outlines one of his two criticisms thus:

> *Also, the book's McGuffin does not acknowledge the debt owed to our present-day fMRI and/or EEG-based machines using AI that are on the road to reproducing dream visuals. (For example, see Miyawaki et al., 2008, Visual Image Reconstruction from Human Brain Activity using a Combination of Multiscale Local Image Decoders; Horikawa et al., 2013, Neural Decoding of Visual Imagery During Sleep; Horikawa, 2015, 2017).*

Nice, I thought, a work of science fiction being critiqued for not quoting its sources. The real and 'academic' world intertwine again with a work of fiction—worlds collide and leak, universes mesh, reality is an unruly beast, at best.

As for its reception in South Africa, the book was favourably reviewed, although feedback appears to be mainly from white readers and reviewers. The enduring legacy of apartheid is a literary bifurcation—with black writers galvanising around a decolonising agenda given the endurance of white gatekeepers within the literary establishment (Mgqolozana, 2016).

And that was one of my intended points in writing *Azanian Bridges*—apartheid may have gone, but its source and legacy still leaks corrosively all over our current world. We need to be vigilant and active in challenging this, in our constant fight for Martin Luther King's 'Dream', half a murdered century old now. Stephen Lawrence's murder, closer to British homes is—even though a quarter of a century ago—still bleeding. How, then, do we heal this? (Patel & Keval, 2018).

(b) *Anneke*: The audience I engage with is often different from where I originally collected data. This way the stories continue, by finding new applications and meanings. For example, recently I gave a talk based on the mentioned psychiatric patient study to an autobiographical writing group. The group consisted of volunteers who support patients in a mental health care institution in writing their life story. After the talk we exchanged ideas about incorporating the *Letter from the Future* into their autobiographical writing procedure, either at the beginning of the process (to better understand the purpose patients saw in creating an autobiography) or at the end (to help keep the life-story open to the future).

Differences became apparent in the group, concerning the value of openness to the patient's own unique experiences and how to serve them best. Based on knowledge from my own and other's research, I could help them reflect on various strategies and the pros and cons of these strategies for the values they hold dear. Based on their vast knowledge about the lifeworld of patients in distress, they could help me see what a continued dialogue with these patients, based on their letters, could look like. For example, one very experienced existential counsellor brought to the fore the importance of letters with only intentional language (e.g. I hope, I wish) and without depiction of a future situation imagined as if already realised (see Sools et al., 2015, for more details about six letter types including intentional ones). She made clear how voicing intent is an important part of the process of finding new meaning. Sharing knowledge with an audience thus served to mutually create new insights in an ongoing process of knowledge production.

Just Doing It: Ten Steps for Turning Story Seeds into Trees

Everyone lives surrounded by stories—our sense of who we are is itself a storied experience (Brockmeier & Carbaugh, 2001). We all carry within us the capacity to create stories. When running a story-writing workshop, these may be helpful steps to bear in mind (Bolton et al., 2006).

1. Meet in a safe space and lay ground rules of respect (and confidentiality if needed) for all the stories to be created and heard.

2. Emphasise we create stories out of events all the time, so all are storytellers.
3. If necessary, remove critical (self) censors about what is a 'good' and a 'bad' story—stories have intrinsic value, in both being made and being told.
4. Choose (or imagine) a main character (or 'protagonist').
5. What do they want to be different, from how things are now (values and desire)?
6. Plot a sequence of events to show them either achieving this (overcoming obstacles: 'happy' ending) or failing ('tragedy'). If failing, what might they have done differently to experience success? Or what else needs to be different?
7. Share stories and listen respectfully.
8. Create a group/community of stories, centring around a theme or identity, seeking positive changes, via storying them into existence.
9. Witness and celebrate new possibilities—self-publishing, internet stories and so on.
10. Keep writing—stories of hope, resistance and change.

References

Abensour, M. (1999). William Morris: The politics of romance, trans. In M. Blechman (Ed.), *Revolutionary romanticism: A drunken boat anthology*. City Lights Books.

Adichie, C. (2009). The danger of a single story. *TED Talks*. https://www.ted.com/talks/chimamanda_adichie_the_danger_of_a_single_story

Arenson, K. (2018). Fiction with an authentic ring of an imagined future South Africa, if still under the boot of Apartheid. *Amazon.com* Retrieved April 26, 2018, from https://www.amazon.com/gp/customer-reviews/R1A6QNT609TJNW/ref=cm_cr_dp_d_rvw_ttl?ie=UTF8&ASIN=B01B1E9P7M

Bloch, E. (1986). *The principle of hope*. Basil Blackwell.

Bolton, G., Field, V., & Thompson, K. (2006). *Writing works: A resource handbook for therapeutic writing workshops and activities*. Jessica Kingsley Publishers.

Bohlmeijer, E. T. (2007). *De verhalen die we leven. Narratieve psychologie als methode*. Amsterdam: Boom.

Booker, C. (2004). *The Seven Basic Plots*. Continuum.

Brockmeier, J. (2013). Fact and fiction: Exploring the narrative mind. In M. Hatavara, L.-C. Hyden, & M. Hyvarinen (Eds.), *The travelling metaphor of narrative*. John Benjamins.

Brockmeier, J., & Carbaugh, D. (2001). *Narrative and identity*. John Benjamins Publishing Company.

Butler, J. (2004). *Precarious life: The power of mourning and violence*. Verso.

Cain, R. (2018). How Neo-liberalism is damaging your mental health. *The Conversation*. Retrieved December 10, 2018, from http://theconversation.com/how-neoliberalism-is-damaging-your-mental-health-90565

Dam, R., & Siang, T. (2017). The power of stories in building empathy. *Interaction Design Foundation*. Retrieved from April 26, 2018, from https://www.interaction-design.org/literature/article/the-power-of-stories-in-building-empathy

DiAngelo, R. (2018). *White Fragility*. Beacon Press.

Eddo-Lodge, R. (2017). *Why I'm no longer talking to white people about race*. Bloomsbury.

Georgakopoulou, A. (2006). The other side of the story: Towards a narrative analysis of narratives-in-interaction. *Discourse Studies, 8*(2), 235–257.

Gergen, K. J. (2015). From mirroring to world-making: Research as future forming. *Journal for the Theory of Social Behaviour, 45*(3), 287–310.

Glaveanu, V. (2018). The possible as a field of inquiry. *Europe's Journal of Psychology, 14*(3), 519–530.

Goodwin, A. (2017). The representation of clinical psychologists in contemporary literary fiction. *Clinical Psychology Forum, 291* (March), 49–53.

Goffman, E. (1959). *The presentation of self in everyday life*. Doubleday.

Hayes, G. (2000). The struggle for mental health in South Africa: Psychologists, apartheid and the story of Durban OASSSA. *Journal of Community and Applied Social Psychology, 10*, 327–342.

Hofmann, W., & Nordgren, L. F. (2016). *The psychology of desire*. The Guilford Press.

Josselson, R. (2004). The hermeneutics of faith and the hermeneutics of suspicion. *Narrative Inquiry, 14*(1), 1–28.

Masilela, J. (2015). The long and short project: Getting South Africans to read. *Mail & Guardian*. Retrieved April 25, 2018, from https://mg.co.za/article/2015-03-26-long-and-short-of-it

McDonald, P. (2009). *The literature police: Apartheid censorship and its cultural consequences*. Oxford University Press.

Melges, F. T. (1982). *Time and inner future. A temporal approach to psychiatric disorders*. John Wiley and Sons.

Mgqolozana, T. (2016). How can we decolonise South African literature? *Mail and Guardian*. https://mg.co.za/article/2016-03-14-author-mgqolozana-how-can-we-decolonise-sa-literature

Nelson Mandela Foundation. (2007). *Rivonia 'Treason Trial' speech*. Retrieved April 30, 2018, from http://db.nelsonmandela.org/speeches/pub_view.asp?pg=item&ItemID=NMS010&txtstr=prepared%20to%20die

Nunn, K. P. (1996). Personal hopefulness: A conceptual review of the relevance of the perceived future to psychiatry. *British Journal of Medical Psychology, 69*(3), 227–245. https://doi.org/10.1111/j.2044-8341.1996.tb01866.x

Ochs, E., & Capps, L. (2001). *Living narrative: Creating lives in everyday storytelling*. Harvard University Press.

Patel, N., & Keval, H. (2018). Fifty ways to lose your … racism. *Journal of Critical Psychology, Counselling and Psychotherapy, 18*(2), 61–79.

Psychologists Against Austerity. (2015). *Briefing Paper*. https://psychagainstausterity.files.wordpress.com/2015/03/paa-briefing-paper.pdf

Ryman, G. (2013). The Mundane Manifesto: *SF Genics*. Retrieved December 10, 2018, from https://sfgenics.wordpress.com/2013/07/04/geoff-ryman-et-al-the-mundane-manifesto/

Ryman, G. (2017, March). Nick Wood: 100 African Writers of SFF. *Strange Horizons*. Retrieved December 10, 2018, from http://strangehorizons.com/non-fiction/100african/nick-wood/

Salvatore, S. (2016). Cultural psychology of desire. In J. Valsiner, G. Marsico, N. Chaudhary, T. Sato, & V. Dazzani (Eds.), *Psychology as the science of human being. Annals of theoretical psychology, Vol 13*. Springer.

Schiff, B., McKim, A. E., & Patron, S. (2017). *Life and narrative: The risks and responsibilities of storying experience*. Oxford University Press.

Seligman, M. E. P., Railton, P., & Baumeister, R. F. (2013). Navigating into the future or driven by the past. *Perspectives on Psychological Science, 8,* 119–141.

Shawl, N., & Ward, C. (2005). *Writing the other: A practical approach*. Aqueduct Press.

Sools, A. (2012). 'To see a world in a grain of sand': Towards future-oriented *what-if* analysis in narrative research. *Narrative Works, 2*(1). Retrieved December 10, 2018, from https://journals.lib.unb.ca/index.php/NW/article/view/19500/21152

Sools, A. (2020). Back from the future: A narrative approach to study the imagination of personal futures. In *International Journal of Social Research Methodology*, (Vol. 23, pp. 451–465). Routledge. https://doi.org/10.1080/13645579.2020.1719617

Sools, A., & Mooren, J. H. M. (2012). Towards narrative futuring in psychology. Becoming resilient by imagining the future. *Graduate Journal of Social Science, 9,* 203–226.

Sools, A., Triliva, S., & Filippas, T. (2017). The role of desired future selves in the creation of new experience: The case of Greek unemployed young adults. *Style, 51*(3), 318–336.

Sools, A., Triliva, S., Fragkiadaki, E., Tzanakis, M., & Gkinopoulos, T. (2018). The Greek referendum vote of 2015 as a paradoxical communicative practice: A narrative, future-making approach. *Political Psychology, 39*(5), 1141–1156.

Sools, A., Tromp, T., & Mooren, J. H. M. (2015). Mapping letters from the future: Exploring narrative processes of imagining the future. *Journal of Health Psychology, 20,* 350–364.

Sools, A. M., Mooren, J. H. M., & Tromp, T. (2013). Positieve gezondheid versterken via narratieve toekomstverbeelding. In E. T. Bohlmeijer, L. Bolier, G. Westerhof, & J. A. Walburg (Eds.), *Handboek positieve psychologie. Theorie, onderzoek, toepassingen*. BOOM.

Squire, C. (2012). Narratives and the gift of the future. *Narrative Works, 2*(1), 67–82.

Streeby, S. (2018). *Imagining the future of climate change*. University of California Press.

Sue, D. W. (2015). *Race talk and the conspiracy of silence*. Wiley.

Witherspoon, D. J., Wooding, S., Rogers, A. R., Marchani, E. E., Watkins, W. S., Batzer, M. A., & Jorde, L. B. (2007). Genetic similarities within and between human populations. *Genetics, 176*(1), 351–359.

Wood, N. (2006). In search of South African science fiction. *Vector Magazine, 247*. One World, Many Stories. https://vector-bsfa.com/2006/08/09/one-world-many-stories/

Wood, N. (2016). *Azanian bridges*. NewCon Press.

Wood, N., & Patel, N. (2017). On addressing 'Whiteness' during clinical psychology training. *South African Journal of Psychology, 47*(3), 280–291.

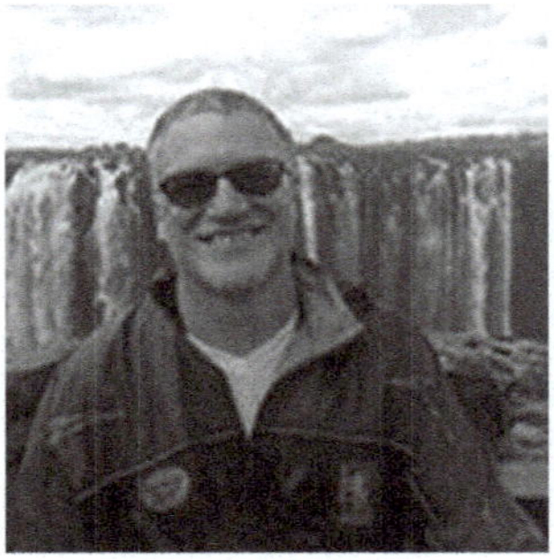

Nicholas Wood I am a South African–trained clinical psychologist with clinical and training experience from South Africa, Aotearoa New Zealand, and the United Kingdom. My training focus is on developing anti-racist practice and incorporating disability and mental health issues (amongst other intersectional axes) as continuum experiences, applicable to everyone, at one time or another. I am thus interested in challenging binary or dichotomous experiences of reality, as well as the hidden and depersonalising ideologies of power, such as patriarchal Whiteness and neo-liberal capitalism. To help me do this, I write stories, and I am lucky enough to have had a good number of them published. I am the author of a science fiction anthology (Learning Monkey and Crocodile; 2019) and my second science fiction novel (Water Must Fall; a decolonising climate catastrophe) was published in 2020.

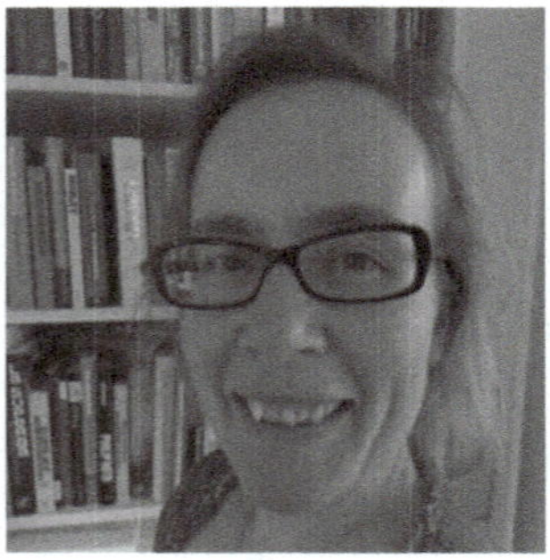

Anneke Sools (PhD) is an assistant professor at the department of Psychology, Health and Technology at the University of Twente (UT) and Program Director of the UT Storylab. Sools is the recipient of the 2018 Early Career Award from the AERA Narrative SIG. She received a MSc Degree in Psychology of Culture and Religion from the University of Nijmegen. Her MSc thesis was awarded the Professor Halkes Thesis Award in 2001. For some years she has been a member of the advisory board of the ANRP (Association for Narrative Research and Practice, formerly CNR) and a member of the steering committee of the international conference Narrative Matters. She is also on the advisory board of EQUIP (Association of European Qualitative Researchers in Psychology). In 2010 she founded the Dutch Network for Narrative Research together with Floor Basten from Campus Orléon. For her current research on how people construct hopeful futures in social and societal situations where possibilities are under pressure (e.g. chronic illness, precarious employment, pandemic conditions, and at risk youth) she collaborates with researchers, professionals and artists in the Netherlands, Greece, the UK, Estonia, and Finland.

29

The Legacy of Art Making: Agency, Activism and Finding the World

Olivia Sagan

In my narrative research with people with enduring mental illness I explore the 'is-ness' of mental distress, its loneliness and trajectory as well as the powerfully creative ways people find not only to manage illness but meaning in it and understand it as part of their very human-ness.

Routinely humbled by people's unique stories and ways of making sense, taking stock and giving account, I am nevertheless concurrently aware that these unique stories are constructed within a given socio-political moment and interlocked with a particular cultural landscape. Drawing on Hannah Arendt amongst other phenomenologists and psychoanalytic philosophers, I ask in my work to what extent illness, distress and loneliness are socially constructed and reproduced as part of neoliberal 'homelessness'—a state vital to uber economies in which the welfare state is reduced to a set of outsourced commodities in a drop-down menu—and in which mental health policy is marked by a sustained shift away from public-collective values to objectives that are private-individualistic and profit motivated.

This chapter is dedicated to Ingrid Andrew

O. Sagan (✉)
Edinburgh, UK
e-mail: OSagan@qmu.ac.uk

C. Walker et al. (eds.), *The Palgrave Handbook of Innovative Community and Clinical Psychologies*, https://doi.org/10.1007/978-3-030-71190-0_29

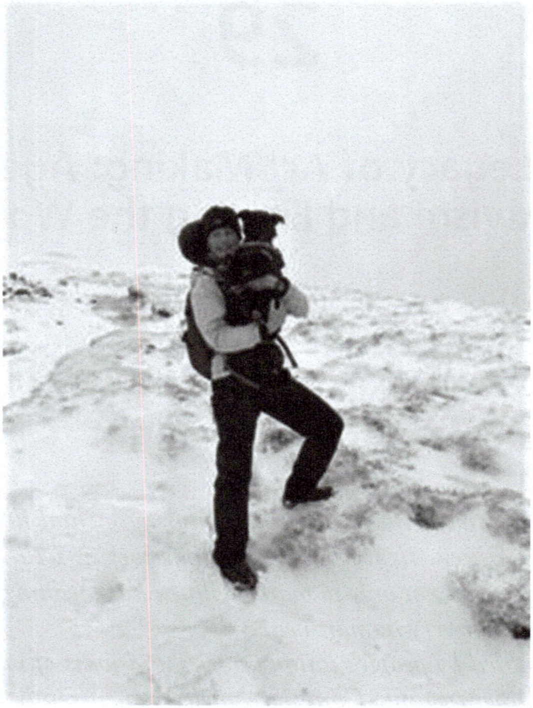

Legacy of Art Making: Finding the World

Arts in Health has become an umbrella term both for a variety of creative interventions in health settings and for a disciplinary arena in which the borders of psychology, therapy and community practice are blurred and sometimes contested (Broderick, 2011). Research into the impact on mental health of arts activities has identified a range of benefits for well-being and community engagement (McLean et al., 2011; Putland, 2012; Lewis et al., 2016; Stickley, 2010; White, 2009), yet the arena remains relatively under-theorized (Raw et al., 2012).

A set of principles can broadly be seen to be in operation in these interventions, including an adherence to democratic and supportive processes of participation, a recognition of the value of narratives of experience and the non-medicalization of the individual. There is often too, a tacit recognition that the nature of psychological distress is complex and that understanding it requires individual biographies to be seen as embedded within a given socio-economic climate and culture and that therefore such work is nestled within a social rather than biomedical health paradigm.

In such practices, the roles of patient and expert are repositioned as participant and facilitator and thus relationships are renegotiated with reflexive activity being positioned in some settings, as a foregrounded strand of the work. As such, Arts in Health practices, while varied, share an allegiance, albeit one often not articulated, to Freirean and feminist pedagogy of discomfort (Boler & Zembylas, 2003), where learning is experiential and collaborative, holding the potential to be transformative.

Within this paradigm, shared creative activity becomes a channel through which to nurture individual and group consciousness raising, civic engagement and activism. Arts in Health activity can therefore offer processes of engagement and reflection substantively different to clinical therapeutic work which focuses on the individual and couches illness and emotional distress within the person. Creative activity in community contexts therefore shares values and practices with critical clinical and community psychology, offering other ways to examine distress, to support, to 'hear' and to galvanize.

This chapter looks at the potential for such work to help forge agency, a new relationship with others and a reimagining of community. It suggests that an Arendtian 'loss of world' (Arendt, 1968) that is experienced in times of mental illness may shift to a subtle 'finding of world' through art making. Drawing on interpersonal psychoanalytic understandings that position the person in a web of relationship with other(s), the chapter suggests how this occurs but also why this kind of outcome poses challenges for researchers.

The Challenge of Evidencing Efficacy and Legacy

Arts in Health practitioners largely maintain a commitment to gathering evidence of efficacy (Clift, 2012). Yet within an audit culture that often requires reducing of complex human processes to numerical indicators for purposes of management, sustainability and control, there is understandable tension regarding the best way to measure impact (Boydell et al., 2016) and to negotiate the "constant friction between selecting methods that fit the stringent requirements of health research and methods that adequately capture the true essence and impact of the art involved" (Fancourt & Joss, 2015, pp. 1–2). Metrics provided through, for example, the Randomised Control Trial (RCT) are acknowledged to be important in the battle for continued funding in a climate of austerity wherein the focus is shifting more and more to finding ways of limiting the financial burden on the health care system rather than on facilitating health (Teghtsoonian, 2009).

In such a climate, where what can be counted stands a better chance of being delivered, measurement is an inevitable requirement—part of a parcel of tools and instruments in the commodification of mental health (Esposito & Perez, 2014) within the neoliberal context (Bell, 2013). Van Lith et al. (2013) raise the ongoing concerns within the field regarding the veracity and appropriateness of such measures, however, concluding their useful critical review by recognizing the value of mixed-method studies in further validating the existing evidence-base, while Raw et al. (2012) stress the value of an inter-disciplinary approach.

One of the findings regarding participation in Arts in Health activities in the existing evidence base points to arts activity facilitating a sense of belonging, community involvement and identity. As observed by Parr (2012, p. 8) art practice can be "an important 'stepping stone' into wider social geographies". This sense of involvement and empowerment and a precipitating of community activism is one of the most elusive outcomes to evidence, however, not least because of the invariably slow and nuanced processes involved.

This chapter focuses on biographic narrative interviews with artist participants within a project provided for and with adults with histories of mental distress. It hopes to throw light on how a visual arts practice (in this case) is perceived to be instrumental in people reconstructing their identity and connecting with others in new ways often hallmarked by a narrative of resistance and a move towards community activism. It goes on to explore a shift reported from the profound sense of 'loss of world', isolation, stigma and withdrawal so often reported by sufferers of mental distress to a connection with others and a regained sense of world. It explores ways in which art works to nurture or reinforce a sense of I and of others, and suggests that Arts in Health practice may constitute a pedagogy of discomfort (Boler & Zembylas, 2003) that lays a path towards a legacy of sustainable critical community engagement and activism.

Methodology

This chapter draws on a project in which artists with experiences of enduring mental health difficulties collaborated in the making of a film about their practice. In so doing, they interviewed each other and/or gave interviews, in some cases over a prolonged period of time. The interviews explored their lives, their art making and their mental well-being. The project and its data are described elsewhere (Sagan, 2011, 2012, 2014, 2017b) but are here revisited to explore only one theme of the work. This is the theme of the legacy of involvement in art making in terms of agency and community activism. This theme has clear implications for those of us working in clinical and community practice who have recognized the importance to our well-being and flourishing, of agency, meaning and connection with others.

The methodology of the larger study is described in detail elsewhere (Sagan, 2014, 2017b) as are the practical and ethical challenges of a multi-level project, in which participation ran from partial to immersed and activity from directed to negotiated (Sagan, 2011, 2014). This section will only describe, therefore, the process of collecting the biographic narrative data obtained, as it is pertinent to the case being forwarded.

In total, approximately sixty people gave full-length interviews which were recorded and transcribed verbatim. Some offered more than one interview and in some cases written accounts were also provided, sometimes much later—in three cases years after the project itself had ended. In most, but not all cases, people also provided examples of their visual art, speaking around these or directly about them. Approximately five people were still in touch with the researcher in one way or another at the time this chapter was being written in 2018. Where new data has been drawn on for this chapter, renewed consent has been obtained.

Participants in this project were all formally diagnosed as having a mental illness, with diagnoses including schizophrenia, borderline personality disorder (BPD), dissociative identity disorder (DID), obsessive-compulsive disorder (OCD), chronic depression, bipolar disorder, psychosis and anxiety. Most (but not all) disagreed with their diagnosis and/or the DSM (5) (American Psychiatric Association, 2013) definitions and categories which did not resonate with their experiences.

A manner of "coparticipatory creativity" (Bradfield, 2012, p. 267) was aspired to for the interviews with the interview being literally an "inter-view" (Kvale, 1999, p. 101). Significant time was allocated to the building of rapport and ensuring clear discussion took place about boundaries, consent and ownership. Some participants reported on the components of the interview process having been a restorative experience for them, with the free-associative element (Hollway & Jefferson, 2000), in which participants were not tied to particular questions or themes but free to digress as broadly as they wished, being useful. Interviews were analysed according to the principles of thematic analysis (Braun & Clarke, 2006) which offered the flexibility to approach and interpret the data through a phenomenological lens, staying close to the lived experience and entirety of the biographic account. Interpretation and understanding drew on an iterative process of analysis, rereading and refining, moving attentively between the descriptive and the interpretative processes.

Influenced by feminist onto-epistemological principles, narrative work of this type continues to highlight the value of reflexive, first-person accounts that function as a resource on which people can draw as part of their rescripting and narrative rebalancing. As such the approach holds particular currency for work with adults experiencing the compound injuries of mental distress, the silencing and voicelessness of traumatic pasts, and futures commonly presaturated in the language of deficit. The deliberate 'slowness' of the narrative interview and the flexibility to return to the participant should s/he wish to elaborate on something after having had time to reflect, coupled with the freedom to present and talk about the artworks themselves, lent a special opportunity for people to consider and reflect upon their lives, their art making, and emergent sense of self. It was only through this kind of unhurried and reflective process that it was possible for people to consider and articulate subtle changes in their agentic self and identify any nuanced developments in their political awareness.

Narratives of Art Making

The biographic narrative data suggests that making art, using imagery and imagination, identifying the emotion of the exploration, along with the genuine shock and sometimes delight of depiction, were each intensely personal process. These processes were spoken of variously as connecting with parts of oneself—discovering hitherto denied or unknown parts and reintegrating these into a new configuration of self now. And while this chapter cannot go into each experience of integration in detail, it is important to point out that this integration of self, or imagined parts of self, was a precursor, possibly a predictor, of a person's ability to reimagine her/his connection with others and society more broadly. As Yarif describes:

> It felt…feels like there is a "wholer" me now…like I got myself together…and I could reach out to others better now…

The narrative of another participant, Yelena, whose words are shared by many of her co-participants, echoes Ricoeur's (1991) words on discovery and memory, a process of striking out ahead *and* looking back—and a bringing together of both in the art making:

> Art brings me into contact with sides of my personality that are surprising, and it's a journey…an exploration that is exciting. It creates better understanding and connection to people and the world around me. It's a discovery as well as a memory.

Jude describes how:

> I remember one drawing in particular that I did. It was about a walk in a forest—it was about the experience of it, which I had actually forgotten as it was many years before…it made me remember the experience of that walk, and why I was walking there, what I was escaping (pause) it was humbling and frightening to go back there. But it, [the drawing] helped me have an in to talking about that experience…and I brought it to the group, and we talked it through (pause) and in a way, out…it led to us doing a joint work on 'places we've escaped from'. It was powerful stuff. Upshot was, a bit of me had been faced, together with others.

Jude went on to describe other work created with this group and how it led to a broader project of community activism when a public space, deemed safe by users, was under threat of closure by local government. It was no coincidence, perhaps, that the subject of space and place, identified through his work as so important, became the focus, now, of his attention and new activism. Jude reflected on how *"all that, started years ago now, with my drawing of the forest…like some dormant seed… (laughs)"*. In this case, art making was the catalyst for wider activism with a clear objective, working with others in the hope of thwarting the removal of services. The process was not always so direct, of course, with other testimonies describing or alluding to a slower and more subtle process wherein people experienced a recognition of lost and a subsequent 'found'. The 'foundness' through art making was the experience that precipitated a connection with others. As Hailey put it:

> I felt I was bringing more of myself, to the group. It was…not a new self…but a newly discovered one. I reached out, (makes scare marks, smiling) and felt I could make things happen (laughs, quizzically).

For reasons of brevity the data cannot be more fully presented here, but such testimonies, emerging frequently in interviews with art makers with long-term mental distress, represent no small feat, given that mental illness is hallmarked by withdrawal, by an oft-described deep sense of meaninglessness and vacuity, spoken of here by Tobias:

> …I completely disconnected myself…I think it was because I felt so disconnected from the world; the world didn't feel particularly real.

The dynamic interface of art, psychological well-being and personal explorations into what it means to be ethically responsible to ourselves and to others is nuanced. It is characterized by small calibrations of self, perceived validation by others and emotional experience occurring over time and in a non-linear manner, classically hard to detect, let alone measure. The narrative identity developed, one of the "far-reaching transformations of self and identity that can happen through art" (Akerman & Ouellette, 2012, pp. 384–385) is also part and parcel of people's experience of, and in some cases resistance to, recovery. Whilst it is beyond the scope of this chapter to enter into the topic of recovery, it must be said that reference to recovery, its politics and more often its processes ran through the interviews. Despite criticisms of a focus in the recovery discourse on the individual and medicalized, neoliberal notions of individual responsibility (Harper & Speed, 2014), the language and tools of recovery nevertheless appeared to be an animating thread in people's lives. Ricoeurian (1991) ontological reframing of narrative presents this as dynamic over time—with a configuring and reconfiguring of narrative making sense of experience and providing alternative courses of possible action. For Ricoeur, reflective movement forward and back, collecting, remembering and meaning making, is part and parcel of narrative balancing. And it was this process that people appeared to be describing as aided by their art making—a process that helped them come to a new sense of their identity and to reflect on the role of recovery (or rejection of it) within it. The making of art emerged as of paramount importance in people's rescripting, being the medium for not only reflection, but analysis, discomfort, reparation and moving on.

It is worth considering, then, how people make the move from the dark, atomized vacuum of deep mental distress, to feeling seen by others and in turn seeing them and developing an openness to engaging with them and a broader community. There are implications for community-based practices and the role of these in supporting mental well-being and directing people's sometimes newfound energies into collective action for the betterment of communities.

Discussion

In *The Human Condition* (1958), Hannah Arendt describes how modernity is characterized by a *loss of the world*, meaning the restriction or elimination of the public sphere of action and speech in favour of the private world of introspection and the private pursuit of economic interests. It is also posited as the "deprivation for certain groups of their place in the world and their naked exposure to the exigencies of life" (Arendt, 1958, pp. 254–255). This Arendtian loss of world with its loneliness and disconnection from others can help to give us a sense of what it is that people suffer through experiences of profound mental distress. Characterized by a deprivation of durable material structures and lasting institutions—a sense of belonging, of community—that are the preconditions for political speech and action, this loss of world renders us politically and socially impotent. This picture of inaction and disenfranchisement is just as apposite in today's reign of neoliberalism[1] and its pervasive practices.

Within neoliberalism the mentally distressed individual is doubly isolated, once through the features of their experience and twice through a cultural context wherein we are all increasingly atomized and rendered voiceless and in which health, including mental health, is commodified (Esposito & Perez, 2014). The narratives of mental distress in this and other studies are characterized by descriptions of the inclination to draw in and lose touch with the world and are accompanied, as in the Arendtian depiction, by a vulnerability through this disconnection and isolation, to being hijacked by totalitarian ideologies. These offer spurious promises to repair the loss and to fill the void—with goods, idols, medications, therapeutic interventions.

Within the neoliberal socioeconomic discourse of individualism, we are all rendered dislocated from wider civic and community engagement and distinct developments in mental health policy are marked by a "motivated shift away from public-collective values to private-individualistic ones" (Barnett, 2005, p. 7). The discourse of psychological distress and a reframing of the 'service user' within neoliberalism have further reinforced notions of individualism and personal responsibility (Brown & Baker, 2013)—locating our 'illness' in personal weakness and fault and its 'cure' increasingly in biomedical responses and behavioural change.

This socioeconomic order and its discourse, along with the hallmarks of mental distress itself, stigma (Thornicroft et al., 2016), isolation, loneliness and a "sense of disconnection, dissociation from society at large" (Rokach, 2014, p. 147), suggest the production of a particularly isolated, doubly distressed person. One study (Sagan, 2017a) reported on the added pressures many adults with mental distress felt within contemporary discourse of recovery and 'responsibilization' wherein individuals are subject to increased surveillance and expected to take moral responsibility to be healthy, productive, committed, employable and successful. As noted by Cosgrove and Karter (2018, p. 669), "at the very moment that neoliberal policies transfer

[1] Ward and England (2007) suggest that it is more productive to speak of 'neoliberalization' as an incomplete process rather than reifying it as a monolithic entity.

responsibility to individuals, there is a simultaneous increase in surveillance in order to reinstall certain patterns of human behavior".

Noticeable too is the irony of the existing rhetoric of connection (with broader economic prosperity and objectives) parallel to a regime of austerity in which many opportunities for connection and interpersonal exchange ceased to exist. It is a discourse notably confusing, simultaneously warning of the perils of isolation *and* touting independence. Given the pressures towards atomization, political impotence and isolation, it is important to look at any means by which a connection to the world can in some sense be restored to people experiencing long-term mental distress and any means by which people experiencing this deep isolation can find voice and a connection to others. One means appears to be through the making of art, which was reported as leading to an array of activity which could fall under the umbrella of 'activism'. This activism ranged from people taking vocal issue with their medical and medicalized treatment and seeking better therapeutic care to joining local community pressure groups and even mass international campaigns. So how does this happen—how does art work?

Most people interviewed did not get into an art practice with the aim of connecting with others. In fact, for some, it began as an inherently solitary activity at one's kitchen table, perhaps, or at least, one that was carried out alone even if others were present. There was indeed frequently an element of escape and refuge inferred in the motivations described.

Through a sustained practice, however, particularly as noted by those involved with an art practice for several years or more, the initial introspective stage bore fruit, as in more traditional art therapy where one externalizes, through, for example, symbol, medium, colour and composition—residue of one's internal conflicts. The memory and discovery noted earlier, with a gradual move towards a better integration of past experiences sometimes troubling or harrowing, enabled a dialogue with the self to open and the Ricoeurian process of configuring and reconfiguring of narrative to gain force. The process further unfolded as people disclosed, exhibited, showed others their works and parts of themselves and in turn were *seen* (Sagan & Sochos, 2016). Psychoanalyst Thomas Ogden (1992, p. 209) observed how, "paradoxically, 'I-ness' is made possible by the other", while for Wright (2009, p. 49) artistic activity offers no less than "a way of realizing and restoring the self". These subtle intrapsychic shifts breathed through in the way people talked about "*seeing myself…everything that happened, differently*" (Chloe) and how then the articulation of these changes and the narrative and symbolism developed to speak of them joined them in a dialogue with others. This was a process that often made them feel, in Tobias's words, "*seen, recognised, validated*".

With a self under restoration, as it were, through a reconfigured narrative identity, it is then possible to imagine more than one position to be known from and from which to know others and an other. Froggett and colleagues (2011, p. 41) conceptualized an 'aesthetic third' in which an art work provides a third object between the artist and others—one that can be shared. They claim that "By animating, or re-animating, a link between individual and the cultural field, it enhances their relational capacity" (2011, p. 92). This work suggests there is a role within community psychology hitherto identified yet little explored, for a broadening of the work we do to include working with cultural artefacts in all their modalities, along with cultural events and institutions.[2]

Here's Chloe describing how:

> It was no longer just about me—my pictures of the sewing, when they were discussed, moved from me and my thoughts to others, how they made them feel, and how we, they…were all (laughs) stitched up!…although that wasn't how I'd thought of it, on my own, like…

This simple (yet complexly arrived at) shared activity, out of isolation and internalized thinking drew on the medium of making art and the products of it and moved from thereon, in many cases to shared collective action within art groups and beyond. Ruth, an artist and mental health service user, went on to develop an art project with others and describes how pivotal this coming to be seen as something other than 'mentally ill' or 'a survivor' can be:

> …we had an opening of an exhibition [the other week] and for the first time ever [and] suddenly their family could see them as somebody else not as someone who unfortunately has a mental health condition but actually somebody who's capable of doing things and doing things well and they can feel more engaged with…and that's quite often some of the feedback we get back from people, that they can start having different conversations with people…

For Hannah Arendt, loneliness and alienation from the meaningful nexus of relations that constitute the common world form the other side of political belonging. In her phenomenology a person reveals herself through the flux of her actions and speeches, with one's presence immediately *counting* if others see, hear and touch it. It is equally dependent on the presence and recognition of and from others. This, Arendt argues, is essential for political belonging and action.

[2] This chapter is limited to exploring the making of art, but its consumption and encounter, dialogically enjoyed, also offer fertile ways in which we might connect with others and reimagine ourselves.

Conclusion: Finding the World

Participation in art activity can strengthen ties within groups and communities and enhance people's sense of civic belonging (Kelaher et al., 2013), but this happens neither instantly nor easily. Neither is it necessarily sustained in a linear progression towards deeper involvement and activism. But what this chapter tries to show is that there are subtle shifts in one's own narrative identity and sense of an other and of others that can occur through the making of art. In this sense, art making can not only restore the self, as in Wright's (2009) schema, but restore the world. It can offer a way in to material structures, to institutions, networks and processes which become accessible, malleable and owned through a (re)invigorated sense of self, other and community. It might be speculated too that this forging of connection may lead to a more sustainable activism—rooted as it is in one's very narrative identity and arrived at through an intrinsically motivated process. Community psychology is alive to exploring ways and means through which we might enhance and nurture interpersonal experiments by engaging people in activities that challenge and add meaning to their lives. Whether these be art making, gardening, running or painting, this chapter suggests that what is gained by such 'simple' activity can be quite profound. As argued by Stuckey and Nobel (2010, p. 254):

> Globalization, bringing with it the need to embrace the broad cultural diversity around how personal and societal philosophies interoperate, will put a premium on finding more effective ways to create and share meaning and meaningfulness. This need for meaning and relevance in daily experience has long been recognized as one of the fundamental driving forces in artistic creation and engagement.

Phenomenological psychoanalytic thought with its close attention to lived experience, deep understanding of our internal workings and the impact that culture and political structure have on us has much to offer in our daily work on the chalk face of community psychology. In the last two decades psychoanalytic thinking, often lambasted by community-oriented practitioners for its traditional focus on individual pathology, has moved "towards a stronger intersubjective orientation" (Bohleber, 2013, p. 799), not least because we have come to grasp how fundamental to mental well-being is the ability for relational interplay. This, along with its incisive understanding of the interface between creativity and our mental well-being, makes it well placed to be of use to community psychology.

Arendt's work, now regularly being revisited by contemporary scholars, is still poignant and relevant. It offers a useful conceptual framework for exploring complex human experience on the borders of mental reparation, belonging, agency and personal transformation and a means by which we can critically reconsider our community participatory interventions, particularly important at a time of neoliberalism.

The case made in this chapter is that for many people experiencing various forms of mental distress art making has a particular and unique role to play. Histories of mental distress and isolation, here conceptualized as a loss of the world, often lead to further stymied engagement with others. This chapter suggests that an art practice has characteristics which may offer a route to self-exploration and a narrative rebalancing which can derail a trajectory of further loss of world, disenfranchisement and vulnerability to the dominant discourses of neoliberalism.

Furthermore, the features of a visual art practice, whereby people show themselves and come to be seen, fulfil an intrapsychic role. These elements together have been indicated in people's experience of moving on from an art practice sometimes deemed 'private' to shared thinking, community working and sometimes various forms of activism. It is finally argued that such a journey is sustained because it is rooted, first and foremost, in an intrapersonal dialogue, one that 'takes stock'—often addressing past trauma and epistemic injustices (Fricker, 2010) through the narrative rebalancing that was described when people spoke of the journey of discovery and recovery, precipitated or supported by an art making practice.

There are risks in narrative approaches to understanding mental distress (see inter alia, Fisher & Lees, 2015) and certainly some of our approaches have their critics. Russo and Beresford (2015, p. 156), for example, raise legitimate concerns about first-person narratives as data being "colonised or reduced to a new area for academic activity". Yet, undoubtedly, the ascendancy of the first-person lived experience has done much to challenge prevalent biomedical definitions. These have gradually yielded some of their former dominance and this has helped trigger and underpin the move to patient-centred care (Keogh, 2013).

Phenomenological narrative approaches offer a nuanced and sensitive means by which to capture the small shifts over time in a person's story about herself—suspending for our attention calibrations which, while subtle and otherwise unnoticed or overlooked, can nevertheless have seismic effects in the ways in which a life is perceived and lived. Ricoeur (1991, p. 30) suggests that hearing a "story not yet told" offers the possibility of producing a better story, "more bearable and more intelligible". In the eruptions of 'something else', where something beyond words and consciousness emerges, the teller, the artist, is jolted into a new way of thinking. In making art, this told story does not initially use words, but finds itself narrated through the journey of recovery and discovery—at first perhaps a solitary one—which is art making. And this narrative then moves forward and out to others. Here's Tam, with whom we end:

> You get to a point when the purge is over. My art stopped throwing up them nasties…turning over the past, and it…started connecting, kind of building with it…a new me…that [me] thought 'right. What needs to be done?' (makes gesture of rolling up sleeves).

References

Akerman S, Ouellette SC. (2012). What Ricoeur's hermeneutics reveal about self and identity and aesthetic experience. *Theory & Psychology, 22*(4), 383–401.

American Psychiatric Association. (2013). *Diagnostic and statistical manual of mental disorders* (5th ed.). American Psychiatric Publishing.

Arendt, H. (1958). *The human condition*. University of Chicago Press.

Arendt, H. (1968). *Men in dark times*. Harcourt, Brace and World.

Barnett, C. (2005). The consolations of "Neoliberalism". *Geoforum, 36*(1), 7–12.

Bell, D. (2013). *Mental Illness and its Treatment Today*. Centre for Health and the Public Interest (CHPI). Retrieved January 20, 2018, from https://chpi.org.uk/wp-content/uploads/2013/12/David-Bell-analysis-Mental-illness-and-its-treatment-today.pdf

Bohleber, W. (2013). The concept of intersubjectivity in psychoanalysis: Taking critical stock. *International Journal of Psychoanalysis, 94*, 799–823.

Boler, M., & Zembylas, M. (2003). Discomforting truths: The emotional terrain of understanding difference. In P. Trifonas (Ed.), *Pedagogies of difference: Rethinking education for social change*. Routledge Falmer.

Boydell, K. M. et al. (2016). Arts-based health research and academic legitimacy: transcending hegemonic conventions'. *Qualitative Research, 16*(6), 681–700. https://doi.org/10.1177/1468794116630040.

Bradfield, B. (2012). Intersubjectivity and the knowing of inner experience: Finding space for a psychoanalytic phenomenology in research. *Journal of Humanistic Psychology, 53*(3), 263–282.

Braun, V., & Clarke, V. (2006). Using thematic analysis in psychology. *Qualitative Research in Psychology, 3*(2), 77–101. https://doi.org/10.1191/1478088706qp063oa

Broderick, S. (2011). Arts practices in unreasonable doubt? Reflections on understandings of arts practices in healthcare contexts. *Arts & Health, 3*(2), 95–109.

Brown, B. J., & Baker, S. (2013). *Responsible citizens: Individuals, health and policy under neoliberalism*. Anthem Press.

Clift, S. (2012). Creative arts as a public health resource: Moving from practice-based research to evidence-based practice. *Perspectives in Public Health., 132*(3), 120–127.

Cosgrove, L., & Karter, J. M. (2018). The poison in the cure: Neoliberalism and contemporary movements in mental health. *Theory & Psychology, 28*(5), 669–683.

Esposito, L., & Perez, F. M. (2014). Neoliberalism and the commodification of mental health. *Humanity & Society, 38*(4), 414–442.

Fancourt, D., & Joss, T. (2015). Aesop: A framework for developing and researching arts in health programmes. *Arts & Health, 7*(1), 1–13.

Fisher, P., & Lees, J. (2015). Narrative and mental health: Preserving the emancipatory tradition. *Health, 20*(6), 599–615.

Fricker, M. (2010). *Epistemic injustice. Power and the ethics of knowing*. Oxford University Press.

Froggett, L., Farrier, A., & Poursanidou, K. (2011). The Who Cares? Research: What can Museums do for Health and Wellbeing: A study of the Renaissance North West Programme. Retrieved from http://www.gmcvo.org.uk/sites/gmcvo.org.uk/files/Who%20Cares%20Report%20FINAL.pdf

Harper, D., & Speed, E. (2014). Uncovering recovery: The resistible rise of recovery and resilience. In E. Speed, J. Moncrieff, & M. Rapley (Eds.), *De-Medicalizing Misery II*. Palgrave Macmillan.

Hollway, W., & Jefferson, T. (2000). *Doing qualitative research differently: Free association, narrative and the interview method*. London: SAGE.

Kelaher, M., Dunt, D., Berman, N., Curry, S., Joubert, L., & Johnson, V. (2013). Evaluating the health impacts of participation in Australian community arts groups. *Health Promotion International, 29*(3), 392–402.

Keogh, B. (2013). *Review into the quality of care and treatment provided by 14 hospital trusts in England*. NHS.

Kvale, S. (1999). The psychoanalytic interview as qualitative research. *Qualitative Inquiry, 5*(1), 87–113.

Lewis, L., Tew, J., Ecclestone, K., & Spandler, H. (2016). Mutuality, wellbeing and mental health recovery. Exploring the roles of creative arts adult community learning and participatory arts initiatives: Connected Communities. Retrieved January 20, 2018, from https://www.wlv.ac.uk/media/departments/research/documents/CC-Short-Final.pdf

McLean, J., Woodhouse, A., Goldie, I., Cyhlarova, E., & Williamson, T. (2011). *An evidence review of the impact of participatory arts on older people*. Mental Health Foundation.

Ogden, T. H. (1992). *The matrix of the mind: Object relations and the psychoanalytic dialogue*. London: Karnac Books.

Parr, H. (2012). The arts and mental health: Creativity and inclusion. In T. Stickley (Ed.), *Qualitative research in arts and mental health: Contexts, meanings and evidence* (pp. 1–21). PCCS Books.
Putland, C. (2012). Arts and health—A guide to the evidence. *Background Document Prepared for the Arts and Health Foundation Australia*. Retrieved January 12, 2018, from https://www.instituteforcreativehealth.org.au/sites/default/files/evidence-guidefinal.pdf
Raw, A., Lewis, S., Russell, A., & Macnaughton, J. (2012). A hole in the heart: Confronting the drive for evidence-based impact research in arts and health. *Arts and Health., 4*(2), 97–108.
Ricoeur, P. (1991). Life in quest of narrative. In D. Wood (Ed.), *On Paul Ricoeur: Narrative and interpretation*. Routledge.
Rokach, A. (2014). Loneliness of the Marginalized. *Open Journal of Depression, 3*, 147–153. https://doi.org/10.4236/ojd.2014.34018.
Russo, J., & Beresford, P. (2015). Between exclusion and colonisation: Seeking a place for mad people's knowledge in academia. *Disability & Society, 30*(1), 153–157.
Sagan, O. (2011). Thou Art: The multiple gaze of audio-visual, community-based participatory research. *Journal of Applied Arts & Health, 2*(2), 125–136.
Sagan, O. (2012). Connection and reparation: Narratives of art practice in the lives of mental health service users. *Counselling Psychology Quarterly, 25*(3), 239–249.
Sagan, O. (2014). *Narratives of arts practice and mental wellbeing: Connection and reparation*. Routledge.
Sagan, O. (2017a). Narratives of loneliness and mental ill health in a time of neoliberalism. Chapter 8. In O. in Sagan & E. Miller (Eds.), *Narratives of loneliness: Multidisciplinary perspectives of the 21st century*. Routledge.
Sagan, O. (2017b). Kunst virker: små justeringer af erkendelsen og genoprettelsen af selvet. In A. Jensen (eds.), *Kultur og Sundhed—en antologi*. DK: Turbine Akademisk
Sagan, O., & Sochos, A. (2016). Group attachment through art practice: A phenomenological analysis of being seen and showing. *Therapeutic Communities: The International Journal of Therapeutic Communities, 37*(2), 45–56.
Stickley, T. (2010). The arts, identity and belonging: A longitudinal study. *Arts & Health., 2*(1), 23–32.
Stuckey, H. L., & Nobel, J. (2010). The connection between art, healing, and public health: A review of current literature. *American Journal of Public Health, 100*(2), 254–263.
Teghtsoonian, K. (2009). Depression and mental health in neoliberal times: Acritical analysis of policy and discourse. *Social Science and Medicine, 69*, 28–35.
Thornicroft, G., Mehta, N., Clement, S., Evans-Lacko, S., Doherty, M., Rose, D., Koschorke, M., Shidhaye, R., O'Reilly, C., & Henderson, C. (2016). Evidence for effective interventions to reduce mental health related stigma and discrimination: Narrative overview. *The Lancet Psychiatry, 387*(10023), 1123–1132.

Van Lith, T., Schofield, M. J., & Fenner, P. (2013). Identifying the evidence-base for art-based practices and their potential benefit for mental health recovery: A critical review. *Disability & Rehabilitation, 35*(16), 1309–1323.

Ward, K., & England, K. (2007). Introduction: Reading neoliberalization. In K. England & K. Ward (Eds.), *Neoliberalization* (pp. 1–22). Blackwell.

Wright, K. (2009). *Mirroring and attunement: Self-realization in psychoanalysis and art*. Routledge/Taylor & Francis Group.

White, M. (2009). *Arts development in community health: A social tonic*. Radcliffe.

30

We Tell Our Own Stories: Older Adults as Expert Researchers

Erin Elizabeth Partridge

Working alongside older adults as partners gives me great hope for our community and clinical and research practices moving forward. I have found older adults to be excellent co-investigators and co-creators. They share so generously from their lived experiences, and when empowered to innovate, they come up with brilliant ideas. As we explore methods with more inclusive potential, we can address the complex problems facing our world today. On a personal note, the work is fulfilling and inspiring in ways I never could have imagined during the early stages of my career. I am ever humbled by the willingness of my older adult partners to ask hard questions, to share the sometimes messy, painful parts of life, and to engage in deep inquiry.

E. E. Partridge (✉)
Elder Care Alliance, Alameda, CA, USA

Department of Art Therapy, Dominican University of California, San Rafael, CA, USA

C. Walker et al. (eds.), *The Palgrave Handbook of Innovative Community and Clinical Psychologies*, https://doi.org/10.1007/978-3-030-71190-0_30

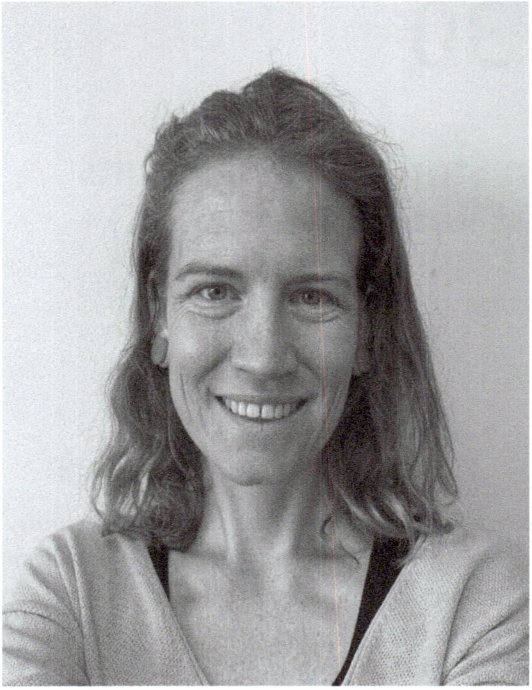

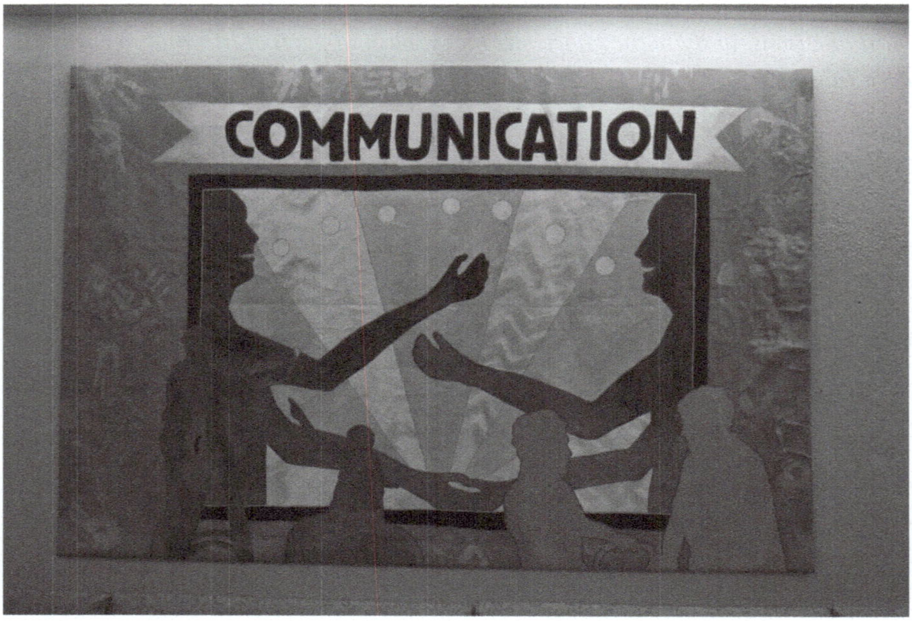

Fig. 30.1 Communication mural. The mural was painted on unstretched canvas and then stretched and hung when complete, in order to enable more people to participate

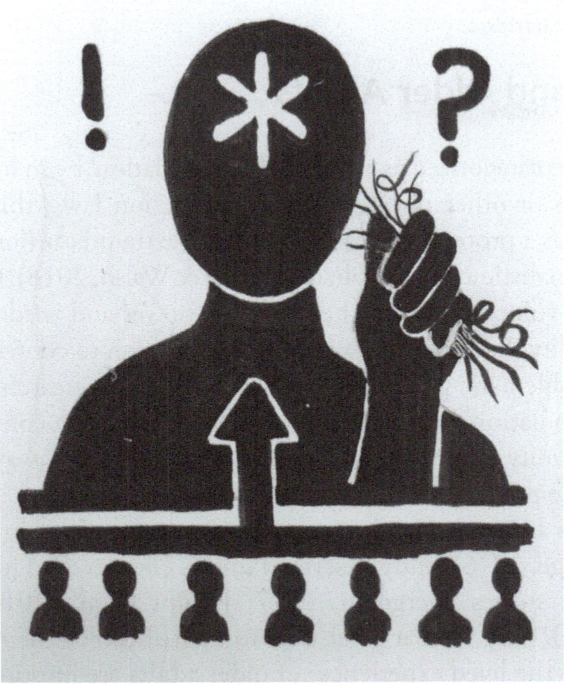

Fig. 30.2 Traditional research dynamics. In traditional research methods, the researcher holds the methods tightly. The researcher has the initial ideas, asks the questions, and receives recognition for the produced knowledge. The research subjects provide data, but do not receive anything back. The barrier between researcher and research subjects is strong; the relationship is unidirectional

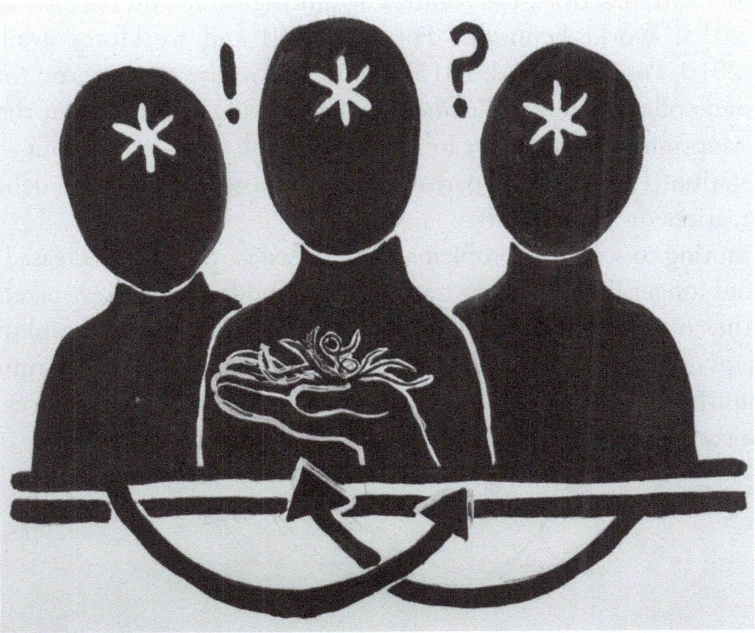

Fig. 30.3 Participatory research dynamics. In this model of research, the researcher and participants are on the same level; they share in the inquiry, findings, and knowledge creation. The researcher offers methods with an open hand. Data and knowledge flow in an omnidirectional manner between stakeholders

Research and Older Adults

Older adults are categorized as a 'vulnerable population' by many institutional research boards or other research subject protection laws; this classification can be viewed as a protective measure ensuring extra precautions, or it can be viewed as paternalistic and infantilizing (Kwan & Walsh, 2018). Characterizing older adults as vulnerable strips them of their power and wisdom—eliminating the possibility that they have valuable information to contribute and reinforcing the problematic power structure of traditional research methods. The 'vulnerable population' lens spills out beyond the research context into clinical and community contexts as well; older adults are shut away, left out, and protected to the point of being silenced.

When elders are empowered to serve as co-researchers, as in the Amplified Elders (Partridge, 2016) study described in this chapter, and involved in telling their own stories (Bergman, 2017; Houpt et al., 2016; Mcleod & Ricketts, 2013), they have a great deal to contribute to their communities and to society. The lived experiences of older adults are important when trying to address issues of ageism (Applewhite, 2016; Levy & Macdonald, 2016) and aging experience; though historically considered to be more favorable in collectivist cultures, a recent meta-analysis revealed more nuanced attitudes incorporating traditions as well as economic and demographic realities (North & Fiske, 2015). When considering how to approach and transform elder care practices, the realities of shifting care contexts (Schoenborn et al., 2013; World Economic Forum, 2012) and workforce availability (Parks, 2010; Poo & Conrad, 2015) require innovative practices on the individual and collective levels. Technology can provide solutions, but the troubling adoption of robotic care and personal devices without careful consideration (Parks, 2010; Sparrow, 2016) imposes limiting and dehumanizing practices on older adults.

Attempting to solve the problems of increased care acuity, decreased workforce, and longer lifespan using traditional methods, we cut key stakeholders out of the conversation. Ethical, person-centered practices and revolutionary or perhaps even disruptive strategies create opportunities for transforming our communities. We need to stop silencing older adults and create spaces where their voices are heard and their requests are met with action.

Interrogating Traditional Research Methods

The criticism and reimagining of research is part of a larger conversation about the "need to resist colonialist, sterile research impulses" (Ellis et al., 2011) of past practices. The recent reconsideration of the ubiquitous 'Word Gap' research in education where the research methodology, presence of the researcher, and underlying assumptions may have had a significant impact on the study outcome (Baugh, 2017; Gilkerson et al., 2017; Sperry et al., 2018) is just one example of heavily circulated research that did not stand up to a more nuanced investigation. While there is certainly a place for traditional methods in the spectrum of social science research, the history of categorizing certain methods as more valid, accurate, truthful, useful, or worthwhile has led to a narrow understanding of human life. We need to 'destabilize' (Fine, 2018, p. 6) past practice to create space for other ways of knowing.

Participatory research with older adults. As I worked to develop my research ideas early in my doctoral program, I knew I wanted to work with something related to the field of aging. My clinical experience was filled with so many rich anecdotes and case studies I wanted to better understand. I came into the program full of drive and fire to 'prove' the efficacy of art therapy with this population through a large, quantitative study. Through the process of writing papers and critiquing past practices, the themes bubbling to the surface were about agency, voice, and expertise—themes far more difficult to quantify and suggesting alternative research methods. Some of the questions I was thinking about were as follows: How are the older adult participants considered by the researchers? What accommodations were made to account for those who may not be able to express themselves through conventional research tools? Who is qualified to speak about the experience of aging?

I also thought about my experiences working with older adults each day; I had a different level of access and connection than an outside researcher would. Instead of a liability or negatively biasing influence, I came to see myself as an embedded ethnographer. Over time, this shifted to a true sharing of the documentation and inquiry process with the older adults I spent each day with.

Amplified Elders Study

As a result of critical analysis of existing practices, reviewing the literature, and an ethical commitment to empowering older adults, my dissertation study involved participatory art-based inquiry (Partridge, 2016). The study was designed to take a holistic look at communication in elder care settings—both in the moment and by tapping into the knowledge of the older adults—how can they inform and teach through their ideas about communication? The following sections will cover the research study with a focus on the challenges to traditional methods and ways to inspire new thinking about research.

Research questions. The Amplified Elders study operated under the assumption that older adults have important knowledge to share about their experiences, needs, and preferences in communication. This assumption placed the older adults in a more empowered role than traditional work with elders; instead of framing aging as a problem with implications for communication practice, this research framed aging as an asset providing a window into longitudinal experiences of communication. The study inquired into the capability of digital art images to express communication experiences and the use of community mural-making as data synthesis.

Methodology. This study was open to older adults in assisted living, skilled nursing, and memory care in four buildings in California operated by a nonprofit organization. Staff, volunteers, and family members were also able to participate. Participants were invited to create an image about their communication experiences and answer a series of semi-structured interview questions. The questions covered their experiences of communication, asked them to define both good and bad communication, asked them about their experiences of communication in the elder care setting, and asked them about their belief in art or visual images as a form of communication. Older adult participants in one of the assisted living communities were also invited to participate in data analysis and in creating a mural as a visual summary of the results.

Use of technology. This study utilized a relatively new, immersive computer system, the Sprout by Hewlett Packard. It was loaned to the researcher's university with no strings attached, just a curiosity about how it could be used as an art-making tool in art therapy. The tool, a touch-based system involving both scanning and mark-making capability, enabled a larger number of participants to express themselves. The tool does not require holding a paintbrush or marker and it may paradoxically seem less intimidating than traditional art tools. Artists and non-artists participated in this study and only one or two of the sixty participants made any statements about not being creative or artistic.

Art-based methods. Art-based methods using a technology tool created a more equal meeting ground for participants; Delbanco (2011) described the ways art and image making is a human drive that does not decrease with advancing age. The simple, touch-activated system eliminated the need for cognitive tracking of multiple steps while maintaining the tactile stimulation of physical art making; though no paint was involved, using fingers to make marks stimulates the participants similar to the expressive, emotive properties of finger painting (Hinz, 2009; Lusebrink, 2004, 2010). The resulting images, whether the participant could verbally supplement their image or not, contained a great deal of insight into communication preferences and experiences.

Researcher reflexive process. Throughout the research process, the researcher engaged in a reflexive art process, similar to the directive given to individual participants. The researcher utilized the digital art tool to create an image after every individual interaction, representing herself, the participant(s), and the communication as she perceived it. These images served two purposes in the study. The first was to create a visual record of the communication experience within the research process itself—an in situ measurement of interaction. The second was to bracket her creative biases and excitement about the technology. The tool can allow for expressive mark making, but most participants chose to limit their use of color and marks. Creating and exploring with the tool between data collection sessions lessened the impulse to suggest participants to use more colors or create more complex images. Making her own images allowed the researcher to maintain an open, receiving stance toward the images created by participants.

Results. The results of this study confirmed the hypotheses; participants were able to use digitally created images to express their communication experiences and were able to provide important insight into communication in the elder care settings. The research revealed an interesting distinction between the elder participants and the younger staff or family participants; older adults tended to create images with positive messages and to reflect positive experiences of communication, while younger people more often created images referencing elder decline and the need to adapt communication to address the decline. In the verbal interviews, older adults tended to give metaphoric or abstract examples, while staff and family members shared specific communication experiences with individual people. The majority of participants across all categories reported an improvement in their communication over their lifespan. Because of the participatory nature of the study design data concentrated into several emergent themes beyond the specific questions about communication: power, technology, and simplicity.

Emergent themes. Several interesting themes surfaced in the verbal and art-based data from individual and group processes during the research. The first emergent theme was about power, specifically as it pertains to culture, ethnicity, language use, and discrimination. Participants discussed the way these issues impact communication along with their individual experiences of racism, ageism, and discrimination. The existence of bias and discrimination can impact the oppressed person's communication; one resident described the racism she faced and how it caused difficulty in her interpersonal communication: "I don't know what it was about me but it just didn't go right. The reason I see is racism. Because I am Mexican, they thought I couldn't have a good mind" (Amplified Voices participant). She described struggling to understand for many years and then coming to realize the problem was with the other person. They related their past experiences to the current political and social climate and worried aloud that if things do not change, the research findings would be the same in five years if the process was replicated. In addition to life-long discrimination, participants discussed experiences of age-related bias. Ageism and the use of elderspeak (Kemper & Harden, 1999; Lubinski, 2010; O'Connor & St. Pierre, 2004; Williams et al., 2003) often inspired participants to mimic the negative communication they witnessed, using voice intonation and gesture as they described their experiences. One elder described how she needed to understand the context to avoid misjudging her peers:

> So even though [peer]'s manner seemed overbearing to us from what we could hear at the next table it really had a purpose that we didn't understand until long afterwards…I judged her as having bad or unsuccessful communication, and being bossy and overbearing with her finger in every pie. But it's from the point of view. Point of view makes a big difference. (Amplified Voices participant)

Many participants spoke to this idea—considering point of view or learning to think about other peoples' perspectives while communicating. Related to ageism and the care environment, many older adults discussed the different power dynamics in the care relationship; they expressed gratitude for good care while also acknowledging that their care needs often meant they were reliant upon or at the mercy of their care providers or family.

A second emergent theme in the data was about technology; participants discussed both the benefits and risks of technology in human life, particularly in reference to communication. In the communication context, it came up most often as a concern; participants worried it was preventing good communication skills or increasing experiences of isolation. They specifically brought up tone of voice and eye contact as important aspects of communication negatively impacted by technology use. During the mural process, the focus was more on the potential benefits of technology as well as the novel experience of using new technology tools. One elder summarized this emergent theme: "We need technology, but not overdone" (Amplified Voices participant).

The third emergent theme, simplicity, came from data throughout the study. Participants laughed aloud when asked to describe good communication; they described it as simple or a basic skill. The older adults involved in the mural creation used simplicity as the editing lens for their design ideas, wanting to make their image as powerful and communicative as possible. One of the individual digital images from an older adult participant and her verbal description of her image exemplifies the use of simplicity in the communication context. She chose to represent the communication between her and her sister, also a resident in the community. Her sister had significant medical and cognitive limitations to verbal communication, but the participant did not identify those limitations as barriers to connection. She drew one line, connecting her figure to her sister: "Nothing is very complicated, I know that. It comes from my heart. Like if I'm saying it and it is going to her? I would draw it from my mouth to her heart" (Amplified Voices participant). The hands of her figure are reaching toward the sister figure, but are not fully extended. These types of small, simple details stood out to the elder co-researchers; they often commented on the importance of the little details like a hand reaching out or figures being tilted toward each other.

For all the emergent themes, the researcher noted them in the verbal and art-based data prior to meeting with the elder co-researchers. The researcher did not introduce the emergent themes to the elder co-researchers; they identified the same themes, often using similar words, without prior knowledge. This finding supports the importance of these emergent themes in understanding communication in elder care settings.

Mural as data analysis and data communication. The mural creation occurred over several weeks of work with older adult co-researchers. The initial phase involved a tour of local murals in the neighborhood, several discussion groups about the history and meaning of murals as sociopolitical and community statements. After the conclusion of all individual data collection, the co-researchers looked at all the individual digital images and discussed what they saw in the images. They sorted and re-sorted the images based on observations about figure proximity, tone of the communication, and gesture. As they discussed ways to create a mural about communication, they talked about wanting to teach through a positive message while addressing some of the emergent themes, especially rebalancing power and emphasizing simplicity. They decided to create a mural within a mural, with people communicating about the process of creating the mural—much like the experience they were currently involved in. Prior to finalizing their design, they wanted feedback from older adults in memory care. One of the memory care participants confirmed the success of the design:

> I think the composition is fulfilled. It has to be taken slowly, but assuredly. You have to fight for every figure and form. I think it's doing a pretty good following of itself, rather than trying to attach something to it or trick into it. (Amplified Voices participant)

The image they designed and then painted on the large mural panel depicts two simple figures in a frame, communicating via touch, gesture, eye contact, and speech; their mouths are opened and up-turned to show the speech is positive and spoken aloud. In the foreground of the image, four silhouetted figures are communicating about the mural within a mural: two older adults on the right side and an elder in a wheelchair directing a young person standing on a ladder painting. As a final touch, they invited people to add their contribution to the mural by painting their hands and putting some handprints on the edge of the mural (Fig. 30.1).

Throughout the mural process, they demonstrated their interest in and commitment to understanding the research questions. They discussed their communication experiences in the moment and made observations about the way the design and painting process enabled them to engage in ongoing inquiry. Thought charts and graphs quantifying elements of the individual images were included in the final research document, the mural tells a more eloquent and holistic story about the research process and findings.

When the mural was complete, we held an event in the community to celebrate the conclusion of our inquiry and to honor the older adult co-researchers. During the event, we unveiled the mural and the co-researchers described each element and what it meant to them. They shared the relationship between their initial ideas and the group composition. They took ownership over the data communication, both in the image and in the presentation to their peers in the community. The mural continues to be a discussion point, and the co-researchers often refer to it in their daily conversations with each other.

Communicating research results. Though they wanted to attend my dissertation defense, the distance and timing precluded this option. As a work-around, I did the same presentation for the residents in one of the assisted living buildings. Again, they surprised me. I assumed I would lose people to boredom and dozing off once the lights were dimmed and I started going through slides with charts and tables. Instead, it was a standing room only in our big community room. Their questions were insightful and they chattered excitedly to each other over some of the more interesting findings. All too often, participants in research are kept out of the final results, unless they go hunting for subsequent publications. For these co-researcher-participants, seeing our findings formatted into a presentation with tables, bullet points, and charts signaled to them: you are part of something, you are creating knowledge.

After the research concluded, the older adult participants in one community had the opportunity to speak directly to stakeholders within the technology company who supplied the digital art tool we utilized. Instead of the usual practice, where the researcher or clinician translates for or operates as an intermediary, the participants spoke directly to people who were responsible for the piece of technology they used. With the exception of internally facilitated market research, consumers rarely have the opportunity to speak directly with the creators or providers of tools, services, or technology they consume. One resident expressed interest in serving as an ongoing test subject or in maintaining a connection with the tech developers: "I can tell you what it is like to bumble around with this thing." The elders felt strongly about talking to the technology industry directly, which is part of why we partnered with Hewlett Packard on a white paper and an article in their magazine (HP Development Company, 2016).

For my part, I hold very close to my heart the weight of presenting on behalf of my co-researchers. Though it is my name in conference proceedings, I remain mindful about describing it as 'our' research. I keep the participants updated when I apply to present at conferences, when those submissions are accepted, and provide updates about the conference proceedings afterward. We continue to discuss their ideas about what the research means and who they want to talk to next.

Research implications. This study was limited to the use of group and individual art therapy in care communities in one US state; participants self-selected or were referred by staff members to the study and may not be a representative sample, and not all participants were able to participate in all parts of the study; the researcher and participants were aware of the potential threats to validity and limitations of this study. The goal was less to achieve one generalizable data set, but rather to do a deep, rich exploration of the lived experience. This study incorporated several methods to ensure validity, most importantly, involving the elders in all aspects of the study, including discussion of emergent themes and study results. Their exact phrasing and language was utilized to illustrate different themes and findings from the study. The research results suggest a need for continued involvement of older adults in research. The study confirmed the elders' ability to provide rich data about their experiences and their ability to use a variety of participatory methods to communicate their experiences.

Research Findings Informing Practice

The findings of the Amplified Voices study have informed the practices of the organization in support of the communities we serve. Efforts to address specific issues included explicitly addressing following up on requests as an expression of the company values. Emphasis on simple, human-to-human communication practices are implemented in our new employee training, regular staff meetings, and definitions of best practices. In response to their enthusiastic participation in this research and queries from student researchers, I developed a decision tree for future research projects; part of the decision tree includes explicit requirements that future researchers demonstrate an awareness about and methods to protect against ageist language and behavior in their writing, methods, and research protocols. It also ensures we prioritize our time and resources to focus on mutually beneficial partnerships. As we continue to engage with stakeholders in the technology field, we will be intentionally involving older adults in these conversations.

All too often, best practices are defined in contexts outside the lived experiences of the populations. The perceived necessity of large, quantitative data to secure funding and drive clinical and community work negates the wisdom of those who are immersed in the experience of that same population, either as a member or as a close ally. Best practice may not be measurable using traditional means to evaluate or quantify; empowering clinicians and clients to collaboratively study, design, implement, and evaluate best practice can result in more responsive, inclusive work.

The increasing accessibility of data and data collection tools means that many populations are no longer passive research subjects. The old model of a blank-slate research subject who passively receives the designed-on-high-research protocol no longer exists. This is not a failure or a shortcoming but a change to celebrate. The older adult participants fully embraced their new roles as researchers and, even two years post study conclusion, continue to refer to 'our' research and assume a confident posture when meeting student researchers or interacting with community groups. The elders have inspired new ways to think about research and the terms used. In a discussion about research gatekeepers, residents created a collaborative image about gatekeepers and concluded that the research gatekeeper is not always adversarial. One older adult mused aloud, "Maybe the gatekeeper is there to welcome us in."

Their interactions also opened the door for considering new and innovative ways to solve problems in their daily lives. An assisted living resident reached out through email with a technology solution to a broken statue outside the building:

> Why can't we use a 3-D printer to make new "prayer hands" for our front yard Handless Mary? We could make several copies so as to have extras on hand ready to use when the next episode of vandalism occurs. Better yet, let's choose a petite old lady resident with the most worn, crooked, and gnarled hands to serve as the model. I believe the contrast of a young Mary with ancient, overworked prayer hands would be thought-provoking. I have a very capable consultant up my sleeve. (Personal Communication, October 31, 2017)

Her language demonstrates a subtle but evident empowerment; instead of asking 'could we' or 'is it possible to…' she put the workload back onto me—she knows this is possible and that it is a good solution. Her words are a challenge; she is asking me to prove her wrong. Another older adult shared her recent insight into the way that participating in research projects and creating visual images as a form of knowledge has shifted her daily thinking: "We're of the old school; I am still finding it hard to accept the background, but I am working on it. In each new image, I work on it." She described the way that looking at the full context instead of just the identified problem has assisted her with the struggles in her life. Her role as a researcher goes beyond the research context into her whole life. The experience of speaking back and speaking up has empowered the residents to voice their opinions in more effective and nuanced ways; they recently questioned a proposal for new chairs in the dining room by stating they do not want or need new chairs, they would rather see money go to other projects, and proposing a compromise of cleaning and reupholstering the existing chairs. They have reimagined themselves as problem-solvers and, more importantly, see themselves as equal stakeholders in their living environment. After several discussions about current events and their desire to get involved, they asked for assistance in establishing a group social media account in order to add their voices to the dialogue.

Increasingly, technology companies are proposing hardware and software solutions to the problem of aging. Their approaches often assume problems where they do not exist or assign importance to problems older adults are not concerned about. In a discussion group with older adults in assisted living, they repeatedly suggested that technology stakeholders come and ask about what their real problems are and also what they are excited about: "Why don't they make us better hearing aids and teeth? Those things impact us every day!" They were excited to try out some virtual reality headsets, but disappointed when use required removing their glasses; they correctly observed that the tool was not built with them in mind.

The Future of Research

Though this chapter emphasizes the importance of participatory, inclusive research practices and questions traditional methods, these same traditional methods absolutely have a place in the greater universe of research. We need large, quantitative studies. We need to do replication studies and meta-analyses. We should continue working on developing and validating measures to use with different populations. However, when researchers are so attached to the methods they lose sight of the population or when the methods as theorized on paper are not relevant in the lived experience, we need to stop and question what we are doing and whether alternative methods would be better suited to the situation. In the worst-case scenario, participants have no power in the research process (Fig. 30.2). In the reimagined future, participants are involved stakeholders in the inquiry (Fig. 30.3).

Research needs in the field of art therapy are applicable to many fields of study in social science and community work. My deepest hope is that we can find some balance as a field. When we get too wrapped up in our fears of legitimacy or proving our merit, we miss the opportunity to celebrate the unique strengths our field brings to inquiry. I have witnessed students struggling to 'prove' not hypotheses but professionalism. The art therapy field is not alone in this fragmentation; Dweck (2017) identified some related problems in the field of psychology and called for a re-enriching of the field to ensure longevity and student interest. When we use our research as a means to justify our existence, we further marginalize the powerful work we do and we miss out on opportunities to bring the wisdom contained in the creative process. Our processes have the ability to empower, to illuminate, and to equalize. Art process with a focus on empowerment is "an emancipatory process in service of a collectively politicized movement towards global citizenship" (Mcleod & Ricketts, 2013, p. 26). Our allegiances in research can do both—establish our legitimacy as scientific researchers as well as active collaborators in client empowerment. I urge students and professionals to recommit to research as an invitation into inquiry rather than a means to stake out territory.

References

Applewhite, A. (2016). *This chair rocks: A manifesto against ageism*. Thorndike Press, A part of Gale, Cengage Learning.

Baugh, J. (2017). Meaning-less differences: Exposing fallacies and flaws in "The Word Gap" hypothesis that conceal a dangerous "language trap" for low-income

American families and their children. *International Multilingual Research Journal, 11*(1), 39–51. https://doi.org/10.1080/19313152.2016.1258189

Bergman, S. (2017). *Lives Well Lived.* USA. http://www.lives-well-lived.com/

Delbanco, N. (2011). *Lastingness: The art of old age.* Grand Central Pub.

Dweck, C. (2017). Is psychology headed in the right direction? Yes, no, and maybe. *Perspectives on Psychological Science, 12*(4), 656–659. https://doi.org/10.1177/1745691616687747

Ellis, C., Adams, T. E., & Bochner, A. P. (2011). Autoethnography: An overview. *Forum: Qualitative Social Research, 12*(1), 345–357.

Fine, M. (2018). *Just research in contentious times: Widening the methodological imagination.* Teachers College Press.

Gilkerson, J., Richards, J. A., Warren, S. F., Montgomery, J. K., Greenwood, C. R., Kimbrough Oller, D., Hansen, J. H. L., & Paul, T. D. (2017). Mapping the early language environment using all-day recordings and automated analysis. *American Journal of Speech-Language Pathology, 26*(2), 248. https://doi.org/10.1044/2016_AJSLP-15-0169

Hinz, L. (2009). *Expressive therapies continuum: A framework for using art in therapy.* Routledge.

Houpt, K., Balkin, L. "Ariella", Broom, R. H., Roth, A. G., & Selma. (2016). Anti-memoir: Creating alternate nursing home narratives through zine making. *Art Therapy, 33*(3), 128–137. https://doi.org/10.1080/07421656.2016.1199243

HP Development Company. (2016). *Dr. Erin Partridge: Sprout by HP offers new possibilities.* http://h20195.www2.hp.com/v2/GetDocument.aspx?docname=4AA6-8503ENW

Kemper, S., & Harden, T. (1999). Experimentally disentangling what's beneficial about elders peak from what's not. *Psychology and Aging, 14*(4), 656–670. https://doi.org/10.1037/0882-7974.14.4.656

Kwan, C., & Walsh, C. A. (2018). Ethical issues in conducting community-based participatory research: A narrative review of the literature. *The Qualitative Report, 23*(232), 369–386. https://nsuworks.nova.edu/tqr/vol23/iss2/6/

Levy, S. R., & Macdonald, J. L. (2016). Progress on understanding ageism. *Journal of Social Issues, 72*(1), 5–25. https://doi.org/10.1111/josi.12153

Lubinski, R. (2010). Communicating effectively with elders and their families. *The ASHA Leader, 15*(3), 12–15. https://doi.org/10.1044/leader.FTR2.15032010.12

Lusebrink, V. B. (2004). Art therapy and the brain: An attempt to understand the underlying processes of art expression in therapy. *Art Therapy, 21*(3), 125–135. https://doi.org/10.1080/07421656.2004.10129496

Lusebrink, V. B. (2010). Assessment and therapeutic application of the Expressive Therapies Continuum: Implications for brain structures and functions. *Art Therapy, 27*(4), 168–177. https://doi.org/10.1080/07421656.2010.10129380

Mcleod, H., & Ricketts, K. (2013). "In between the fireflies": Community art with senior women of Chinese heritage around issues of culture, language and storytelling. *International Journal of Education Through Art, 9*(1), 23–39. https://doi.org/10.1386/eta.9.1.23_1

North, M. S., & Fiske, S. T. (2015). Modern attitudes toward older adults in the aging world: A cross-cultural meta-analysis. *Psychological Bulletin, 141*(5), 993–1021. https://doi.org/10.1037/a0039469

O'Connor, B. P., & St. Pierre, E. S. (2004). Older persons' perceptions of the frequency and meaning of elderspeak from family, friends, and service workers. *International Journal of Aging and Human Development, 58*(3), 197–221.

Parks, J. A. (2010). Lifting the burden of women's care work: Should robots replace the "human touch"? *Hypatia, 25*(1), 100–120. https://doi.org/10.1111/j.1527-2001.2009.01086.x

Partridge, E. E. (2016). *Amplified voices: Art-based inquiry into elder communication* (Doctoral dissertation). Notre Dame de Namur University. http://webinfo.ndnu.edu:8080/login?url=http://search.proquest.com.webinfo.ndnu.edu:8080/docview/1845857392?accountid=25323

Poo, A., & Conrad, A. (2015). *The age of dignity: Preparing for the elder boom in a changing America*. The New Press.

Schoenborn, N. L., Arbaje, A. I., Eubank, K. J., Maynor, K., & Carrese, J. A. (2013). Clinician roles and responsibilities during care transitions of older adults. *Journal of the American Geriatrics Society, 61*(2), 231–236. https://doi.org/10.1111/jgs.12084

Sparrow, R. (2016). Robots in aged care: A dystopian future? *AI and Society, 31*(4), 445–454. https://doi.org/10.1007/s00146-015-0625-4

Sperry, D. E., Sperry, L. L., & Miller, P. J. (2018). Reexamining the verbal environments of children from different socioeconomic backgrounds. *Child Development.* https://doi.org/10.1111/cdev.13072

Williams, K., Kemper, S., & Hummert, M. L. (2003). Improving nursing home communication: An intervention to reduce elderspeak. *The Gerontologist, 43*(2), 242–247.

World Economic Forum. (2012). *Global population ageing: Peril or promise? Global Agenda Council on Ageing Society.*

31

'We Can Speak but Will There Be Any Change?' Voices from Blikkiesdorp, South Africa

Rashid Ahmed, Abdulrazak Karriem, and Shaheed Mohammed

Blikkiesdorp is a symbol of the degeneration of living standards of the poor and marginalised both nationally and globally. It emphasised for us the need to work collectively to transform social conditions and respond to contexts like Blikkiesdorp. Psychology as a discipline and mental health service provision specifically is detached from the community, and this was an attempt to bridge this divide. It was an attempt to merge theory and practice, pool collective resources, and challenge disciplinary boundaries. We tried to acknowledge the context of power and the extent to which participatory and inclusive processes with communities could help address structural power and facilitate social change. Within mental health provision specifically, it helped to illustrate that helping responses can move out of the narrow confines of individual mainstream theory and praxis. While we remain

---

R. Ahmed (✉)
Department of Psychology, University of the Western Cape,
Cape Town, South Africa
e-mail: rasahmed@uwc.ac.za

A. Karriem
Institute for Social Development, University of the Western Cape,
Cape Town, South Africa
e-mail: akarriem@uwc.ac.za

S. Mohammed
Workers International Vangaurd League, Cape Town, South Africa
e-mail: workersinternational@gmail.com

C. Walker et al. (eds.), *The Palgrave Handbook of Innovative Community and Clinical Psychologies*, https://doi.org/10.1007/978-3-030-71190-0_31

uncertain about the benefit to the community, it was a very rich learning experience for us as a team. We hope to continue working together for a very long time.

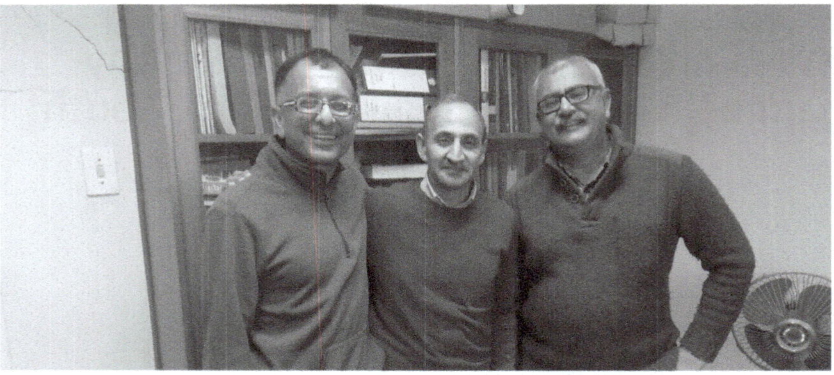

There are many differences between mainstream clinical and community and critical psychology approaches, and the extent to which interventions could be considered emancipatory is one of the key issues that differentiate critical perspectives from mainstream perspectives. This broad question serves as a departure point for this chapter. Drawing on a community intervention that we were all part of, we consider both from our and the communities perspective, whether we were able to achieve this aim of emancipatory work.

In trying to identify our aims for the chapter, our main aim was to facilitate and highlight the experiences of displaced communities. At the very least we hoped to let the 'community speak' and to raise awareness and generate support for their ongoing struggle. However, the extent to which this occurred is the primary focus of this chapter. For a complex set of reasons (which we shall explore later) we argue that we fell far short of this aim of letting the community speak. We argue that the failure to achieve this aim occurred through a combination of errors we made, but also reflects the global challenges of developing a more critical clinical and community psychology in diverse contexts. While the primary focus identified above is crucial, the struggle for social justice is broader than specific communities and issues, and a secondary aim was also to incorporate reflections from others who were also involved in the project to inform future work. The reasons for the focus on the latter, and the apparent tension between these two aims, we address by asking who benefitted the most from the intervention. Certainly one of the key unanswered questions throughout the project, and which we explore more fully in the chapter is the extent to which we feel the intervention benefitted the communities we worked with.

We found Fryer's (2017) approach to writing as a method of resistance and liberation a helpful way of framing our approach to this chapter. While we are aware of academic conventions, we agree that the potential surveillance and regulation that Fryer (2017) identifies and the extent to which this may constrain a social justice agenda. Fryer (2017) argues that even for those who position themselves as critical psychologists, the current parameters of academic scholarship may constrain critical thought and our research may serve to reproduce ideas and practices that maintain rather than challenge existing inequalities. All writing, including this piece of work then, should aim to be subversive and be clearly grounded in a social justice agenda.

Drawing on this approach (Fryer, 2017), we reflect on our experiences of the project and make explicit our positions and views. We also see this as a collective piece of work that draws from the experiences of community members as well as the many students involved in the project. We refer to ourselves by name in the chapter, Rashid Ahmed (RA), Razak Karriem (RK) and Shaheed Mohamed (SM). We are also aware of the extent to which our voice may be louder than the communities we chose to work with, as well as the students, and the limitations thereof. Within these limitations we hope that the chapter will not only facilitate a broader engagement with some of the issues we raise, but more importantly be beneficial to the communities we worked with as well as other displaced communities.

Blikkiesdorp and the Struggle for Housing in Cape Town, South Africa

South Africa is a new democracy and was characterised by the system of apartheid. While there is different descriptions of South African society, the conceptualisation of South African society as 'racial capitalism' (Wolpe, 1990) is particularly helpful because it characterises South Africa as being marked by two huge inequities, namely race and class. However, inequities and exclusion span many areas, including gender (Kiguwa, 2004), and South African society is best conceptualised as consisting of intersecting and numerous inequities. One explanation that stresses both the continuities and discontinuities of the apartheid era has focused on the national pursuit of a free-market economy in the post-apartheid era. Both the lack of success in transforming post-apartheid inequities, as well as some of the new challenges that have occurred, are theorised to emerge from the location of the South African economy in global capitalism and the consequences of its neo-liberal economic policy (Bond, 2014).

In 1994, South Africa's ruling party, the African National Congress (ANC), came to power on its election slogan, 'A Better Life for All'. The ANC government has made important strides in tackling the apartheid legacy of social marginalisation by providing access to social services such as housing, electricity and schooling, among others; however, poverty and inequality still remain widespread and access to basic services remains poor (Karriem & Hoskins, 2016). A recent report found that South Africa was still one of the most unequal countries in the world and that poverty levels had increased between 2011 and 2015 as an additional 2.5 million South Africans dropped into poverty (World Bank, 2018). The large majority of the previously disadvantaged still reside in areas created under the previous dispensation, with enormous challenges to ensure the more equitable distribution of resources. For example, a bifurcated health system persists with a private healthcare and relatively well-functioning system for the rich, and a state-funded, poorly resourced, inaccessible system for the poor (Coovadia et al., 2009; Seedat et al., 2009).

South Africa's housing backlog was 1.5 million houses in 1994 and has grown to 2 million, and the number of informal settlements shot up from 300 to more than 2000 over the same period (Muller, 2017). The City of Cape Town (CCT) and other city governments have resorted to establishing Temporary Relocation Areas (TRAs) to house those who need housing, along with those who have been displaced through natural disasters or who have lost their accommodation through an inability to pay their rentals or rates. Blikkiesdorp (Tin Can Town) was established as a response to a fire that destroyed the shacks of 3000 households in the Joe Slovo informal settlement in the neighbourhood of Langa in 2005. The majority of these people were housed 20 km away in Blikkiesdorp in the township of Delft, along with those who had been evicted by the City of Cape Town's Anti-Land Invasion Unit (ALIU) (Levenson, 2017; Millstein, 2014). The CCT had promised the Blikkiesdorp 'community' that they would be allocated public housing within six months. Twelve years later most families, living in precarious conditions, are still waiting: what was 'temporary' has become a Permanent Relocation Area. The Blikkiesdorp TRA houses are constructed from corrugated iron sheets and fall far short of national and international conventions for adequate housing (Baqutayan et al., 2015; UN-Habitat, 2012). These terrible, overcrowded living conditions have led to serious health, social and psychological problems and contradict former Minister of Housing Tokyo Sexwale's injunction that "human settlements must be places where people can play, stay and pray. They should be green, landscaped communities, pleasant places where people live, learn and spend leisure time" (Medani, 2017).

Poor access to basic services such as housing, sanitation, healthcare and so on has generated widespread service delivery protests in rural and urban areas, leading Peter Alexander (2010) to characterise South Africa as the "protest capital of the world". In the city of Cape Town, the waiting list to get access to a house has grown to 320,160 (Payi, 2017) which may be a conservative estimate based on official applications. Section 26 of the South African Constitution states, "Everyone has the right to have access to adequate housing"; however, the long housing waiting list has meant that the poor's right to housing will likely never be realised in their lifetime. To address this, many homeless have organised themselves into organisations to occupy urban land to meet their needs for shelter. While some have succeeded, most occupiers are violently evicted by the Anti-Land Invasion Unit (ALIU). It is this combination of increasing inequities and poverty but also vigorous civic participation and resistance that forms the backdrop for the project.

Background and History of the Project

The project was initiated in 2011 and is viewed as having multiple locations, with one location for the project being the professional training programme for clinical psychologists at the University of the Western Cape. We all teach on the module called Contextual Psychology, which along with a module called Community Psychology, is categorised as the Community Psychology component of the programme. The emphasis in the contextual module is largely experiential and theoretical, with a small practical component, while the community psychology module is primarily a more practical intervention based course. The community project for the latter is often a rural outreach project that involves the facilitation of psycho-educational workshops and is facilitated by other colleagues. One reason for including a small practical component to the contextual course is to bridge the theory-practice divide and to expose students to alternative intervention modalities (relative to primarily psycho-educational interventions). The module is a very short one (12–14 hours in total). These slots are used for seminars and the project work is completed outside of this time. The project is a voluntary component of the course and is chosen each year in consultation with the students. For example, in 2017, while there was a strong desire and commitment to be involved with the project, students felt unable to manage the demands of the training programme as well as contribute to the project.

The three co-facilitators of the project also teach on the course. SM's lectures focus on the global and national context of capitalism, and RK's lectures focus on social movements in South Africa and globally. Both emphasise the role of activism and the role of social movements in social transformation. RA's lectures could be conceptualised as a critical-community psychology approach and focus on critical self-reflexivity in terms of professional roles, responsibilities and values. The course develops the theme that helping as a professional can encompass many actions outside of, and complementary to individual therapeutic help.

RA's training and disciplinary location is in clinical psychology, RK is currently a lecturer in Development Studies, and SM is currently an activist with Workers International Vanguard League. While never explicitly articulated, until a recent meeting that was held to discuss the chapter, all three shared a commitment to social justice and a vision of a transformed society in terms of both oppression and exploitation. All of us agree that involvement in community and other struggles is part of both academic and private citizenship and these boundaries are interchangeable. This is one reason why the project is considered as having multiple locations, in that involvement in the project was also part of private citizenship and also occurred outside of the confines of professional and work roles. A more important reason as well is that SM is an activist whose involvement with the communities we worked with preceded his involvement in the teaching programme of the university.

In 2011 SM suggested the community project be with the people of Blikkiesdorp, a community in which he had been involved. Blikkiesdorp was and remains a Temporary Residence Area, with the community involved in a struggle with the city to secure permanent housing. In consultation with the community, but particularly in the light of resource constraints such as funding and the availability of students and ourselves, a small intervention was agreed upon. It was felt that a report that documented the communities' experiences of the psychological consequences from living in Temporary Residence Areas would be a manageable project.

Focus group interviews were held with members and the outcome was the completion of a report in 2011 titled "Psychological consequences of displacement: The experiences of the people of Blikkiesdorp" (Fell et al., 2011). In 2012 the project continued and it was felt that it would be helpful to include a similar community (Happy Valley) and document their experiences as well. The integrated findings were presented at the 30th International Congress of Psychology (ICP) held in Cape Town in 2012 with the title "The impact of displacement on community cohesion in Blikkiesdorp" (Mohammed et al., 2012), and members of the community were present at the presentation. The report got some coverage and was included by the Integrated Regional Information Networks (IRIN) in a report titled "The psychological strain of living in Tin Can town" (Corcoran, 2012).

In 2013 the students again agreed to continue with the project but the focus was a bit broader by this time. Rather than mainly focusing on the negative psychological and other consequences of living in TRAs, there was a stronger and clearer argument that the housing conditions in these communities violated, both national and international conventions and rights to decent housing. Presentations focused both on the plight of these communities and on the responses psychologists need to make to assist displaced communities. This was located in a broader debate about how to transform professional roles, responsibilities and values. Dissemination took the form of a Continuing Professional Development (CPD) seminar through the Psychological Society of South Africa (PSYSSA). The seminar focused on the experiences of these communities, but combined this with questions about the responses psychologists can make to these kinds of community struggles, in a workshop titled "Challenges facing temporary residence communities in Cape Town: What can we do?" (Mohammed et al., 2013). For 2014 and 2015 the project was put on hold, due to RA not teaching the module, because of his focus on his own research.

In 2016 the class again agreed to continue with the project. It was decided that social media dissemination might be a better option to raise awareness and mobilise support. In consultation with the community it was agreed that a short documentary clip be completed. The documentary clip was completed in 2016 and screened at two PSYSSA CPD seminars titled "The plight of the people of Blikkiesdorp: Social responsibility and social action", held on 25 November 2016 and 20 June 2017, respectively (PSYSSA Western Cape CPD Seminar, 2016, 2017). It again focused on the plight of the community as well as a consideration of the responses psychologists need to make. Even though both SM and the community members were unable to attend, the original aim of the screening was to obtain feedback from the community as well as others present and find a way forward. A follow-up meeting has not yet been scheduled. This brief chronological overview identifies the chequered and challenging course of the project and our reflections below analyse some of the reasons for this.

Reflections on the Project

In this section, we reflect on some of the issues and challenges that emerged. Our focus is confined largely to how we understood what we did, some of the challenges and issues associated with what we did and a consideration of whether the project could be considered emancipatory and for whom.

From the perspective of both the facilitators and students it was clear that this was an intervention project. The research conducted was secondary to the intervention; the research was solely for the benefit of the community and viewed by the facilitators as part of a broader mobilisation of community members to use the information for various forms of social action. Furthermore, drawing on Prilleltensky's (2001, 2010) terminology, the intervention was viewed as transformative, rather than ameliorative.

Prilleltensky and Prilleltensky (2003) argue that ameliorative work can be understood as work done as professional psychologists or others that alleviates human suffering more directly, like a therapeutic intervention, while transformative work also addresses and transforms the social conditions that cause human suffering. This distinction can be thought of as existing on a continuum with a complex relationship between the two. We believe it is only important to alleviate human suffering more directly and immediately, but also to intervene with the structures that create and reproduce human suffering. We believed that through advocacy for suitable housing, we would alleviate human suffering through trying to improve the social conditions associated with some of this suffering. We agreed therefore that we could take on multiple roles and that some form of advocacy or activism was crucial for the project. All the co-authors to some degree drew from critical social theories and a shared view that larger economic and political processes impact on communities, and local community struggles are part of a larger social transformation agenda. However, while there were many points of consensus, some of the differences that emerged, both between the co-authors, between the students and the co-authors, as well as within the student cohort were both revealing and challenging.

While it is acknowledged that there was a diversity of positions, two key issues remained a consistent thread throughout the project. First, there was debate about the extent to which this form of intervention fell outside of the boundaries of even community psychology, with some students verbalising that the intervention was 'political'. The second more challenging issue was the extent to which many students felt that the various forms the project took did not address individual distress, as well as the necessity for interventions that more directly address distress in these communities (such as individual psychotherapy or other group interventions). One of the consistent themes in class discussions throughout the project was the strong resonance with individual and community narratives of distress that emerged.

We felt that these challenges were indicative of the broader context within which psychology is taught and practised as we discuss below. Nonetheless, we were able to utilise these challenges to reflect on and challenge our worldviews. We saw the need to more directly address human suffering as a reflection of the extent to which the community struggles had resonated with us and the students, and the desire therefore to make a compassionate response to this suffering. Without this exposure, we do not believe that material covered in the course would have impacted or challenged us as much. Framing helping as a continuum of responses in the course may have helped, but this tension we believe will always be there with any form of intervention. The view that the intervention was 'political' we framed as part of a broader worldview that 'everything is political'. As outlined in our position we made it clear to students that professional helping and presenting psychology as a 'science' are political acts rather than neutral positions and we did not distinguish between these acts and political activism. While these may have helped mediate these tensions for some students, we argue that these are challenges we all have to grapple with in all the work that we do and pertain to some of what we explore below.

The module includes exposure to social movements and articulates a paradigm that clearly locates even social action as a helping response at the outset. Furthermore, the challenges identified above emerged in spite of a shared understanding of the importance of context on human behaviour and more importantly a shared commitment to social justice amongst all the students and the co-authors. Why then this disjuncture between a strong resonance with the struggles of these communities, but a difficulty in appreciating the potential utility of advocacy or activism?

We argue that in spite of these strong shared values and similarities, the impact of mainstream clinical psychology on positionality should not be underestimated. The focus in clinical psychology training programmes remains primarily on individual deficit and pathology, and individual psychotherapy is promised as the most viable solution. The extent to which this maintains and reproduces particular understandings of human subjectivity and social change should not be underestimated. Even those who embrace the view that community psychology interventions should be transformative, rather than ameliorative (Prilleltensky, 2001, 2010) may struggle to question and transcend disciplinary boundaries. For example, the practical component of the community psychology part of the course that involves psycho-educational workshops resonated far more with many students and was often perceived as being more beneficial to communities. This difference seemed to also parallel the differences between the co-authors as well, in the extent to which for RK and SM grassroots mobilisation could far more easily be foregrounded and implemented, relative to RA. RK and SM were quite clear: it was this kind of activism that not only empowered people but also alleviated human suffering. RA on the other hand, while also holding this view, found it less easy to so strongly embrace activism.

The decolonising lens is a more recent one (Seedat & Suffla, 2017; Adams et al., 2017) and perhaps both echoes and extends what emerged in South Africa as the 'relevance of psychology debate' in the 1980s (e.g. Dawes, 1985, 1986) and more recently (Long, 2014, 2016; Long & Foster, 2013). It suggests that some of the issues in clinical psychology discussed above are not specific to clinical psychology or a branch of psychology but how 'western scientific' thinking is dominant. It implies that even for those like ourselves who position themselves as critical psychologists, we may still be privileging certain knowledges and practices over others and may not be aware of how strongly an individual rather than collective narrative and other dominant narratives are being reproduced. RA's and some of the students responses then reflect the extent to which this colonial legacy entrenches ways of seeing and being (Bulhan, 2015). It is then this confluence of both an individualistic and internal, subjective narrative orientation most evident in clinical psychology, rather than other fields of psychology, as well as the failure to more critically interrogate the colonial lens, that might help explain some of the differences that were observed. While we explore later the decolonisation debate within the context of higher education institutions, the question it raises is the extent to which clinical psychology training specifically can house more subversive forms of engagement, and the wisdom of our decision to locate the project within the professional training programme.

The research component of the project also raised several challenges. We were quite clear that it was an intervention project but because of the research component, the project could also be categorised as community-based participatory research (CBPR). Certainly the extent to which CBPR is considered an orientation, rather than a method, the focus on giving voice to marginalised communities and a foregrounding of the social justice agenda (Horowitz et al., 2009), evident in the project, would suggest that it can be considered a form of CBPR. However, we question the utility of this categorisation for several reasons. First, in CBPR action is often linked to some kind of research, but for the project research it was not essential for the intervention. Both from our theoretical perspectives, but also from a moral and social justice perspective, involvement and action were imperative. Research was, therefore, viewed as a strategy to facilitate particular intervention outcomes, rather than being necessary to inform social action. Second, the outcomes of CBPR are often confined to narrow parameters such as geographical location or specific actions more directly linked to research outcomes. While we chose to work with a particular community, for many reasons, it was always conceptualised as a broader local and global struggle against the inequality associated with capitalism. Therefore even with the prominence of the extent to which we focused on giving voice, an intervention grounded in social theory might be the most accurate description of the project. Certainly, the research-action boundary may be more ambiguous and fluid than current conceptualisations allow, and it is this ambiguity that may allow for more liberatory enactments.

In addition to our conceptualisation of the project as an intervention with multiple locations, there was also a more conscious decision not to register it as research project. Like the global context, higher education institutions in South Africa are shaped by a neo-liberal agenda that emphasise research outputs over critical or liberatory scholarship, cost-saving managerial solutions to educational and social issues and reward systems that promote compliance and individual advancement, over collective engagement and social justice goals (Fryer, 2017; Vally & Motala, 2017; Pennington et al., 2017). We believe that the danger of submitting it for institutional registration would have increased surveillance and regulation, may have required modification of project goals and would have potentially transformed an intervention project into an outcome-based research project. While ethics committees remain important for oversight and very necessary, the very narrow parameters that ethical issues are confined to potentially constrain emancipatory work. They do not prevent parachute research that is exploitative rather than equal and compassionate, individual advancement over community well-being, and are generally not constituted to engage with the value-laden and contested nature of science and research. Even community psychology is a far cry from the call to develop shared definitions of ethical guidelines with communities (Serrano-Garcia, 1994). It is this benchmark that was far more important to us, and it was this aspect that we feel should have been more clearly articulated and agreed to with the community. Beyond a conscious recognition of power and other ethical issues, as well as a stated commitment to social justice, a discussion of and an agreement on ethics should have been more explicitly articulated and agreed to with the community.

The characterisation of the research aspect of the project may be far less important than an evaluation of the advantages and disadvantages of not framing it as a research endeavour in the conventional sense. Certainly one of the tensions that formed the backdrop of this chapter is the extent to which we wanted to give voice to the community. Even for a text positioned outside of mainstream theory and practice, we were uncertain about how a chapter that focused primarily on our 'empirical findings' would be received. While we believe that we took steps to ensure scientific rigour, we feel some of the qualitative data from the interviews and focus groups would not have met the criteria for qualitative research. Would it therefore have helped to ensure that aspects of the research did meet the criteria in terms of a particular methodology? While this might permit dissemination in spaces such as academic journals, would this have benefitted the community? A crucial question therefore is the extent to which our findings are less valid and therefore also less useful. While academic spaces like journals are important spaces for engagement, we argue that they may not only constrain community voices, but have also militated against some of the progress made on the project. While the option of using funding more subversively exists (e.g. to benefit a community, rather than primarily an institutional neo-liberal agenda) the funding gains may be offset by the narrow focus on research outputs.

Did the Community Benefit?

The tension we highlighted at the beginning of the chapter is one that we struggled with throughout the project. Did our shared vision of and commitment to social justice, translate into benefits for the community? In evaluating their work on community asset mapping, Lazarus et al. (2017) provide a framework for emancipatory community work. For work to be considered emancipatory, they argue it should address power dynamics, promote human rights and transformation for social justice, include a contextual analysis of person in context and enable voice. Included under these critical benchmarks are areas often emphasised in CBPR such as collaboration and trust, local capacity building, empowerment and sustainability (Horowitz et al., 2009). We consider below the extent to which we were able to achieve some of these aims, but more importantly the extent to which our interventions benefitted the community.

As discussed the module focuses on analysing people in context, and there was a clear commitment to social justice and transformation from the three co-authors and the students as well as the values promoted in the course. This was evident throughout the project and manifested in different ways. Within the context of structural power between the community, and us, there was a constant awareness of power dynamics and we believe we succeeded in creating a spirit of trust and a relatively equal partnership. For example, we were welcomed into the community, able to re-establish the project even after absences and some community members verbalised how they felt part of the project. At the ICP 2012 presentation, the community members who attended were able to express their viewpoints as well as disagree with both what we presented and the viewpoints of some of the other delegates. Project decisions were made together and we believe that SM's involvement with the community prior to the project helped build this spirit of trust and partnership. Community entry was gained through the elected residents committee for the area and all decisions were made in consultation with the committee.

There was also an acute awareness of marginalisation and the importance of enabling voice. Certainly one of the more helpful outcomes of the project was the extent to which voice was enabled and the extent to which attention was drawn to community's plight. Even though the documentary was screened only twice (for some of the reasons we explore in this chapter), it resonated strongly with many of those who attended, the students who compiled the video and the three co-facilitators. We do intend to continue in creating further spaces for the documentary through our networks and teaching. SM recently met with the representatives of the community at which the documentary was viewed by them. The representatives agreed that the documentary be disseminated to publicise their struggles and for it to be included as part of this text.

While an analytical lens and a social justice value system are critical for any intervention, these can only serve as a starting point and the acid test is the extent to which these translate into social change. We concur with Fox (2003) that while awareness is good, action is even better. For this project, then, transformation could be understood as a contribution to the local communities' struggles, extending this to other related struggles (other TRA communities) and finally connecting specific struggles like housing to broader and intersecting struggles (e.g. the privatisation of social welfare, education and healthcare) in South Africa and globally. Given the receptivity of participants at the presentations and workshops on the plight of the community, at the very least a modest aim would have been for this symbolic support to be translated into more tangible outcomes for the community, and this did not happen for the reasons we explain in this chapter.

While there was no agreed upon timeframe for getting the feedback and in particular the documentary to the community, the long delays were not beneficial. They potentially erode trust and may mean outcomes are less useful for the purposes they were intended to serve. Furthermore, the failure to maintain an ongoing presence as well as the absence of a commitment beyond the year would militate against the development of partnerships. While SM's ongoing work with the community helped to some degree in maintaining continuity and trust, this had to be complemented by the project teams continued presence and ability to deliver agreed outcomes. Furthermore, in the focus on the outcomes, insufficient attention was paid to process issues such as capacity building and joint responsibility for delivering the outcomes.

Relative to the community there were potentially more benefits to other role-players like us, the students and participants at the presentations and workshops, rather than community members. For the students, in terms of teaching and learning outcomes, our belief is that involvement in the project facilitated a kind of engagement that is not possible only through seminars. The exposure to and solidarity with the lived experiences of the marginalised facilitated an engagement with the roles, responsibilities and values of psychologists that the classroom environment would have been unable to provide. Similarly, some participants at the presentations and workshops strongly verbalised a need for social, political action for and with the community. Some participants verbalised the need for actions such as using social media to develop a petition against the City of Cape Town's policy of dumping the homeless in Temporary Relocation Areas. Others proposed actively supporting social movement mobilisations in pressuring the City of Cape Town into meeting homeless people's constitutional right to housing. The workshops then succeeded in foregrounding the importance of social action even by psychologists.

Certainly, these are important achievements. The extent to which psychologists do not step outside of mainstream parameters is evident (Fox, 2003) and these kinds of engagements remain crucial for the profession. However, we were left with two questions. First, how much of this engagement translates into transformed practice, and our fear is similar to Fox (2003) who suggests that not much has changed in the profession. Fox (2003) argues that for students with a strong commitment to social justice, psychology may not be the best location, with other fields and professions offering more possibilities of realising a social justice vision. Second, the symbolic support shown for the communities has to translate into some form of tangible support for the community's struggles. Certainly, part of the answer, perhaps the larger part, to the latter question has to do with choices we made and on reflection now, what we could have done differently as we reflect below. However, we believe the reservations we are expressing about the benefits to the community as well as other role-players have to be located within the broader neo-liberal context that shapes choice.

Any partnership between an academic partner and the community takes place within a context of broader neo-liberal policies that is a serious threat to critical thought and collective engagement (Fryer, 2017). We highlight some of the more important challenges that affected not only our project, but remain important for future work. The impact of these policies on knowledge production is immense as institutions and academics negotiate this minefield, and it has impacted on areas like curricula, critical thinking, teaching and learning, and community involvement. Given the emphasis often on research outputs in the form of accredited publications, this can impact on other equally important areas like community engagement. While this is not a linear process, nor uncontested, it has impacted on all institution's. At the University of the Western Cape we have seen it in the institutions attempts to integrate its characterisation and identity in the 1980s as the 'Home of the Left', to its position and identity presently as a 'research-intensive institution', and with all the attendant complexities, contestations and contradictions that this process involves.

The student tagline, "Free, de-colonial and quality education" (Pennington et al., 2017), captures the profound impact of these policies on the higher education sector. The student protests of 2015 and 2016 brought to the fore not only the privatisation of education, but also the absence of transformation in curricula. It is a reflection of the dominance of Euro-American thought and the failure to engage with local knowledge and facilitate social justice. The critical questioning of the relevance of psychology for a country marked by racial and economic inequality in the early 1980s referred to as the relevance debate (e.g. Anonymous, 1986; Dawes, 1985, 1986; Cooper & Nicholas, 1990) questioned the legitimacy of psychological theory and practice. By comparison, in the current neo-liberal climate, psychology not only has gained legitimacy, but is also evaluated and lauded for the extent to which the criteria set by the metropole and Northern dominance can be emulated. Long (2014) argues that two discourses emerge in the discussions about relevance in South Africa: a market discourse that positions psychology as a globally competitive, internationally recognised and financially enriching enterprise, and a social relevance discourse that engages with historical inequities, but not surprisingly, it is the former that dominates. Clinical psychology in particular is marked by discourses like evidence-based models and manualised treatment approaches like CBT based on international best practices. The accent on narrow definitions of professional competence and the premium on professional and career advancement further serve to remove its sphere of influence from the collective to the individual, and modes of helping that retain the status quo. Not surprisingly then the opportunities for creativity and working towards a more compassionate and humane society and the public good seems like a bridge too far.

Both RA and RK have been involved in the University of the Western since the late 1980s and have witnessed the shift referred to by Long as the emergence of a 'market discourse' (2014). Alongside more radical understandings of terms like relevance, social justice and community engagement, there has been an emergence of understandings that have commodified and subsumed even these terms within the broader market discourse. This we do not understand as our institution's 'failure' but a challenge all institutions face in keeping a more radical agenda alive. It reflects the profound global changes in higher education and the expansion of neo-liberal ideas and practice that have turned education into a commodity, rather than a public good.

At the project level, there were many consequences from these shifts and a few are highlighted here. First it is the market discourse and the ascendancy of the neo-liberal agenda that may help explain the relatively poor interest in the seminars and workshops at which the work was presented. It is likely that this kind of work is seen as an anomaly now, rather than an approach that would have gained far more traction and support in the earlier eras referred to above. We also struggled to balance relevance with other demands, and it was relevance and specifically the project that always came second best. While the binary we created between research and social action may partially explain this, it is also a much broader issue currently emerging in different forms such as debates about the role of public intellectuals in transformation, and issues like the research versus service delivery ethical dilemma in CBPR (Simon et al., 2007). Our struggle was to find space for relevant work within a context that seriously challenges this vision and implementation, and places a high premium on publications that bring in revenue and improve individual research profiles. We believe that the decision to focus on other research activities and perspectives by some of us impacted on project outcomes. Finally, in spite of a partnership, the geographical and class divide between the university setting and the community still remained. There were many reasons and manifestations of this. For example, the community was unable to attend some of the presentations and needed financial support for transport to some of the presentations that they were able to attend, and all presentations took place at university-associated settings. While partnerships can bridge these divides, the concern was the extent to which community voice was limited and restricted to these settings, and as a consequence, more beneficial to the academic, rather than community partners.

What Now?

The choice and opportunity to reflect primarily on our challenges we believe is helpful, but do not want this critique to constrain liberatory work especially for those new to the profession. In spite of some of our reservations about the potential benefit to the community, we would all still again choose to work with the community in this way. This process has renewed our commitment and helped us to learn from our mistakes. While acknowledging our role in the choices we made and learned from, our reflections are located in the broader neo-liberal context that serves to undermine liberatory work.

While we fell short of our aims and question the extent to which we helped the community, the lessons learned are invaluable. We concur that, in spite of our reservations, we would again undertake a similar project, but make a far more concerted effort to prioritise the project over other competing demands like our own research. Even with the constraints of work and personal lives, the project should have come first. We remain quite clear that the benefits to conceptualising and implementing it as an intervention project far outweigh the gains that may have come from developing it as an institutionally regulated research project. We would definitely retain it as an intervention rather than a research project with multiple locations. There were advantages to locating the project in the clinical training programme, and the utilisation of student resources as well as the teaching and learning outcomes was important gains.

While a range of compassionate helping responses are necessary in the current climate, work that takes us out of current comfort zones and extends into activism would be a big achievement. All shades and kinds of activism are necessary in our profession in the current global political climate that threatens our world. It is essential that we complement ameliorative with transformative interventions. While we believe that mainstream clinical psychology is most in need of this kind of engagement it may also be the space in which projects like these get least traction for the reasons we have explored earlier.

The project also succeeded in reaffirming a commitment we all need to make towards greater transformative rather ameliorative work. We believe many opportunities exist for liberatory and subversive activities, as our work has also illustrated, even though we have not elaborated on this. For example, the benefit to students and the challenge to their worldviews is an important gain in transforming the discipline. Finally, and this is perhaps the most important lesson, we needed to pay as much attention to building capacity and cementing inclusive and equal partnerships as we did to achieving outcomes like the reports and documentaries. If we had perhaps the communities could speak and be heard.

Conclusion

The initial plan for this chapter given the exciting and liberating brief given for the book was some sort of collaboration with the people of Blikkiesdorp and the failure to achieve this aim is symptomatic of the challenges we faced throughout the project. We have argued that in spite of our stated commitment to liberatory work we fell far short of this aim. We remain unsure about the extent to which we did facilitate voice for the community. More importantly, there was a disjuncture between our commitment to and ability to facilitate voice and generate corresponding benefits for the communities we worked with. Certainly part of the explanation lies in the choices we made and the binaries we may have created. However, we have argued that the larger part has to do with the context in which all current work is located. Higher education limitations, implementation of neo-liberal agenda and the individual, internal subjective narrative perhaps most evident in clinical psychology remain huge challenges for liberatory work. While these challenges are daunting, the large number of social protests in South Africa and globally also attest to the strength of human agency and resistance. While we may not have succeeded in fully utilising this agency, it is a belief in this agency that should guide emancipatory work and it is our belief in this potential that may be one of our success stories for the project. In the documentary that we include as part of this chapter we hope that both the narratives of damage and despair in response to damaging social conditions co-exist with narratives of hope and agency that could be mobilised for transformation. Finally, the objectives and clear positioning of the parameters of this text developed by the editors allowed us to write in a way that we have not been able to before. To paraphrase Steve Biko we have written what we liked and this in itself has been liberatory.

Acknowledgements While we take responsibility for any errors in the text, this has genuinely been a collective undertaking. Thanks to all the students who contributed so much to the project over the years, and to all the administration and support staff, especially Renee Klink. Thanks also to the editors for creating this opportunity for us. The biggest acknowledgement is to the communities we worked with. We are deeply grateful to all of you. If you wish to support the community in any way, or want to have acess to the documentary referred to in the chapter, please contact any of the authors. As expressed earlier this started out as the main purpose of the project and chapter. (Please note this is an essential change and must be included. This was the main purpose of the chapter being written)

References

Adams, G., Ordóñez, L. G., Kurtiş, T., Molina, L. E., & Dobles, I. (2017). Notes of decolonizing psychology: from one Special Issue to another. *South African Journal of Psychology, 47*(4), 531–541. https://doi.org/10.1177/0081246317738173

Alexander, P. (2010). Rebellion of the poor: South Africa's service delivery protests—A preliminary analysis. *Review of African Political Economy, 30*(123), 25–40.

Anonymous. (1986). Some thoughts on a more relevant or indigenous counselling psychology in South Africa: Discovering the socio-political context of the oppressed. *Psychology in Society, 76*, 21--26.

Baqutayan, S., Raji, F., & Ariffin, A. (2015). The impact of housing conditions on the emotion, behaviour, and psychological wellbeing of middle-income groups. *Journal of Sustainable Development, 8*(8), 1913–9071.

Bond, P. (2014). *Elite transition: From apartheid to neoliberalism in South Africa*. Pluto Press.

Bulhan, H. A. (2015). Stages of colonialism in Africa: From occupation of land to occupation of being. *Journal of Social and Political Psychology, 3*(1), 239–256.

Cooper, S., & Nicholas, L. J. (Eds.). (1990). *Psychology and apartheid*. Vision/Madiba.

Coovadia, H., Jewkes, R., Barron, P., Sanders, D., & McIntyre, D. (2009). The health and health system of South Africa: Historical roots of current public health challenges. *Lancet, 374*, 817–834.

Corcoran, B. (2012, October 30). The psychological strain of living in Tin Can Town. Irin. http://www.irinnews.org/report/96656/psychological-strain-living-tin-can-town

Dawes, A. (1985). Politics and mental health: The position of clinical psychology in South Africa. *South African Journal of Psychology, 15*, 55–61.

Dawes, A. (1986). The notion of relevant psychology with particular reference to Africanist pragmatic initiatives. *Psychology in Society, 5*(1), 28–48.

Fell, B., Menette, C., Elkington, E., Towfie, S., Drummond, S., & Charles, W. (2011). Psychological consequences of displacement: The experiences of the people of Blikkiesdorp. Unpublished Report, University of the Western Cape, Cape Town.

Fox, D. R. (2003). Awareness is good, but action is better. *The Counselling Psychologist, 31*(3), 299–304.

Fryer, D. (2017). Writing as an engaged method of resistance and liberation. In M. Seedat, S. Suffla, & D. J. Christie (Eds.), *Emancipatory and participatory methodologies in peace, critical and community psychology* (pp. 19–31). Springer International Publications.

Horowitz, C. R., Robinson, M., & Seifer, S. (2009). Community-based participatory research from the margin to the mainstream: Are researchers prepared? *Circulation, 119*(19), 2633–2642.

Karriem, A., & Hoskins, M. (2016). From the RDP to the NDP: A critical appraisal of the developmental state, land reform and rural development in South Africa. *Politikon: South African Journal of Political Studies, 43*(3), 325–343.

Kiguwa, P. (2004). Feminist critical psychology in South Africa. In D. Hook (Ed.), *Critical psychology* (pp. 278–315). UCT Press.

Lazarus, S., Taliep, N., & Naidoo, A. V. (2017). Community asset mapping as a critical participatory research method. In M. Seedat, S. Suffla, & D. J. Christie (Eds.), *Emancipatory and participatory methodologies in peace, critical and community psychology* (pp. 45–59). Springer International Publications.

Levenson, Z. (2017). Precarious Welfare States: Urban Struggles over housing delivery in post-apartheid South Africa. *International Sociology, 32*(4), 474–492.

Long, W. (2014). Understanding 'relevance' in psychology. *New Ideas in Psychology, 35*, 28–35.

Long, W. (2016). On the Africanization of psychology. *South African Journal of Psychology, 46*(4), 429–431.

Long, W., & Foster, D. (2013). The changing face of "relevance" in South African Psychology. *PINS, 45*, 3–16.

Medani, S. (2017). Backyard Shacks and Brick houses: A real promise of SA's property market. Retrieved March 25, 2018, from https://www.biznews.com/sa-investing/2017/08/28/real-picture-sa-property-market/

Millstein, M. (2014). Information and the mediation of power in Delft, Cape Town. *Nordic Journal of African Studies, 23*(2), 100–119.

Mohammed, S., Karriem, A., & Bawa, U. (2013). CPD Seminar: Challenges facing temporary residence communities in Cape Town: What can we do? Department of Psychology, University of the Western Cape, Cape Town, South Africa.

Mohammed, S., Fell, B., Menette, C., Drummond, S., Charles, W., Towfie, S., & Ahmed, R. (2012). The impact of displacement on community cohesion in Blikkiesdorp. 30th International congress of psychology, 22–27 July, Cape Town. p. 171, South Africa.

Muller, J. (2017, February 24). Human Settlements: Housing scores big. Retrieved March 25, 2018, from https://www.businesslive.co.za/fm/features/2017-02-24-human-settlements-housing-scores-big/

Payi, B. (2017, July 23). R80bn needed for housing crisis. *Weekend Argus*.

Pennington, A., Mokose, M., Smith, M. N., & Kawanu, Z. (2017). Neoliberalism and the crisis in higher education in South Africa, New Agenda. *South African Journal of Social and Economic Policy, 64*, 28–32.

Prilleltensky, I. (2001). Value-based praxis in community psychology: Moving toward social justice and social action. *American Journal of Community Psychology, 29*(5), 747–778.

Prilleltensky, I. (2010). Child wellness and social inclusion. *American Journal of Community Psychology, 46*(*1–2*), *283–249*.

Prilleltensky, I., & Prilleltensky, O. (2003). Reconciling the Roles of Professional Helper and Critical Agent in Health Psychology. *Journal of Health Psychology, 8*(2), 243–246.

PSYSSA Western Cape. (2016). *CPD Seminar: The plight of the people of Blikkiesdorp: What can we do?* Medical Research Council.

PSYSSA Western Cape. (2017). *CPD Seminar: The plight of the people of Blikkiesdorp: Social responsibility and social action.* Department of Psychology.

Seedat, M., & Suffla, S. (2017). Community psychology and its (dis)contents, archival legacies and decolonisation. *South African Journal of Psychology, 47*(4), 421–431.

Seedat, M., Van Niekerk, A., Jewkes, R., Suffla, S., & Ratele, K. (2009). Violence and injuries in South Africa: Prioritising an agenda for prevention. *Lancet, 374*(9694), 1011–1022.

Serrano-Garcia, I. (1994). The ethics of the powerful and the power of ethics. *American Journal of Community Psychology, 22*(1), 1–20.

Simon, C., Mosavel, M., & van Stade, D. (2007). Ethical challenges in the design and conduct of locally relevant international health research. *Social Science & Medicine, 64*(9), 1960–1969.

UN-Habitat. (2012). State of the World's Cities 2012/2013. Retrieved October 3, 2018, from http://mirror.unhabitat.org/pmss/listItemDetails.aspx?publicationID=3387

Vally, S., & Motala, E. (2017). Education, training and work under neoliberalism in South Africa: Toward alternatives. *Education as Change, 21*(3), 20.

Wolpe, H. (1990). *Race, class and the apartheid state.* Africa World Press.

World Bank. (2018). *Overcoming poverty and inequality in South Africa: An assessment of drivers, constraints and opportunities.* World Bank.

32

Conclusion

Carl Walker, Sally Zlotowitz, and Anna Zoli

The authors in this book have responded to the array of political, social and economic injustices that frame distress. In order to do so they reoriented their practice to confront, resist, challenge and sometimes subvert the psychologising that has been criticised for strengthening oppressive structures. Instead, the projects and approaches reframed distress practices around human rights, creativity, political activism, social change, space and place, systemic violence, community transformation, resource allocation and radical practices of disruption and direct action. In so doing they address Martin-Baro's challenge to make meaningful contributions to the problems of the day (Martin-Baro, 1994).

Several key questions arose for us as editors reading these contributions. Why did the people try these new approaches? How did they manage to carve out space to undertake work that moved beyond the mainstream and what challenges do we find ourselves facing as we reflect on the implications for what is possible going forward?

C. Walker (✉) • A. Zoli
School of Applied Social Science, University of Brighton, Brighton, UK
e-mail: c.j.walker@brighton.ac.uk; a.zoli@brighton.ac.uk

S. Zlotowitz
MAC-UK & Art Against Knives, London, UK

C. Walker et al. (eds.), *The Palgrave Handbook of Innovative Community and Clinical Psychologies*, https://doi.org/10.1007/978-3-030-71190-0_32

Why Are People Trying New Approaches?

We believe that a key element driving much of the work in this book was a recognition among our authors of the complex nature of distressing experiences and the often invisible routinised misery inflicted upon people through structural arrangements. To 'know' the complex nature of suffering requires individual biographies to be embedded in the larger matrix of culture, history and political economy, which cannot be understood simply through the intrapsychic biomedical lens.

The work contained within sought to realise versions of wellbeing that were inherently social and relational. Rather than understand it as a set of entities to be acquired or internalised qualities of individuals, there was a commitment to an understanding of wellbeing as sets of effects produced in specific times, places and circumstances (Atkinson, 2013). The approaches mobilised in this book often used, as a start, the idea that distress results from complex and embodied arrays of social experiences that are embedded within specific historical, cultural, political and economic settings.

To explain and act upon distress, it was important to embed individual biographies in the larger matrix of culture, history and political economy. That what have been discussed as 'symptoms' that need treatment, can often be usefully understood as the attempts of everyday people to control, deflect or ignore the pain that accompanies these. Many of the projects in this book recognise that social inequality has a powerful effect on mental and physical health (Cromby et al., 2012; Friedli, 2009; Marmot, 2010; Mirowsky & Ross, 2003; Read & Sanders, 2010; Wilkinson & Pickett, 2009) and that attempts to act on suffering means that we can no longer ignore the effects of such social inequalities. The long-term impact of racism, bullying, poverty, inequality and the corrosive effects of dysfunctional families, social worlds and political regimes are reasons why people become distressed (Ussher, 2011; Dillon et al., 2012). There was a recognition that counselling focussed solely on individual change is insufficient when interventions do not address external barriers or the challenges presented by policies and practices (Toporek, 2018). Experiences of distress are inseparable from material, social environmental, socioeconomic and cultural contexts and patterns of emotional difficulties always reflect prevailing social and cultural discourses (Johnstone et al., 2018; Kleinman et al., 2012).

Moreover, suffering is something that most people find difficult to grasp. It is not a natural phenomenon that we can identify and measure but a social status that we extend or withhold, usually through formal diagnosis (Morris,

1997). The link between poverty and mental distress is not due to a singular variable of 'income' (Harper, 2016). Living in poverty is more stressful, with fewer buffers, so challenges are more likely to be catastrophic. People living in poverty have less control over their lives, and live with lower status, often accompanied by shame, powerlessness and stigma (Wilkinson & Pickett, 2009). Poor wellbeing is consistently associated with markers of social inequality such as unemployment, low income and impoverished education (Harper, 2016; Cromby et al., 2012; Walker, 2007).

Indeed the premise that experiences of distress are inseparable from material, social environmental, socioeconomic and cultural contexts frame a number of the attempts within the book to grapple with, and to challenge, the prevailing mainstream diagnostic practice. Carolyn Kagan and colleagues (2011) suggest that diagnoses of 'mental illness' often invisibilise the way that distal, proximal social conditions transform people's social identity to the extent that employment is restricted and people are perceived as a threat, become ghettoised by a label and locked into a social identity (Kagan et al., 2011). In Chap. 5, 'Taking a Position Within Powerful Systems', James Randall, Sarah Gunn and Steven Coles explore the way that psychiatric discourses rooted in the biomedical and biopsychosocial models are structurally embedded within service design throughout the UK and determine service provision, access to help and support, research grants and overwhelmingly shape policy and legislation. They foreground the importance of psychologists continuing to develop alternative conceptual frameworks and practices to counter individualising and arguably pathologising constructs of 'disorder' and 'mental illness' in ways that allow practitioners to become increasingly outwardly looking and focus efforts on changing the underlying socio-materialist conditions that shape psychological distress. Indeed their clear message is to recalibrate clinical psychology to address inequality, discrimination and social injustice as a matter of course.

If, as Paul Farmer (1997) suggests, various large-scale social forces come to be translated into personal distress and disease where people's life choices are structured by sexism, racism and grinding poverty, then it makes sense why, in Chap. 3, 'Growing a Movement: Psychologists for Social Change', Psychologists for Social Change, a national activist network of UK psychologists, suggest the need for a huge range of campaigns to shift the focus from the personal to the structural patterns of emotional distress.

Some of the chapters in this book focussed on the need to both challenge and move beyond the narrow identity politics of distress that has been obscuring the way that structural violence metes out injuries of vastly different severity. For instance, in Chap. 23, 'Collaborating with Social Justice Activists in Ghana's Fight Against Modern Day Slavery: A Case Study of Challenging Heights', Kate Danvers highlights the need for systemic changes, rather than medicalising people's problems. Following her own identity as a values-led practitioner, Kate worked with a community-based child rights NGO in Ghana to develop rehabilitation practices for trafficked children and this work is the focus of her chapter in this book. This chapter and others contained within highlight how suffering is less a condition than an event within the context of a larger surrounding plot; the outcome of a series of preceding acts (Morris, 1997).

The Practice of Innovating

Moving on from the recognition of the importance of socially and relationally locating suffering and distress, a series of chapters in this book sought to sketch out what a more 'action-oriented' psychology (Burton & Gomez Ordonez, 2009) could look like. It was clear from the contributions and projects embarked upon by the practitioners and psychologists in this book that there are many different ways to perform action orientation. For some, this included more activist-oriented work that directly sought to challenge, subvert and repel specific forms of oppression, marginalisation and the broader realities mediated by the schemata, discourses, practices and relays of power capable of shaping circumstances of distress. In this regard, Tod Sloan and John Brush explored the way that psychology could support activism. They outlined and explored the specific emotional and personal challenges that frequently arise in activist organising, and suggest specific interventions that those trained in psychology may attempt to support and enhance activism within social movements.

In Chap. 7, 'Statactivism and Critical Community Psychology: Using Statistical Activism to Resist Injustice in the NHS and Higher Education', Carl Walker and Anna Zoli focus on statactivist projects in the south of England where the researchers sought to subvert problematic models of social accountability through a public survey on local health commissioning and privatisation and a National Senior Management Survey (Erickson et al., 2020) that challenged the narrow metrics of HE managerialism via a national league table of senior management teams. This project sought to answer Montero's (2009) call for methods that are specifically related to conscientisation. Montero noted that these are difficult to find or even non-existent because, while the mode of community psychology developed in many countries has openly manifested social transformation as the ultimate goal, what is not clear is the way in which that goal is to be obtained. This chapter and others contained within started to sketch out what some of these methods could look like.

One of the biggest challenges that the UK is facing is generating the conditions for a vision of public health that is founded on successful preventative community-oriented approaches to wellbeing. Many disparate community settings, spaces and projects can offer alternative social worlds where people can feel that they belong to a group and where different criteria of worth may be applied making possible positive identities and status. People can experience relationships of mutual support either formally or informally within these settings where loss, guilt, isolation, social marginalisation and stigmatisation can be ameliorated by the psychological sense of community, role models, practical information, ideas on coping, opportunity to help others and mutually supportive relationships (Walker et al., 2017). These can be settings where people have opportunities to experiment with social roles, imagine alternative futures, develop agency and active citizenship, where discourses of disability, victimhood, powerlessness and dependence can, for some, become recognition, belonging and a sense of control (Solomon et al., 2001).

Some of the chapters in this book point to the importance of these disparate community settings, spaces and projects that can offer alternative social worlds. For instance, Charlotte Wilcox and Rebecca Graber, in Chap. 11, '"We the Marlborough": Elucidating Users' Experience of Radical, Informal Therapeutic Practices Within a Queer Community Pub', highlight the Marlborough Pub, a vibrant social and creative centre of the LGBTQIA+ (and especially trans and nonbinary) community in Brighton, UK. A 2016 MindOut award recognised the radical practices that support mental distress among community members who often desire support but are disincentivised from accessing traditional talking therapies. This pub was a community space that offered a space/place for reciprocity, interconnectedness, embodiment and complex experiences of mental (ill/)health. This echoes research which outlines the way that connectedness, rebuilding positive identities, often within context of stigma and discrimination, hope and finding meaning are central to experiences of recovery (Tew et al., 2011).

Ootes et al. (2013) outline the way that certain notions of space appear in the objectives of mental healthcare and these entail particular notions of citizenship. Objects and space are co-produced and the sense of being 'out of place' in care settings is due to all sorts of discontinuities between people's own places and care settings. A sense of 'being in place' is understood as important to people and speaks to citizens' relationships with other people and groups. This can take the form of community spaces like the Marlborough Pub but also more intimate relational experiences. The 'Options' project by Hannah Denton, Mark Haydon-Laurelut, Duncan Moss, Angela Paterson Foster and Jan Shepherd showed the way that innovation could come within the therapeutic framework. 'Options' is a locally developed brief therapy intervention that draws on ideas from systemic and narrative therapy as well as community psychology and uses a reflecting team in order to challenge traditional therapeutic norms.

In Chap. 30, 'We Tell Our Own Stories: Older Adults as Expert Researchers', Erin Elizabeth Partridge and The Elder Care Alliance discuss their research and inquiry where older adults serve as co-researchers and leaders in defining research agendas. The initial art-based study, 'Amplified Elders', involved the elders in data analysis and established the possibility for adopting a researcher identity. Subsequent work created opportunities for older adults to speak directly to decision-makers in health care and technology, and use social media as a knowledge dissemination platform. The team concluded that creative, participatory approaches are an essential way to explore new possibilities for the future as well as to subvert and interrogate conventional practice.

Challenges in Trying to Innovate

The various projects, research, activism and approaches outlined in this book are important moves in the journey away from pathologising and individualising approaches to the way that people suffer. However, we have to unpack this notion of 'innovative' uncritically offered in the title of the book.

A problem with making claims about stretching the boundaries of a discipline, of newness and of being radical is that we are all positioned on different continua of practice. For some people, some of the projects will look edgy, innovative and evidence a commitment to politicising the personal. However, for others, some of these pieces of work will appear wilfully and inherently conservative, staid and accommodationist. Moreover, we might experience an uncomfortable need to shuffle in our seat if we are asked how our work meaningfully contributes to decolonising our communities when our institutional arrangements continue to produce relations that are asymmetrically structured through configurations of gender, race and class that are naturalised through everyday living.

In Chap. 8, 'Reflexively Interrogating (De)colonial Praxes in Critical Community Psychologies', Nick Malherbe, Shahnaaz Suffla and Mohamed

Seedat make the point that while much critical community psychology scholarship argues for forms of epistemological rupture that dislocate social hegemony and espouse emancipatory ideals, its focus on the continued salience of coloniality in the subjugation of 'Other' knowledges and ways of life remains uneven. Their chapter explores the way that the decolonial turn in psychology is increasingly evident in contributions from the Global South that seek to make visible the structures of power, and mainstream 'ways of knowing' that continue to produce alienated people. However, on the whole there remains a dearth of work examining the imminent contradictions, regressions and unevenness inherent in decolonising work. One's positionality and intersecting cultural identities influence the ways in which we encounter or participate in structural inequality. A temptation in social justice work is the tendency to allow deficit narratives to describe those who are affected by injustice. Here we can perpetuate a saviour approach to addressing inequity as well as reinforce the notion of the individual as the source of the problem as opposed to the role of an unjust system (Toporek, 2018). The reader can judge the degree to which this is evident in this text.

The chapters contained within this book only fleetingly take on the spectre of coloniality in our institutions. Moreover, much of the work in these chapters could be criticised for being embedded within what Fryer and McCormack (2010) call the 'briefcase war', where the drafting and enacting of policy, the relaying of problematic discourses, the relays of structural oppression, including politicians, policymakers, bureaucrats, teachers, lecturers, psychiatrists, psychologists, therapists and social workers, eschew the notion that structural oppression is being intentionally waged by malevolent individual agents. Rather, in the words of Iris Marion Young (1989, p. 272), '[o]ppression designates disadvantage and injustice; some people suffer not because a tyrannical power intends to keep them down but because of the everyday practices of well-intentioned liberal society'.

Most versions of community psychology would claim to be critical in the sense that they claim a commitment to 'liberation' of people from pathogenic, socially unjust enslavement through social and structural intervention which 'empowers'. However, Fryer and Fox (2015) remind us that in the Frankfurt School of Marxist intellectuals what is meant by 'critical' is an approach that tries to understand a social reality through introduction of another, more penetrating and comprehensive frame of reference. It has been suggested that much of the action of community psychologists is politically conservative, ideologically problematic and acritical in theorisation, and in reality constitutes an accommodationist position seeking greater influence within the mainstream fraternity. There is accommodationism in the projects in this book but there is also a resolute commitment to journeying away from accommodationism into edgy, challenging and uncomfortable spaces of practice. Moreover, we sense a commitment to challenging the dominant discourses in the mainstream psychologies that can appear natural, deny their own partiality and maintain their authority by appealing to a much peddled 'psy common sense'.

Power itself can be overt or covert, subtle or blatant. It can afford people multiple identities as people engage in domination or resist domination. Individuals will come into contact with externalised forces that they will often internalise, desires are embedded in norms and regulations and experience is shaped by the prescriptions of the day. Agency and personal power are not completely erased but these 'floating discourses' exist and are profoundly influential. This makes social change work incredibly challenging. In Chap. 31, '"We Can Speak but Will There Be Any Change?" Voices from Blikkiesdorp, South Africa', Rashid Ahmed, Abdulrazak Karriem and Shaheed Mohammed reflect on the struggles of communities living in temporary residence areas (TRAs) in South Africa. They note that, in spite of the extent to which they believed they were able to step outside of the parameters of mainstream clinical psychology, the translation to community gains of their particular project was very little. They highlight the power of constraints on all researchers, practitioners and activists trying to create a more socially just world. For them, the devastating impact of neo-liberal economic policies and the increasing ascendancy and dominance of mainstream psychology in South Africa and globally made social justice work impossible.

While the chapters in this book make a good case for psychologist's greater involvement in human rights issues, we have to be mindful of the argument for their reduced involvement in human rights. We constantly need to reflect on psychology's role in perpetuating systems that infringe people's human rights (Kinderman, 2007).

We need to guard against the uncritical acceptance of community as a 'spray-on' solution where social rupture is sacrificed for a limited vision of community rebuilding. Too often our work is reduced to simplistic new age notions of individual power (Gridley & Turner, 2010).

Moreover, it is useful to recognise that, while this book evidences a commitment to models of suffering and distress which are relational, critical, political and structural, much of the inherent theorising of subjectivity remains conservative. A glance at the work of anthropologist Tim Ingold (2015), for instance, highlights a degree of radical thinking that averts us from presupposing the mind of the individual as an externally bounded entity, instead committing to lives and minds as open-ended processes whose most outstanding characteristic is that they carry on. Ingold (2015) discusses performed sociality where 'the form of a thing does not stand over it or lie behind it but emerges from mutual shaping, within a gathering of forces, both tensile and frictional' (p. 24). Here, social life lies not in the accretion of distinct blobs but in the correspondence of lines. For Ingold (2015), real life humans inhabit a fluid reality in which nothing is the same one moment to the next and nothing repeats, where finding a place and holding fast in a fluid medium presents its greatest challenge, and where the metaphorical, and literal, commitment to understanding human beings as lines opens levels of possibility still beyond the reach of much of the psychologies.

Final Thoughts

Poverty infiltrates deeply, through the structuring and limiting of social relationships to shame, sadness and the fear of social difference and marginalisation. We are living in a time of new ideological landscapes of poverty as deficit and dependency (Ridge, 2013), where even childhood poverty has been privatised into families. More than ever we need new ways to understand the operation of complicated social apparatuses (Miller & Rose, 2008). The work contained within this book to a large degree recognises these challenges and constitutes a progressive step away from the 'little engineers of the human soul and their mundane knowledges' (p. 5) where a narrow commitment to the hegemony of mainstream psychiatry and psychology masks colonial discourses and practices, and hence resolutely resists the politicisation of suffering.

The community psychologist Isaac Prilleltensky noted that 'cholera wasn't eradicated by developing new treatments, rather it was eradicated by improving drains back in pre-Victorian times' (Nelson & Prilleltensky, 2010, p. 85). It is this structural frame of reference that we will need to develop if we are to start to seriously impact suffering. The projects contained within this book constitute a much-needed attempt to start to build such a frame of reference.

References

Atkinson, S. (2013). Beyond components of wellbeing:the effects of relational and situated assemblage. *Topoi 32*, 137–144.

Burton, M., & Gomez Ordonez, L. H. (2009). Liberation psychology—Another kind of critical psychology. In M. Montero & C. Sonn (Eds.), *Psychology of liberation—Theory and applications*. Springer.

Cromby, J., Harper, D., & Reavey, P. (2012). *Psychology, mental health and distress*. Palgrave Macmillan.

Dillon, J., Johnstone, L., & Longden, E. (2012). Trauma, dissociation, attachment and neuroscience: A new paradigm for understanding severe mental distress. *Journal of Critical Psychology, Counselling and Psychotherapy, 12*(3), 145–155.

Erickson, M., Hanna, P., & Walker, C. (2020). The UK higher education senior management survey: A statactivist response to managerialist governance. *Studies in Higher Education*. https://doi.org/10.1080/03075079.2020.1712693

Farmer, P. (1997). On suffering and structural violence: a view from below. About suffering: voice, genre and moral community. In Kleinman, A, Das, V, Lock, M., Introduction. Social suffering. University of California Press.

Friedli, L. (2009). *Mental health, resilience and inequalities*. World Health Organization.

Fryer, D., & Fox, R. (2015). Community psychology—Subjectivity, power, collectivity. In I. Parker (Ed.), *Handbook of critical psychology*. Routledge.

Fryer, D., & McCormack, C. (2010). *The war without bullets: Socio-structural violence from a critical standpoint*. Paper presented at 3iccp Puebla June 3–5.

Gridley, H., & Turner, C. (2010). Gender, power and community psychology. In G. Nelson & I. Prilleltensky (Eds.), *Community psychology*. Red Globe Press.

Harper, D. (2016). Beyond individual therapy. *The Psychologist, 29*, 440–444. https://thepsychologist.bps.org.uk/volume-29/june/beyond-individual-therapy

Ingold, T. (2015). *The life of lines*. Routledge.

Johnstone, L., Boyle, M. with Cromby, J., Dillon, J., Harper, D., Kinderman, P., Longden, E., Pilgrim, D., & Read, J. (2018). The Power Threat Meaning Framework: Towards the identification of patterns in emotional distress, unusual experiences and troubled or troubling behaviour, as an alternative to functional psychiatric diagnosis. Leicester: British Psychological Society. https://www1.bps.org.uk/system/files/userfiles/Division%20of%20Clinical%20Psychology/public/INF299%20PTM%20Main%20web.pdf.

Kagan, C. Burton, M. Duckett, P. Lawthom, R., & A. Siddiquee. (2011). Critical Community Psychology: Critical Action and Social Change. BPS Blackwell Textbooks.

Kinderman, P. (2007). Human rights and applied psychology. *Journal of Community and Applied Social Psychology, 17*, 218–228.

Kleinman, A. (2012). Rebalancing academic psychiatry: why it needs to happen – and soon. *The British Journal of Psychiatry, 201*, 421–422.

Marmot, M. (2010). *Fair society, healthy lives: The Marmot Review executive summary*. The Marmot Review. http://www.parliament.uk/documents/fair-society-healthy-lives-full-report.pdf

Martin-Baro, I. (1994). *Writings for a liberation psychology*. Harvard University Press.

Miller, P., & Rose, N. (2008). *Governing the present*. Polity Press.

Mirowsky, J., & Ross, C. E. (2003). *Social causes of psychological distress* (2nd ed.). Aldine de Gruyter.

Montero, M. (2009). Methods for liberation: Critical consciousness in action. In M. Montero & C. Sonn (Eds.), *Psychology of liberation—Theory and applications*. Springer.

Morris, D. (1997). About suffering: voice, genre and moral community. In Kleinman, A, Das, V, Lock, M., Introduction. Social suffering. University of California Press.

Nelson, G., & Prilleltensky, I. (eds.). (2010). Community psychology: In pursuit of liberation and well-being. Palgrave Macmillan.

Ootes, S. T. C., Pols, A. J., Tonkens, E. H., & Willems, D. L. (2013). Where is the citizen? Comparing civic spaces in long terms mental healthcare. *Health & Place, 22*, 11–18.

Read, J., & Sanders, P. (2010). *A straight talking introduction to the causes of mental health problems*. PCCS Books.

Ridge, T. (2013). 'We are all in this together'? The hidden costs of poverty, recession and austerity policies on Britain's poorest children. *Children & Society, 27*, 406–417.

Solomon, M., Pistrang, N., & Barker, C. (2001). The benefits of mutual support groups for parents of children with disabilities. *American Journal of Community Psychology, 29*(1), 113–132.

Tew, J., Ramon, S., Slade, M., Bird, V., Melton, J., & Le Boutillier, C. (2011). Social factors and recovery from mental health difficulties: A review of the evidence. *British Journal of Social Work, 42*(3), 1–18.

Toporek, R. (2018). Strength, solidarity strategy and sustainability. The counselling psychologists guide to social action. *European Journal of Clinical Pharmacology, 7*(1), 90–110.

Ussher, J. M. (2011). *The madness of women: Myth and experience*. Routledge.

Walker, C. (2007). *Depression and globalisation*. Springer.

Walker, C., Hanna, P., & Hart, A. (2017). *A community psychology approach to wellbeing*. Palgrave Macmillan.

Wilkinson, R., & Pickett, K. (2009). *The spirit level: Why more equal societies almost always do better*. Allen Lane. For slides see: tinyurl.com/5s6vqjl

Young, I. M. (1989). Polity and group difference: A critique of the idea of universal citizenship. *Ethics, 99*, 250–274.

Index[1]

A

Abuse/abused, 62, 84, 241, 302, 360, 362, 404, 418, 431, 434, 438, 447–470, 475, 477, 486, 487, 489, 508, 530
Accommodationist, 122, 133, 658
Accompaniment, 26, 145–148, 153, 350, 490, 491
Accountability, 9, 122, 123, 126, 127, 129, 130, 150, 242, 377, 396, 507, 537, 656
Action-oriented, 3, 60, 102, 132, 179–196, 270, 433, 443, 490, 656
Action research, 21, 94, 126, 130, 139, 196, 240, 241, 313, 314, 317, 318, 433, 438, 508, 509, 591
Activist groups, 2, 3, 17, 21, 24, 25, 43, 48, 52, 53, 59, 69, 91, 102–108, 112, 113, 117, 230
Advocacy, 21, 52, 350, 367, 379, 380, 387–389, 393–395, 397, 413–415, 483–484, 488, 490, 491, 638, 639
Agency, 10, 23, 31, 36, 59, 75, 141, 143, 151, 153, 245, 319, 357, 370, 377, 429, 443, 489, 490, 498–516, 522, 534, 556, 586, 597–610, 619, 648, 657, 660
Agriculture, 331–333, 336, 338, 339, 341, 482
Amelioration/ameliorative, 306, 349–351, 365, 369, 404, 484, 487, 488, 638, 639, 647
Amplified Elders study, 618–625, 658
Annan, Kofi, 474, 480
Anti-social, 143
Anxiety, 47, 58, 72, 79, 104, 110, 170, 236, 246, 280, 359, 360, 366, 418, 514, 569, 582, 583, 601
Apartheid, 53, 144, 302, 350, 449–451, 456, 503, 505, 508, 509, 579, 581, 583, 584, 586, 588, 591, 633, 634
Arendt, H., 139, 521, 522, 597, 599, 604, 607, 609
Art making, 597, 604, 606, 607n2, 608, 620, 621

[1] Note: Page numbers followed by 'n' refer to notes.

C. Walker et al. (eds.), *The Palgrave Handbook of Innovative Community and Clinical Psychologies*, https://doi.org/10.1007/978-3-030-71190-0

Austerity, 2, 3, 12, 13, 21, 26, 35, 37–41, 43–46, 52, 53, 62, 132, 139, 145, 180, 181, 185–187, 195, 229, 243, 334, 342, 370, 408, 522, 526, 529, 537, 551, 559–573, 580, 582, 599, 606
Autonomy, 31, 34, 90, 115, 141, 151, 336, 362, 438, 501, 508
Azanian Bridges, 577, 582, 584, 586, 589–591

B

Balance, 41, 45, 48, 53, 90, 104, 109, 226, 235, 271, 285–286, 288–290, 292–295, 310, 362, 380, 531, 535, 569, 628, 646
BAME, *see* Black, Asian and Minority Ethnic
Bedroom tax, 56, 57
Belonging, 203, 211, 282, 434, 453, 461, 463, 464, 526, 535, 536, 600, 605, 607–609, 657
Benefits system, 44, 57, 62, 71
Biomedical, 8, 69, 72, 73, 79, 85, 90, 92, 598, 605, 609, 654, 655
Black, Asian and Minority Ethnic (BAME), 20, 72, 88, 89, 278
Brexit, 26, 43, 228
Brush, John, 18, 656

C

Capitalist/capitalism, 5, 6, 10, 114, 133, 144, 342, 633, 635, 641
Challenging Heights, 302, 473–491
The clinic/clinical practice, 4, 8, 18, 39, 51–65, 69, 70, 78, 83, 85, 87, 95
Clinicians, 8, 69, 70, 74, 78–84, 86–88, 91–93, 162, 216, 286, 293, 566, 573, 626
Co-constructed/co-construction, 84, 186, 310, 312, 426–443, 513, 514
Collaborative/collaboration, 17, 36, 38, 44, 53, 84, 87–89, 93, 102, 159–175, 189, 191, 194, 196, 228, 229, 235, 240, 242, 243, 246–249, 261, 267–270, 272, 273, 279, 296–297, 302, 307–309, 313, 314, 319, 335–337, 349, 357, 359, 364, 396, 411, 413, 418, 502, 513, 514, 524, 524n1, 549, 551, 555, 556, 599, 626, 642, 648
Collective power/people power, 31, 41, 42, 201
Collective solidarity, 10
Colonialism/colonial/colonising, 5, 116, 121, 141–143, 147, 148, 449, 456, 499, 505, 640, 661
Community based participatory action research (CBPAR), 380, 388, 389, 395, 397, 509
Community cohesion, 20, 148, 228, 536, 636
Community psychology festival, 25, 39, 140, 223–236
Community Psychology Section (CPS), 224, 225, 235, 349, 491
Compassion, 112, 289, 363, 450, 455, 486, 522, 525–527, 525n2, 525n3, 530, 533, 559–573
Conflict, 38, 69, 72, 78, 82, 91, 105, 213, 249, 253, 302, 339, 340, 367, 371, 426–429, 432, 434, 435, 441, 442, 452, 483, 488, 507, 537, 566, 582, 584, 606
Converge, 140
Conversation, 28, 39, 112, 127, 152, 153, 159–175, 190, 196, 232, 235, 249, 251, 315, 326, 383, 392, 404, 409, 450, 451, 489,

504, 506, 508, 607, 618, 619, 624, 626
Coproduction/co-production, 9, 87, 140, 226, 248, 255, 256, 426, 429, 439–442, 521, 531–532, 535, 538, 549, 551–552
Creative/creativity, 12, 21, 25, 71, 85, 107, 115, 140, 142, 148, 165, 215, 225, 228, 229, 240, 242, 245–250, 253–256, 260–263, 266, 268, 271, 273, 286, 293, 318, 360, 416–420, 427, 429, 430, 435–443, 469, 511, 521–522, 524, 527, 532–535, 545, 549–555, 559–573, 589, 597–599, 608, 620, 621, 628, 645, 653, 657, 658
Critical community psychology (CCP), 5, 9, 59, 121–133, 141–155, 225–227, 231, 241, 293, 327–329, 332, 337, 342, 349–351, 353, 354, 357, 364, 366, 367, 369–371, 404–421, 636, 658, 659
Critical consciousness, 350, 377, 379, 500, 504–506

D

Debtors, 182, 185, 188–194
Debt Resistance UK, 22
Decolonial/decolonising, 12, 94, 115, 117, 139, 141–155, 499, 500, 505, 510, 515, 516, 591, 640, 658, 659
Define Normal, 239–256
Dementia, 528, 571
Denaturalisation, 145, 146, 148, 152
Depression, 23, 70, 72, 279, 280, 560, 601
Disabled/disability/disabilities, 2, 3, 35, 40, 45, 62, 89, 166, 297, 301, 305, 319, 321, 332–336, 338, 341, 404–421, 434, 657
Discourse, 7, 39, 40, 43, 61, 71–73, 85, 93, 123, 124, 132, 148, 180, 182, 186–188, 194, 218, 243, 248, 277, 279, 280, 302, 357, 377, 396, 397, 442, 480, 489, 505, 528, 581, 586, 589, 604–606, 645, 646, 654–657, 659, 661
Discriminate/discrimination, 45, 72, 74, 82, 203, 333, 349, 350, 362, 375, 376, 378, 383, 384, 388, 389, 427, 434, 439, 449, 452, 528, 621, 622, 655, 657
Disobedience, 139, 142, 147, 149–155, 506
Displaced, 19, 22, 434, 632–634, 637
Disruptive, 12, 112, 125, 139–140, 151, 152, 203, 451, 454, 618
Distress, 2–6, 8, 12, 17, 21, 23, 27, 34, 35, 37, 39, 40, 43, 45, 47, 69–79, 81–85, 88–95, 139, 161, 201, 203, 205, 206, 213, 214, 216, 218, 219, 226, 233, 249, 250, 260–263, 265, 266, 268, 270, 272, 273, 278–280, 283, 293, 327–342, 350, 452, 473, 488, 491, 524, 526, 530, 531, 534–537, 559, 569, 571, 572, 582, 587, 592, 597–600, 602–606, 609, 638, 653–657, 660
Dominant discourse/narrative/culture, 10, 18, 270–272, 302, 369, 379, 383, 552, 589, 609, 640, 660

E

Earth, 282, 288, 292, 328, 332, 531
Ecology/ecological, 11, 27, 105–108, 113, 312, 329, 332, 333, 339, 379, 547, 548

Economic crisis, 194, 338
Efficacy, 565, 599–600, 619
Emotional wellbeing, 40, 561
Empowerment, 94, 121, 133, 216, 243, 248, 253, 271, 297, 301, 310, 349, 377, 379, 380, 389, 481, 482, 498–516, 529, 531, 549, 585, 589, 600, 627, 628, 642
Environment/environmental, 23, 34, 36, 52, 53, 58, 70, 74, 76, 78, 80–82, 88, 90, 92, 93, 102, 169, 174, 195, 211, 248, 267, 271, 284, 285, 290, 292, 308, 317, 321, 327, 328, 330–332, 337, 342, 407, 428, 438, 442, 451, 457, 487, 488, 501, 506, 508, 547, 551, 553, 563, 568, 571, 572, 622, 627, 644, 654, 655
Epistemic justice /injustice, 5, 21, 23–24, 38, 94, 103, 114, 121–133, 152, 226, 243, 245, 271, 305, 320, 321, 352, 375, 380, 397, 456, 482, 489, 491, 504, 535, 537, 572, 609, 653, 655, 656, 659
Ethnocentric, 182, 186–190
Ethnography, 330
Eurocentric, 10, 71, 280, 293, 294
Extremism, 52

F

Far right groups, 51
Feminist, 2, 590, 599, 602
Food bank, 34, 54, 58, 62, 560
Foreclosure, 179–196
Foucault, M., 71, 348, 407, 480
Framing, 188, 249, 272, 620, 633, 639, 641

G

Gender/gendered, 43, 61, 153, 154, 203, 210, 215, 216, 226, 230, 357, 433–435, 438, 441, 499, 528, 633, 658
Gentrification, 3, 21, 22, 218, 381
Governance, 93, 133, 179, 302, 376, 377, 381, 428–429, 491
Grassroots, 21, 47, 52, 63, 89, 101–103, 114, 148, 181, 187, 340, 474–475, 479, 490, 506, 639

H

Happiness, 78, 203, 217, 270, 271, 326
Healing, 106, 117, 140, 201, 203, 207, 215, 216, 229, 277–294, 452, 453, 469, 470, 531, 536
Health providers, 126, 219, 382, 383, 385–389, 391–394, 396
Hegemonic, 123, 142, 146, 151, 152, 180, 182, 187, 369, 498, 512
Hermeneutic circle, 160–162
Heteronormativity/heteronormative, 204, 207, 215
HIV/AIDS, 354, 355, 434, 527, 536
Homeless (ness), 3, 12, 22–25, 47, 54–56, 61, 62, 241, 551–552, 554, 556, 597, 635, 644
Housing activists, 17, 19–21, 25
Housing instability/insecurity/secure housing, 20, 21, 23, 25, 45, 70
Human rights, 2, 12, 22, 428, 474, 477, 488, 490, 642, 653, 660

I

Ideological/ideology, 2, 5, 89, 103, 124, 132, 142, 187–188, 190, 204, 406, 502, 504, 522, 569, 570, 605, 661

Imagination, 142, 418, 449, 580, 582, 587, 588, 602
Indigenisation/indigenous, 10, 116, 117, 145–146, 148, 152, 279, 280, 293–295, 434, 499, 501, 503, 506, 509–511, 515, 584, 590
Individualisation/individualizing/individualistic, 1, 4–6, 38, 73, 79, 103, 167, 186, 270, 271, 273, 418, 640, 655, 658
Innovation, 5, 6, 11, 59, 60, 419–421, 534, 658
Intervention, 4–7, 17, 45, 76, 90, 94, 105, 109, 112, 139, 148, 149, 151, 162, 163, 166, 169, 175, 180, 182, 190, 191, 228, 267, 270, 277–280, 282, 283, 286, 293–297, 302, 306, 310, 319, 328, 329, 340, 351, 354–357, 362–364, 367, 368, 382, 384, 386, 396, 411, 417, 442, 454, 475, 479, 487, 488, 490, 498, 503, 522, 534, 535, 537, 538, 547, 564, 572, 598, 605, 609, 632, 635, 636, 638–643, 647, 654, 656, 658, 659
Isolation, 40, 62, 94, 104, 243, 250, 521, 526–528, 532, 536, 537, 553, 563, 571, 600, 605–607, 609, 622, 657

J

Jannah tree, 8, 140, 277–295
Job Seekers Allowance, 57

K

Knowledge production, 498, 499, 502, 510, 511, 516, 592, 644
Knowledges, 5, 7–9, 24, 26, 31, 38–42, 44, 45, 48, 59, 64, 85, 87, 92, 122, 124, 126, 127, 133, 140–143, 145–147, 149, 152–154, 160, 163, 166, 167, 182, 186, 201, 203, 204, 219, 225, 226, 242, 243, 247, 250, 255, 270, 272, 281, 288, 294, 296, 307, 308, 320, 327, 333, 347–350, 352, 354, 358, 363, 366, 369, 370, 379, 388, 389, 396, 407, 411, 414, 416–420, 433, 435, 442, 473, 488, 490, 498, 499, 502, 502n1, 503, 506, 508, 510–514, 516, 524, 528, 535–537, 545, 549, 553, 555, 572, 573, 586, 592, 617, 620, 623, 625, 627, 640, 644, 645, 658, 659, 661

L

Label/labelling, 69, 70, 72–74, 76–78, 80, 81, 88, 170, 211, 242, 336, 338, 405, 406, 409, 413, 417, 418, 454, 522, 530, 655
Learning disabilities (LD), 166, 297, 301, 302, 305, 334, 404–421, 525
LGBTQIA+, 202–205, 202n1, 210, 211, 215, 218, 219, 657
Liberation psychology, 6, 9, 36, 78, 124, 132, 351, 377–380, 395, 480, 484
Lived experience, 7, 8, 20, 25, 34, 40, 55, 59, 62, 85, 203–205, 207, 217, 226, 262, 333–338, 513, 547, 549, 553, 554, 588, 601, 608, 609, 615, 618, 625, 626, 628, 644

M

Mainstream, 1, 4, 6–9, 36, 54, 59, 64, 89, 125, 132, 140, 142–146, 149, 179, 180, 204, 225, 226, 230, 236, 249, 253, 254, 277–279, 294, 303, 350, 356, 418, 434, 491, 511, 534, 569, 631, 632, 639, 641, 644, 647, 653, 655, 659–661
Mapping, 302, 380, 384–387, 436–438, 503, 507, 553, 555, 642
Marginalisation/marginalised, 1, 3, 9, 11, 12, 19–28, 59, 63, 85, 125, 152, 201, 202, 207, 219, 232, 243, 278, 280, 302, 327–342, 365, 368, 370, 376, 378, 381, 383, 389, 407, 413, 418, 426–443, 498–501, 503, 506, 511, 515, 522, 538, 545, 547, 586, 628, 631, 634, 640, 643, 644, 656, 657, 661
Marketisation, 2, 18, 129–130, 132, 273
The Marlborough Pub, 201, 202, 206, 657, 658
Martín-Baró, I., 2, 36, 76, 78, 124, 132, 195, 377, 479, 480, 653
Medicalising/medicalisation, 71, 85, 167, 242, 250, 473, 537, 656
Mental distress, 12, 17, 34, 35, 39, 40, 43, 47, 72, 73, 76, 89, 94, 95, 139, 203, 206, 226, 233, 260–263, 265, 266, 272, 273, 327–342, 522, 536, 538, 597, 600, 602–606, 609, 655, 657
Mental health awareness, 6, 534
Mental health professionals, 28, 69, 71, 85, 93, 180, 247, 253, 568
Mental health provision, 139, 534, 631
Metaphor/metaphorical, 8, 72, 140, 167, 172, 212, 267, 277–294, 451, 536, 548, 661
The Midlands Psychology Group, 76, 77
Migrants, 189, 297, 301, 332, 333, 337–339, 341, 428
Movements, 2, 10–12, 17, 18, 27, 28, 31–49, 52, 89, 101–118, 123, 143, 182, 186, 188, 189, 191–195, 207, 210, 213, 227, 230, 255, 265, 271, 288, 291, 297, 301, 327, 328, 341, 417, 428, 432, 436, 454, 474–475, 479–489, 491, 535, 537, 538, 587, 589, 590, 604, 628, 636, 639, 644, 655, 656
Mural, 266, 616, 620, 622–624
Muslim, 140, 190, 277, 279–281, 286, 536

N

Narrative interviews, 600, 602
Narrative research, 448, 590, 597
National Health Service (NHS), 8, 28, 44, 82, 90, 121–133, 164, 171, 241, 242, 254–256, 273, 278, 279, 283, 294, 473, 474, 491, 524n1, 525, 525n3, 534, 537, 538, 560–564, 568, 569, 571, 572, 656
Neoliberalism/neoliberal, 2, 3, 8, 21, 89, 121, 123, 133, 142, 144, 145, 151, 179, 180, 185–187, 189, 196, 204, 218, 243, 270, 342, 351, 376, 477, 522, 526, 569, 570, 597, 600, 604, 605, 609, 633, 641, 642, 644–648, 660
Neurodivergence, 112
Non-diagnostic, 77, 78, 83, 92–94
Norms, 27, 78, 109, 113, 144, 207, 210, 213, 216, 217, 278, 294, 306, 308, 309, 312, 319, 321,

376, 379, 434, 438, 439, 512, 569, 658, 660

O

Objectify/objectifying, 246, 250
Older adults, 504, 522, 525, 527, 531, 532, 549, 553–555, 615–628, 658
Oppression, 36, 43, 59, 102, 104, 111, 115, 124, 132, 141, 189, 203, 204, 215, 270, 302, 329, 350, 377–379, 396, 407, 418, 419, 455, 479, 501, 502, 504, 636, 656, 659
Options model, 159, 166
Othering, 261, 265

P

Participation, 101, 107, 109, 112, 114, 117, 121, 124–127, 133, 140, 151, 186, 191, 230, 232, 234, 242, 248, 272, 279, 281, 296, 305, 307, 312, 321, 328, 340, 341, 350, 353, 359, 365, 367, 377, 380, 396, 397, 409, 419, 432, 457, 504, 506, 511, 514, 516, 521, 534, 598, 600, 601, 608, 626, 635
Participatory action research (PAR), 24, 269, 448–450, 454, 469, 509, 549
Peer support, 26, 89, 203, 204, 356, 563
Permaculture, 327–329, 331, 332, 338, 342
Personalization, 311–312
Personal stories/experiences, 4, 19, 31, 55, 70, 102, 122, 146, 159, 189, 196, 201–219, 226, 241, 261, 277, 304, 347, 377, 407, 429, 447, 473, 526, 531, 547, 560, 582, 598, 615, 632, 654
Person centered/person-centered, 303, 304, 306–309, 314, 316, 317, 319, 320, 534, 618
Person-centered review (PCR), 297, 301, 304–321
Photography, 12, 405, 417, 420, 550, 551, 555
PhotoVoice, 389, 392–393
Place-making/place making, 522, 553–556
Polarisation, 51, 52, 228
Policy making, 125, 382
Political activism, 8, 12, 17–18, 31, 164, 196, 217, 639, 653
Political context, 3, 38, 92, 329, 342, 349, 430, 481, 581
Positivist, 1, 8, 186, 269, 572
Poverty, 2, 3, 7, 8, 11, 13, 17, 36, 45, 47, 54, 55, 61, 62, 82, 94, 241, 261, 270, 302, 351, 354, 376, 377, 382, 426, 428, 431, 433, 435, 438, 442, 443, 452, 476, 477, 480–482, 499, 503, 506, 509, 510, 525, 528, 529, 550, 559, 560, 634, 635, 654, 655, 661
Power, 2, 22, 31, 52, 77, 109, 122, 140, 161, 195, 201, 226, 247, 265, 285, 303, 339, 348, 377, 407, 443, 451, 480, 498, 526, 552, 569–570, 618, 631, 656
Praxis/praxes, 36, 59, 122, 124, 125, 132, 133, 141–155, 181, 182, 187, 190, 195, 240, 242, 254, 255, 261, 273, 329, 333, 340, 342, 378, 380, 395, 499, 502–503, 506–509, 515, 521, 631, 658
Prisoners, 297, 301, 332, 333, 335–338, 335n5, 341

Privatisation, 21, 125–127, 132, 180, 218, 477, 537, 562, 563, 643, 645, 656
Process, 8, 22, 35, 55, 72, 106, 121, 146, 160, 182, 204, 225, 240, 267, 278, 304, 327, 349, 377, 407, 426, 454, 477, 498, 528, 547, 570, 598, 619, 631, 638, 660
Protest/protesting, 39, 42, 51, 53, 70, 79–81, 88–95, 105, 148, 182, 195, 505, 530, 551, 635, 645, 648
Psychiatric, 2–4, 18, 43, 70–74, 76, 77, 80, 82, 90, 93, 95, 140, 161, 196, 204, 246, 249, 250, 252, 253, 255, 261, 354, 355, 580, 587, 592, 655
Psychoanalytic, 454, 522, 597, 599, 608
Psychologists for Social Change (PSC), 7, 17, 31–49, 474, 491, 535, 655
Psychologists for Social Responsibility (Psysr), 103
Psychologizing, 180
Psy professionals, 17, 18, 521, 522
Public engagement, 85, 126, 127
Public space, 65, 180, 182, 190–193, 389, 603

Q

Qualitative, 131, 166, 182, 185, 186, 189, 190, 196, 205, 247, 330, 420, 429, 430, 432, 442, 443, 561, 572, 642
Queer listening, 207, 212–215, 219

R

Radical, 2, 4, 9, 12, 103, 104, 114, 115, 117, 124, 132, 139–140, 144, 160, 181, 187, 201–219, 242, 254, 255, 302, 306, 329, 335, 339, 342, 371, 484, 586, 653, 657, 658, 660
Recognition, 4, 144, 147, 195, 202–204, 206, 207, 210, 211, 214–216, 242, 278, 352, 377, 393, 536, 549, 555, 563, 598, 603, 607, 641, 654, 656, 657
Recovery in the Bin (RITB), 2, 89
Reflecting team (RT), 160, 162, 163, 168, 658
Reflexivity/reflective, 10, 26, 49, 139, 154, 155, 173, 180, 188, 196, 207, 236, 272, 295, 308, 313, 333, 348–371, 383, 419, 430–431, 450, 454, 469, 498, 501, 502, 504–506, 508, 511, 513, 514, 516, 602, 604
Regeneration, 19, 25, 396
Rehabilitation, 451, 473, 475, 484–488, 525, 532, 656
Re-memberment, 143, 151
Resistance, 12, 20, 41, 85, 88, 94, 118, 124, 141, 142, 145, 148, 151, 201, 217, 219, 273, 339, 357, 379, 501, 505, 509, 510, 522, 554, 593, 600, 604, 633, 635, 648
Responsibilization, 605
Roma communities, 375, 377–379, 382, 383, 386, 391–396

S

Safeguarding, 4, 241, 271, 312
Safety, 23, 71, 133, 148, 211, 212, 216, 217, 231, 249, 296, 302, 416, 437, 447–470, 476, 485, 500, 503, 513
St John of God (SJOG), 524–528, 525n2, 532, 533
Saviour, 146, 659

Science fiction (SF), 577–582, 590, 591
SCRATCHMAPS, 500, 503–504, 506–510, 513, 514
Self, 12, 114, 151, 167, 205, 207, 210–217, 271, 280, 283, 285–286, 293, 353, 455, 464, 470, 528n4, 571, 577, 582, 583, 593, 602–604, 606–608
Self-advocacy, 415–417
Self-harm, 3, 246, 250
Self-help, 73, 88, 528
Self-improvement, 8
Sexuality, 210, 215, 404, 414, 416, 417, 580
Shame, 40, 161, 171, 186, 212, 216, 217, 219, 271, 294, 352, 487, 527, 560, 655, 661
Slacktivism/slacktivist, 52
Slavery, 53, 104, 435, 449, 473–491
Smail, D. J., 4, 35, 36, 53, 75, 77, 78, 91–93, 160–162, 172, 227, 570
Small groups, 55, 106, 115, 245, 267, 280, 331, 367, 528, 553
Social action, 35, 61, 63, 65, 113, 146, 351, 363, 368, 637–640, 644, 646
Social attitudes, 530, 560
Social campaign, 31
Social change, 7n1, 12, 13, 17, 26, 53, 59, 60, 88, 89, 93, 94, 102, 103, 114, 125, 133, 149, 196, 329, 330, 333, 340, 342, 474, 480, 484, 491, 500, 501, 513, 521–522, 547, 577, 631, 639, 643, 653, 655, 660
Social cleansing, 20, 21
Social constructionist/constructionism, 159, 160, 162, 166, 309
Social context, 1, 8, 34, 40, 63, 65, 76, 547
Social determinant, 6, 12, 28, 36, 406, 535
Social-economic inequality, 3
Social factors, 73, 250, 530
Social inclusion, 243, 304–321, 328, 333, 534, 536, 538
Social inequality, 3, 17, 36, 122, 329, 342, 427, 502, 526, 537, 563, 654, 655
Social justice/injustice, 8–10, 17, 21, 34, 36, 43, 53, 63, 65, 78, 113, 121, 140, 146, 147, 153, 186, 189, 225, 227–229, 235, 239, 255, 270, 297, 301, 328, 329, 332, 337, 341, 347, 349, 350, 353, 365–367, 369, 375–397, 473–491, 500–502, 504, 506, 512–516, 526, 538, 547, 581, 632, 633, 636, 639–646, 655, 659, 660
Social-materialist, 35, 76, 77, 82, 93
Social media, 25, 26, 34, 37, 39, 42, 48, 51, 52, 54, 55, 59, 64, 85, 128, 205, 282, 294–296, 440, 483, 561, 627, 637, 644, 658
Social narrative, 31
Social role valorisation (SRV), 307
Socio-political, 3, 36, 72, 92, 94, 179–196, 227, 396, 578, 597, 623
Solidarity, 4, 10, 20, 26, 31, 39, 41–43, 45, 48, 104, 105, 111, 117, 162, 172, 181, 186, 187, 204, 236, 337, 350, 536, 644
Spaces, 3, 10, 12, 17, 25–27, 37, 38, 45, 53, 54, 65, 109, 113, 117, 126, 127, 129, 132, 133, 139–140, 142, 151, 152, 160–162, 164, 166, 167, 169, 171–175, 186, 189–191, 195, 196, 201–205, 207, 210–213, 215, 217, 218, 225, 227, 229–231, 246–248, 255, 280, 311–312, 318, 331–333, 337, 341, 347, 348, 356, 366, 380,

382, 388, 389, 391–394, 396, 397, 404, 408, 409, 414, 416, 419, 421, 430, 436–438, 451, 469, 505, 509, 510, 513, 515, 521, 522, 536, 537, 545–556, 564, 571, 573, 582, 584, 587, 589, 590, 592, 603, 618, 619, 642, 643, 646, 647, 653, 657, 658, 660
Special educational need or disability (SEND), 297, 301, 304–321
Speculative fiction, 590
Spiritual, 8, 72, 113, 114, 224, 277–294, 500, 503, 529–531, 534, 571
Statactivism, 18, 121–133, 656
Stereotype, 382, 409, 417–420, 507, 527, 551
Stewardship, 9, 121, 225, 229, 235, 328, 332, 337, 350, 353, 366, 407, 408
Stigmatisation, 260, 411, 657
Streccapogn, 327–342
Suicide, 3, 94, 250, 478, 531
Survivor, 2, 23, 36, 43, 62, 69, 80, 89, 90, 232, 233, 454, 474, 478–480, 484, 486–491, 607

T

Technology, 277–294, 530, 618, 620–622, 625–627, 658
Temporary accommodation, 3, 22, 23, 25–27, 551
Territorialism, 53
Thematic, 185, 187, 189, 191, 314, 330, 356, 389, 431, 550, 601
Themes, 10, 12, 62, 85, 104, 113, 163, 173, 185, 187, 194, 207–214, 227–229, 246, 247, 250, 269, 271, 273, 278, 280–282, 349, 358, 360, 362, 404, 411, 431, 443, 506, 532, 549, 550, 554, 561, 584, 593, 600, 601, 619, 621–623, 625, 636, 638
Therapeutic spaces, 139, 162, 215, 280
Threat/s, 52, 71, 79, 81, 84, 88, 211, 212, 215–217, 454, 469, 483, 561–563, 565, 566, 569, 573, 579, 603, 625, 644, 655
Trafficking, 302, 449, 476, 477, 479–482, 484–487
Transdiagnostic, 69, 76, 81
Transformative, 12, 78, 117, 125, 140, 215, 256, 262, 270, 272, 297–298, 301–302, 306, 329, 336, 340, 342, 369, 370, 382, 396, 484, 487, 488, 500, 501, 516, 579, 590, 599, 638, 639, 647
Transition Towns (TT), 327–331, 330n3, 333, 339–341
Trauma, 26, 35, 47, 70–72, 74, 76, 77, 80–85, 88, 94, 95, 113, 116–118, 201, 203, 216, 217, 255, 280, 447–470, 474, 475, 486–487, 565, 609
Trust, 10, 44, 106, 107, 109, 111, 174, 216, 249, 267, 273, 341, 391, 456, 480, 515, 532, 537, 548, 568, 584, 642, 643

U

Ukhamba, 150–153, 155
Umoza, 521, 524, 526, 531, 533
Unemployed/unemployment, 2, 40, 94, 148, 179, 297, 301, 332, 333, 338, 341, 354, 381, 382, 413, 432, 452, 482, 508–510, 580, 589, 655

V

Violence, 7, 11, 12, 22, 23, 45, 61, 122, 132, 133, 141–143, 146,

148, 149, 151, 154, 190, 204, 211, 255, 302, 354, 378, 382, 426, 439, 440, 449, 451, 452, 477, 489, 508, 509, 552, 586, 653, 655
Visual methods, 411, 418

W

Walk the Talk, 18, 54–60, 506
Welfare, 2, 11, 34, 35, 54, 55, 61, 71, 180, 342, 377, 382, 396, 477, 529, 561, 643
Wellbeing/well-being, 6, 10, 11, 21, 24, 25, 39, 40, 45, 53, 70, 71, 74, 76–78, 92, 94, 102, 105, 143, 163, 174, 203, 204, 218, 228, 261, 278, 279, 286, 293, 295, 326, 328, 331, 333, 340, 349, 387, 389, 397, 409, 522, 526, 529, 530, 533–537, 545–556, 563, 568–573, 589, 598, 600, 601, 603, 604, 608, 641, 654, 655, 657
Western/westernised, 1, 8, 10, 51, 71–73, 85, 116, 117, 140, 153, 224, 229, 261, 277–280, 293, 294, 302, 329, 347, 369, 482, 483, 486–490, 499, 529–533, 536, 537, 581, 582, 584, 640, 645
Wider collective, 262
Workshops, 39, 85, 105, 106, 114, 227, 229, 231, 326, 333, 334, 337, 338, 341, 355, 404, 405, 411, 419, 429, 430, 450, 455, 505, 507, 508, 511, 535, 553, 554, 582, 583, 585, 590, 592, 635, 637, 639, 643, 644, 646
World Health Organisation (WHO), 6, 36, 376, 525, 553, 554

Y

York St John (YSJ), 260, 262, 265, 266, 269, 271–273
YOUR World, 429–434, 436, 438, 441–443
Youth care and education centre (YCEC), 449, 450, 452–458, 461, 469, 470
Youth narratives, 448

The manufacturer's authorised representative in the EU is Springer Nature Customer Service Centre GmbH, Europaplatz 3, 69115 Heidelberg, Germany. If you have any concerns regarding our products, please contact ProductSafety@springernature.com

Printed and bound by CPI Group (UK) Ltd, Croydon, CR0 4YY
30/09/2026
02225701-0020